Arthritis: Evaluation, Care and Management

Arthritis: Evaluation, Care and Management

Editor: Grenn Jones

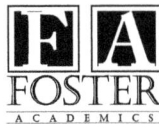

FOSTER
A C A D E M I C S

www.fosteracademics.com

www.fosteracademics.com

FA **FOSTER**
ACADEMICS

Cataloging-in-Publication Data

Arthritis : evaluation, care and management / edited by Grenn Jones.
   p. cm.
Includes bibliographical references and index.
ISBN 978-1-63242-760-1
   1. Arthritis. 2. Arthritis--Diagnosis. 3. Arthritis--Treatment. I. Jones, Grenn.
RC933 .A78 2019
616.722--dc23

Foster Academics,
118-35 Queens Blvd., Suite 400,
Forest Hills, NY 11375, USA

ISBN 978-1-63242-760-1 (Hardback)

Contents

Preface

Over the recent decade, advancements and applications have progressed exponentially. This has led to the increased interest in this field and projects are being conducted to enhance knowledge. The main objective of this book is to present some of the critical challenges and provide insights into possible solutions. This book will answer the varied questions that arise in the field and also provide an increased scope for furthering studies.

All disorders related to the functioning of the joints are categorised as arthritis. The common symptoms of arthritis include reduced motion, joint pain, swelling, stiffness, and redness. Ankylosing spondylitis is one of the most common types of arthritis. It involves the long term inflammation of the joints of the spine, pelvis, shoulder, and hips. Back pain, stiffness in the affected area, eye and bowel problems are some of the common symptoms of ankylosing spondylitis. Medical imaging and blood tests are two of the common ways of diagnosis. Arthritis treatment methods include the use of disease-modifying antirheumatic drugs (DMARDs), pain replacements and anti-inflammatory drugs, joint replacements, etc. This book elucidates the concepts and innovative models around prospective developments with respect to arthritis care and management. It includes some of the vital pieces of work being conducted across the world, on various topics related to arthritis. This book will serve as a reference to a broad spectrum of readers.

I hope that this book, with its visionary approach, will be a valuable addition and will promote interest among readers. Each of the authors has provided their extraordinary competence in their specific fields by providing different perspectives as they come from diverse nations and regions. I thank them for their contributions.

Editor

The plasma biomarker soluble SIGLEC-1 is associated with the type I interferon transcriptional signature, ethnic background and renal disease in systemic lupus erythematosus

João J. Oliveira[1†], Sarah Karrar[2†], Daniel B. Rainbow[1,3], Christopher L. Pinder[2], Pamela Clarke[1], Arcadio Rubio García[1,3], Osama Al-Assar[3], Keith Burling[4], Sian Morris[5], Richard Stratton[5], Tim J. Vyse[2], Linda S. Wicker[1,3], John A. Todd[1,3] and Ricardo C. Ferreira[1,3*] iD

Abstract

Background: The molecular heterogeneity of autoimmune and inflammatory diseases has been one of the main obstacles to the development of safe and specific therapeutic options. Here, we evaluated the diagnostic and clinical value of a robust, inexpensive, immunoassay detecting the circulating soluble form of the monocyte-specific surface receptor sialic acid binding Ig-like lectin 1 (sSIGLEC-1).

Methods: We developed an immunoassay to measure sSIGLEC-1 in small volumes of plasma/serum from systemic lupus erythematosus (SLE) patients ($n = 75$) and healthy donors ($n = 504$). Samples from systemic sclerosis patients ($n = 99$) were studied as an autoimmune control. We investigated the correlation between sSIGLEC-1 and both monocyte surface SIGLEC-1 and type I interferon-regulated gene (IRG) expression. Associations of sSIGLEC-1 with clinical features were evaluated in an independent cohort of SLE patients ($n = 656$).

Results: Plasma concentrations of sSIGLEC-1 strongly correlated with expression of SIGLEC-1 on the surface of blood monocytes and with IRG expression in SLE patients. We found ancestry-related differences in sSIGLEC-1 concentrations in SLE patients, with patients of non-European ancestry showing higher levels compared to patients of European ancestry. Higher sSIGLEC-1 concentrations were associated with lower serum complement component 3 and increased frequency of renal complications in European patients, but not with the SLE Disease Activity Index clinical score.

Conclusions: Our sSIGLEC-1 immunoassay provides a specific and easily assayed marker for monocyte–macrophage activation, and interferonopathy in SLE and other diseases. Further studies can extend its clinical associations and its potential use to stratify patients and as a secondary endpoint in clinical trials.

Keywords: Soluble SIGLEC-1, Biomarker, Autoimmunity, Type I interferon, Interferonopathy

* Correspondence: ricardo.ferreira@well.ox.ac.uk
†João J. Oliveira and Sarah Karrar contributed equally to this work.
[1]Department of Medical Genetics, JDRF/Wellcome Diabetes and Inflammation Laboratory, NIHR Cambridge Biomedical Research Centre, Cambridge Institute for Medical Research, University of Cambridge, Cambridge, UK
[3]JDRF/Wellcome Diabetes and Inflammation Laboratory, Wellcome Centre for Human Genetics, Nuffield Department of Medicine, NIHR Oxford Biomedical Research Centre, University of Oxford, Roosevelt Drive, Oxford, UK
Full list of author information is available at the end of the article

Background

The type I interferon (IFN) pathway was identified as a central feature of the autoimmune disease systemic lupus erythematosus (SLE) when IFN-α was first detected at high levels in patients' sera [1]. Since this initial observation, the development of SLE-like clinical manifestations in patients treated with IFN-α for different malignancies pointed to the involvement of IFN-α in the aetiology of the disease [2]. Furthermore, naturally occurring anti-IFN-α antibodies in SLE patients have been shown to be associated with milder forms of the disease [3]. The identification of a constitutive IFN transcriptional signature comprising hundreds of IFN-regulated genes (IRGs) in peripheral blood from a subset of SLE patients [4, 5] suggested that the IFN signature could be used as a clinical biomarker to stratify patients with autoimmune and inflammatory diseases in which type I IFNs are known to play a pathogenic role, referred to as the interferonopathies. Nevertheless, the precise link between the IFN signature and molecular subtypes of disease or with broader disease severity scores has been put into question [6]. With the development of more sophisticated high-throughput genomic tools, it has become apparent that the IFN signature is a complex composite marker, which can be further stratified into several distinct signatures that are better predictors of disease subtype [7]. Longitudinal analyses have revealed that the IFN signature is highly variable over time as a result of alterations in blood composition caused by therapy or progression of the disease [7, 8]. This is particularly relevant to IFN-driven diseases, as IFN-α is known to significantly alter the relative distribution of immune cell types in blood, which can severely compromise the diagnostic potential of the whole blood IFN signature [8] and lead to the observed lack of correlation between the signature and disease activity over time [9, 10].

These findings have led to the investigation of other potential cell-type specific biomarkers that could be better predictors of disease severity or clinical subtypes. One such IFN-regulated marker that has shown promise for the stratification of SLE patients is sialic acid binding Ig-like lectin 1 (SIGLEC-1) [11–13]. SIGLEC-1 is a cell-adhesion molecule involved in the initial contacts with sialylated pathogens and mediates phagocytosis and endocytosis of pathogens, thereby promoting efficient immune responses to limit infection [14]. Unlike the canonical IFN transcriptional signature, which is a composite of many genes expressed at different levels in different immune cells, SIGLEC-1 is expressed exclusively in cells of the myeloid lineage, namely tissue-resident macrophages and monocyte-derived dendritic cells [15, 16]. In blood, expression of surface SIGLEC-1 is restricted to CD14$^+$ monocytes, and has been previously reported to be increased in several other autoimmune diseases, including

rheumatoid arthritis [17], systemic sclerosis (SSc) [18] and primary biliary cirrhosis [19]. In addition, a recent study has shown that increased SIGLEC-1 expression on the surface of monocytes was a predictor of congenital heart block during pregnancy in children from Ro/SS-A autoantibody-positive mothers [20].

These data support the use of SIGLEC-1 as a potential cell-type specific biomarker for the stratification of patients with an overt type I IFN response. However, assay of surface SIGLEC-1 requires intact cells and flow cytometry, features that are not conducive for the development of a high-throughput, inexpensive biomarker assay, ideally detectable in plasma/serum. Here we show that a circulating form of SIGLEC-1 can be detected in serum/plasma, and develop a robust and inexpensive immunoassay to measure its concentration. Furthermore, we provide evidence that the concentration of soluble SIGLEC-1 (sSIGLEC-1) is associated with the patient's ancestry and with renal involvement in SLE patients. Therefore, sSIGLEC-1 is a new circulating plasma/serum biomarker of type I IFN activity in systemic autoimmune, inflammatory and infectious diseases that can be used accurately and conveniently in large numbers of samples, and could be used in clinical trials of drugs modulating the IFN signalling pathway for patient stratification and as a secondary endpoint.

Methods

Participants

Discovery cohort (cohort 1) study participants included 34 SLE patients (median age 39 years, range 20–72 years; 32/34 female) recruited from Guy's and St Thomas' NHS Foundation Trust. All patients satisfied ACR SLE classification criteria and were allocated a disease activity using SLEDAI-2K at the time of sampling. Patients were recruited from a clinic in which the severity of disease was such that none of the patients was on high-dose oral corticosteroids (> 15 mg/day) or B-cell depleting therapy. Healthy volunteers matched for age and sex (n = 24; median age 43 years, range 25–60 years; 23/24 female) were recruited from the Cambridge BioResource.

A replication cohort (cohort 2) of 41 SLE patients (median age 52 years, range 21–82 years; 38/41 female) and 490 healthy volunteers (median age 48 years, range 18–78 years; 320/490 female) was recruited from the Cambridge BioResource. The SLE patients were recruited specifically for this study outside their regular clinic visits, and were otherwise well at the time of bleeding. No additional disease information or ancestry data were available for this cohort of patients.

To investigate the association between sSIGLEC-1 with ancestry and clinical manifestations, a third independent cohort (cohort 3) of SLE patients (n = 656; median age 45 years, range 15–82 years; 592/655 female, one unknown) was recruited from multiple collaborative centres in the UK (St Thomas's Hospital, Newcastle Hospital, City Hospital Sunderland, City Hospital Birmingham, Royal Hallamshire Hospital, Hammersmith Hospital, West Middlesex Hospital and Basildon Hospital). Most patients were of European ($n = 370$), South East Asian ($n = 134$), African/Afro-Caribbean ($n = 94$) and Far East Asian ($n = 19$) ancestries. Twenty-three patients were of other minor ancestry groups (including Middle Eastern, Maori and Fiji ancestry) and 16 had missing ancestry information. The history of patients' clinical manifestations since their disease diagnosis up to the time of their visit is summarised in Table 1.

A cohort of systemic sclerosis (SSc) patients ($N = 99$), stratified into patients with limited cutaneous SSc ($N = 50$) or diffuse SSc ($N = 49$), and a matching cohort of healthy donors ($N = 50$) were recruited from the Royal Free Hospital, UCL, London. All patients had a definite diagnosis of SSc according to the 2013 ACR/EULAR SSc classification criteria [21].

All samples and information were collected with written and signed informed consent after approval from the relevant research ethics committees (REC numbers 05/Q0106/20, 07/H0718/49 and 08/H0308/153; and NHS Health Research Authority, NRES Committee London-Hampstead, HRA, REC number 6398, Investigating the pathogenesis of systemic sclerosis).

Flow cytometry

SIGLEC-1 expression was measured in peripheral blood mononuclear cells (PBMCs) from 34 SLE patients and 24 healthy donors from the discovery cohort. PBMCs were thawed in a 37 °C water bath, resuspended in X-VIVO 15 (Lonza) + 1% heat-inactivated, filtered, human AB serum (Sigma) and immunostained for 30 min at room temperature. SIGLEC-1 expression on CD14$^+$

monocytes was determined using fluorochrome-conjugated antibodies against CD14 (Clone M5E2; BioLegend) and SIGLEC-1 (Clone 7–239; BioLegend). Immunostained samples were acquired using a BD LSR Fortessa (BD Biosciences) flow cytometer, and data were analysed using FlowJo (Tree Star). Dead cells were excluded based on the eFluor780 Fixable Viability Dye (eBiosciences).

Soluble SIGLEC-1 time-resolved fluorescence immunoassay

Plasma/serum sSIGLEC-1 concentrations were measured using a non-isotopic time-resolved fluorescence (TRF) assay based on the dissociation-enhanced lanthanide fluorescent immunoassay technology (DELFIA; PerkinElmer). Duplicate test plasma/serum samples diluted 1:10 in assay buffer (PBS, 0.05% Tween-20, 10% FCS) were incubated for 2 h at room temperature and then at 4 °C overnight in 96-well EIA/RIA plates (Corning) coated with 1 µg/ml mouse monoclonal anti-human SIGLEC-1 capture antibody (AB18619; Abcam). Sample detection was performed using a biotinylated sheep polyclonal detection antibody (BAF5197; R&D Systems) diluted to a final concentration of 200 ng/ml. Following incubation with the secondary antibody, europium-labelled streptavidin (PerkinElmer) was added and the concentration of antigen was measured by the amount of disassociated europium that is fluorescent at 615 nm after excitation at 320 nm.

Quantification of test samples was obtained by fitting the readings to a human recombinant SIGLEC-1 (R&D Systems) serial dilution standard curve on each plate ($r^2 > 0.995$). To maintain assay consistency, the recombinant protein was aliquoted and stored at -80 °C immediately following reconstitution and a fresh aliquot from the same lot was used for each assay.

Table 1 Summary of the history of clinical manifestation of the SLE patients in cohort 3

Phenotype	EUR		Non-EUR			
	N	Affected patients, n (%)	N	Affected patients, n (%)	OR^a (95% CI)	P value^b
Renal	320	75 (24.4%)	243	81 (33.3%)	1.60 (1.11–2.32)	0.01
Neurological	330	36 (10.9%)	244	42 (17.2%)	1.67 (1.05–2.74)	0.03
Haematological	366	185 (50.5%)	268	106 (39.6%)	0.65 (0.47–0.89)	0.007
dsDNA positivity	370	143 (38.6%)	270	83 (30.7%)	0.70 (0.51–0.98)	0.04
Admission rate^c	351	140 (39.9%)	196	86 (43.9)	1.20 (0.84–1.71)	0.31
Biologics ever needed^d	332	23 (6.9%)	239	12 (5.0%)	0.70 (0.34–1.43)	0.33

Summary of available clinical history for the 656 study participants from cohort 3 since their disease diagnosis and up to the time of their visit. Data were stratified by study cohort

CI confidence interval, EUR patients of European ancestry, non-EUR patients of non-European ancestry, SLE systemic lupus erythematosus

^{a}Odds ratio (OR) in non-European patients

^{b}P values calculated using Pearson's chi-squared test

^{c}Admission defined as any patient requiring hospital admission specifically for SLE in the 5 years prior to and including the date of their clinic visit at which the blood sample was taken

^{d}Patients treated with biologic drugs at any time since their disease diagnosis

The lower limit of detection of the assay was set as 2x background levels in each plate and corresponded to an average of 1.29 ng/ml across all plates. Samples with measurements below the limit of detection (6/589) were set to 1.29 ng/ml. Assay specificity was confirmed using a biotinylated sheep polyclonal isotype control (R&D Systems). Technical variation was assessed in duplicate measurements of all samples (average CV = 5.0%). Samples with CV > 30% between duplicates (10/589) were excluded from the analysis. To evaluate potential matrix effects, we diluted a sample with high sSIGLEC-1 concentration with assay medium and showed a linear titration between 1:2 and 1:16 dilutions (r^2 = 0.94).

IFN-α_{2b} single-molecule digital ELISA assay

Circulating levels of IFN-α_{2b} were measured by Single-Molecule Array (SIMOA) digital ELISA (Quanterix) according to the manufacturer's instructions. IFN-α detection was achieved using mouse anti-IFN-α monoclonal antibodies: a neutralising antibody (clone MMHA—capture) and an anti-IFN-α antibody raised against an IFN-α_{2b} antigen (clone 7 N41—detection). Cross-reactivity to the other IFN-α subtypes was not assessed. Measurements were performed in plasma samples, which had never been previously thawed, from the 41 SLE patients of cohort 2.

Type I IFN transcriptional signature in PBMCs

RNA from 34 SLE patients and 24 age and sex-matched healthy donors in cohort 1 and from 41 SLE patients and 41 age and sex-matched healthy donors in cohort 2 was extracted from freshly isolated PBMCs stored in TRIZOL immediately after collection, using the Direct-zol RNA Mini-Prep kit (Zymo Research) following the manufacturer's instructions. The RNA concentration was measured by NanoDrop (Thermo Fisher Scientific), and 50 ng of total RNA were hybridised with a custom NanoString CodeSet (NanoString Technologies), containing 56 IRGs previously identified as discriminative of the IFN signature [22]. Expression levels were assessed using an nCounter Flex instrument (NanoString Technologies). Data were processed using the nSolver Analysis Software following normalisation to the geometric mean of positive control spike-ins and the gene expression of eight housekeeping genes.

Expression of 56 IRGs previously identified as discriminative of the IFN signature [22] were assessed, with a custom NanoString CodeSet (NanoString Technologies), using RNA from 34 SLE patients and 24 age and sex-matched healthy donors in cohort 1 and from 41 SLE patients and 41 age and sex-matched healthy donors in cohort 2.

A quantitative metric of the IFN signature was generated using principal component analysis by projection of the expression of the 56 IRGs onto the first principal component (PC1), which was found to explain 86.3% of the variance of this dataset. A complete list of the 56 IRGs and respective NanoString probe sequences is presented in Additional file 1.

Statistical analyses

Statistical analyses were performed using Prism software (GraphPad) and R software (https://www.r-project.org). Given that most phenotypes showed moderate to strong right skew that violated the assumption of normality, the phenotypes were log-transformed before statistical testing and all reported values refer to the geometric mean of the respective measurements.

Cohorts 1 and 2

The association of sSIGLEC-1 and measured immune parameters in cohorts 1 and 2 was performed using two-tailed non-parametric Mann–Whitney tests. Correlation analyses were performed using linear regression on the log-transformed data.

Cohort 3

All statistical analyses with the clinical data available for the 656 patients from cohort 3 were performed using R software. Association between ancestry and sSIGLEC-1 concentration was assessed using a two-tailed Student's t test. The odds ratio (OR) of each clinical parameter (history of admission within 5 years; ever having suffered with renal, haematological or neurological disease; requiring biological therapy or active corticosteroid use to control disease) in European and non-European patients was assessed by Pearson's chi-squared test.

Patients were divided into groups based on sSIGLEC-1 serum level centiles (< 50th centile, 51st–74th centile, 75th–95th centile and > 95th centile). Association of each group and clinical parameters was performed using a logistical regression model. Patients of European and non-European ancestry were analysed separately as ethnicity was a major confounding factor.

Association of the sSIGLEC-1 concentration with other serological parameters of disease (levels of C3 and C4 measured within 3 months of the visit at the patient's local centre/hospital, anti-dsDNA antibody titres and C-reactive protein) and the estimated glomerular filtration rate (eGFR) were assessed using linear regression on the log-transformed data. Association of sSIGLEC-1 concentration and renal disease activity was also determined, based on the clinical notes documentation, at the time of the sample collection and the last documented episode of active nephritis. Comparison of the different disease activity groups was done using two-tailed Student's t tests comparing the mean sSIGLEC-1 concentration of each group to the control group of patients who never developed renal complications.

Results

Soluble SIGLEC-1 assay development

To investigate whether we could detect SIGLEC-1 expression levels in peripheral blood, we developed an immunoassay based on TRF to measure the concentrations of the circulating form of the receptor, which we refer to as sSIGLEC-1. Although *SIGLEC1* is predicted to encode a soluble protein isoform, it has not been previously shown that such a soluble protein can be detected in plasma/serum.

We found that sSIGLEC-1 was detected in the circulation, with concentrations ranging from 1.29 to 276.1 ng/ml in plasma/serum samples from healthy donors and SLE patients. Technical variation of the assay was found to be very low, as assessed by two independent measurements of the same plasma sample from 23 healthy donors performed 308 days apart (median CV = 4.8%, $r^2 = 0.91$; Fig. 1a), indicating minimal inter-assay variability. Similarly, biological sSIGLEC-1 levels were found to be very stable (CV = 11.8%, $r^2 = 0.67$; Fig. 1b) in 19 healthy donors bled at two separate visits (median time between visit 378 days, range 239–519 days), with only two donors showing physiological differences (CV > 20%) between visits, likely due to viral infections [22]. Of note, one donor showed high concentrations of sSIGLEC-1 on the first visit (28.3 ng/ml), which were maintained 343 days after the initial measurement (23.4 ng/ml; Fig. 1b), suggesting that, in addition to viral and possibly non-viral infections, genetic factors regulate the sSIGLEC-1 levels.

To expand the applicability of the sSIGLEC-1 immunoassay, we also developed an electrochemical luminescence-based (ECL) assay on the Meso Scale Discovery (MSD) platform, using the same detection antibodies and experimental protocol. The assay working range was found to be 0.5–1000 ng/ml, with an approximate 92% recovery of recombinant SIGLEC-1 protein spiked into serum samples. Stability of the assay over time was assessed using three pools of serum samples with increasing sSIGLEC-1 concentrations that were measured over six different assays run over a 2-day period. Assay stability was consistent with the TRF assay, with CVs of 7.7%, 5.6% and 8.5% for the low, medium and high QC pools, respectively (Fig. 1c). Furthermore, we found a very high concordance between the TRF and ECL assays ($r^2 = 0.78$; Fig. 1d), as assessed by measuring a subset of 41 SLE patients on both platforms, using two independent serum aliquots.

Soluble SIGLEC-1 levels are correlated with the surface SIGLEC-1 expression on CD14$^+$ monocytes

Currently, the surface expression of SIGLEC-1 on monocytes has been suggested as a sensitive cell-type specific biomarker for SLE in blood [13]. To investigate the relationship between surface and soluble SIGLEC-1 levels, we immunophenotyped the expression of this protein on the surface of CD14$^+$ monocytes in PBMCs collected from a discovery cohort (cohort 1) of 34 SLE patients and 24 matched healthy donors (Fig. 2a). Consistent with previous findings [12, 13], we found that the surface expression of SIGLEC-1 was increased in CD14$^+$ monocytes from SLE patients compared to healthy controls ($P = 1.4 \times 10^{-4}$; Fig. 2b). However, we found bimodal expression of the surface SIGLEC-1 among SLE patients, with 10 subjects (10/34, 29%; Fig. 2b) presenting low levels of protein expression, similar to the ranges observed in healthy donors, and the rest presenting much higher levels, rarely observed in healthy volunteers (Fig. 2a, b).

We found a strong correlation between the surface expression of SIGLEC-1 on monocytes and the concentration of sSIGLEC-1 in plasma samples from the same donors, particularly among SLE patients ($r^2 = 0.73$, $P = 7.9 \times 10^{-10}$; Fig. 2c). The distribution of sSIGLEC-1 levels recapitulated the same bimodal distribution of the surface SIGLEC-1 expression on SLE patients, ranging from 'low normal' physiological levels observed in healthy donors to the very high levels observed in a subset of patients (Fig. 2c).

Association of sSIGLEC-1 with the IFN transcriptional signature and SLE Disease Activity Index

To assess whether sSIGLEC-1 was associated with the IFN signature, we measured the transcription of 56 IRGs previously found to recapitulate the IFN signature [22]. We found that sSIGLEC-1 levels were significantly correlated with the IFN transcriptional signature in PBMCs from SLE patients ($r^2 = 0.67$, $P = 2.9 \times 10^{-9}$; Fig. 3a). The correlation was also observed in healthy donors ($r^2 = 0.34$, $P = 2.8 \times 10^{-3}$; Fig. 3a), albeit to a lower extent. These findings were replicated in an independent cohort (cohort 2) of 41 SLE patients ($r^2 = 0.46$, $P = 1.2 \times 10^{-6}$; Fig. 3b), confirming that sSIGLEC-1 is a marker of the peripheral IFN signature. The lower correlation in the replication cohort is consistent with a lower overall disease severity— and concomitant lower sSIGLEC-1 levels—of the patients in the replication cohort, who were recruited outside their regular clinic visits.

Recently, a single-molecule digital ELISA assay has been shown to detect IFN-α at femtomolar levels in the circulation even from healthy individuals [23]. Consistent with its potent biological activity, over a third of the SLE patients showed very low IFN-α_{2b} concentrations (< 10 fg/ml; Fig. 3c), which were close to the reported limit of detection. In our hands, the assay showed good reproducibility (CV = 4.1% between replicates), indicating that it is sensitive to detect even low concentrations of IFN-α_{2b}. We found a significant correlation between the concentrations of IFN-α_{2b} in plasma and sSIGLEC-1 ($r^2 = 0.27$, $P = 5.1 \times$

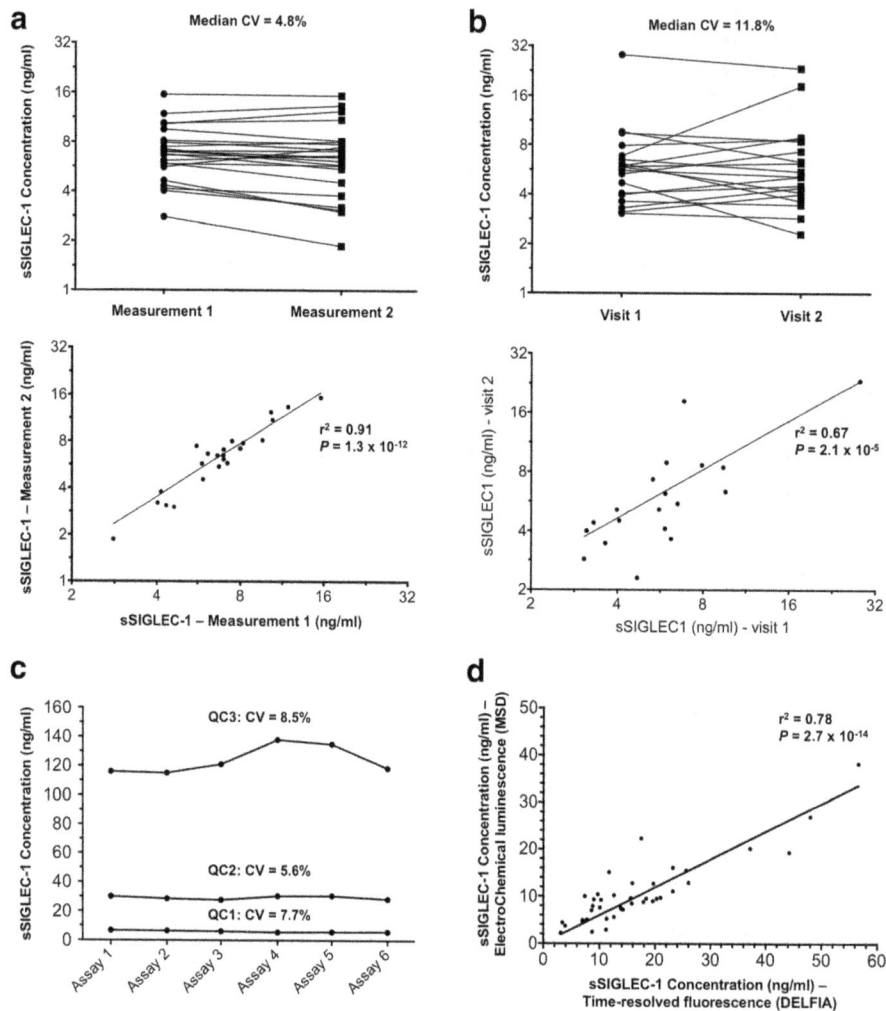

Fig. 1 sSIGLEC-1 stability and assay performance. **a** Data depict the inter-assay (technical) variation of the time-resolved fluorescence (TRF) sSIGLEC-1 immunoassay. Data were obtained from the measurement of the same plasma sample from 23 healthy donors on two independent assays, performed 308 days apart. **b** Data depict the intra-individual (biological) variation of sSIGLEC-1 concentration between two visits of the same donor. Longitudinal variation was assessed in 19 independent healthy donors using plasma samples collected at each separate visit. Median time between visits was 378 days (minimum = 239 days, maximum = 519 days). **c** Technical variation of the electrochemical luminescence (ECL) sSIGLEC-1 immunoassay using the Meso Scale Discovery (MSD) platform. Assay stability was assessed in three reference quality control (QC) pools of serum samples with increasing sSIGLEC-1 concentrations (QC1 = 6.0 ng/ml, QC2 = 29.2 ng/ml and QC3 = 123.9 ng/ml), measured in each assay over a 2-day period. **d** Correlation between TRF (DELFIA) and ECL (MSD)-based immunoassays. Measurements were performed in independent serum aliquots from a subset of 41 SLE patients from cohort 3. P values were calculated by linear regression. CV coefficient of variation, DELFIA dissociation-enhanced lanthanide fluorescent immunoassay, sSIGLEC-1 soluble sialic acid binding Ig-like lectin 1

10^{-4}; Fig. 3c) as well as the IFN signature ($r^2 = 0.34$, $P = 5.6 \times 10^{-5}$; see Additional file 2), although both were less pronounced than the observed correlation between sSIGLEC-1 and the IFN transcriptional signature.

In our sample of 34 SLE patients from the discovery cohort, sSIGLEC-1 concentrations and the SLE Disease Activity Index (SLEDAI) were not correlated ($r^2 = 0.10$, $P = 0.07$; Fig. 3d). This result is consistent with previous evidence showing a lack of association of other common serological disease markers, including various intra-nuclear autoantibodies, elevated B-cell activating factor of the tumour necrosis factor family (BAFF)

levels and hypocomplementaemia, as well as the whole blood IFN signature, with disease activity scores such as the SLEDAI [6].

Increased sSIGLEC-1 concentration is associated with renal involvement

Having assessed that sSIGLEC-1 is an IFN-regulated marker that can be detected in the circulation, we next investigated its potential as a clinical biomarker in SLE. Similarly to surface SIGLEC-1 expression, sSIGLEC-1 concentrations were markedly increased in SLE patients (10.4 ng/ml, 95% CI 8.8–12.2) compared to healthy

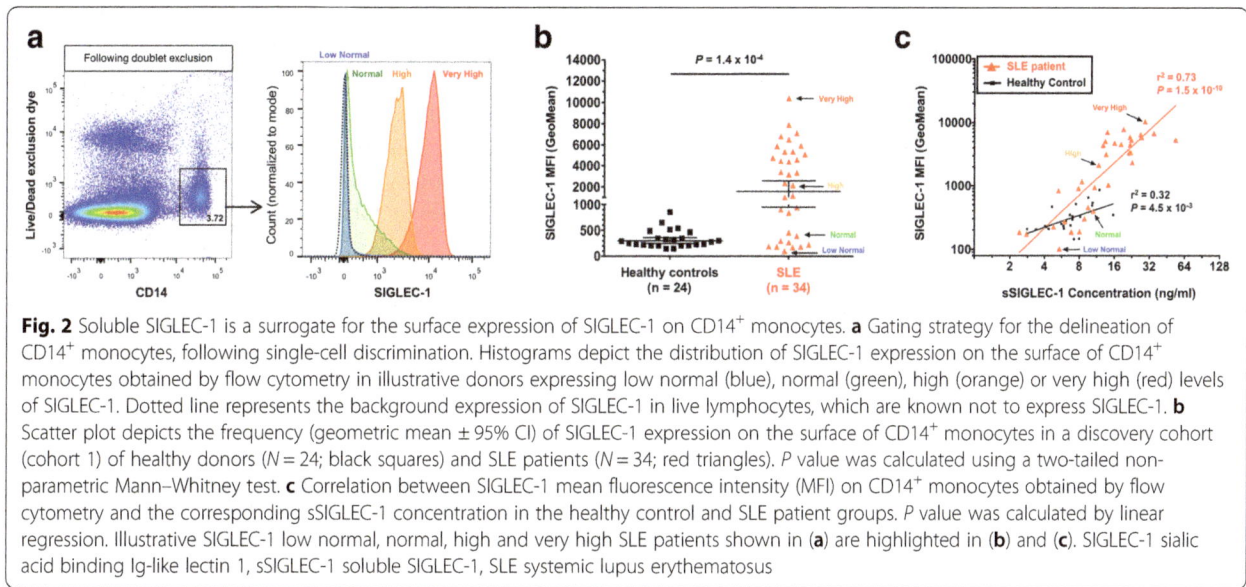

Fig. 2 Soluble SIGLEC-1 is a surrogate for the surface expression of SIGLEC-1 on CD14$^+$ monocytes. **a** Gating strategy for the delineation of CD14$^+$ monocytes, following single-cell discrimination. Histograms depict the distribution of SIGLEC-1 expression on the surface of CD14$^+$ monocytes obtained by flow cytometry in illustrative donors expressing low normal (blue), normal (green), high (orange) or very high (red) levels of SIGLEC-1. Dotted line represents the background expression of SIGLEC-1 in live lymphocytes, which are known not to express SIGLEC-1. **b** Scatter plot depicts the frequency (geometric mean ± 95% CI) of SIGLEC-1 expression on the surface of CD14$^+$ monocytes in a discovery cohort (cohort 1) of healthy donors (N = 24; black squares) and SLE patients (N = 34; red triangles). P value was calculated using a two-tailed non-parametric Mann–Whitney test. **c** Correlation between SIGLEC-1 mean fluorescence intensity (MFI) on CD14$^+$ monocytes obtained by flow cytometry and the corresponding sSIGLEC-1 concentration in the healthy control and SLE patient groups. P value was calculated by linear regression. Illustrative SIGLEC-1 low normal, normal, high and very high SLE patients shown in (**a**) are highlighted in (**b**) and (**c**). SIGLEC-1 sialic acid binding Ig-like lectin 1, sSIGLEC-1 soluble SIGLEC-1, SLE systemic lupus erythematosus

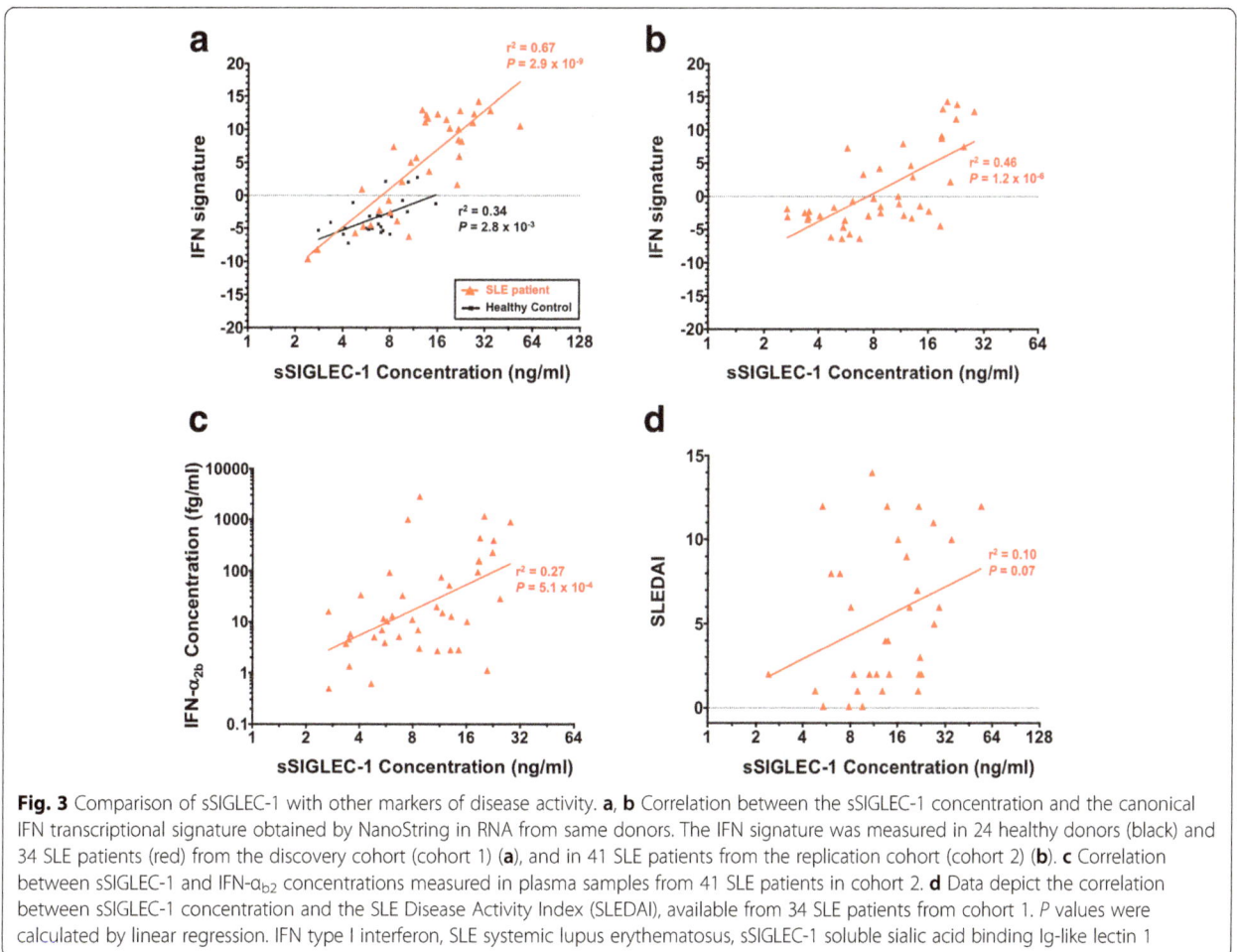

Fig. 3 Comparison of sSIGLEC-1 with other markers of disease activity. **a**, **b** Correlation between the sSIGLEC-1 concentration and the canonical IFN transcriptional signature obtained by NanoString in RNA from same donors. The IFN signature was measured in 24 healthy donors (black) and 34 SLE patients (red) from the discovery cohort (cohort 1) (**a**), and in 41 SLE patients from the replication cohort (cohort 2) (**b**). **c** Correlation between sSIGLEC-1 and IFN-α_{b2} concentrations measured in plasma samples from 41 SLE patients in cohort 2. **d** Data depict the correlation between sSIGLEC-1 concentration and the SLE Disease Activity Index (SLEDAI), available from 34 SLE patients from cohort 1. P values were calculated by linear regression. IFN type I interferon, SLE systemic lupus erythematosus, sSIGLEC-1 soluble sialic acid binding Ig-like lectin 1

controls (5.78 ng/ml, 95% CI 5.5–6.0, $P = 9.6 \times 10^{-12}$; Fig. 4a) in the combined discovery and replication cohorts of 75 SLE patients and 504 healthy donors. In addition to SLE, we also assessed sSIGLEC-1 concentrations in a cohort of SSc patients ($n = 50$ presenting with limited cutaneous and 49 with diffuse cutaneous SSc), another systemic autoimmune disease where type I IFN and overt monocyte/macrophage activation have been suggested to play an important aetiological role [18, 24]. Consistent with previous data showing an increased expression of SIGLEC-1 on the surface of CD14$^+$ monocytes in SSc patients [18], we found evidence for an increased

concentration of sSIGLEC-1 in serum samples from SSc (8.49 ng/ml, 95% CI 8.5–10.5) compared to matched healthy controls (7.07, 95% CI 6.7–8.6, $P = 8.3 \times 10^{-3}$; Fig. 4b). The distribution of sSIGLEC-1 in SSc was similar to the SLE patients and the increased concentrations were maintained in both patients with limited cutaneous SSc or diffuse SSc ($P = 0.02$ and $P = 0.05$, respectively; Fig. 4b).

To assess the potential clinical application of sSIGLEC-1, we measured sSIGLEC-1 levels in serum from 656 SLE patients with available clinical information (cohort 3). We observed that the concentrations of sSIGLEC-1 were

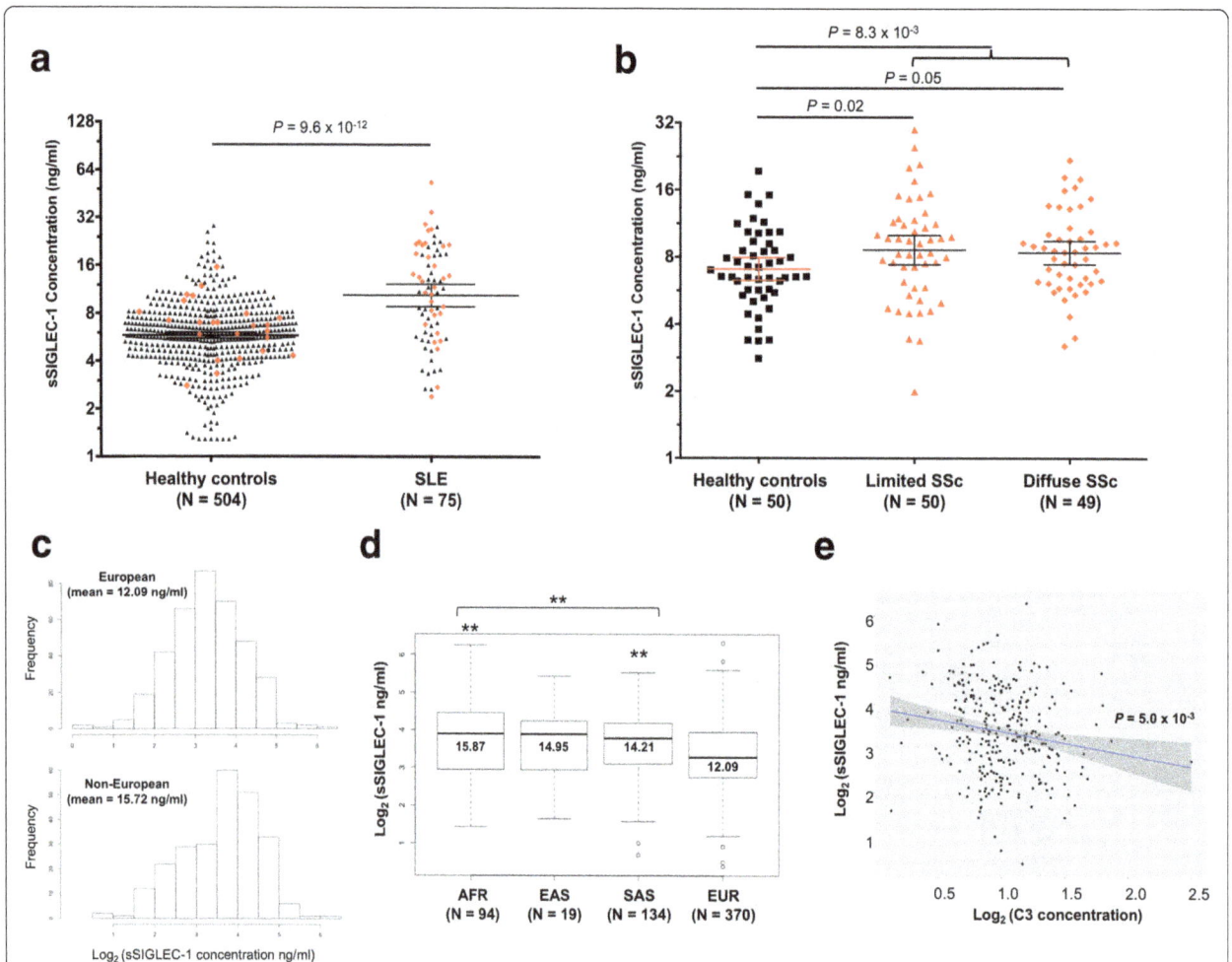

Fig. 4 Association of sSIGLEC-1 with ancestry and serological markers of SLE. **a** Scatter plots depict the frequency (geometric mean ± 95% CI) of sSIGLEC-1 concentrations in healthy donors ($N = 504$) and SLE patients ($N = 75$). Red diamonds, 24 healthy donors and 34 SLE patients from cohort 1 for which we have generated additional immunophenotyping and transcriptional data. P value was calculated using a two-tailed non-parametric Mann–Whitney test. **b** Scatter plots depict the frequency (geometric mean ± 95% CI) of sSIGLEC-1 concentrations in serum samples from a cohort of 99 systemic sclerosis (SSc) patients (red) and 50 healthy donors (black). SSc patients were stratified into patients displaying limited ($N = 50$) or diffuse ($N = 49$) cutaneous disease manifestation. **c** Histograms depict the distribution of sSIGLEC-1 concentrations in European and non-European SLE patients from cohort 3. **d** Box plots depict the distribution of sSIGLEC-1 concentrations in SLE patients stratified by ancestry group. Mean sSIGLEC-1 levels are indicated for each population. Twenty-three patients of additional minor ancestry groups (including Middle Eastern, Maori and Fiji) were included in the non-European population for the combined analysis. P values were calculated using Pearson's chi-squared test comparing the concentration of sSIGLEC-1 in patients of non-European and European ancestry. **e** Association between sSIGLEC-1 concentrations and serum complement component 3 (C3) levels. P value was calculated by linear regression. **$P < 0.01$. AFR African/Afro-Caribbean, EAS East Asian, EUR European, SAS South East Asian, SLE systemic lupus erythematosus, SSc systemic sclerosis, sSIGLEC-1 soluble sialic acid binding Ig-like lectin 1

significantly higher in non-European patients (15.7 ng/ml, 95% CI 13.52–17.92) compared to those of European ancestry (12.1 ng/ml, 95% CI 11.25–12.94, $P = 2.7 \times 10^{-3}$; Fig. 4c). Soluble SIGLEC-1 levels were similarly elevated among the different non-European populations (Fig. 4d), and were therefore combined into a single group to increase statistical power. Increased disease severity—and particularly incidence of renal disease—has been documented in patients of non-European ancestry [25–27]. In agreement with this observation, in our study, non-European SLE patients presented with an increased history of renal complications (Table 1), thus suggesting that the increased sSIGLEC-1 concentrations reflected the increased disease severity in non-European patients.

In addition to the ancestry-related changes, we found that sSIGLEC-1 levels were associated with lower levels of serum complement component 3 (C3) ($P = 5.0 \times 10^{-3}$; Fig. 4e), but not with other common serological markers of SLE such as C-reactive protein or anti-nuclear auto-antibody levels (see Additional file 3). This association was observed in both European and non-European patients and remained present even when adjusting for the presence of nephritis. Furthermore, we found that increased sSIGLEC-1 concentrations were associated with a history of renal disease in the combined patient population ($P = 0.01$; Table 2). Although the number of patients with active nephritis was limited in our study, we found that sSIGLEC-1 concentrations were strongly associated with duration of renal disease, with significantly higher levels observed in patients with active renal disease, and gradually declining with time (Fig. 5a), likely reflecting improved disease management since the last episode of active nephritis. The risk of renal complications/nephritis in patients with very high concentrations of sSIGLEC-1 was much more pronounced in European patients (OR = 1.65) compared to non-European patients (OR = 1.16; Table 2), and was maintained after adjusting for the

association of sSIGLEC-1 with low C3 and C4 levels, which are predictors for renal disease (OR = 1.96, 95% CI 1.10–3.45; $P = 0.021$). Since sSIGLEC-1 could be physiologically excreted through the kidney, we also investigated whether increased sSIGLEC-1 concentrations could be associated with decreased kidney function in patients with renal disease. We found no evidence for an association between kidney function, as measured by the patients' estimated glomerular filtration rate (eGFR), and sSIGLEC-1 concentration (Fig. 5b). The association of sSIGLEC-1 and renal nephritis was maintained after adjusting for the effect of eGFR (OR = 1.49, 95% CI 1.02–2.17; $P = 0.04$). These data suggest that decreased renal function in patients with renal nephritis does not fully explain the association with increased sSIGLEC-1 concentrations observed in this study.

In addition to the association of sSIGLEC-1 with renal complications, we also observed a similar trend towards increased risk of haematological complications in patients with high concentrations of sSIGLEC-1, although not reaching statistical significance in our analysis (OR = 1.35, $P = 0.09$; Table 2). Further supporting the potential use of sSIGLEC-1 as a biomarker of disease severity, a higher frequency of patients with high levels of sSIGLEC-1 had a history of treatment with biologics (OR = 1.20, $P = 0.04$ in the combined population; Table 2), usually associated with patients with poor disease management who have not responded to standard treatment options. This remained the case even when we adjusted for history of renal complication as a confounding factor for biologics use.

Discussion

Recent advances in medical research have led to the development of a breadth of novel treatment options. The characterisation of biomarkers that identify the exact pathophysiological mechanism underpinning the clinical manifestations in each patient has thus become a

Table 2 Association of sSIGLEC-1 with clinical parameters of SLE

Clinical parameter	Combined			EUR			Non-EUR		
	N (total)	OR[a] (95% CI)	P value[b]	N (total)	OR[a] (95% CI)	P value[b]	N (total)	OR[a] (95% CI)	P value[b]
Renal (nephritis)	156	1.53 (1.10–2.15)	0.01	75	1.65 (1.09–2.52)	0.02	81	1.16 (0.60–2.25)	0.67
Haematological	291	1.35 (0.95–1.92)	0.09	185	1.34 (0.80–2.20)	0.25	106	1.28 (0.72–2.25)	0.4
Biologics[c]	35	1.20 (1.01–1.42)	0.04	23	1.18 (0.90–1.18)	0.19	12	0.95 (0.70–1.23)	0.71
Neurological	78	1.01 (0.76–1.34)	0.95	36	0.87 (0.63–1.18)	0.37	42	0.83 (0.39–1.76)	0.64
Admission	226	1.18 (0.81–1.71)	0.39	140	145 (0.90–2.37)	0.13	86	0.60 (0.30–1.21)	0.16
Corticosteroid use	302	0.98 (0.69–1.41)	0.96	174	0.96 (0.57–1.57)	0.86	128	0.88 (0.49–1.56)	0.35

Association of sSIGLEC-1 concentration with clinical parameters recorded from SLE patients occurring since their disease diagnosis and up to the time of their visit
CI confidence interval, *EUR* patients of European ancestry, *non-EUR* patients of non-European ancestry, *SLE* systemic lupus erythematosus, *sSIGLEC-1* soluble sialic acid binding Ig-like lectin 1
[a]Odds ratio (OR) calculated on the group of patients with sSIGLEC levels > 95th percentile
[b]P values were calculated in each group using a logistical regression model, where the SLE patients were divided into groups based on sSIGLEC1 serum level centiles (< 50th centile, 51st–74th centile, 75th–95th centile and > 95th centile)
[c]Patients treated with biologic drugs at the time of visit

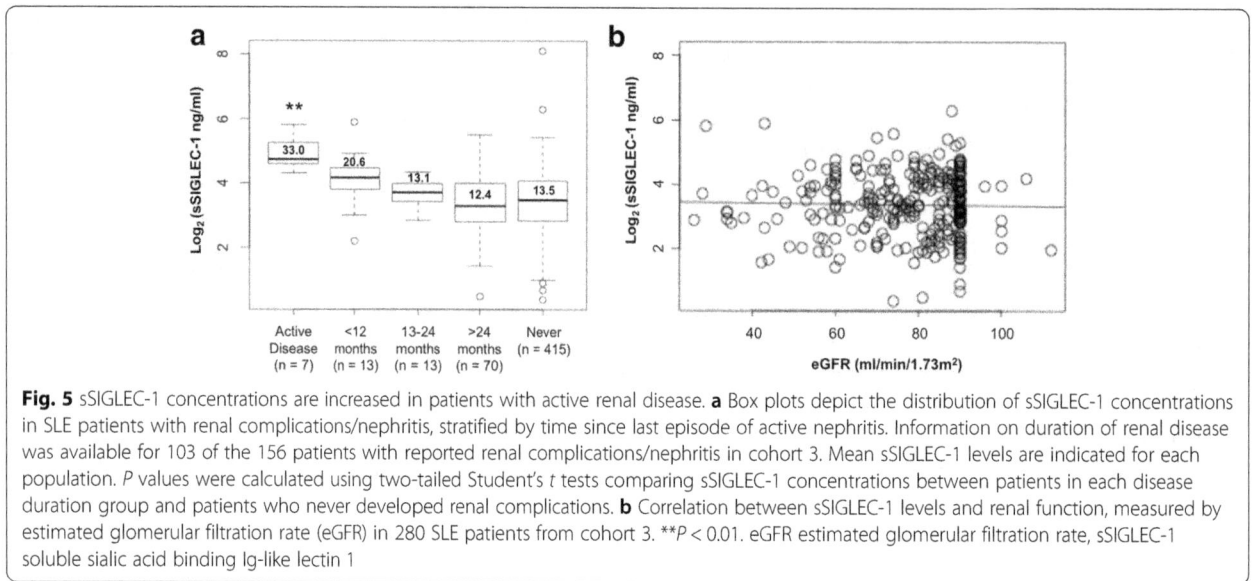

Fig. 5 sSIGLEC-1 concentrations are increased in patients with active renal disease. **a** Box plots depict the distribution of sSIGLEC-1 concentrations in SLE patients with renal complications/nephritis, stratified by time since last episode of active nephritis. Information on duration of renal disease was available for 103 of the 156 patients with reported renal complications/nephritis in cohort 3. Mean sSIGLEC-1 levels are indicated for each population. P values were calculated using two-tailed Student's t tests comparing sSIGLEC-1 concentrations between patients in each disease duration group and patients who never developed renal complications. **b** Correlation between sSIGLEC-1 levels and renal function, measured by estimated glomerular filtration rate (eGFR) in 280 SLE patients from cohort 3. **$P < 0.01$. eGFR estimated glomerular filtration rate, sSIGLEC-1 soluble sialic acid binding Ig-like lectin 1

priority to allow the advent of a truly personalised medicine approach to human complex diseases. In systemic autoimmune and inflammatory diseases, chronic IFN signalling has been shown to be directly involved in the pathogenesis of the diseases, most notably in SLE [28]. This observation has led to the development of therapeutic strategies to target IFN-α, which are currently being tested in the clinic [29, 30]. There is therefore an urgent need to develop robust and sensitive biomarkers to identify patients with an active IFN response who would be more likely to benefit from anti-IFN-α therapy.

In the present study, we show that a circulating form of the surface-bound SIGLEC-1 receptor can be detected in human plasma/serum, and developed a sensitive immunoassay to measure the circulating concentrations of sSIGLEC-1. To our knowledge we are the first to detect the presence of a soluble SIGLEC-1 isoform in humans. Our current data do not allow us to determine the origin of sSIGLEC-1, and further work is needed to assess whether the soluble isoform is generated through alternative splicing or by proteolytic shedding of the membrane-bound receptor. A key feature of this bioassay is the limited sample requirements, making it amenable—as compared to a flow cytometric assay of surface SIGLEC-1— to screen large numbers of samples. We therefore propose that quantification of sSIGLEC-1 using our immunoassay is an alternative to flow cytometric endpoints, or the classical IFN signature or its PCR-analysed surrogate [6], and will result in a more robust, simpler and less expensive measure of SIGLEC-1 expression and the IFN signature.

Other plasma/serum IFN-regulated biomarkers have been described in the literature, most notably IFN-α and IFN-γ-inducible protein 10 (IP-10) [12]. However, the protein stability, cell-type specificity and much higher concentrations of sSIGLEC-1 are major practical

advantages of our immunoassay. Moreover, measuring all 16 different IFN-α subtypes currently requires access to naturally occurring high-affinity anti-IFN-α antibodies that are not readily available [23], which in combination with the much lower sample requirement compared to the SIMOA assay makes the sSIGLEC-1 assay ideally suited for high-throughput screening, including the retrospective testing of samples collected from completed clinical studies or cohorts for flares of IFN signalling and/or response to treatment of large cohorts and retrospective studies. Recently, a study has reported that plasma concentrations of presepsin (PSEP), a product of CD14+ monocyte cleavage, is increased in patients with SLE and other autoimmune and inflammatory diseases [31]. Although the study was limited to a small sample size and available clinical data, the wide spread of PSEP levels measured in SLE patients and the suggested association with disease activity are consistent with our data and support a role for activated monocyte/ macrophages in the aetiology of SLE and other related autoimmune diseases. Further work will be required to investigate the relation between sSIGLEC-1 and PSEP, and the putative diagnostic and/or prognostic value of using a combination of biomarkers associated with exacerbated monocyte activation for the clinical stratification of patients with a systemic activation of the innate immune system.

Clinically, we identified marked ancestry-related differences in sSIGLEC-1 levels among SLE patients, which were consistent with the higher disease severity in patients of non-European ancestry. In agreement with this hypothesis, sSIGLEC-1 levels were also associated with lower levels of C3, a classical serologic marker of the disease. Furthermore, our data provide evidence that high sSIGLEC-1 levels could be predictive of active renal and haematological complications, particularly in patients of European ancestry.

These findings clearly underscore the importance of large, well-characterised, clinical cohorts to estimate the confounding effects of ancestry. In this study we had access to very limited numbers of non-European healthy controls, which prevented us from investigating whether steady-state sSIGLEC-1 levels could also be altered in populations of non-European ancestry. However, the association of sSIGLEC-1 concentrations with overall increased disease severity was consistently maintained in both groups of patients. A possible explanation for the more modest predictive capacity observed in non-European patients is an increased disease heterogeneity, which could reflect a reduced dependency on the type I IFN pathway for disease severity and late-stage organ damage in this group of patients. A limitation of this study was the number of available patients with active disease manifestations—namely, nephritis—which reduced the power to investigate the predictive capacity of high sSIGLEC-1 levels for the identification of patients with active disease. Further work will now be required to validate these findings in additional autoimmune and inflammatory diseases associated with a chronic activation of the innate immune system using large and clinically well-characterised patient populations, as well as to extend the findings to non-European cohorts.

There has been considerable interest in developing drugs targeting the IFN-α signalling pathway to treat conditions associated with chronic IFN signalling. Our assay could also have utility in clinical trials; for example, for the selection of patients who could benefit the most from such inhibition of IFN-α. Conversely, IFN-α is also one of the most used compounds in cytokine therapy. However, its immunomodulatory properties may result in various autoimmune manifestations, with reported incidence of 4–19% in patients undergoing IFN-α therapy [32]. We therefore hypothesise that these adverse events may be avoided if the background IFN signature is known and therapy is adjusted to avoid the excessive IFN signalling known to be a factor in the promotion of secondary autoimmunity in these patients. Moreover, it has been recently suggested that the detection of an IFN signature in peripheral blood is associated with poor response to both B-cell depleting therapy (rituximab) and anti-IL-6R treatment (tocilizumab) in rheumatoid arthritis patients [33, 34]. These data suggest that sSIGLEC-1 could be useful in prediction to therapeutic responses, and supports a broader application of this assay in the context of patient stratification for clinical trials.

Conclusions

In this study we report the development of a sensitive immunoassay to detect circulating concentrations of sSIGLEC-1 in plasma/serum. Taken together, our findings suggest that sSIGLEC-1 is a marker of monocyte and macrophage activation, which is critically implicated in the progression of several autoimmune and inflammatory diseases, such as SLE and SSc. In combination with additional available IFN-regulated biomarkers, the sSIGLEC-1 bioassay could help improve our capacity to dissect the molecular and clinical heterogeneity of complex conditions associated with an overt IFN response, and identify subsets of common and rare autoimmune and inflammatory diseases, collectively classified as interferonopathies. We have also shown that increased sSIGLEC-1 concentrations could, with further studies, have a clinical application in predicting increased risk of developing renal complications, one of the most severe clinical complications of SLE.

Additional files

Additional file 1: Table S1. Custom NanoString probe sequences used to measure expression of the 56 IFN-regulated genes defining the transcriptional IFN signature in this study and eight housekeeping genes used to normalise expression levels between donors.

Additional file 2: Figure S1. Concentration of IFN-α_{b2} is associated with the IFN transcriptional signature. Data depict correlation between plasma IFN-α_{b2} concentration and transcriptional IFN signature in 41 SLE patients from cohort 2.

Additional file 3: Figure S2. Association of sSIGLEC-1 with serological markers of SLE. **a, b** Data depict the association of sSIGLEC-1 concentrations with C-reactive protein (CRP) levels (**a**) and with disease-specific anti-nuclear autoantibody (ANA) titres (**b**). P values were calculated by linear regression.

Abbreviations

ACR: American College of Rheumatology; C3: Serum complement component 3; CI: Confidence interval; CV: Coefficient of variation; DELFIA: Dissociation-enhanced lanthanide fluorescent immunoassay; ECL: Electrochemical luminescence; ELISA: Enzyme-linked immunosorbent assay; IFN: Type I interferon; IP-10: IFN-γ-inducible protein 10; IRG: Type I interferon regulated genes; OR: Odds ratio; PBMC: Peripheral blood mononuclear cell; SIGLEC-1: Sialic acid binding Ig-like lectin 1; SLE: Systemic lupus erythematosus; SLEDAI: SLE Disease Activity Index; SSc: Systemic sclerosis; sSIGLEC-1: Soluble SIGLEC-1; TRF: Time-resolved fluorescence

Acknowledgements

The authors gratefully acknowledge the participation of all NIHR Cambridge BioResource volunteers, and thank the NIHR Cambridge BioResource centre and staff for their contribution. They thank the National Institute for Health Research and NHS Blood and Transplant. The authors thank Neil Walker and Helen Schuilenburg from the Cambridge Institute for Medical Research, University of Cambridge for data management. They thank members of the Cambridge BioResource SAB and management committee for their support and the National Institute for Health Research Cambridge Biomedical Research Centre for funding. The authors also thank Helen Stevens, Gill Coleman, Sarah Dawson, Simon Duley, Meeta Maisuria and Sumiyya Mahmood from the Cambridge Institute for Medical Research, University of Cambridge for preparation of DNA and PBMC samples. They also thank Emma Jones from AstraZeneca for the use of the NanoString instrument and Claudia Gonzalez-Lopez from the Weatherall Institute of Molecular Medicine, Oxford, for the use of the Simoa HD-1 analyser.

Funding

This work was funded by the JDRF (9-2011-253), the Wellcome (WT061858/ 091157) and the National Institute for Health Research Cambridge Biomedical Research Centre. This research was also funded/supported by the National Institute for Health Research Biomedical Research Centre based at Guy's and St Thomas' NHS Foundation Trust and King's College London. RCF is funded by a JDRF Advanced post-doctoral fellowship (2-APF-2017-420-A-N).

Authors' contributions
JAT and RCF conceived the study. TJV, LSW, JAT and RCF designed the experiments. JJO, DBR, CLP, PC, OA-A, KB and RCF performed the experiments. JJO, SK, ARG, KB and RCF analysed the data and interpreted the results. SK, SM, RS and TJV provided patient samples. RCF wrote the manuscript with input from all co-authors. All authors read and approved the final manuscript.

Consent for publication
Not applicable.

Competing interests
JJO is an employee of GlaxoSmithKline pharmaceuticals. The other authors declare that they have no competing interests.

Author details
[1]Department of Medical Genetics, JDRF/Wellcome Diabetes and Inflammation Laboratory, NIHR Cambridge Biomedical Research Centre, Cambridge Institute for Medical Research, University of Cambridge, Cambridge, UK. [2]Division of Genetics and Molecular Medicine and Division of Immunology, Infection and Inflammatory Disease, King's College London, Great Maze Pond, London, UK. [3]JDRF/Wellcome Diabetes and Inflammation Laboratory, Wellcome Centre for Human Genetics, Nuffield Department of Medicine, NIHR Oxford Biomedical Research Centre, University of Oxford, Roosevelt Drive, Oxford, UK. [4]NIHR Cambridge Biomedical Research Centre, Core Biochemical Assay Laboratory, Cambridge, UK. [5]UCL Centre for Rheumatology and Connective Tissue Diseases, UCL Medical School, Royal Free Hospital Campus, Rowland Hill Street, London, UK.

References
1. Preble OT, Black RJ, Friedman RM, Klippel JH, Vilcek J. Systemic lupus erythematosus: presence in human serum of an unusual acid-labile leukocyte interferon. Science (80). 1982;216:429–31.
2. Obermoser G, Pascual V. The interferon-α signature of systemic lupus erythematosus. Lupus. 2010;19:1012–9.
3. Morimoto AM, Flesher DT, Yang J, Wolslegel K, Wang X, Brady A, et al. Association of endogenous anti-interferon-α autoantibodies with decreased interferon-pathway and disease activity in patients with systemic lupus erythematosus. Arthritis Rheum. 2011;63:2407–15.
4. Baechler EC, Batliwalla FM, Karypis G, Gaffney PM, Ortmann WA, Espe KJ, et al. Interferon-inducible gene expression signature in peripheral blood cells of patients with severe lupus. Proc Natl Acad Sci U S A. 2003;100:2610–5.
5. Bennett L, Palucka AK, Arce E, Cantrell V, Borvak J, Banchereau J, et al. Interferon and granulopoiesis signatures in systemic lupus erythematosus blood. J Exp Med. 2003;197:711–23.
6. Kennedy WP, Maciuca R, Wolslegel K, Tew W, Abbas AR, Chaivorapol C, et al. Association of the interferon signature metric with serological disease manifestations but not global activity scores in multiple cohorts of patients with SLE. Lupus Sci Med. 2015;2:e000080.
7. Banchereau R, Hong S, Cantarel B, Baldwin N, Baisch J, Edens M, et al. Personalized Immunomonitoring uncovers molecular networks that stratify lupus patients. Cell. 2016;165:551–65.
8. Strauß R, Rose T, Flint SM, Klotsche J, Häupl T, Peck-Radosavljevic M, et al. Type I interferon as a biomarker in autoimmunity and viral infection: a leukocyte subset-specific analysis unveils hidden diagnostic options. J Mol Med. 2017;95:753–65.
9. Landolt-Marticorena C, Bonventi G, Lubovich A, Ferguson C, Unnithan T, Su J, et al. Lack of association between the interferon-α signature and longitudinal changes in disease activity in systemic lupus erythematosus. Ann Rheum Dis. 2009;68:1440–6.
10. Petri M, Singh S, Tesfasyone H, Dedrick R, Fry K, Lal PG, et al. Longitudinal expression of type I interferon responsive genes in systemic lupus erythematosus. Lupus. 2009;18:980–9.
11. Biesen R, Demir C, Barkhudarova F, Grün JR, Steinbrich-Zöllner M, Backhaus M, et al. Sialic acid-binding Ig-like lectin 1 expression in inflammatory and resident monocytes is a potential biomarker for monitoring disease activity and success of therapy in systemic lupus erythematosus. Arthritis Rheum. 2008;58:1136–45.
12. Rose T, Grützkau A, Hirseland H, Huscher D, Dähnrich C, Dzionek A, et al. IFNα and its response proteins, IP-10 and SIGLEC-1, are biomarkers of disease activity in systemic lupus erythematosus. Ann Rheum Dis. 2013;72:1639–45.
13. Rose T, Grützkau A, Klotsche J, Enghard P, Flechsig A, Keller J, et al. Are interferon-related biomarkers advantageous for monitoring disease activity in systemic lupus erythematosus? A longitudinal benchmark study. Rheumatology. 2017;56:1618–26.
14. O'Neill ASG, van den Berg TK, Mullen GED. Sialoadhesin—a macrophage-restricted marker of immunoregulation and inflammation. Immunology. 2013;138:198–207.
15. Hartnell A, Steel J, Turley H, Jones M, Jackson DG, Crocker PR. Characterization of human sialoadhesin, a sialic acid binding receptor expressed by resident and inflammatory macrophage populations. Blood. 2001;97:288–96.
16. Izquierdo-Useros N, Lorizate M, Puertas MC, Rodriguez-Plata MT, Zangger N, Erikson E, et al. Siglec-1 is a novel dendritic cell receptor that mediates HIV-1 trans-infection through recognition of viral membrane gangliosides. PLoS Biol. 2012;10:e1001448.
17. Xiong Y-S, Cheng Y, Lin Q-S, Wu A-L, Yu J, Li C, et al. Increased expression of Siglec-1 on peripheral blood monocytes and its role in mononuclear cell reactivity to autoantigen in rheumatoid arthritis. Rheumatol. 2014;53:250–9.
18. York MR, Nagai T, Mangini AJ, Lemaire R, van Seventer JM, Lafyatis R. A macrophage marker, Siglec-1, is increased on circulating monocytes in patients with systemic sclerosis and induced by type I interferons and toll-like receptor agonists. Arthritis Rheum. 2007;56:1010–20.
19. Bao G, Han Z, Yan Z, Wang Q, Zhou Y, Yao D, et al. Increased Siglec-1 expression in monocytes of patients with primary biliary cirrhosis. Immunol Investig. 2010;39:645–60.
20. Lisney AR, Szelinski F, Reiter K, Burmester GR, Rose T, Dörner T. High maternal expression of SIGLEC1 on monocytes as a surrogate marker of a type I interferon signature is a risk factor for the development of autoimmune congenital heart block. Ann Rheum Dis. 2017;76:1476–80.
21. van den Hoogen F, Khanna D, Fransen J, Johnson SR, Baron M, Tyndall A, et al. 2013 classification criteria for systemic sclerosis: an American College of Rheumatology/European League Against Rheumatism collaborative initiative. Ann Rheum Dis. 2013;72:1747–55.
22. Ferreira RC, Guo H, Coulson RMR, Smyth DJ, Pekalski ML, Burren OS, et al. A type I interferon transcriptional signature precedes autoimmunity in children genetically at risk for type 1 diabetes. Diabetes. 2014;63:2538–50.
23. Rodero MP, Decalf J, Bondet V, Hunt D, Rice GI, Werneke S, et al. Detection of interferon alpha protein reveals differential levels and cellular sources in disease. J Exp Med. 2017;214:1547–55.
24. Wu M, Assassi S. The role of type 1 interferon in systemic sclerosis. Front Immunol. 2013;4:266.
25. Petri M, Perez-Gutthann S, Longenecker JC, Hochberg M. Morbidity of systemic lupus erythematosus: role of race and socioeconomic status. Am J Med. 1991;91:345–53.
26. Alarcón GS, McGwin G Jr, Petri M, Ramsey-Goldman R, Fessler BJ, Vilá LM, et al. Time to renal disease and end-stage renal disease in PROFILE: a multiethnic lupus cohort. PLoS Med. 2006;3:e396.
27. Bruce IN, O'Keeffe AG, Farewell V, Hanly JG, Manzi S, Su L, et al. Factors associated with damage accrual in patients with systemic lupus erythematosus: results from the Systemic Lupus International Collaborating Clinics (SLICC) Inception Cohort. Ann Rheum Dis. 2015;74:1706–13.
28. Hooks JJ, Moutsopoulos HM, Geis SA, Stahl NI, Decker JL, Notkins AL. Immune interferon in the circulation of patients with autoimmune disease. N Engl J Med. 1979;301:5–8.
29. Lauwerys BR, Ducreux J, Houssiau FA. Type I interferon blockade in systemic lupus erythematosus: where do we stand? Rheumatol. 2014;53:1369–76.
30. Oon S, Wilson NJ, Wicks I. Targeted therapeutics in SLE: emerging strategies to modulate the interferon pathway. Clin Trans Immunol. 2016;5:e79.
31. Tanimura S, Fujieda Y, Kono M, Shibata Y, Hisada R, Sugawara E, et al. Clinical significance of plasma presepsin levels in patients with systemic lupus erythematosus. Mod Rheumatol. 2017:1–7. https://doi.org/10.1080/14397595.2017.1408755.
32. Ioannou Y, Isenberg DA. Current evidence for the induction of autoimmune rheumatic manifestations by cytokine therapy. Arthritis Rheum. 2000;43:1431–42.
33. Raterman HG, Vosslamber S, de Ridder S, Nurmohamed MT, Lems WF, Boers M, et al. The interferon type I signature towards prediction of non-response to rituximab in rheumatoid arthritis patients. Arthritis Res Ther. 2012;14:1–10.

2

MRI-detected osteophytes of the knee: natural history and structural correlates of change

Zhaohua Zhu[1,2], Changhai Ding[1,2,3], Weiyu Han[1], Shuang Zheng[2], Tania Winzenberg[2,4], Flavia Cicuttini[3] and Graeme Jones[2*]

Abstract

Backgroud: The natural history of semi-quantitative magnetic resonance imaging (MRI)-detected osteophytes (MRI-detected OPs) has not been described and it is unknown whether knee structural abnormalities can predict MRI-detected OP change over time. Thus, the aim of current study is to describe the natural history of knee MRI-detected OP, and to determine if knee structural abnormalities are associated with change of MRI-detected OP in a longitudinal study of older adults.

Methods: Randomly selected older adults ($n = 837$, mean age 63 years) had MRI at baseline and 413 of them had MRI 2.6 years later to measure MRI-detected OP, cartilage defects, cartilage volume, bone marrow lesions (BMLs), meniscal extrusion, infrapatellar fat pad (IPFP) quality score/maximum area and effusion-synovitis.

Results: Over 2.6 years, average MRI-detected OP score increased significantly in all compartments. The total MRI-detected OP score remained stable in 53% of participants, worsened ($\geq$ 1-point increase) in 46% and decreased in 1%. Baseline cartilage defects (RR, 1.25–1.35), BMLs (RR, 1.16–1.17), meniscal extrusion (RR, 1.22–1.33) and IPFP quality score (RR, 1.08–1.20) site-specifically and independently predicted an increase in MRI-detected OP (p values all $\leq$ 0.05), after adjustment for covariates. Presence of IPFP abnormality was significantly associated with increased MRI-detected OPs but became non-significant after adjustment for other structural abnormalities. Total (RR, 1.27) and suprapatellar pouch effusion-synovitis (RR, 1.22) were both associated with increased MRI-detected OPs in the lateral compartment only (both $p < 0.04$).

Conclusion: Knee MRI-detected OPs are common in older adults and are likely to progress. The association between baseline structural abnormalities and worsening MRI-detected OPs suggest MRI-detected OP could be a consequence of multiple knee structural abnormalities.

Keywords: Osteoarthritis, Magnetic resonance imaging, Osteophyte, Natural history

Background

Osteoarthritis (OA) is a major contributor to overall disability in Western populations. Osteophytes (OPs) have long been viewed as a defining structural feature of knee OA [1] and a fundamental sign of disease incidence and progression [2]. They are associated with radiographic joint space narrowing, subchondral sclerosis, and cartilage defects in both tibiofemoral and patellofemoral compartments [3, 4]. The size and extent of OP formation is routinely used for classifying the stage of OA [5].

Conventional radiographs remain the gold standard for assessment of OPs [6], but the association between presence of knee OPs on radiographs and symptoms is poor [7]. Two-dimensional conventional radiographs may miss the extent and size of OPs [8]. On the other hand, magnetic resonance imaging (MRI) is a non-invasive multiplanar tomographic modality that can assess many knee osteoarthritic changes [9]. Studies suggest that MRI can assess OPs

---
* Correspondence: Graeme.Jones@utas.edu.au
[2]Menzies Institute for Medical Research, University of Tasmania, Hobart, TAS, Australia
Full list of author information is available at the end of the article

with much greater sensitivity than radiographs and in locations that are not easily visualised by conventional radiography due to its ability to provide three-dimensional information [10–12]. Our recent study reported that MRI-detected OPs are highly prevalent in older adults (85% vs 10% radiographic OPs prevalence) and can independently and site-specifically predict increases in cartilage defects, BMLs and loss of cartilage volume, and worsening knee pain over time, suggesting MRI-detected OPs are clinically relevant [13].

As far as we know, there are seldom longitudinal studies [14–16] investigating the relationship between MRI-detected OPs and clinical changes of OA. Sowers et al. found that large MRI-detected OPs were associated with increased odds of knee pain and reduced physical function [14]. Hakky et al. measured OP volume using MRI and observed significant positive correlation between OP volume and cartilage thickness loss [16]. In the latest study, MRI-detected OPs in a group of patients with end-stage OA scored using the Whole-Organ Magnetic Resonance Imaging Score (WORMS) grading system, those with a MRI-detected OP score of more than 30 have about threefold higher risk of undergoing total knee arthroplasty [15]. Based on the Chingford study, the natural history of radiographic OA is that of very slow progression [17]. However, the natural history of semi-quantitative MRI-detected OPs has not been described and it is unknown whether knee structural abnormalities, including cartilage defects, bone marrow lesions (BMLs), meniscal extrusion, infrapatellar fat pad (IPFP), and effusion-synovitis, can predict MRI-detected OP change over time. Hence, the aims of this study were to describe the natural history of knee MRI-detected OP, and to determine if knee structural abnormalities are associated with change of MRI-detected OP in a longitudinal study of older adults.

Methods
Participants
This study was from the Tasmania Older Adult Cohort (TASOAC) Study, a population-based, ongoing, prospective longitudinal cohort study which was designed to identify the genetic, environmental, and biochemical factors associated with the development and progression of OA at multiple sites. Participants between 50 and 80 years old were randomly selected from the electoral roll in Southern Tasmania (population 229,000) with an equal number of men and women (response rate 57%). Participants were excluded if they were institutionalized or had contraindications to MRI. The Southern Tasmania Health and Medical Human Research Ethics Committee approved the study, and written informed consent was obtained from all participants. Baseline examinations were made between February 2002 and September 2004, and follow-up measures were made at approximately 2.6 years later. This study consisted of 837 participants who had both knee MRI and radiographic scans at baseline.

Anthropometrics
Weight was measured using electronic scales (nearest 0.1 kg), with shoes, socks and bulky clothing removed. Height was measured using a stadiometer (nearest 0.1 cm), with shoes, socks and headgear removed. Body mass index (BMI) was calculated using height and weight (kg/m^2).

Magnetic resonance imaging
MRI scans of the right knees were performed on two occasions and imaged in the sagittal plane on a 1.5-T whole body magnetic resonance unit (Picker, Cleveland, OH, USA) using a commercial transmit-receive extremity coil. The image sequences used are listed as follows: (1) T1-weighted fat-saturation 3D gradient recall acquisition in the steady state; flip angle 30°; repetition time 31 ms; echo time 6.71 ms; field of view 16 cm; 60 partitions; 512×512 matrix; acquisition time 11 min 56 s; one acquisition. Sagittal images were obtained at a partition thickness of 1.5 mm and an in-plane resolution of 0.31×0.31 (512×512 pixels); (2) T2-weighted fat-saturation 3D fast spin echo, flip angle 90, repetition time 3067 ms, echo time 112 ms, field of view 16 cm, 15 partitions, 228×256-pixel matrix; sagittal images were obtained at a partition thickness of 4 mm with a between-slices gap of 0.5 to 1.0 mm. The image database was transferred to an independent computer workstation using the software program Osirix (University of Geneva, Geneva, Switzerland) as previously described [18, 19].

MRI-detected osteophytes
MRI-detected OPs were measured by ZZ using a combination of Whole-Organ Magnetic Resonance Imaging Score (WORMS) and the Knee Osteoarthritis Scoring System (KOSS) [9, 20]. OPs were defined as focal bony excrescences, seen on sagittal, axial or coronal images, extending from a cortical surface. Size was measured from the base (distinguished from that of adjacent articular cartilage with a normal MRI appearance) to the tip of the OP [11] at each of the following 14 sites: the anterior (a), central weight bearing (c) and posterior (p) margins of the femoral condyles and tibial plateaus, and the medial (M) and lateral (L) margins of the patella [20] (Fig. 1). OPs were graded as follows: grade 0, absent; grade 1, minimal (< 3 mm high); grade 2, moderate (3–5 mm); grade 3, severe (> 5 mm) [9]. The sum total score of each individual site in the relevant compartment (or whole knee) was regarded as the OP score in that compartment (or whole knee).

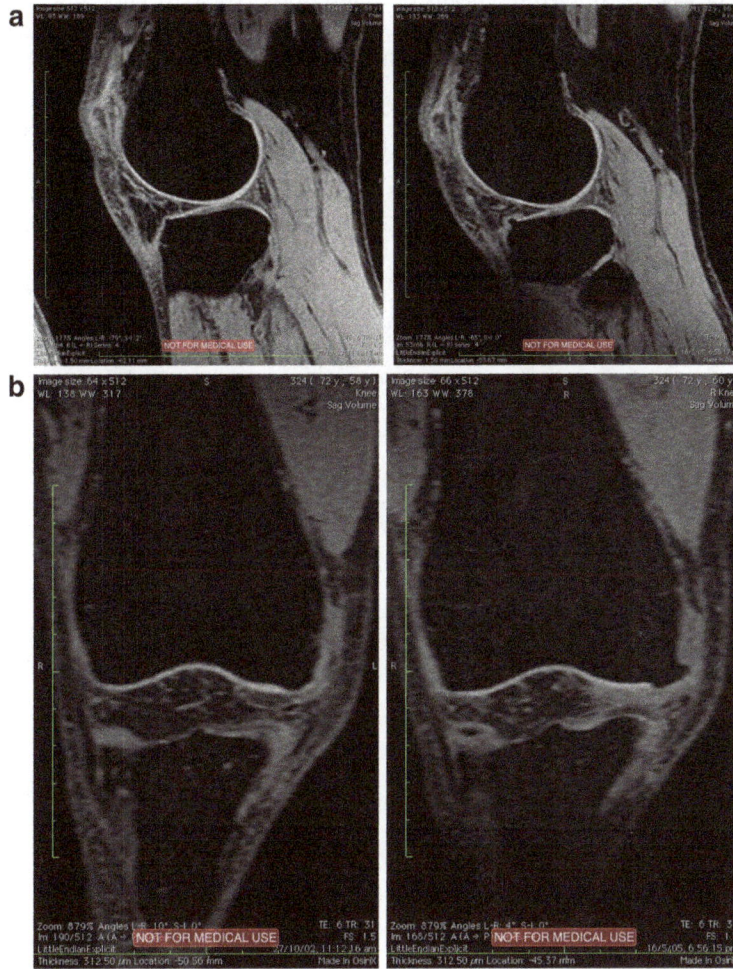

Fig. 1 Sample images show magnetic resonance imaging (MRI)-detected osteophyte (OP) progression. **a** Tibial MRI-detected OP increases from baseline to follow up (wider arrow indicates follow-up MRI-detected OP). **b** Femoral MRI-detected OP increases from baseline to follow up (wider arrow indicates follow-up MRI-detected OP)

MRI-detected OP score ≥ 1 was considered as OP present. An increase in the MRI-detected OP score from baseline to follow up at any site was defined as a change of ≥ 1 at the site. MRI-detected OPs were remeasured by ZZ and WH in 40 randomly selected participants, with a 4-week interval, to calculate intra-observer and inter-observer reliabilities. Intra-observer reliability (expressed as intraclass correlation coefficients, ICCs) was 0.94–0.97 and inter-observer reliability was 0.90–0.96 [21].

Cartilage defects

Cartilage defects were graded by CD at the medial tibial, lateral tibial, medial femoral, lateral femoral and patellar regions as previously described [22] as follows: grade 0, normal cartilage; grade 1, focal blistering and low-signal intensity change with an intact surface and bottom; grade 2, irregularities on the surface or bottom and loss of thickness

< 50%; grade 4, full-thickness cartilage loss with exposure of subchondral bone [23]. The highest score of each individual site in the relevant compartment (or whole knee) was regarded as the cartilage defect score in that compartment (or whole knee). The presence of cartilage defects was defined as a cartilage defect score ≥ 2 at any site. An increase in cartilage defects was defined as a change in cartilage defects ≥ 1. Intra-observer reliability was 0.89–0.94 and inter-observer reliability was 0.85–0.93 [22].

Cartilage volume

Knee cartilage volume was measured on T1-weighted images by a single trained observer at baseline as previously described [23, 24]. The volumes of individual cartilage plates (medial tibial, lateral tibial, medial femoral, lateral femoral and patellar) were isolated from the total volume by manually drawing disarticulation contours around the cartilage boundaries on a section by section basis. These data were resampled by means of bilinear and cubic interpolation (area of 312×312) μm and 1.5 mm thickness, continuous sections) for the final 3D rendering. Changes in cartilage volume were calculated as:

Percentage change per annum = [(Follow-up volume − Baseline volume)/Baseline cartilage volume]/Time between 2 scans in years × 100.

The coefficients of variation (CVs) for cartilage volume measures were 2.1% to 2.6% [23, 24].

Bone marrow lesions

Subchondral bone marrow lesions (BMLs) were defined as a discrete area of increased signal adjacent to the subcortical bone on T2-weighted MRI and were scored at the medial tibial, lateral tibial, medial femoral, lateral femoral, medial patellar and lateral patellar regions using a modified version of WORMS: grade 0, absence of BML; grade 1, area < 25% of the region; grade 2, area between 25% and 50% of the region; grade 3, area > 50% of the region [20]. The highest score of each individual site in the relevant compartment (or whole knee) was regarded as the BML score in that compartment (or whole knee). An increase in BMLs was defined as a change in BMLs ≥ 1. The inter-observer reliability of this BML scoring system was assessed by randomly selecting 40 subjects with BMLs and having their MRI scans re-read by another observer. The ICCs for inter-observer reliability were also excellent (0.73–0.95) [25, 26].

Meniscal extrusion

Meniscal extrusion was assessed by a trained observer on T1-weighted MRI as previously described [27]. The proportion of the menisci affected by full extrusion was scored on the medial and lateral edges of the tibiofemoral joint space using a semi-quantitative scale. The extent of meniscal extrusion, not including the osteophytes, was evaluated for the anterior, middle and posterior horns of the menisci with 0, no extrusion; 1, partial extrusion and 2, complete extrusion with no contact with the joint space (severe). The intra-observer and inter-observer correlation coefficient ranged from 0.85 to 0.92 [28].

Infrapatellar fat pad

The infrapatellar fat pad (IPFP) was measured both semi-quantitatively and quantitatively. IPFP maximum area was measured by manually drawing disarticulation contours around the IPFP boundaries on a secton-by-section T2-weighted MR image, using the software program Osiris (University of Geneva). The maximal area was selected to represent the IPFP size. One observer graded the IPFP area in all MRI examinations. The intra-class correlation coefficient was 0.96 for intra-observer reliability and was 0.92 for inter-observer reliability [29]. The IPFP quality score was assessed semi-quantitatively according to its signal intensity alteration, which was defined as discrete areas of increased signal within IPFP: grade 0, no signal intensity alteration; grade 1, < 10% of the region has altered signal intensity; grade 2, 10–20% of the region; grade 3, > 20% of the region. Intra-observer and inter-observer reliability was high (intra-class correlation coefficient of 0.90 and inter-class correlation coefficient of 0.89, respectively) [30]. Presence of IPFP abnormality was defined as a signal intensity alteration score ≥ 1.

Effusion-synovitis

Knee effusion-synovitis at baseline was defined as the presence of intra-articular fluid-equivalent signal on T2-weighted MRI. We measured effusion-synovitis in the following subregions: (1) suprapatellar pouch, extending superiorly from the upper surface of the femur; (2) central portion, lying between the central femoral and tibia condyles, around the ligaments and menisci; (3) posterior femoral recess, lying behind the posterior portion of each femoral condyle and the deep surface of the lateral and medial heads of the gastrocnemius; (4) subpopliteal recess, lying posteriorly between the lateral meniscus and the popliteal tendon. Effusion-synovitis in each subregion was scored from 0 to 3 in terms of the estimated maximal distention of the synovial cavity: 0, normal; 1 < 33% of maximum potential distention; 2, 33–66% of maximum potential distention; 3, > 66% of maximum potential distention [20]. The two independent observers scored images blinded to participant information. The intra-class reliability and the inter-class reliability in different subregions was 0.63–0.79 [31].

Statistical analysis

Student's t test or the chi-square (χ^2) test was used to compare means or proportions between participants with or without an increase in total knee MRI-detected OPs. The paired t test was used to compare means between baseline and follow-up MRI-detected OPs in different compartments. Crude and adjusted log binominal regression was used to examine the longitudinal associations between increases in MRI-detected OPs (dependent variable), and baseline knee BMLs, cartilage defects, meniscal extrusion, effusion-synovitis and IPFP (independent variables), with age, sex, BMI and all the structural abnormalities as covariates. All statistical analyses were performed in Stata version 12.0 for Windows (StataCorp, College Station, TX, USA) [12]. A p value < 0.05 (two-tailed) or a 95% confidence interval (CI) not including a value of 1.00 was considered statistically significant.

Results

Characteristics of the study population

A total of 1099 participants aged between 51 and 81 (mean 63) years were recruited to the TASOAC study of whom 837 had radiographs and MRI scans taken at baseline. The current study consists of a sample of 413 participants who had completed MRI scans at baseline and follow up. MRI scans were discontinued after this follow up due to decommissioning of the scanner. As reported previously [13], participants who did not complete follow-up MRI measures were similar to the remainder of the cohort in terms of demographics, smoking status, cartilage defects, BMLs, cartilage volume and radiographic OA at baseline. The characteristics of participants grouped by whether they had an increase or no increase in total knee MRI-detected OPs over 2.6 years of follow up are shown in Table 1. Participants with an increase in MRI-detected OPs over 2.6 years had significantly higher baseline BMI, MRI-detected OP score, cartilage defect score, BML score, meniscal extrusion score, total and suprapatellar effusion-synovitis score and IPFP quality score.

Natural history of MRI-detected OPs

The changes in MRI-detected OP scores by site over 2.6 years are presented in Fig. 2: 413 participants had completed follow-up MRI scans, 83%, 69%, 77%, and 53% of these participants had stable MRI-detected OP scores in the medial tibiofemoral, lateral tibiofemoral, patellar and total knee, respectively. Of these participants, 17%, 30%, 23% and 46% had increased MRI-detected OP scores in the medial tibiofemoral, lateral tibiofemoral, patellar and total knee, respectively. Of the 413 participants (86%) who completed follow up, 356 had knee MRI-detected OPs at baseline. Of these participants, 48% persisted in total MRI-detected OP size, 51% increased in total MRI-detected OP size, and only 1% decreased in total MRI-detected OP size. At baseline, MRI-detected OPs were absent in a total of 57 participants, of whom 11 (19%) developed new OPs. Over 2.6 years, the average MRI-detected OP scores in all compartments increased significantly (Fig. 3).

Factors associated with an increase in MRI-detected OPs

Table 2 gives the association between baseline BMLs, cartilage defects, meniscal extrusion and increases in MRI-detected OPs over 2.6 years. Higher baseline BML scores and meniscal extrusion scores in medial tibiofemoral, lateral tibiofemoral and total compartments were significantly associated with increased MRI-detected OPs in the corresponding compartments, after adjustment for age, sex and BMI. These associations remained after further adjustment for baseline MRI-detected OPs and other structural abnormalities, except for the

Table 1 Characteristics of participants at baseline

	Stable or decreased OPs N = 222	Increased OPs N = 191	p
Age (years)	62.2 ± 7.3	62.9 ± 7.0	0.30
Female (%)	53	47	0.22
BMI (kg/m^2)	**26.9 ± 3.9**	**28.5 ± 4.9**	**< 0.01**
Baseline total cartilage defect score (0–4)	**1.48 ± 0.73**	**2.13 ± 1.03**	**< 0.01**
Baseline total BML score (0–3)	**0.33 ± 0.56**	**0.59 ± 0.78**	**< 0.01**
Baseline total tibial CV (ml)	5.11 ± 1.22	5.08 ± 1.13	0.80
Baseline meniscal extrusion score (0–2)	**0.13 ± 0.36**	**0.27 ± 0.51**	**< 0.01**
Total effusion-synovitis score (0–3)	**1.90 ± 0.67**	**2.08 ± 0.81**	**0.01**
Suprapatellar effusion-synovitis score (0–3)	**1.53 ± 0.64**	**1.76 ± 0.84**	**0.01**
Central portion effusion-synovitis score (0–3)	1.56 ± 0.71	1.65 ± 0.77	0.19
Posterior femoral recess effusion-synovitis score (0–3)	0.66 ± 0.79	0.76 ± 0.78	0.14
Subpopliteal recess effusion-synovitis score (0–3)	**0.60 ± 0.79**	**0.78 ± 0.94**	**0.04**
IPFP area (cm^2)	7.6 ± 1.2	7.7 ± 1.3	0.18
Presence of IPFP abnormality (%)	75%	82%	0.10
IPFP quality score (0–6)	**1.45 ± 1.21**	**2.12 ± 1.64**	**< 0.01**
Baseline total OP score (0–36)	**2.80 ± 3.45**	**7.62 ± 7.70**	**< 0.01**

The two-tailed t test was used to examine differences between means, and the χ2 test was used for proportions (percentages). Significant differences are shown in bold. Mean ± SD except for percentages

BMI body mass index, BM: bone marrow lesion, OP osteophyte, CV cartilage volume, IPFP infrapatellar fat pad

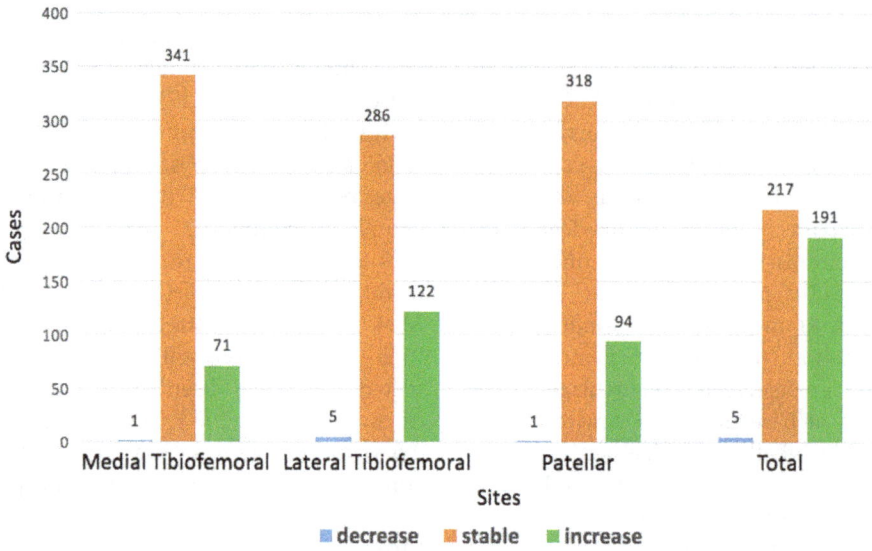

Fig. 2 Change in magnetic resonance imaging (MRI)-detected osteophyte (OP) scores by site over 2.6 years. Total score was calculated by summing medial tibiofemoral (tibfem), lateral tibiofemoral and patellar scores

associations with BMLs in the lateral tibiofemoral and patellar compartments. Higher baseline cartilage defect score in the medial tibiofemoral, lateral tibiofemoral and total compartments was significantly associated with increased MRI-detected OPs in the corresponding compartments, after adjustment for age, sex and BMI, and remained significant after further adjustment for baseline MRI-detected OPs and other structural abnormalities.

Table 3 shows the associations between baseline effusion-synovitis, IPFP and increased MRI-detected OPs over 2.6 years. Baseline total and suprapatellar effusion-synovitis scores were significantly associated with increases in total MRI-detected OP after adjustment for age, sex and BMI, but this did not persist after

further adjustment for baseline OPs, BMLs and cartilage defects. Baseline effusion-synovitis score was not associated with increased medial MRI-detected OPs. In the lateral tibiofemoral compartment, baseline total, suprapatellar and central portion effusion-synovitis were significantly associated with increased MRI-detected OPs after adjustment for age, sex and BMI. The associations with total effusion-synovitis and suprapatellar effusion-synovitis but not central portion effusion-synovitis remained after further adjustment.

Baseline IPFP quality scores were significantly associated with increases in total MRI-detected OPs both before and after adjustment for covariates. In the medial tibiofemoral compartment, baseline IPFP quality score and presence of

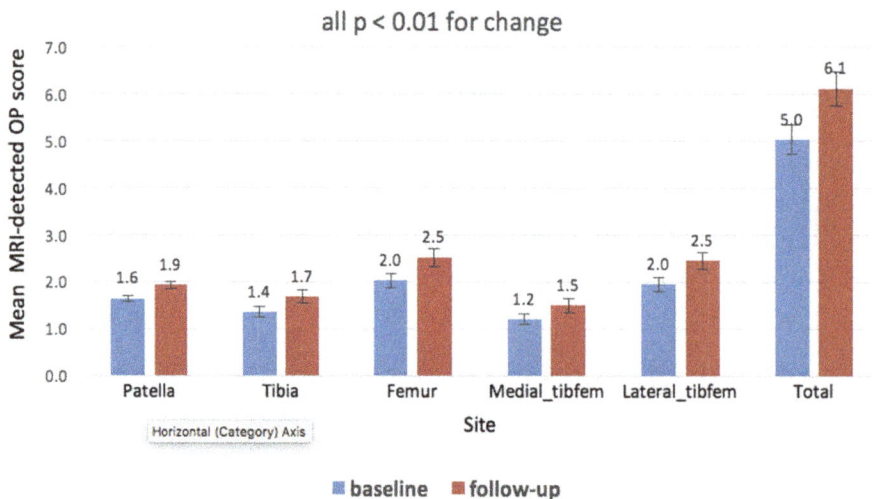

Fig. 3 Average magnetic resonance imaging (MRI)-detected osteophyte (OP) scores increased significantly in all compartments over 2.6 years

Table 2 Site-specific association with increase in MRI-detected OPs over 2.6 years

	Multivariable* RR (95% CI)	Multivariable** RR (95% CI)
Increase in MRI-detected OPs (yes or no)		
Medial BMLs	1.37 (1.19, 1.58)	1.17 (1.02, 1.35)
Lateral BMLs	1.81 (1.11, 2.97)	1.11 (0.84, 2.40)
Patellar BMLs	1.16 (1.02, 1.33)	1.14 (0.94, 1.37)
Total BMLs	1.30 (1.19, 1.42)	1.16 (1.03, 1.31)
Medial cartilage defects	1.39 (1.25, 1.54)	1.30 (1.16, 1.45)
Lateral cartilage defects	1.42 (1.26, 1.61)	1.35 (1.21, 1.51)
Patellar cartilage defects	1.34 (1.22, 1.47)	1.25 (1.13, 1.38)
Total cartilage defects	2.19 (1.71, 2.80)	1.33 (1.20, 1.46)
Medial meniscal extrusion	1.39 (1.12, 1.71)	1.24 (1.00, 1.55)
Lateral meniscal extrusion	1.50 (1.27, 1.79)	1.33 (1.14, 1.56)
Total meniscal extrusion	1.40 (1.17, 1.69)	1.22 (1.01, 1.47)

Dependent variable: increases in magnetic resonance imaging (MRI)-detected osteophytes (OPs) (yes or no) in the same compartment as each exposure. Independent variables: baseline bone marrow lesions (BMLs), cartilage defects, meniscal extrusion (per grade)
*Adjusted for age, sex and body mass index
**Further adjusted for other structural abnormalities and baseline OP scores. Bold denotes statistical significance

IPFP abnormality was significantly associated with increased MRI-detected OPs after adjustment for age, sex and BMI, but only IPFP quality score remained significant after further adjustments. IPFP quality scores and presence of IPFP abnormality were significantly associated with increased MRI-detected OPs in the lateral tibiofemoral compartment after adjustment for age, sex and BMI, but only IPFP quality scores persisted after further adjustment. IPFP maximum area was not associated with increased MRI-detected OPs in any compartments (Table 3).

Discussion

To the best of our knowledge, this is the first study to describe the natural history of MRI-detected OPs and structural factors associated with this change. In this older adult sample, MRI-detected OPs were common, progressed in nearly half of participants over 2.6 years and rarely regressed. Baseline BMLs, cartilage defects, meniscal extrusion, presence of IPFP abnormality and effusion-synovitis were associated with worsening MRI-detected OPs, suggesting MRI-detected OPs are consequences of knee structural abnormalities.

Previous studies showed that knee MRI-detected OPs are far more common than OPs detected by conventional radiographs. One study reported that MRI-detected OPs were present in 60% of older persons without radiographic OA [32], and another found that the prevalence of MRI-detected OPs was 72% among middle-aged women [14]. Our current study is largely in

line with these studies, with MRI-detected OPs present in 85% of a community-based older population. We also found that 51% of those participants who had MRI-detected OPs at baseline progressed over time, compared with only 19% of those with no MRI-detected OPs at baseline. Hart et al. investigated the natural history of grade-1 OPs measured by radiography in a 10-year follow-up knee study and reported that 62% of participants graded at baseline with a "doubtful" OP went on to develop confirmed radiographic knee OA compared with only 22% of controls with no sign of disease [33]. In our current cohort, 46% of all participants had increased total knee MRI-detected OPs over 2.6 years. Leyland et al. reported the annual cumulative incidence of radiographic knee OA was 2.3% between baseline and year 15, and participants with a Kellgren-Lawrence score of 1 were four times more likely to experience worsening by year 15 compared with participants with a baseline grade 0 [17]. These findings indicate that early OP formation on radiographs can be used as an early marker of initiation of disease process and when identified by primary healthcare provider, should warrant further action. It is reasonable to hypothesize that the same is true for MRI-detected OP based on this paper and our recent report [13]. The apparently higher rate of change in MRI-detected OPs raises the possibility of MRI being used instead of x-rays for monitoring OP progression.

Correlation between cartilage damage and MRI-defined OPs has been reported previously [34]. But few other studies have examined the associations of IPFP abnormality and effusion-synovitis with MRI-detected OP progression. One cross-sectional study suggested, unsurprisingly, that greater size of MRI-detected OPs related to severity of radiographic OA [32]. Another cross-sectional study revealed that MRI-detected OPs were weakly associated with synovitis or joint effusion but not correlated with Kellgren-Lawrence score [35]. Hill et al. reported that change in synovitis correlated with change in knee pain, but not loss of cartilage [36]. The only longitudinal study to be published revealed significant associations between MRI-detected OP volume and cartilage thickness loss but did not investigate associations with other structures [16]. In the current study, baseline BMLs, cartilage defects, meniscal extrusion, IPFP abnormality and effusion-synovitis were associated with worsening MRI-detected OPs over time, but presence of IPFP abnormality, IPFP maximum area, effusion-synovitis in the central portion, posterior femoral recess and subpopliteal recess were not independently associated with worsening MRI-detected OPs over time. Although the underlying structural mechanisms are largely unknown, these findings reinforce the evolving concept that knee OA is a

Table 3 Associations between baseline effusion-synovitis/IPFP and increased MRI-detected OPs over 2.6 years

	Multivariable* RR (95% CI)	Multivariable** RR (95% CI)
Increased total MRI-detected OP (yes or no)		
Total effusion-synovitis	**1.23 (1.05, 1.45)**	1.08 (0.94, 1.24)
Suprapatellar effusion-synovitis	**1.25 (1.09, 1.45)**	1.08 (0.92, 1.64)
Central portion effusion-synovitis	1.11 (0.96, 1.29)	1.06 (0.94, 1.20)
Posterior femoral recess effusion-synovitis	1.14 (0.97, 1.33)	1.05 (0.93, 1.19)
Subpopliteal recess effusion-synovitis	**1.15 (1.03, 1.29)**	1.07 (0.97, 1.18)
IPFP quality score (0–6)	**1.17 (1.10, 1.24)**	**1.08 (1.01, 1.15)**
IPFP maximum area (cm^2)	1.04 (0.93, 1.16)	1.03 (0.93, 1.14)
IPFP abnormal change (yes/no)	1.21 (0.91, 1.60)	0.91 (0.69, 1.22)
Increased medial MRI-detected OP (yes or no)		
Total effusion-synovitis	1.25 (0.91, 1.73)	1.13 (0.84, 1.51)
Suprapatellar effusion-synovitis	1.31 (0.96, 1.80)	1.15 (0.89, 1.48)
Central portion effusion-synovitis	1.14 (0.83, 1.58)	1.02 (0.75, 1.39)
Posterior femoral recess effusion-synovitis	1.10 (0.83, 1.46)	1.01 (0.76, 1.33)
Subpopliteal recess effusion-synovitis	1.22 (0.99, 1.52)	1.09 (0.88, 1.34)
IPFP quality score (0–6)	**1.40 (1.24, 1.57)**	**1.20 (1.06, 1.37)**
IPFP maximum area (cm^2)	0.96 (0.77, 1.20)	0.96 (0.78, 1.19)
IPFP abnormal change (yes/no)	**3.17 (1.31, 7.65)**	1.87 (0.73, 4.79)
Increased lateral MRI-detected OP (yes or no)		
Total effusion-synovitis	**1.40 (1.13, 1.75)**	**1.27 (1.03, 1.57)**
Suprapatellar effusion-synovitis	**1.37 (1.22, 1.68)**	**1.22 (1.01, 1.47)**
Central portion effusion-synovitis	**1.24 (1.00, 1.53)**	1.16 (0.97, 1.40)
Posterior femoral recess effusion-synovitis	1.18 (0.97, 1.43)	1.08 (0.91, 1.28)
Subpopliteal recess effusion-synovitis	1.12 (0.96, 1.31)	1.08 (0.94, 1.25)
IPFP quality score (0–6)	**1.29 (1.19, 1.40)**	**1.19 (1.08, 1.30)**
IPFP maximum area (cm^2)	1.02 (0.89, 1.18)	1.05 (0.91, 1.21)
IPFP abnormal change (yes/no)	**1.87 (1.15, 3.03)**	1.40 (0.87, 2.25)

Dependent variable: increases in magnetic resonance imaging (MRI)-detected osteophytes (OPs) (yes or no). Independent variables: baseline effusion-synovitis
IPFP intrapatellar fat pad
*Adjusted for age, sex and body mass index
**Further adjusted for bone marrow lesions, cartilage defects and baseline OPs. Significant differences are shown in bold

whole-organ disease and that most structures are involved, including cartilage, meniscal, effusion-synovitis, subchondral bone and IPFP.

This study also found that participants with higher BMI had a higher rate of OP progression, which is in line with previous studies [37, 38]. The increased loading may have altered the biomechanics of the knee joints and accelerated the progression of OP, while a sedentary lifestyle may contribute to rapid progression of both BMI and OPs [39].

Although cartilage damage and OP formation are not perfectly correlated [40], joint space narrowing, which is a surrogate of cartilage damage, has been reported to be highly associated with the presence of OPs [41]. In animal models, OPs have been found to develop at sites of

adjacent cartilage loss [42]. This is consistent with the current finding that cartilage defects at baseline site-specifically predicted an increase in MRI-detected OPs over 2.6 years.

In an older population sample, a fair proportion (61%) of the participants with meniscal abnormalities had no knee pain [43]. However, meniscal pathology is associated with the development of radiographic OA [44–46]. The existence of meniscal damage in a compartment appears to be a factor affecting the progression of OPs. Moreover, a study suggested that the mechanical stimuli in certain compartments may translate to factors on a cellular level or autonomous biochemical stimuli that initiate the process of OP formation [40, 47]. Felson et al. suggested that OPs are not directly involved in disease progression but might serve as markers of the location and severity of the pathologic process [8]. Our study found that BMLs, cartilage defects, meniscal extrusion, IPFP abnormality and effusion-synovitis were the structural risk factors for worsening MRI-detected OP, suggesting that MRI-detected OP could be a result of other osteoarthritic structural abnormalities. On the other hand, it should be noted that MRI-detected OPs were also found to consistently and independently predict changes in knee cartilage, BMLs and cartilage volume, and the need to undergo total knee replacement (TKA) [13, 15]. It is thought that subchondral bone expansion leads to splitting of cartilage and is potentially a precursor to formation of cartilage defects [22, 48]. Combined with our current findings, these studies indicate that OP formation is involved in the OA disease pathway and can be both a risk factor and a consequence of knee OA progression, suggesting the processes are not independent but are linked.

A combination of WORMS and KOSS for the measurement of OPs was employed in the present study. These two grading systems are validated instruments, which have good reliability to assess OPs semi-quantitatively on MRI [9, 20]. The WORMS grading system has the advantage of subdividing the whole knee into different subregions, which includes both marginal and central OPs, but its OP grading scale is more subjective. On the other hand, the KOSS grading system has the advantage of a quatitative OP grading scale for each subregion. The reliability of our measures was excellent.

Strengths of this study included the random selection of participants for the cohort from a community, with a large sample size. On the other hand, there are some potential limitations in our study. First, follow-up MRI scans were only available in 413 out of 837 participants due to decommissioning of the MRI scanner. However, there were no significant differences in demographic factors, ROA, baseline cartilage defects and BMLs between the current study sample and the rest of the cohort. Second, using a higher field-strength magnet than 1.5 T might be marginally more sensitive in detecting OPs; however, as reported previously [49], the results are unlikely to be markedly different as this benefit is modest. Third, the reproducibility for measurement of MRI-detected OPs was good rather than excellent, which may contribute to underestimation of the associations.

Conclusion

Knee MRI-detected OPs are common in older adults and are likely to progress. The associations between baseline structural abnormalities and worsening MRI-detected OPs suggest MRI-detected OPs could be a consequence of multiple knee structural abnormalities.

Abbreviations
BMI: Body mass index; BML: Bone marrow lesion; ICCs: Intraclass correlation coefficients; IPFP: Infrapatellar fat pad; KOSS: Knee Osteoarthritis Scoring System; MRI: Magnetic resonance imaging; OA: Osteoarthritis; OP: Osteophyte; ROA: Radiographic osteoarthritis; TASOAC: Tasmania Older Adult Cohort Study; TKA: Total knee arthroplasty; WORMS: Whole-Organ Magnetic Resonance Imaging Score

Acknowledgements
The authors thank the participants who made this study possible, and acknowledge the role of the staff and volunteers in collecting the data, particularly research nurses Boon C and Boon P. Warren R assessed MRIs and Dr Srikanth V and Dr Cooley H assessed radiographs.

Patient consent
Obtained.

Funding
This study was funded by the National Health and Medical Research Council of Australia (302204), the Tasmanian Community Fund (D0015018), the Arthritis Foundation of Australia (MRI06161) and the University of Tasmania Institutional Research Grants Scheme (D0015019).

Authors' contributions
ZZ had full access to all the data in the study and takes responsibility for the integrity of the data and the accuracy of the data analysis. Study design: FC and GJ. Acquisition of data: ZZ, CD, LL, WH and GJ. Analysis and interpretation of data: ZZ, LL, WH, SZ, FC, TW, GJ and CD. Manuscript preparation and approval: ZZ, LL, WH, SZ, FC, TW, GJ and CD.

Consent for publication
Not applicable.

Competing interests
The authors declare that they have no competing interests.

Publisher's Note

Springer Nature remains neutral with regard to jurisdictional claims in published maps and institutional affiliations.

Author details
[1]Clinical Research Centre, Zhujiang Hospital, Southern Medical University, Guangzhou, Guangdong, China. [2]Menzies Institute for Medical Research, University of Tasmania, Hobart, TAS, Australia. [3]Department of Epidemiology and Preventive Medicine, Monash University, Melbourne, VIC, Australia. [4]Faculty of Health, University of Tasmania, Hobart, TAS, Australia.

References
1. Spector TD, Hart DJ, Byrne J, Harris PA, Dacre JE, Doyle DV. Definition of osteoarthritis of the knee for epidemiological studies. Ann Rheum Dis. 1993; 52(11):790–4.
2. Felson DT, McAlindon TE, Anderson JJ, Naimark A, Weissman BW, Aliabadi P, Evans S, Levy D, LaValley MP. Defining radiographic osteoarthritis for the whole knee. Osteoarthr Cartil. 1997;5(4):241–50.
3. Boegard T, Rudling O, Petersson IF, Jonsson K. Correlation between radiographically diagnosed osteophytes and magnetic resonance detected cartilage defects in the tibiofemoral joint. Ann Rheum Dis. 1998;57(7):401–7.

4. Dieppe PA, Cushnaghan J, Shepstone L. The Bristol 'OA500' study: progression of osteoarthritis (OA) over 3 years and the relationship between clinical and radiographic changes at the knee joint. Osteoarthr Cartil. 1997; 5(2):87–97.

5. Kellgren JH, Lawrence JS. Radiological assessment of osteo-arthrosis. Ann Rheum Dis. 1957;16(4):494–502.

6. Lanyon P, O'Reilly S, Jones A, Doherty M. Radiographic assessment of symptomatic knee osteoarthritis in the community: definitions and normal joint space. Ann Rheum Dis. 1998;57(10):595–601.

7. Eckstein F, Wirth W, Hudelmaier MI, Maschek S, Hitzl W, Wyman BT, Nevitt M, Le Graverand MPH, Hunter D, OA Initiative Investigator Group. Relationship of compartment-specific structural knee status at baseline with change in cartilage morphology: a prospective observational study using data from the osteoarthritis initiative. Arthritis Res Ther. 2009;11(3):R90.

8. Felson DT, Gale DR, Elon Gale M, Niu J, Hunter DJ, Goggins J, Lavalley MP. Osteophytes and progression of knee osteoarthritis. Rheumatology (Oxford). 2005;44(1):100–4.

9. Kornaat PR, Ceulemans RYT, Kroon HM, Riyazi N, Kloppenburg M, Carter WO, Woodworth TG, Bloem JL. MRI assessment of knee osteoarthritis: Knee Osteoarthritis Scoring System (KOSS) - inter-observer and intra-observer reproducibility of a compartment-based scoring system. Skelet Radiol. 2005;34(2):95–102.

10. Kwok WY, Kortekaas MC, Reijnierse M, van der Heijde D, Bloem JL, Kloppenburg M. MRI in hand osteoarthritis: validation of the Oslo Hand Osteoarthritis MRI-Scoring Method and association with pain. Osteoarthr Cartilage. 2011;19:S26–7.

11. McCauley TR, Kornaat PR, Jee WH. Central osteophytes in the knee: prevalence and association with cartilage defects on MR imaging. Am J Roentgenol. 2001;176(2):359–64.

12. Katsuragi J, Sasho T, Yamaguchi S, Sato Y, Watanabe A, Akagi R, Muramatsu Y, Mukoyama S, Akatsu Y, Fukawa T, et al. Hidden osteophyte formation on plain x-ray is the predictive factor for development of knee osteoarthritis after 48 months - data from the Osteoarthritis Initiative. Osteoarthr Cartilage. 2015;23(3):383–90.

13. Zhu Z, Laslett LL, Jin X, Han W, Antony B, Wang X, Lu M, Cicuttini F, Jones G, Ding C. Association between MRI-detected osteophytes and changes in knee structures and pain in older adults: a cohort study. Osteoarthr Cartilage. 2017; 25(7):1084–92.

14. Sowers M, Karvonen-Gutierrez CA, Jacobson JA, Jiang Y, Yosef M. Associations of anatomical measures from MRI with radiographically defined knee osteoarthritis score, pain, and physical functioning. J Bone Joint Surg Am. 2011;93(3):241–51.

15. Liu L, Ishijima M, Kaneko H, Sadatsuki R, Hada S, Kinoshita M, Aoki T, Futami I, Yusup A, Arita H, et al. The MRI-detected osteophyte score is a predictor for undergoing joint replacement in patients with end-stage knee osteoarthritis. Mod Rheumatol. 2017;27(2):332–8.

16. Hakky M, Jarraya M, Ratzlaff C, Guermazi A, Duryea J. Validity and responsiveness of a new measure of knee osteophytes for osteoarthritis studies: data from the Osteoarthritis Initiative. Osteoarthr Cartil. 2015;23(12): 2199–205.

17. Leyland KM, Hart DJ, Javaid MK, Judge A, Kiran A, Soni A, Goulston LM, Cooper C, Spector TD, Arden NK. The natural history of radiographic knee osteoarthritis: a fourteen-year population-based cohort study. Arthritis Rheum. 2012;64(7):2243–51.

18. Peterfy CG, Vandijke CF, Janzen DL, Gluer CC, Namba R, Majumdar S, Lang P, Genant HK. Quantification of articular-cartilage in the knee with pulsed saturation-transfer subtraction and fat-suppressed Mr-imaging - optimization and validation. Radiology. 1994;192(2):485–91.

19. Jones G, Ding CH, Scott F, Glisson M, Cicuttini F. Early radiographic osteoarthritis is associated with substantial changes in cartilage volume and tibial bone surface area in both males and females. Osteoarthr Cartilage. 2004;12(2):169–74.

20. Peterfy CG, Guermazi A, Zaim S, Tirman PFJ, Miaux Y, White D, Kothari M, Lu Y, Fye K, Zhao S, et al. Whole-organ magnetic resonance imaging score (WORMS) of the knee in osteoarthritis. Osteoarthr Cartilage. 2004;12(3):177–90.

21. Altman DG. Statistics in medical journals - developments in the 1980s. Stat Med. 1991;10(12):1897–913.

22. Ding CH, Garnero P, Cicuttini F, Scott F, Cooley H, Jones G. Knee cartilage defects: association with early radiographic osteoarthritis, decreased cartilage volume, increased joint surface area and type II collagen breakdown. Osteoarthr Cartilage. 2005;13(3):198–205.

23. Ding C, Cicuttini F, Scott F, Glisson M, Jones G. Sex differences in knee cartilage volume in adults: role of body and bone size, age and physical activity. Rheumatology. 2003;42(11):1317–23.

24. Jones G, Glisson M, Hynes K, Cicuttini F. Sex and site differences in cartilage development - a possible explanation for variations in knee osteoarthritis in later life. Arthritis Rheum-Us. 2000;43(11):2543–9.

25. Raynauld JP, Martel-Pelletier J, Berthiaume MJ, Abram F, Choquette D, Haraoui B, Beary JF, Cline GA, Meyer JM, Pelletier JP. Correlation between bone lesion changes and cartilage volume loss in patients with osteoarthritis of the knee as assessed by quantitative magnetic resonance imaging over a 24-month period. Ann Rheum Dis. 2008;67(5):683–8.

26. Wang J, Antony B, Zhu Z, Han W, Pan F, Wang X, Jin X, Liu Z, Cicuttini F, Jones G, et al. Association of patellar bone marrow lesions with knee pain, patellar cartilage defect and patellar cartilage volume loss in older adults: a cohort study. Osteoarthr Cartilage. 2015;23(8):1330–6.

27. Berthiaume MJ, Raynauld JP, Martel-Pelletier J, Labonte F, Beaudoin G, Bloch DA, Choquette D, Haraoui B, Altman RD, Hochberg M, et al. Meniscal tear and extrusion are strongly associated with progression of symptomatic knee osteoarthritis as assessed by quantitative magnetic resonance imaging. Ann Rheum Dis. 2005;64(4):556–63.

28. Raynauld JP, Martel-Pelletier J, Berthiaume MJ, Beaudoin G, Choquette D, Haraoui B, Tannenbaum H, Meyer JM, Beary JF, Cline GA, et al. Long term evaluation of disease progression through the quantitative magnetic resonance imaging of symptomatic knee osteoarthritis patients: correlation with clinical symptoms and radiographic changes. Osteoporosis Int. 2006;17:S13.

29. Pan F, Han W, Wang X, Liu Z, Jin X, Antony B, Cicuttini F, Jones G, Ding C. A longitudinal study of the association between infrapatellar fat pad maximal area and changes in knee symptoms and structure in older adults. Ann Rheum Dis. 2015;74(10):1818–24.

30. Han W, Aitken D, Zhu Z, Halliday A, Wang X, Antony B, Cicuttini F, Jones G, Ding C. Hypointense signals in the infrapatellar fat pad assessed by magnetic resonance imaging are associated with knee symptoms and structure in older adults: a cohort study. Arthritis Res Ther. 2016;18(1):234.

31. Wang X, Blizzard L, Halliday A, Han W, Jin X, Cicuttini F, Jones G, Ding C. Association between MRI-detected knee joint regional effusion-synovitis and structural changes in older adults: a cohort study. Ann Rheum Dis. 2016;75(3):519–25.

32. Hayes CW, Jamadar DA, Welch GW, Jannausch ML, Lachance LL, Capul DC, Sowers MR. Osteoarthritis of the knee: comparison of MR imaging findings with radiographic severity measurements and pain in middle-aged women. Radiology. 2005;237(3):998–1007.

33. Hart DJ, Spector TD. Kellgren & Lawrence grade 1 osteophytes in the knee-- doubtful or definite? Osteoarthr Cartil. 2003;11(2):149–50.

34. Roemer FW, Guermazi A, Niu JB, Zhang YQ, Mohr A, Felson DT. Prevalence of magnetic resonance imaging-defined atrophic and hypertrophic phenotypes of knee osteoarthritis in a population-based cohort. Arthritis Rheum-Us. 2012;64(2):429–37.

35. Link TM, Steinbach LS, Ghosh S, Ries M, Lu Y, Lane N, Majumdar S. Osteoarthritis: MR imaging findings in different stages of disease and correlation with clinical findings. Radiology. 2003;226(2):373–81.

36. Hill CL, Hunter DJ, Niu J, Clancy M, Guermazi A, Genant H, Gale D, Grainger A, Conaghan P, Felson DT. Synovitis detected on magnetic resonance imaging and its relation to pain and cartilage loss in knee osteoarthritis. Ann Rheum Dis. 2007;66(12):1599–603.

37. Wills AK, Black S, Cooper R, Coppack RJ, Hardy R, Martin KR, Cooper C, Kuh D. Life course body mass index and risk of knee osteoarthritis at the age of 53 years: evidence from the 1946 British birth cohort study. Ann Rheum Dis. 2012;71(5):655–60.

38. Zheng H, Chen C. Body mass index and risk of knee osteoarthritis: systematic review and meta-analysis of prospective studies. BMJ Open. 2015;5(12):e007568.

39. Musumeci G, Aiello FC, Szychlinska MA, Di Rosa M, Castrogiovanni P, Mobasheri A. Osteoarthritis in the XXIst century: risk factors and behaviours that influence disease onset and progression. Int J Mol Sci. 2015;16(3):6093–112.

40. van der Kraan PM, van den Berg WB. Osteophytes: relevance and biology. Osteoarthr Cartil. 2007;15(3):237–44.

41. Boegard T, Rudling O, Petersson IF, Jonsson K. Correlation between radiographically diagnosed osteophytes and magnetic resonance detected cartilage defects in the patellofemoral joint. Ann Rheum Dis. 1998;57(7):395–400.

42. vanOsch GJVM, vanderKraan PM, vanValburg AA, vandenBerg WB. The relation between cartilage damage and osteophyte size in a murine model for osteoarthritis in the knee. Rheumatol Int. 1996;16(3):115–9.

43. Englund M, Guermazi A, Gale D, Hunter DJ, Aliabadi P, Clancy M, Felson DT. Incidental meniscal findings on knee MRI in middle-aged and elderly persons. N Engl J Med. 2008;359(11):1108–15.

44. Sharma L, Chmiel JS, Almagor O, Dunlop D, Guermazi A, Bathon JM, Eaton CB, Hochberg MC, Jackson RD, Kwoh CK, et al. Significance of preradiographic magnetic resonance imaging lesions in persons at increased risk of knee osteoarthritis. Arthritis Rheumatol. 2014;66(7):1811–9.

45. Englund M, Niu J, Guermazi A, Roemer FW, Hunter DJ, Lynch JA, Lewis CE, Torner J, Nevitt MC, Zhang YQ, et al. Effect of meniscal damage on the development of frequent knee pain, aching, or stiffness. Arthritis Rheum. 2007;56(12):4048–54.

46. van Oudenaarde K, Jobke B, Oostveen AC, Marijnissen AC, Wolterbeek R, Wesseling J, Bierma-Zeinstra SM, Bloem HL, Reijnierse M, Kloppenburg M. Predictive value of MRI features for development of radiographic osteoarthritis in a cohort of participants with pre-radiographic knee osteoarthritis-the CHECK study. Rheumatology (Oxford). 2017;56(1):113–20.

47. Blom AB, van Lent PL, Holthuysen AE, van der Kraan PM, Roth J, van Rooijen N, van den Berg WB. Synovial lining macrophages mediate osteophyte formation during experimental osteoarthritis. Osteoarthr Cartil. 2004;12(8):627–35.

48. Davies-Tuck ML, Wluka AE, Wang Y, Teichtahl AJ, Jones G, Ding C, Cicuttini FM. The natural history of cartilage defects in people with knee osteoarthritis. Osteoarthr Cartil. 2008;16(3):337–42.

49. Roemer FW, Lynch JA, Niu J, Zhang Y, Crema MD, Tolstykh I, El-Khoury GY, Felson DT, Lewis CE, Nevitt MC, et al. A comparison of dedicated 1.0 T extremity MRI vs large-bore 1.5 T MRI for semiquantitative whole organ assessment of osteoarthritis: the MOST study. Osteoarthr Cartil. 2010;18(2):168–74.

3

Osteoporosis of the vertebra and osteochondral remodeling of the endplate causes intervertebral disc degeneration in ovariectomized mice

Zhi-feng Xiao[1,2,3†], Jian-bo He[1,2,3†], Guo-yi Su[1,3], Mei-hui Chen[1,2,3], Yu Hou[1,3], Shu-dong Chen[1,3] and Ding-kun Lin[1,2,3*]

Abstract

Background: Studies on the relationship between osteoporosis and intervertebral disc degeneration (IVDD) are inconsistent. Therefore, we assessed whether IVDD is affected by vertebral osteoporosis in ovariectomized mice and investigated the underlying pathogenesis of IVDD related to osteoporosis.

Methods: Thirty healthy female C57BL/6 J mice aged 8 weeks were randomly divided into two groups: a control group (sham operation, $n = 15$) and an ovariectomy group (OVX; bilateral ovariectomy, $n = 15$). At 12 weeks after surgery, the bone quantity and microstructure in the lumbar vertebra and endplate as well as the volume of the L4/5 disc space were evaluated by microcomputed tomography (micro-CT). The occurrence and characteristic alterations of IVDD were identified via histopathological staining. The osteoclasts were detected using tartrate-resistant acid phosphatase (TRAP) staining. Type II collagen (Col II), osterix (OSX), osteopontin (OPN), and vascular endothelial growth factor (VEGF) expression in the intervertebral disc were detected by immunohistochemical analysis.

Results: OVX significantly increased the body weight and decreased the uterus weight. Micro-CT analysis showed that osteoporosis of the vertebra and osteochondral remodeling of the endplate were accompanied by an increase in the endplate porosity and a decrease in the disc volume in the OVX group. Likewise, histological evaluation revealed that IVDD occurred at 12 weeks after ovariectomy, with features of endochondral ossification of the endplate, loose and broken annulus fibrosus, and degeneration of nucleus pulposus. TRAP staining showed that numerous active osteoclasts appeared in the subchondral bone and cartilaginous endplate of OVX mice, whereas osteoclasts were rarely detected in control mice. Immunohistochemical analysis demonstrated that the expression of osterix was significantly increased, notably in the endplate of OVX mice. In addition, Col II was decreased in the ossification endplate and the degenerative annulus fibrosus, where OPN and VEGF expressions were elevated in OVX mice.

(Continued on next page)

* Correspondence: lindingkuntcm@126.com
†Zhi-feng Xiao and Jian-bo He contributed equally to this work.
[1]The Department of Spinal Surgery, The Second Affiliated Hospital of Guangzhou University of Chinese Medicine, No. 111, Dade Road, Yuexiu District, Guangzhou 510120, China
[2]The Laboratory Affiliated to Orthopaedics and Traumatology of Chinese Medicine of Linnan Medical Research Center of Guangzhou University of Chinese Medicine, No. 12, Jichang Road, Baiyun District, Guangzhou 510405, China
Full list of author information is available at the end of the article

(Continued from previous page)

Conclusions: OVX induced vertebral osteoporosis and osteochondral remodeling of the cartilaginous endplate contributing to the angiogenesis and an increase in porosity of the bone-cartilage surface, and also affected the matrix metabolism which consequently had detrimental effects on the intervertebral disc. Our study suggests that preserving the structural integrity and the function of the adjacent structures, including the vertebrae and endplates, may protect the disc against degeneration.

Keywords: Intervertebral disc degeneration, Osteoporosis, Ovariectomy, Endplate, Osteochondral remodeling, Microcomputed tomography,

Background

Lower back pain and spinal compression nerve pain are the major symptoms caused by intervertebral disc degeneration (IVDD) in the clinic [1, 2]. Spinal instability or disability is common in serious IVDD which leads to enormous human suffering and significant socioeconomic losses [3]. Unfortunately, there are no currently effective methods to repair IVDD [4] and disc resection with interbody fusion are often the final choice. Therefore there is an urgent need to explore the key mechanism of IVDD and to develop drugs for its treatment.

It has long been recognized that musculoskeletal degeneration disorders such as osteoporosis, IVDD, and osteoarthritis are a difficult focus in locomotor disease research. An intimate relationship between cartilage and subchondral bone has been proven in recent years. Anatomically, the vertebrae and the intervertebral discs are combined in bundles to form the motion segments of the spine. From the mechanical and biological points of view they are closely linked and are considered as a functional unit [5–7]. Although it is not fully clear whether it precedes or follows nucleus pulposus degeneration, the modic change in the endplate is an important feature of IVDD physiopathology [8]. Therefore, the health of the bone and its attached nonosseous tissues such as cartilage and disc are tightly associated. Research has shown that crosstalk between bone and cartilage is elevated in osteoarthritis where the coupling of bone and cartilage turnover is even aggravated [9–11]. Moreover, remodeling of the subchondral bone microstructure due to osteoporosis could further exacerbate experimental osteoarthritis [12]. All of this suggests that the subchondral bone is an indispensable factor in the process of osteoarthritis. In terms of IVDD, however, there is a lack of research on the pathological mechanisms of subchondral bone in IVDD, and it is also unclear how osteoporosis affects the nonosseous tissues such as the intervertebral disc.

Because of the structural similarities between joint and intervertebral discs [13, 14], it is well known that the intervertebral disc is a nonvascular structure and the exchange of substances between the intervertebral disc and the vertebra depends on the cranial and caudal endplates [15–17]. The endplate contains marrow contact channels which provide nutrients for the intervertebral disc and discharge metabolic waste through diffusion and liquid flow under cyclic loading [4, 18, 19]. Hence, changes in the vertebra microenvironment resulting from rapid bone turnover during vertebral osteoporosis and obstruction of marrow contact channels induced by calcification of the cartilaginous endplate may accelerate IVDD.

Recent studies have provided increasing evidence that osteoporosis is associated with the evolution of IVDD. The osteoporosis of vertebrae in postmenopausal women was correlated with IVDD [20, 21], and sex hormones can affect the severity of IVDD [21–23]. Furthermore, in osteoprotegerin (OPG) knockout mice, ossification occurred in the cartilage endplate and resulted in IVDD [24]. IVDD often occurs with osteoporosis of the vertebrae, indicating that the development of osteoporosis and IVDD might be a coupling process which could explain why postmenopausal women have more lower back pain than men. Some studies have reported the prospect of delaying the course of disc degeneration through improving bone metabolism and vertebral osteoporosis. For example, it was found that alendronate could retard the progression of lumbar IVDD in ovariectomized rats by improving the bone quality [25, 26]. Calcitonin could also suppress intervertebral disk degeneration and preserve lumbar vertebral bone mineral density and bone strength [27]. However, it is still puzzling that some clinical and epidemiological studies have shown that osteoporosis is inversely related to spinal degenerative diseases and IVDD [19, 28, 29]. These studies support osteoporosis in increasing endplate permeability and delaying IVDD [19]. In addition, radiographic features of lumbar disc degeneration were associated with an increased bone mineral density (BMD) in the spine [28, 30]. Thus, the relationship between osteoporosis and IVDD is still controversial and confusing. Consequently, whether a positive correlation exists between osteoporosis and IVDD and how the vertebral body affects the intervertebral disc are still undefined and remain to be further clarified.

Mice are commonly used as an animal model for osteoporosis and intervertebral disc degeneration [31–33]. Many studies have demonstrated that the ovariectomized mouse is a good model for postmenopausal osteoporosis [34]. Thus, the purpose of this study was to determine the roles of postmenopausal osteoporosis in IVDD and to further clarify its underlying mechanism by assessing the detailed pathological changes in L4–L5 spine motion segments including vertebrae, the endplate, and the intervertebral disc in ovariectomized mice.

Methods

Animals and designs

Female C57BL/6 J mice (8 weeks old) were purchased from the Animal Center of Guangzhou University of Chinese Medicine, Guangzhou, China (license number: SCXK (YUE) 2013–0034). The mice were housed in conditions of controlled temperature (22–25 °C) at 40–60% relative humidity with alternate day and night and were allowed food and water freely. The animals were randomly divided into two groups. The mice underwent either sham operation (control group, $n = 15$) or bilateral ovariectomy (OVX group, $n = 15$) while under anesthesia with 4% chloral hydrate at a dose of 400 mg/kg weight via intraperitoneal injection. The body weight of the mice was recorded weekly. The mice were sacrificed at 12 weeks after surgery, and L3–L6 spinal motion segments and hind limbs were harvested for subsequent experiments. All experimental protocols were approved by the Ethics Committee of Guangzhou University of Chinese Medicine and implemented according to the Guide for Use and Care of Animals.

Microcomputed tomography analyses

L3–L6 spinal motion segments were harvested and immediately fixed in 4% neutral paraformaldehyde for 72 h at 4 °C. The samples were washed three times with phosphate-buffered saline (PBS) for 15 min each time. The L4–L5 segment of samples ($n = 6$) was measured by high resolution microcomputed tomography (micro-CT; Skyscan1172) according to a previously described protocol [31]. Briefly, the scanner was set at a voltage of 59 kV, a current of 100uA, and a resolution of 9 μm per pixel to measure the spinal segment. Images were reconstructed and analyzed using NRecon v1.6 and CTAn v1.9 software, respectively. Three-dimensional (3D) reconstruction images were obtained using CTvox v3.0. The coronal images of the L4/5 segment were used to perform 3D histomorphometric analyses of the intervertebral disc and cartilage endplate, while transverse images of L5 vertebrae were used to measure the vertebral body. The region of interest (ROI) of vertebrae, endplates, and intervertebral discs were depicted using CTAn v1.9. A total of 200 or 20 consecutive images of the ROI were respectively used to show the 3D reconstruction of the microarchitecture in the vertebra and endplate. The ROI of the intervertebral disc was shown as the mid-plane coronal images of the L4/5 segment. The disc volume was defined as the ROI covered by the entire invisible space between the L4/5 vertebrae. The cartilage endplate volume was defined as the visible bone plate volume that covers the vertebrae. Three dimensional structural parameters of vertebrae included the total volume of bone mineral density (BMDtv; reflecting bone mass per unit volume), percentage bone volume (bone volume (BV)/total volume (TV)), trabecular number (Tb.N; the inverse of the mean distance between the mid-axes of the structure), trabecular thickness (Tb.Th), trabecular separation (Tb.Sp; the average separation between the mid-axes), trabecular pattern factor (Tb.Pf; measuring the degree of convex surfaces and concave surfaces of the trabecular, where having many concave surfaces represents a well-connected spongy lattice, while more convex surfaces indicates a bad connectedness; the rising value represents the decrease in trabecular connectedness); connectivity density (CONN.D; reflecting the connection in the trabecular, with a lower value indicating increased interruption of the trabecular), and structural model index (SMI; reflecting the proportion of the plate and rod structure of the trabecular with a value range of 0–3 where a higher value indicates an increase in rod-shaped trabecular volume). The parameters of the endplate included the percentage bone volume (BV/TV), number of closed pores (Po.N(cl); representing the number of pores with a closed cavity in the endplate structure), open porosity (PO(op); open pore volume over total pore volume), and total volume of pore space (Po.V(tot)).

Histology and immunohistochemistry examinations

After fixation in 4% neutral paraformaldehyde for 72 h, the dorsal attachment including the vertebral arch/lamina and facet joint were removed from lumbar L4/5 spinal segments ($n = 9$) and were decalcified in 10% EDTA (pH 7.4) for 14 days at room temperature. The tibia received the same process. The samples were then dehydrated and embedded in paraffin. The L4/5 segments were sliced into 4-μm thick sections to perform hematoxylin and eosin (H&E) staining, safranin O and fast green staining, tartrate-resistant acid phosphatase (TRAP) staining, and immunohistochemistry.

H&E and safranin O staining were guided by the instructions of the reagent kits (Servicebio Biological Technology Co. Ltd., China). TRAP staining was handled according to the protocol of the staining kit (Solarbio Science & Technology Co. Ltd., China). Briefly, after dewaxing and hydration, slices were soaked in TRAP staining solution and incubated at 37 °C for 50 min. After washing in tap water, specimens were counterstained by methyl green.

Immunostaining was performed using standard protocols according to the Abcam/Santa Cruz official website (https://www.abcam.cn/protocols/ihc-tissue-processing-protocol and https://www.scbt.com/scbt/zh/resources/protocols/immuno-fluorescence-cell-staining). Briefly, sections were dewaxed and hydrated and then boiled in EDTA antigen repair solution (pH 8.0) for 20 min for antigen retrieval. Tissues were treated with 3% H_2O_2 to block endogenous peroxidase. The sections were then incubated with normal goat serum for blocking and subsequently with primary antibodies including mouse collagen II (Col II; Abcam, 1:200, ab34712), osterix (OSX; Santa Cruz, 1:200, sc-393,060), osteopontin (OPN; Santa Cruz, 1:200, sc-73,631), and vascular endothelial growth factor (VEGF; Santa Cruz, 1:200, sc-7269) at 4 °C overnight. Negative control slices were incubated in PBS without antibodies. For immunohistochemical staining, the rest of the procedures were manipulated according to the PV-6001 Two-Step IHC Detection Reagent instructions. After coloration with 3,3'-diaminobenzidine (DAB) solution (ZSGB-BIO Corporation, China), the sections were counterstained with hematoxylin and the yellow or brown color was considered as positive staining. For the immunofluorescent assay, the slides were incubated with the secondary antibody conjugated with fluorescence-Alexa Fluor® 555 (CST Corporation, USA, #4409) for 1 h avoiding light, followed by counterstaining with 4', 6-diamidino-2-phenylindole (DAPI), and then detected under fluorescence microscopy (Olympus DP80, Japan). Positive staining in the disc was quantified using ImageJ Pro Plus software (Media Cybernetics, Baltimore, MD, USA).

Statistics

All data were analyzed using the paired t test of SPSS 20.0 software (SPSS Inc., Chicago, IL). The comparisons of means were performed between the control and OVX groups. All data were checked for normality and homogeneity of variance and represent the mean ± standard deviation (SD). In all analyses, $p < 0.05$ was considered statistically significant.

Results

Macroscopic observation, body, and uterus weight of OVX mice

The body weight of each animal was measured weekly in both the control and OVX groups. Results showed that the weight of the two groups increased over time, but was more significant in the OVX group from week 2 to week 12 (Fig. 1a; $p < 0.05$). At 12 weeks postsurgery, the abdominal cavity of OVX mice was filled with massive fat deposits and showed an obese body (Fig. 1a). In addition, a lack of estrogen from OVX resulted in atrophy of the uterus and significantly decreased uterus weight of the OVX group compared with the control group (Fig. 1b; $p < 0.05$).

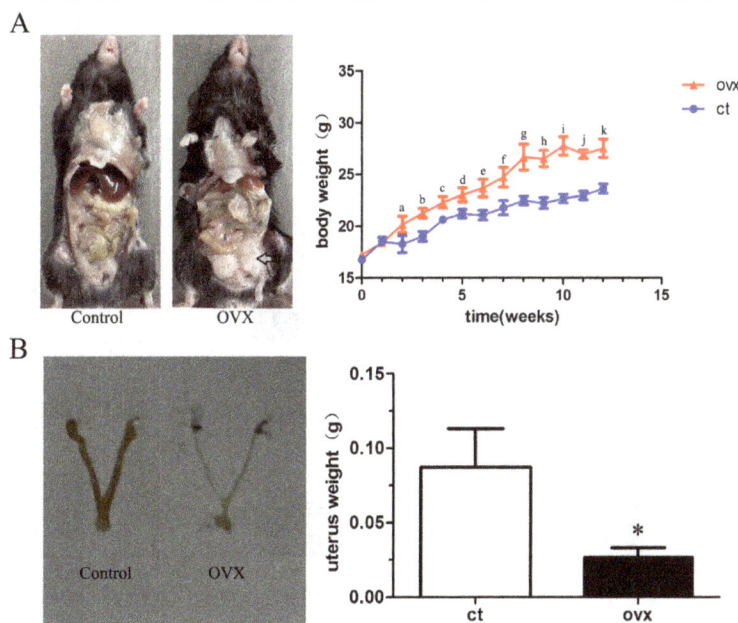

Fig. 1 Gross macrographs and body and uterus weight changes of mice after ovariectomy. **a** There is a remarkable accumulation of fat in the abdominal cavity (black open arrow) and the body weight increase significantly over time in ovariectomized (OVX) mice. **b** The uterus is visibly atrophied in the OVX group and is significant lighter in weight compared with the control (ct) group. Data are shown as mean ± SD; $n = 15$ per group. [a–k]$p < 0.05$ vs control group at 2–12 weeks for body weight; *$p < 0.05$ vs control group for uterus weight

Changes in microarchitecture of the vertebra and endplate as well as increasing porosity lead to narrowing of the disc space in OVX mice

To determine if vertebral osteoporosis and endplate lesions, as well as disc changes, were presented in OVX mice, micro-CT analysis was performed. Sparse trabeculae were displayed in the OVX group (Fig. 2a and Additional file 1: Figure S1). Quantification of the trabecular structures revealed that BMDtv, BV/TV, Tb.N, and Conn.Dn in the OVX group were significantly decreased when compared with the control group (Fig. 2b–d, h; $p < 0.05$), while the Tb.pf and SMI of the OVX group were markedly higher than those of the control group (Fig. 2g, i; $p < 0.05$). Although no significant difference was observed for Tb.Th and Tb.sp. between the two groups, the OVX mice showed a slightly higher value for Tb.sp. (Fig. 2e, f).

Moreover, a large number of cavities was found in the endplate of the OVX group (Fig. 3A and Additional file 1: Figure S1B). To confirm the degree of porosity in the endplate, we examined the micro-CT parameters of the caudal endplate. The parameters showed that the BV/TV and Po.N(cl) were significantly decreased ($p < 0.05$), while the PO(op) and po.V(tot) were significantly increased ($p < 0.05$), suggesting an increasing endplate porosity in the OVX group. Additionally, from the top view of the caudal endplate, there were markedly higher pores on the surface of the endplate in the OVX mice and most of them were located in the central area corresponding to the nucleus pulposus (Fig. 3B-a). Furthermore, the intervertebral disc space of the OVX mice were narrowed (Fig. 3B-b and Additional file 1: Figure S1B). Meanwhile, the OVX group showed a significantly smaller intervertebral disc volume than the control group (Fig. 3B-c; $p < 0.05$).

Osteoporosis with osteochondral remodeling of the endplate causes disc degeneration in OVX mice

To test if the disc space stenosis in the OVX mice was related to osteoporosis and the accelerated osteochondral remodeling, we performed histological studies. H&E staining of tibia further confirmed osteoporosis in the

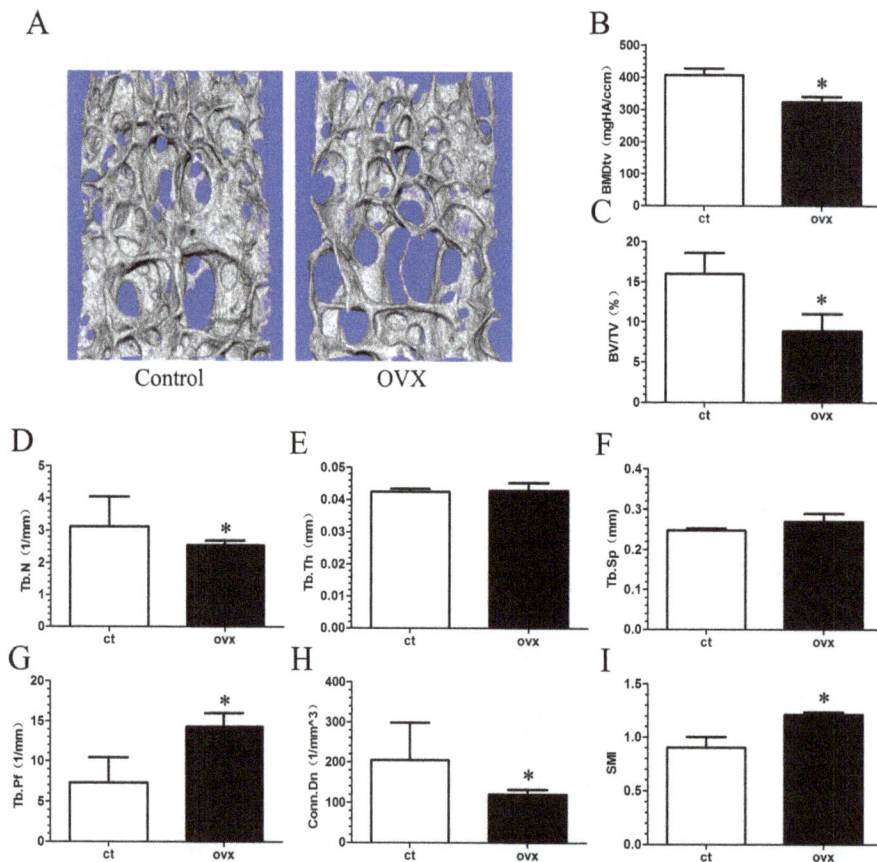

Fig. 2 Changes in L5 total volume of bone mineral density (BMDtv) and microarchitecture parameters of the trabecular bone determined by micro-CT. **a** Representative three-dimensional images of trabecular bone. **b–i** The parameters of L5 trabecular bone. There is markedly decreased BMDtv, bone volume (BV)/total volume (TV), trabecular number (Tb.N; 1/mm), and connectivity density (CONN.D, 1/mm³), and increased trabecular thickness (Tb.Th; mm), and structural model index (SMI) in the ovariectomized (OVX) group when compared with the control (ct) group. Mice were analyzed at 12 weeks post-sham or OVX surgery, $n = 6$ per group. Data are shown as mean ± SD. *$p < 0.05$. Tb.Pf trabecular pattern factor, Tb.Sp trabecular separation

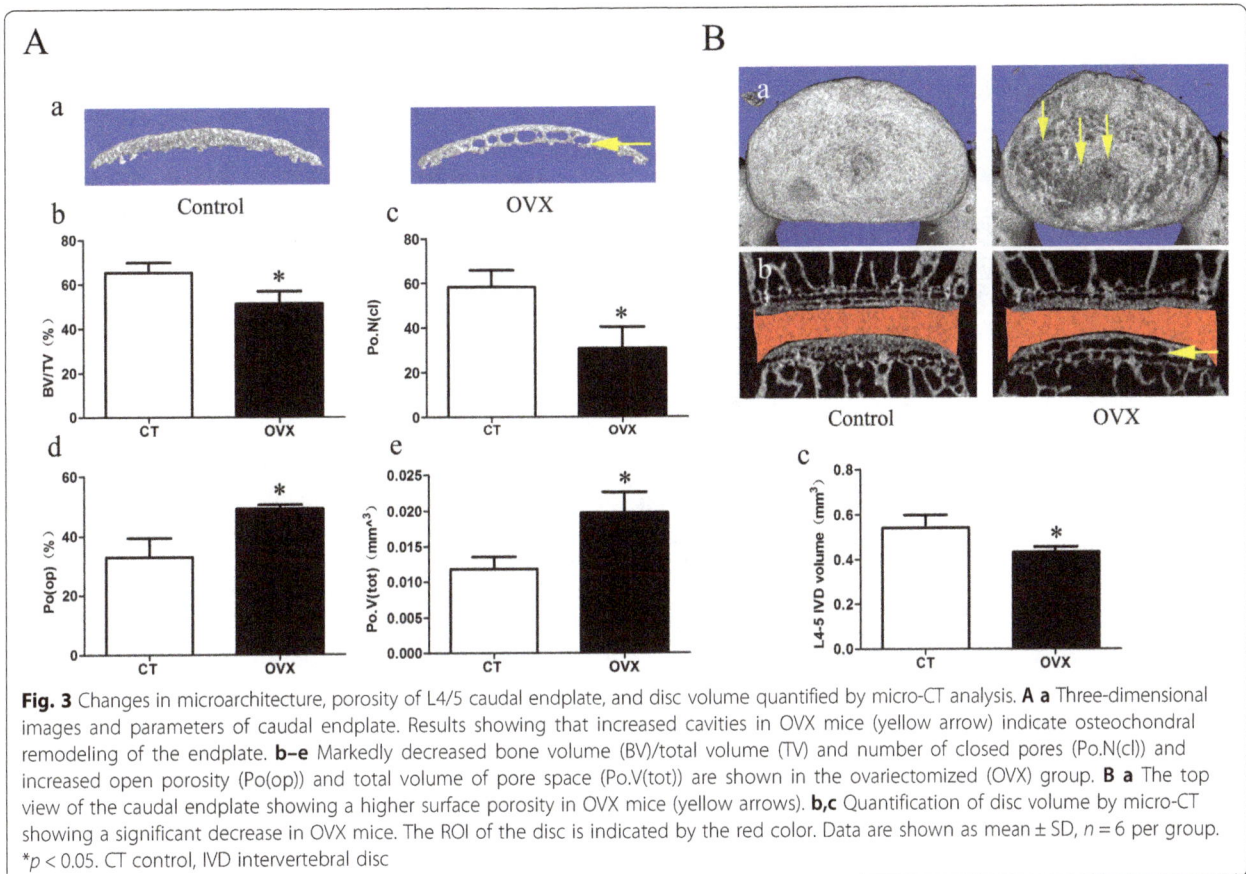

Fig. 3 Changes in microarchitecture, porosity of L4/5 caudal endplate, and disc volume quantified by micro-CT analysis. **A a** Three-dimensional images and parameters of caudal endplate. Results showing that increased cavities in OVX mice (yellow arrow) indicate osteochondral remodeling of the endplate. **b–e** Markedly decreased bone volume (BV)/total volume (TV) and number of closed pores (Po.N(cl)) and increased open porosity (Po(op)) and total volume of pore space (Po.V(tot)) are shown in the ovariectomized (OVX) group. **B a** The top view of the caudal endplate showing a higher surface porosity in OVX mice (yellow arrows). **b,c** Quantification of disc volume by micro-CT showing a significant decrease in OVX mice. The ROI of the disc is indicated by the red color. Data are shown as mean ± SD, $n = 6$ per group. *$p < 0.05$. CT control, IVD intervertebral disc

OVX group, in which trabeculae were sparse and diminished (Fig. 4b). The bone marrow was almost replaced by adipose tissue (Fig. 4b).

Histological findings of the intervertebral disc volume showed that the nucleus pulposus contained abundant notochordal cells surrounded by large zones of extracellular matrix, and the cartilaginous endplates were hyaline cartilages composed of chondrocytes in the control group. In contrast, in the OVX group, the discs showed degenerative changes and reduction in the nucleus pulposus and were comprised of relatively few, clustered doublets of chondrocyte-like cells (Fig. 4a). Proteoglycan loss could be also found in the nucleus pulposus of OVX mice with pale safranin-O staining (Fig. 5). Moreover, ossification of the cartilaginous endplate occurred in the OVX group (Figs. 4a and 5). Safranin O and fast green staining suggested that endplates underwent endochondral ossification at 12 weeks postsurgery, indicated by the erosion of the wavy tidemark (Fig. 5) and green-stained bone matrix surrounding the cavities in OVX mice relative to the control group (Fig. 5). The endplate structure showed damage, further calcification and ossification, and eventually became a bony structure. Bony tissues contained bone marrow, hematopoietic lineage cells, and mineralized bone, and appeared more obvious in the deep zone of the middle

cartilaginous endplate (Figs. 4a and 5). However, the superficial cartilage endplate became markedly thinner and had fewer active cells (Figs. 4a and 5). Furthermore, an increased number of clefts formed in the annulus fibrosus of OVX mice with collagen disarrangement and cell reduction, and even loose and broken lamella (Figs. 4a and 5).

Increasing bone turnover accompanied by osteochondral remodeling exists in OVX mice

TRAP and OSX were detected to reflect the bone turnover of the intervertebral disc volume. TRAP staining showed that many activated osteoclasts were widely located on the trabecular surface of subchondral bone and were significantly increased in the cartilaginous endplate of OVX mice ($p < 0.05$), but there were only a few osteoclasts in the control mice (Fig. 6). Simultaneously, OSX expression was significantly elevated in the OVX mice ($p < 0.05$), especially in the ossification region of the endplate which was consistent with the area of osteoclast activation (Fig. 7).

Decreasing Col II and increasing OPN and VEGF are expressed in the degenerative disc of OVX mice

Immunohistochemistry and immunofluorescence assays were performed to assess the protein levels of Col II, OPN,

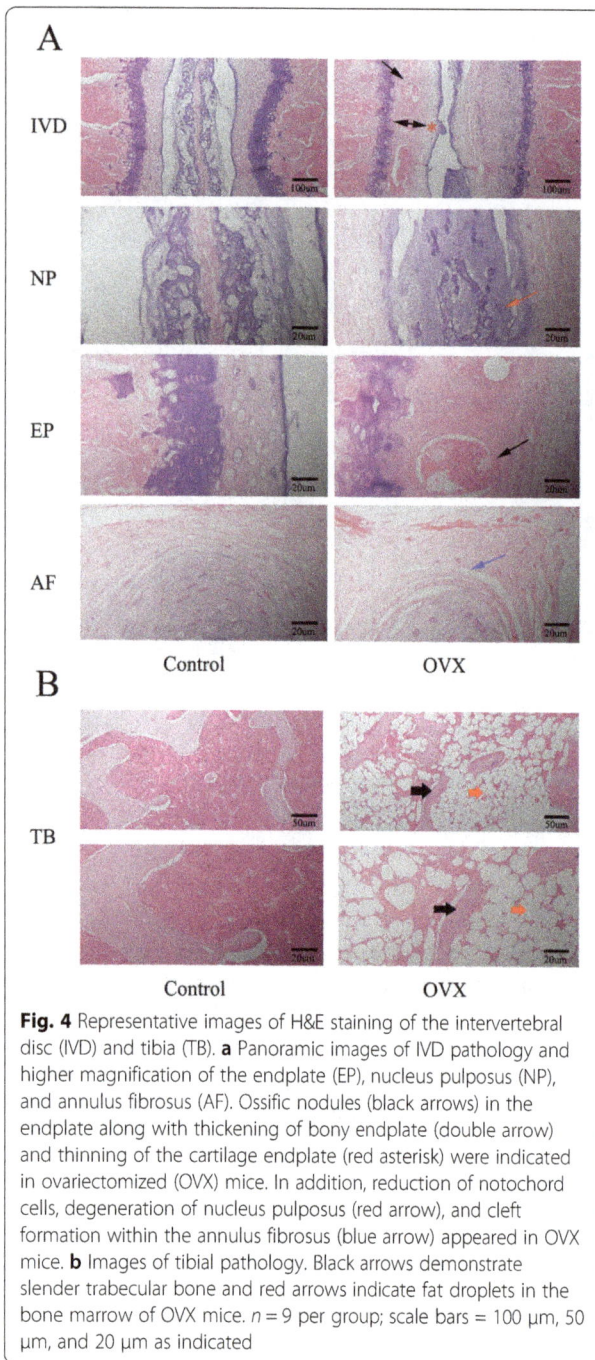

Fig. 4 Representative images of H&E staining of the intervertebral disc (IVD) and tibia (TB). **a** Panoramic images of IVD pathology and higher magnification of the endplate (EP), nucleus pulposus (NP), and annulus fibrosus (AF). Ossific nodules (black arrows) in the endplate along with thickening of bony endplate (double arrow) and thinning of the cartilage endplate (red asterisk) were indicated in ovariectomized (OVX) mice. In addition, reduction of notochord cells, degeneration of nucleus pulposus (red arrow), and cleft formation within the annulus fibrosus (blue arrow) appeared in OVX mice. **b** Images of tibial pathology. Black arrows demonstrate slender trabecular bone and red arrows indicate fat droplets in the bone marrow of OVX mice. n = 9 per group; scale bars = 100 μm, 50 μm, and 20 μm as indicated

and VEGF in the intervertebral disc. As seen in Fig. 8, the changes in the organization of Col II were commonly detected in the cartilage. The expression of Col II is significantly decreased in the discs of OVX mice, especially in the endplate ossified zone and outer layer of the annulus fibrosus, and their spatial arrangement has changed in the remainder of the endplate (Fig. 8). However, OPN (an osteogenic marker protein) and VEGF (a cytokine associated with angiogenesis), which are closely associated with endochondral ossification and rarely expressed in normal

discs, were markedly increased in the endplate and annulus fibrosus in OVX mice (Figs. 9 and 10). Interestingly, decreased Col II expression and increased OPN and VEGF expression was colocalized in the endplate ossified areas and inner annulus fibrosus, suggesting that osteochondral remodeling and abnormal angiogenesis in the avascular soft disc was a coupling process and may be an important link to disc degeneration in OVX mice.

Discussion

IVDD and osteoporosis are the most common degenerative diseases in the spine, both of which are often accompanied with the other. However, the detailed relationship between them is not clear. In the present study, we evaluated the effects of estrogen deficiency on the bone mass and microarchitecture in vertebrae, the microarchitecture and porosity of the endplate, and the histopathology of the adjacent intervertebral disc to elucidate the possible relationship between osteoporosis and IVDD and to explore the superficial mechanism of IVDD associated with osteoporosis.

Our study showed that OVX could cause vertebrae osteopenia. Additionally, OVX promoted bone turnover and osteochondral remodeling at the junction of the vertebra and intervertebral disc, leading to an increased ossification and hypertrophy of the endplate, abnormal pores within the cartilaginous endplate, high porosity between the vertebra and intervertebral disc, and narrowing of the intervertebral disc space. Therefore, OVX exerted a detrimental effect on subchondral bone structure, particularly in the subchondral plate, which was closely related with disorders of the overlying cartilaginous endplate and played a crucial role in the development of IVDD.

At the same time, decreasing proteoglycans in the nucleus pulposus, increasing cracks within the annulus fibrosus, and osteochondral remodeling of the endplate could be also found in the intervertebral disc histomorphology of OVX mice. TRAP staining showed that the osteoclasts in the subchondral bone were significantly increased and particularly appeared in the endplate. The immunohistochemistry showed a corresponding increase in OSX expression, indicating that the ovariectomy induced a fast bone turnover which led to the structural remodeling of the endplate and changes in the porosity. It has been reported that there is a significant correlation between the effective permeability and marrow contact channel or porosity of the endplate [35, 36]. Thus, the increase in permeability induced by postmenopausal vertebral osteoporosis and endplate remodeling might be the most important factor contributing to the lesions of the soft tissue of the intervertebral disc in OVX mice. Additionally, the results of immunohistochemistry showed that OVX weakens the expressions of

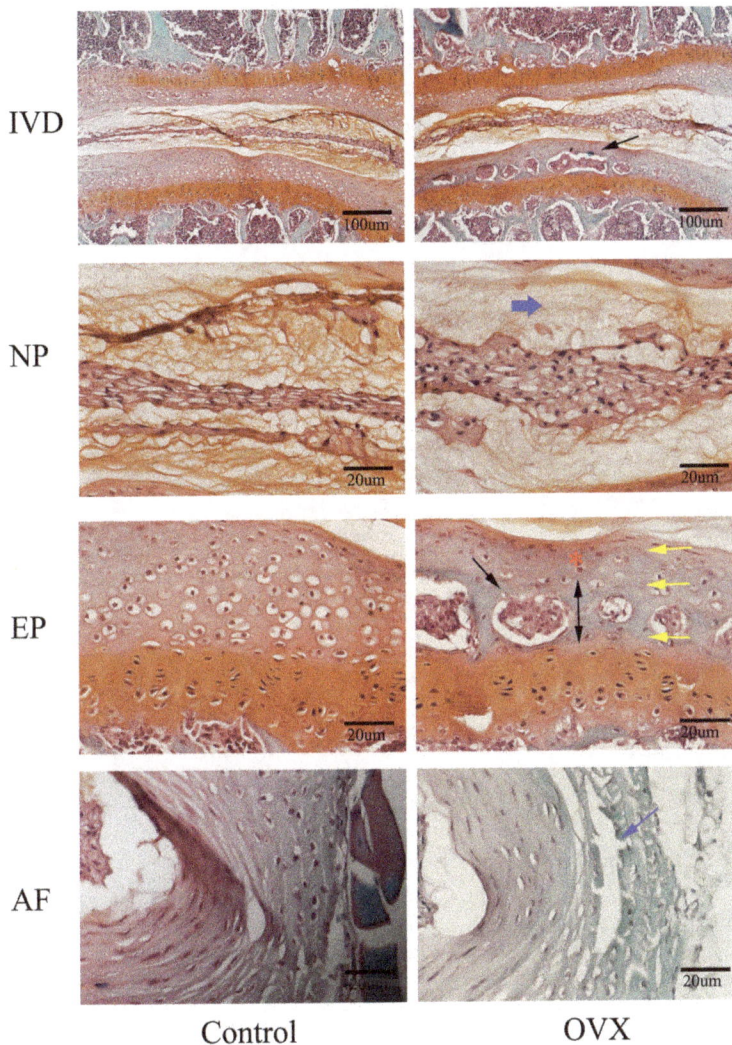

Fig. 5 Representative images of safranin O and fast green staining of the intervertebral disc (IVD). This showed consistent results with H&E staining. Specially, thickening of the bony endplate (EP; double arrow) accompanied by accelerated osteochondral remodeling (black arrows) and duplication of tidemarks (yellow arrow) were displayed more clearly in the EP of ovariectomized (OVX) mice by safranin O fast green staining. Moreover, reduction of aggrecan in the nucleus pulposus (NP), as indicated by a paucity of safranin O staining (blue thick arrow), cleft/crack formation in the annulus fibrosus (AF) (blue arrow), and loss of cells indicate intervertebral disc degeneration in OVX mice. $n = 9$ per group; scale bars = 100 μm and 20 μm as indicated

Col II and upregulates OPN and VEGF expressions in the endplate and annulus fibrosus, suggesting that abnormal ossification and angiogenesis are involved in the process of IVDD related to osteoporosis.

Estrogen as an endocrine hormone influences the metabolism of various tissues and organs in the body, such as the rich collagenous tissues of bone, cartilage, disc, artery, and skin, etc. [23]. It has been clearly shown that a rapid decline of estrogen levels is an important factor for osteoporosis in postmenopausal women. Insufficient estrogen caused by OVX is the common method to mimic postmenopausal status and can effectively induce osteoporosis. Many studies have confirmed that ovariectomy could cause osteoporosis in various animals, such as rats, mice, monkeys, and so forth [25, 32, 37]. In the current study, our results show that ovariotomy caused an increased body weight with abdominal fat accumulation but a decreased uterine weight with a severe atrophy in morphology. Furthermore, a mass of fat in the bone marrow of the tibia and thin trabeculae were observed in OVX mice, which supports that estrogen deficiency may induce adipogenic differentiation of bone marrow stem cells, but not osteogenesis. Moreover, the poorer results for BMDtv and the bone parameters including BV/TV, Tb.N, Tb.pf, CONN.D, and SMI were seen in the L5 vertebra of the OVX group when compared with the control group suggesting a deterioration in bone quality and quantity due to ovariectomy, consistent with previous

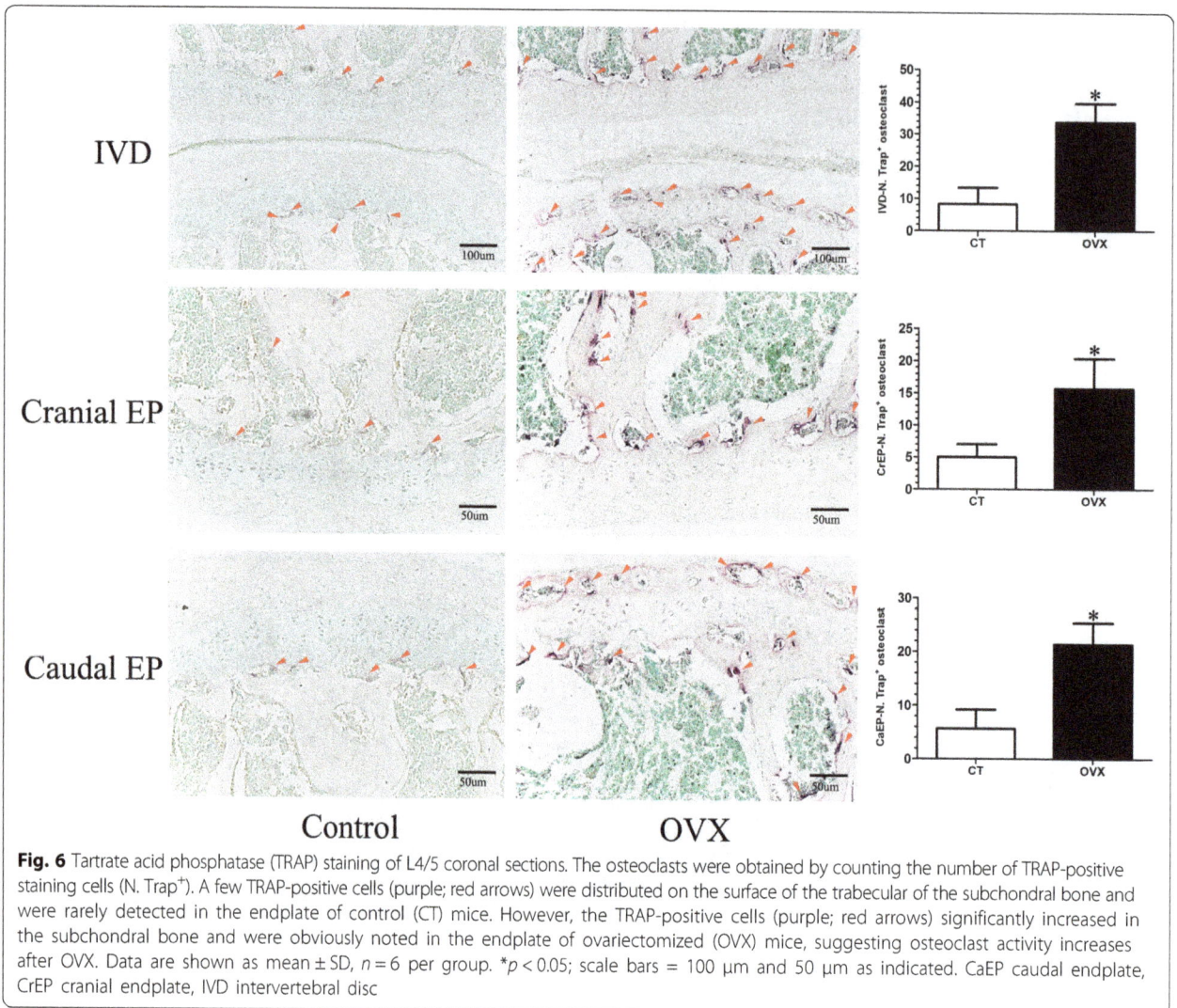

Fig. 6 Tartrate acid phosphatase (TRAP) staining of L4/5 coronal sections. The osteoclasts were obtained by counting the number of TRAP-positive staining cells (N. Trap+). A few TRAP-positive cells (purple; red arrows) were distributed on the surface of the trabecular of the subchondral bone and were rarely detected in the endplate of control (CT) mice. However, the TRAP-positive cells (purple; red arrows) significantly increased in the subchondral bone and were obviously noted in the endplate of ovariectomized (OVX) mice, suggesting osteoclast activity increases after OVX. Data are shown as mean ± SD, $n = 6$ per group. $*p < 0.05$; scale bars = 100 μm and 50 μm as indicated. CaEP caudal endplate, CrEP cranial endplate, IVD intervertebral disc

studies [32, 37, 38]. Progressively, we investigated the effects of OVX on the intervertebral disc. As expected, OVX mice showed increases in the osteochondral remodeling and porosity of the endplate accompanied by decreases in the height and volume of the intervertebral disc, loss of proteoglycans and cells, and the formation of clefts, suggesting that ovariotomy effectively accelerates the deterioration of the endplate and induces IVDD. Considering that the intervertebral disc is avascular, material exchange with the vertebrae mainly relies on the endplate. Thus, it can be speculated that some effects of estrogen on the intervertebral disc are indirect. The initial occurrences of osteoporosis and cartilaginous endplate remodeling and subsequent disorders of intervertebral disc metabolism may be a reasonable explanation for the induction of IVDD by estrogen deficiency.

Many risk factors have been found to be involved in the IVDD process, including age, sex, injury, obesity, genetic predisposition, immune, nutrition, inflammation, and mechanical factors [7, 24, 39]. Increasing evidence indicates that IVDD is associated with the disruption of an intact spinal structure, such as adjacent structures including the vertebra and endplate [14, 16, 17, 22]. In recent years, the important role of subchondral bone in the development of osteoarthritis has been increasingly recognized [40]; in fact, it is the same with IVDD. Changes in vertebral strain energy were correlated with increasing Schmorl's nodes in multilevel lumbar disk degeneration [41]. The changes in vertebral-endplate subchondral bone signal detected by magnetic resonance imaging (MRI) may serve as an 'active discopathy' judgment [8]. Therefore, as the bridge of communication between the vertebra and the intervertebral disc, the integrity of the endplate may be the key factor affecting the intervertebral disc [42, 43], and the deterioration of subchondral bone may be the trigger of IVDD. Interestingly, in some studies, ossification of the endplate with a

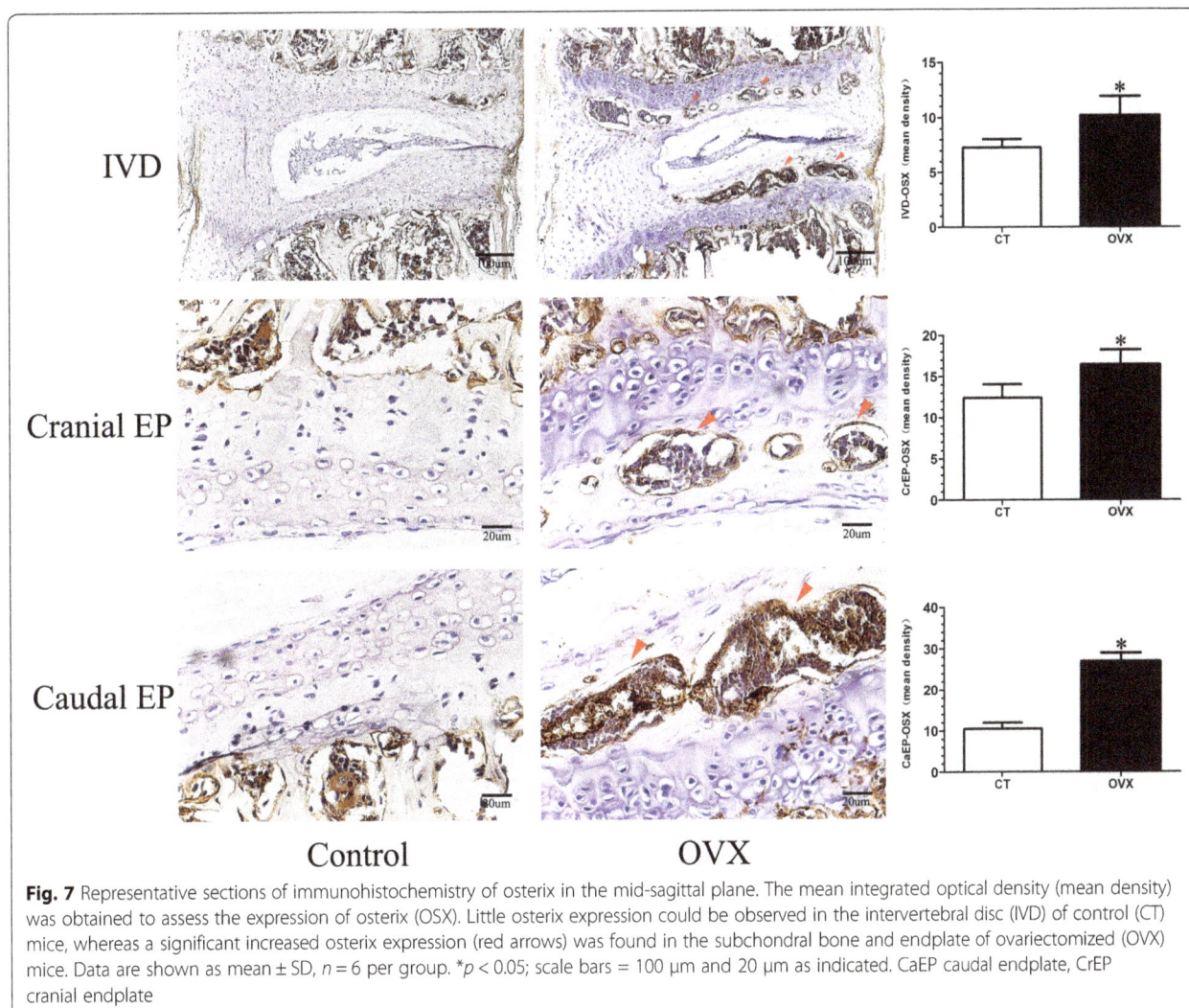

Fig. 7 Representative sections of immunohistochemistry of osterix in the mid-sagittal plane. The mean integrated optical density (mean density) was obtained to assess the expression of osterix (OSX). Little osterix expression could be observed in the intervertebral disc (IVD) of control (CT) mice, whereas a significant increased osterix expression (red arrows) was found in the subchondral bone and endplate of ovariectomized (OVX) mice. Data are shown as mean ± SD, $n = 6$ per group. *$p < 0.05$; scale bars = 100 μm and 20 μm as indicated. CaEP caudal endplate, CrEP cranial endplate

reduction in porosity and permeability accelerated degeneration of the intervertebral disc during the osteoporosis process [17, 38]. It has been shown by a dynamic contrast-enhanced MRI study that ovariectomy induces a decrease in the second wash-in phase, indicating that the diffusion between the vertebra and the disc was impaired as a result of ovariectomy [44]. On the contrary, other studies have concluded that osteoporosis increases the porosity and permeability of the endplate, leading to a delay in disc degeneration [19]. Indeed, these conclusions are derived from the theory that nutrient acquisition of the intervertebral disc relies on endplate permeability. However, our study has found that endplate osteochondral remodeling causes a high endplate porosity/permeability leading to disc degeneration, and this may be associated with antigen exposure, immune inflammation, and loss of nucleus pulposus osmotic pressure in the intervertebral disc due to the increased endplate porosity. TRAP staining showed that a large number of activated osteoclasts appeared in the osteochondral interface of OVX mice, which

indicated the osteochondral remodeling of the endplate. Here, we speculate that the rapid bone turnover caused by OVX should be responsible for the endplate remodeling and the increased porosity which could reflect the high permeability between vertebrae and the intervertebral disc and which is closely associated with disc degeneration. Several studies could support these etiological hypotheses. Rodriguez et al. [36] found that porosity and permeability of the endplate were increased with age and disc degeneration. Osteoprotegerin (OPG) knockdown mice had an increase in neovascularization and expression of inflammatory cytokines in the intervertebral disc, indicating that osteoporosis can induce inflammation and consequently become the cause of disc degeneration [24]. The modic change of the endplate is closely related to back pain [1, 16]. Endplate damage could also lead to decompression of the nucleus pulposus [6]. Furthermore, severe disc degeneration is more common in patients with endplate modic changes, which suggests that modic changes could result in the occurrence and

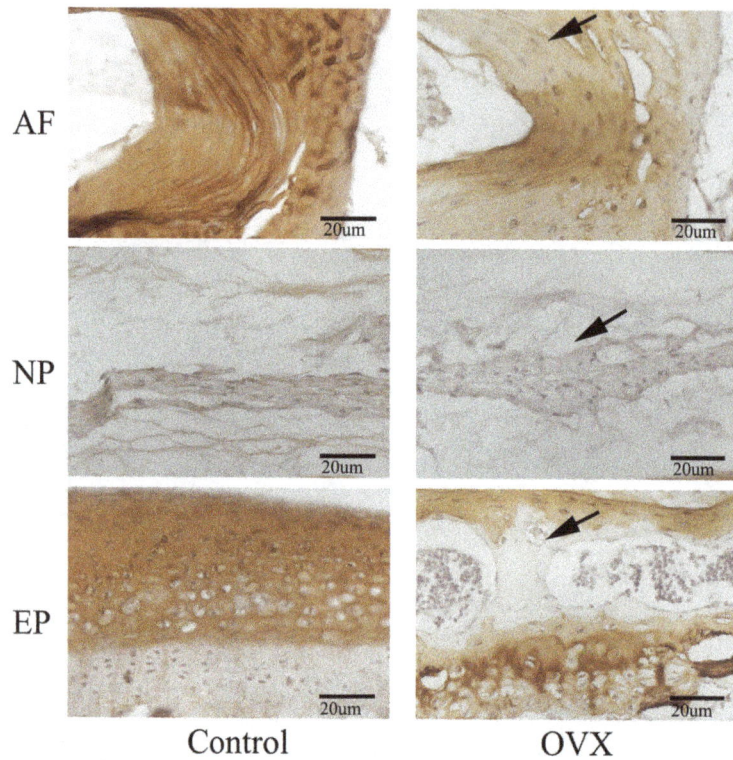

Fig. 8 Representative sections of immunohistochemistry of Col II. Positive immunostaining was noted as brown staining. Black arrows indicate loss of Col II, especially in the ossification area of the cartilaginous endplate (EP) and the outer layer of the annulus fibrosus (AF) in ovariectomized (OVX) mice. $n = 9$ per group; scale bars = 20 μm as indicated. NP nucleus pulposus

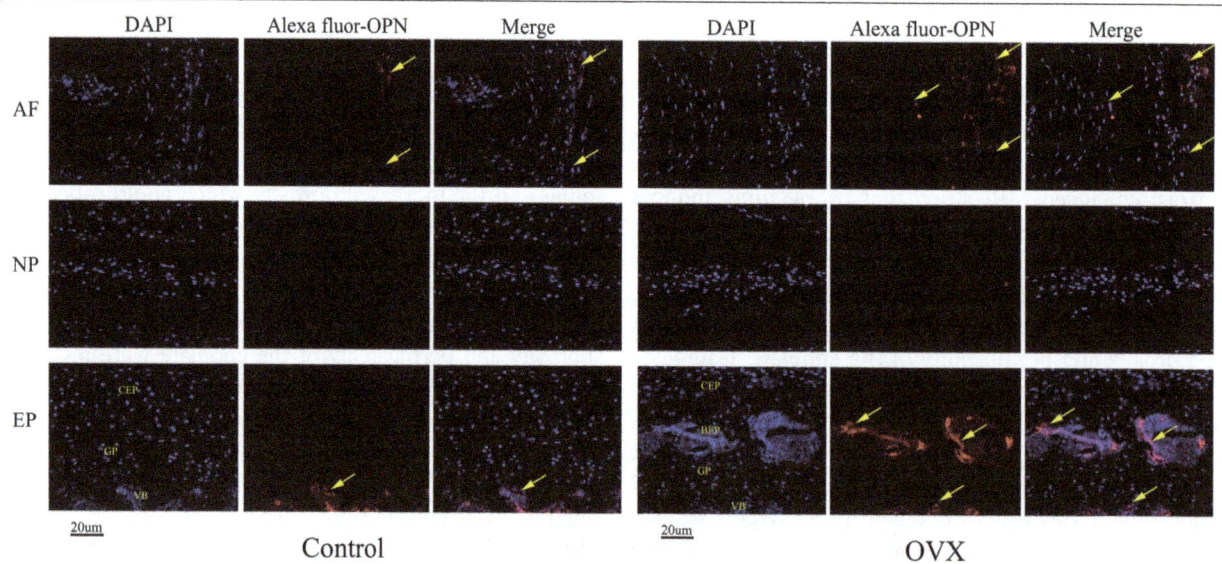

Fig. 9 Immunohistochemical staining of osteopontin (OPN). DAPI stains nuclei blue and OPN expression was detected as red. Both control and ovariectomized (OVX) mice have OPN expression in the vertebral body (VB) and outer annulus fibrosus (AF), but it was almost undetectable in the nucleus. However, remarkable expression of OPN was found in the bony endplate (BEP) and outer AF in OVX mice. Meanwhile, the expression of OPN was also detected in the inner AF. $n = 9$ per group; scale bar = 20 μm as indicated. CEP cartilaginous endplate, EP endplate, GP growth plate, NP nucleus pulposus

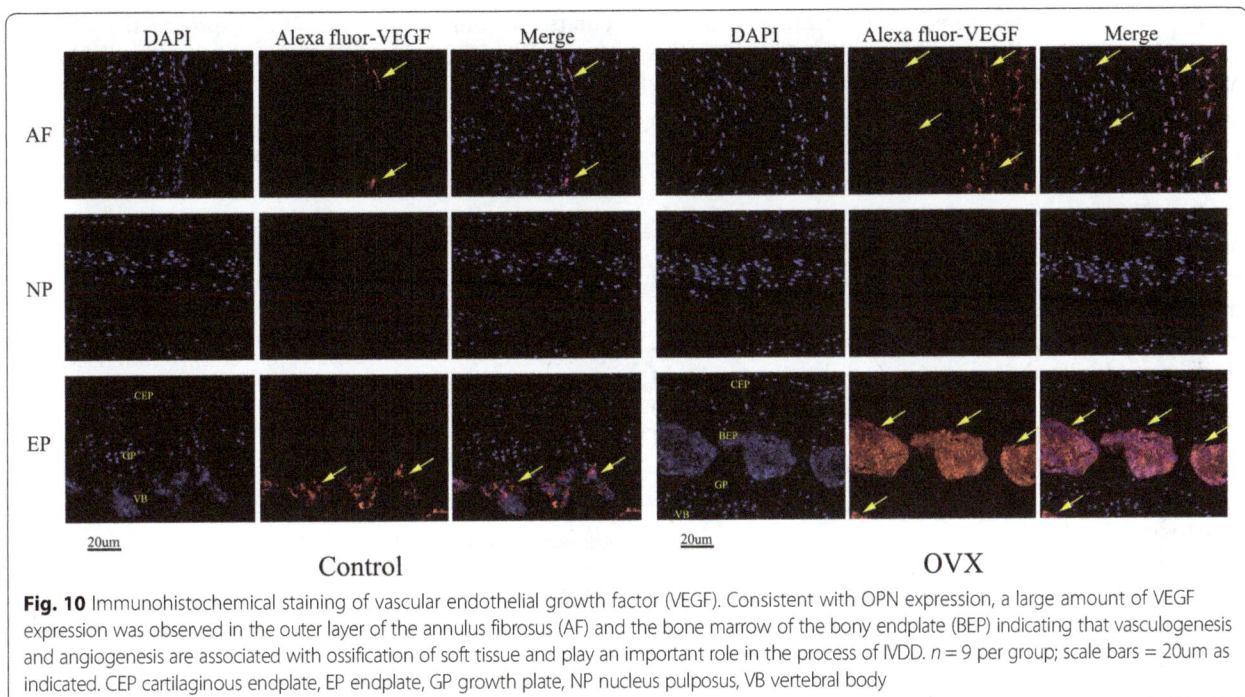

Fig. 10 Immunohistochemical staining of vascular endothelial growth factor (VEGF). Consistent with OPN expression, a large amount of VEGF expression was observed in the outer layer of the annulus fibrosus (AF) and the bone marrow of the bony endplate (BEP) indicating that vasculogenesis and angiogenesis are associated with ossification of soft tissue and play an important role in the process of IVDD. $n = 9$ per group; scale bars = 20um as indicated. CEP cartilaginous endplate, EP endplate, GP growth plate, NP nucleus pulposus, VB vertebral body

development of IVDD [45]. Consistently, we found that remodeling of the endplate led to an increased surface porosity and permeability, which could lead to degeneration of the intervertebral disc.

Yuan et al. [42] successfully developed a rat model of IVDD using the injection of alcohol within the endplate to block the blood vessels. IVDD and osteoporosis can also result in endplate cartilage injury [46], supporting that the intervertebral disc interacts with the vertebra. A finite element analysis showed us that both decreased trabecular core density and IVDD have been suggested to play roles in vertebral fractures. IVDD caused a shift of the load from the nucleus pulposus to the anulus fibrosus, resulting in bone adaptation which was presented as a dramatically reduced density of the trabecular core and an increased density in the vertebral walls [47]. Furthermore, the positive correlation between the thickness of the subchondral bone and the proteoglycan content of the adjacent disc have been found in human cadaveric material, particularly in the region of the nucleus pulposus [48]. Bone responds to a greater hydrostatic pressure exerted by discs with higher proteoglycan content than that by discs with less proteoglycan present, which indicates that vertebral osteoporosis with resultant endplate-bone remodeling could affect the flow of solutes to and from the intervertebral disc by failing to maintain the normal hydrostatic pressure of the nucleus pulposus, resulting in the loss of proteoglycans [48]. Therefore, only by guaranteeing a certain appropriate permeability with the proper microstructure of the subchondral bone, being neither too high nor too low,

could the endplate maintain the specific hydrostatic pressure and balance the microenvironment of the nucleus pulposus to ensure the stability of the intervertebral disc. The endplate might play the role of a biological semipermeable membrane.

Col II is the most abundant collagen in cartilaginous tissues and is often referred to as the major collagen. Therefore, its content is crucial for proper disc function, particularly in the cartilaginous endplate and nucleus pulposus [49]. Our study showed that OVX could effectively weaken Col II expression, especially in the zone of ossification of the endplate, which could be related to OVX-induced osteochondral remodeling. Furthermore, the levels of OPN and VEGF were markedly elevated in the endplate and annulus fibrosus of OVX mice, consistent with the results of IVDD caused by spinal instability [31]. It is noteworthy that colocalized expression of OPN and VEGF were visible in degenerative discs. The molecular pathological changes in the intervertebral disc indicate that ossification and angiogenesis of the intervertebral disc are not to supply more nutrient for disc repair but to accelerate the intervertebral disc fibrosis and ossification.

Osteoclastogenesis is a prerequisite for osteochondral remodeling, and the osteoclast resorption process is required to degrade subchondral bone and cartilage [50]. Our study found a significant increase in osteoclasts in the subchondral bone and cartilaginous endplate of the OVX group, consistent with the previous findings. Interestingly, alendronate and calcitonin can inhibit osteoclast activity and osteochondral remodeling to extenuate

IVDD [26, 27]. Although parathyroid hormone 1–34 has substantial anabolic effects on bone mass and trabecular microarchitecture, nonsignificant effects have not yet been found on disc degeneration [51]. This leads us to suggest that preventing the remodeling of the osteochondral structure caused by the initial osteoclastogenesis after the menopause could be an important aspect in the fight against the occurrence of intervertebral disc degeneration. Furthermore, some reports have confirmed that suppressing osteoclastogenesis and aberrant angiogenesis could blunt IVDD and osteoarthritis [52, 53], which provides further promise for the treatment of IVDD in the future. It may be beneficial to renew the intervertebral disc by balancing bone metabolism and regulating permeability of the endplate.

Conclusions

In summary, this study uncovered the mystery of the deteriorative effects of OVX on IVDD, clearly showing that OVX can induce and accelerate the progression of disc degeneration. The underlying mechanisms could be related to the destruction of the structural integrity and the function of the vertebra and endplate induced by OVX, both of which are essential structures for maintaining disc function. OVX modulates bone turnover and results in osteochondral interface remodeling which could also influences the expressions of Col II, OSX, OPN, and VEGF to stimulate the disc degeneration. It is conceivable that osteoporosis of vertebrae and endplate remodeling resulting from estrogen depletion may affect the bone marrow microenvironment and endplate permeability which subsequently could alter the metabolism and biomechanics of the intervertebral disc. Simultaneously, the reduction in estrogen caused by OVX could also directly affect the metabolism of the intervertebral disc because of the presence of estrogen receptors in the nucleus pulposus. These changes may be a reasonable explanation for disc degeneration related to osteoporosis. However, our observations are preliminary and need to be further confirmed through clinical trials or additional animal experiments. Based on the above results, intervention for osteoporosis and improvement in the vertebral body and endplate structure may be an effective way to retard IVDD; the mechanisms of IVDD related to osteoporosis need to be further studied.

Shortcomings and limitations

There are several limitations for this study. First, the findings from the current study are preliminary because of the limited sample sizes and insufficient evidence. The penetration of the endplate lacks intuitive measurement methods and the porosity of the endplate was defined by an indirect index for assessing permeability. Second, our study lacks investigation at different time

points and thus we cannot observe progressive changes of vertebrae and discs. Third, although some differentially expressed proteins were found using immunohistochemistry, other methods of detection were not used due to research grant limitations and insufficient mice disc tissue.

Abbreviations
BMD: Bone mineral density; BV: Bone volume; Col: Collagen; CONN.D: Connectivity density; CT: Computed tomography; H&E: Hematoxylin and eosin; IVDD: Intervertebral disc degeneration; OPN: Osteopontin; OSX: Osterix; OVX: Ovariectomy; PO(op): Open porosity; Po.N(cl): Number of closed pores; Po.V(tot): Total volume of pore space; ROI: Region of interest; SMI: Structural model index; Tb.N: Trabecular number; Tb.Pf: Trabecular pattern factor; Tb.Sp: Trabecular separation; Tb.Th: Trabecular thickness; TRAP: Tartrate-resistant acid phosphatase; TV: Total volume; VEGF: Vascular endothelial growth factor

Acknowledgments
The authors would like to thank Mr. Fang Yang for helping with micro-CT scanning and analyses, and we thank the Laboratory of Orthopedics and Traumatology of Lingnan Medical Research Center of Guangzhou University of Chinese Medicine for providing associated facilities.

Funding
This study is supported by a National Natural Science Foundation of China (NSFC; grant number 81673992) and the Open Foundation of The National Key Discipline and The Laboratory of Orthopedics and Traumatology of Guangzhou University of Chinese Medicine.

Authors' contributions
All authors made substantial contributions to the data analysis and interpretation, drafting of the manuscript and critical revision of the manuscript for important intellectual content. All authors gave final approval of the version to be published. ZX and DL had full access to all the data in the study and take responsibility for the integrity of the data and the accuracy of the data analysis. Conception and design: DL, ZX, MC, and YH. Collection and assembly of data: ZX, JH, MC, GS, and SC. Analysis and interpretation of the data: GS, YH, MC, ZX, and SC. Manuscript drafting: ZX, JH, DL, MC, and YH. Manuscript revision and supplementary experiments: JH and GS.

Competing interests
The authors declare that they have no competing interests.

Author details
[1]The Department of Spinal Surgery, The Second Affiliated Hospital of Guangzhou University of Chinese Medicine, No. 111, Dade Road, Yuexiu District, Guangzhou 510120, China. [2]The Laboratory Affiliated to Orthopaedics and Traumatology of Chinese Medicine of Linnan Medical Research Center of Guangzhou University of Chinese Medicine, No. 12, Jichang Road, Baiyun District, Guangzhou 510405, China. [3]Guangzhou University of Chinese Medicine, No. 12, Jichang Road, Baiyun District, Guangzhou 510405, China.

References
1. Luoma K, Vehmas T, Kerttula L, Grönblad M, Rinne E. Chronic low back pain in relation to modic changes, bony endplate lesions, and disc degeneration in a prospective MRI study. Eur Spine J. 2016;25(9):2873–81.
2. Izzo R, Popolizio T, D'Aprile P, Muto M. Spinal pain. Eur J Radiol. 2015;84(5): 746–56.
3. Wenig CM, Schmidt CO, Kohlmann T, Schweikert B. Costs of back pain in Germany. Eur J Pain. 2009;13(3):280–6.
4. Paesold G, Nerlich AG, Boos N. Biological treatment strategies for disc degeneration: potentials and shortcomings. Eur Spine J. 2007;16(4):447–68.

5.   Humzah MD, Soames RW. Human intervertebral disc: structure and function. Anat Rec. 1988;220(4):337–56.

6.   Dolan P, Luo J, Pollintine P, Landham PR, Stefanakis M, Adams MA. Intervertebral disc decompression following endplate damage: implications for disc degeneration depend on spinal level and age. Spine (Phila Pa 1976). 2013;38(17):1473–81.

7.   Vergroesen PPA, Kingma I, Emanuel KS, Hoogendoorn RJW, Welting TJ, van Royen BJ, van Dieen JH, Smit TH. Mechanics and biology in intervertebral disc degeneration: a vicious circle. Osteoarthr Cartilage. 2015;23(7):1057–70.

8.   Nguyen C, Poiraudeau S, Rannou F. From Modic 1 vertebral-endplate subchondral bone signal changes detected by MRI to the concept of 'active discopathy'. Ann Rheum Dis. 2015;74(8):1488–94.

9.   Karsdal MA, Bay-Jensen AC, Lories RJ, Abramson S, Spector T, Pastoureau P, Christiansen C, Attur M, Henriksen K, Goldring SR, et al. The coupling of bone and cartilage turnover in osteoarthritis: opportunities for bone antiresorptives and anabolics as potential treatments? Ann Rheum Dis. 2014;73(2):336–48.

10. Yuan XL, Meng HY, Wang YC, Peng J, Guo QY, Wang AY, Lu SB. Bone-cartilage interface crosstalk in osteoarthritis: potential pathways and future therapeutic strategies. Osteoarthr Cartil. 2014;22(8):1077–89.

11. Funck-Brentano T, Cohen-Solal M. Crosstalk between cartilage and bone: when bone cytokines matter. Cytokine Growth Factor Rev. 2011;22(2):91–7.

12. Bellido M, Lugo L, Roman-Blas JA, Castaneda S, Caeiro JR, Dapia S, Calvo E, Largo R, Herrero-Beaumont G. Subchondral bone microstructural damage by increased remodelling aggravates experimental osteoarthritis preceded by osteoporosis. Arthritis Res Ther. 2010;12(4):R152.

13. Shapiro IM, Vresilovic EJ, Risbud MV. Is the spinal motion segment a diarthrodial polyaxial joint: what a nice nucleus like you doing in a joint like this? Bone. 2012;50(3):771–6.

14. Chen S, Fu P, Wu H, Pei M. Meniscus, articular cartilage and nucleus pulposus: a comparative review of cartilage-like tissues in anatomy, development and function. Cell Tissue Res. 2017;370(1):53–70.

15. Kang R, Li H, Ringgaard S, Rickers K, Sun H, Chen M, Xie L, Bunger C. Interference in the endplate nutritional pathway causes intervertebral disc degeneration in an immature porcine model. Int Orthop. 2014;38(5):1011–7.

16. Moore RJ. The vertebral endplate: disc degeneration. Eur Spine J. 2006;153:S333–7.

17. Tomaszewski KA, Adamek D, Konopka T, Tomaszewska R, Walocha JA. Endplate calcification and cervical intervertebral disc degeneration: the role of endplate marrow contact channel occlusion. Folia Morphol (Warsz). 2015; 74(1):84–92.

18. Holm S, Maroudas A, Urban JP, Selstam G, Nachemson A. Nutrition of the intervertebral disc: solute transport and metabolism. Connect Tissue Res. 1981;8(2):101–19.

19. Mattei TA. Osteoporosis delays intervertebral disc degeneration by increasing intradiscal diffusive transport of nutrients through both mechanical and vascular pathophysiological pathways. Med Hypotheses. 2013;80(5):582–6.

20. Lou C, Chen H, Feng X, Xiang G, Zhu S, Tian N, Jin Y, Fang M, Wang C, Xu H. Menopause is associated with lumbar disc degeneration: a review of 4230 intervertebral discs. Climacteric. 2014;17(6):700–4.

21. Wang YJ, Griffith JF. Effect of menopause on lumbar disk degeneration. Radiology. 2010;257(2):319–20.

22. Wang YJ, Griffith JF. Menopause causes vertebral endplate degeneration and decrease in nutrient diffusion to the intervertebral discs. Med Hypotheses. 2011;77(1):18–20.

23. Calleja-Agius J, Muscat-Baron Y, Brincat MP. Estrogens and the intervertebral disc. Menopause Int. 2009;15(3):127–30.

24. Li X, Xue C, Zhao Y, Cheng S, Zhao D, Liang Q, Chen L, Wang Q, Lu S, Shi Q, et al. Deletion of OPG leads to increased neovascularization and expression of inflammatory cytokines in the lumbar intervertebral disc of mice. Spine. 2017;42(1):E8–E14.

25. Luo Y, Zhang L, Wang W, Hu Q, Song H, Su Y, Zhang Y. Alendronate retards the progression of lumbar intervertebral disc degeneration in ovariectomized rats. Bone. 2013;55(2):439–48.

26. Song H, Luo Y, Wang W, Li S, Yang K, Dai M, Shen Y, Zhang Y, Zhang L. Effects of alendronate on lumbar intervertebral disc degeneration with bone loss in ovariectomized rats. Spine J. 2017;17(7):995–1003.

27. Tian FM, Yang K, Wang WY, Luo Y, Li SY, Song HP, Zhang YZ, Shen Y, Zhang L. Calcitonin suppresses intervertebral disk degeneration and preserves lumbar vertebral bone mineral density and bone strength in ovariectomized rats. Osteoporos Int. 2015;26(12):2853–61.

28. Nanjo Y, Morio Y, Nagashima H, Hagino H, Teshima R. Correlation between bone mineral density and intervertebral disk degeneration in pre- and postmenopausal women. J Bone Miner Metab. 2003;21(1):22–7.

29. Miyakoshi N, Itoi E, Murai H, Wakabayashi I, Ito H, Minato T. Inverse relation between osteoporosis and spondylosis in postmenopausal women as evaluated by bone mineral density and semiquantitative scoring of spinal degeneration. Spine. 2003;28(5):492–5.

30. Pye SR, Reid DM, Adams JE, Silman AJ, O'Neill TW. Radiographic features of lumbar disc degeneration and bone mineral density in men and women. Ann Rheum Dis. 2006;65(2):234–8.

31. Bian Q, Jain A, Xu X, Kebaish K, Crane JL, Zhang Z, Wan M, Ma L, Riley LH, Sponseller PD, et al. Excessive activation of TGFbeta by spinal instability causes vertebral endplate sclerosis. Sci Rep. 2016;6:27093.

32. Bonucci E, Ballanti P. Osteoporosis-bone remodeling and animal models. Toxicol Pathol. 2014;42(6):957–69.

33. Martin JT, Gorth DJ, Beattie EE, Harfe BD, Smith LJ, Elliott DM. Needle puncture injury causes acute and long-term mechanical deficiency in a mouse model of intervertebral disc degeneration. J Orthop Res. 2013;31(8):1276–82.

34. Naito Y, Wakabayashi H, Kato S, Nakagawa T, Iino T, Sudo A. Alendronate inhibits hyperalgesia and suppresses neuropeptide markers of pain in a mouse model of osteoporosis. J Orthop Sci. 2017;22(4):771–7.

35. Laffosse JM, Accadbled F, Molinier F, Bonnevialle N, de Gauzy JS, Swider P. Correlations between effective permeability and marrow contact channels surface of vertebral endplates. J Orthop Res. 2010;28(9):1229–34.

36. Rodriguez AG, Slichter CK, Acosta FL, Rodriguez-Soto AE, Burghardt AJ, Majumdar S, Lotz JC. Human disc nucleus properties and vertebral endplate permeability. Spine (Phila Pa 1976). 2011;36(7):512–20.

37. Ren H, Liang D, Shen G, Yao Z, Jiang X, Tang J, Cui J, Lin S. Effects of combined ovariectomy with dexamethasone on rat lumbar vertebrae. Menopause. 2016;23(4):441–50.

38. Ding Y, Jiang J, Zhou J, Wu X, Huang Z, Chen J, Zhu Q. The effects of osteoporosis and disc degeneration on vertebral cartilage endplate lesions in rats. Eur Spine J. 2014;23(9):1848–55.

39. Dario AB, Ferreira ML, Refshauge KM, Lima TS, Ordonana JR, Ferreira PH. The relationship between obesity, low back pain, and lumbar disc degeneration when genetics and the environment are considered: a systematic review of twin studies. Spine J. 2015;15(5):1106–17.

40. Zhen G, Wen C, Jia X, Li Y, Crane JL, Mears SC, Askin FB, Frassica FJ, Chang W, Yao J, et al. Inhibition of TGF-beta signaling in mesenchymal stem cells of subchondral bone attenuates osteoarthritis. Nat Med. 2013;19(6):704.

41. Von Forell GA, Nelson TG, Samartzis D, Bowden AE. Changes in vertebral strain energy correlate with increased presence of Schmorl's nodes in multi-level lumbar disk degeneration. J Biomech Eng-T ASME. 2014;136:0610026.

42. Yuan W, Che W, Jiang Y, Yuan F, Wang H, Zheng G, Li X, Dong J. Establishment of intervertebral disc degeneration model induced by ischemic sub-endplate in rat tail. Spine J. 2015;15(5):1050–9.

43. Maatta JH, Kraatari M, Wolber L, Niinimaki J, Wadge S, Karppinen J, Williams FMK. Vertebral endplate change as a feature of intervertebral disc degeneration: a heritability study. Eur Spine J. 2014;23(9):1856–62.

44. Deng M, Griffith JF, Zhu X, Poon WS, Ahuja AT, Wang YJ. Effect of ovariectomy on contrast agent diffusion into lumbar intervertebral disc: a dynamic contrast-enhanced MRI study in female rats. Magn Reson Imaging. 2012;30(5):683–8.

45. Hu Z, Zhao F, Fang X, Fan S. Modic changes, possible causes and promotion to lumbar intervertebral disc degeneration. Med Hypotheses. 2009;73(6):930–2.

46. Wang L, Cui W, Kalala JP, Van Hoof T, Liu B. Effect of osteoporosis and intervertebral disc degeneration on endplate cartilage injury in rats. Asian Pac J Trop Med. 2014;7(10):796–800.

47. Homminga J, Aquarius R, Bulsink VE, Jansen CTJ, Verdonschot N. Can vertebral density changes be explained by intervertebral disc degeneration? Med Eng Phys. 2012;34(4):453–8.

48. Roberts S, McCall IW, Menage J, Haddaway MJ, Eisenstein SM. Does the thickness of the vertebral subchondral bone reflect the composition of the intervertebral disc? Eur Spine J. 1997;6(6):385–9.

49. Kim KW, Ha KY, Park JB, Woo YK, Chung HN, An HS. Expressions of membrane-type I matrix metalloproteinase, Ki-67 protein, and type II collagen by chondrocytes migrating from cartilage endplate into nucleus pulposus in rat intervertebral discs—a cartilage endplate-fracture model using an intervertebral disc organ culture. SPINE. 2005;30(12):1373–8.

50. Lofvall H, Newbould H, Karsdal MA, Dziegiel MH, Richter J, Henriksen K, Thudium CS. Osteoclasts degrade bone and cartilage knee joint compartments through different resorption processes. Arthritis Res Ther. 2018;20(1):67.

51. Luo Y, Li SY, Tian FM, Song HP, Zhang YZ, Zhang L. Effects of human parathyroid hormone 1–34 on bone loss and lumbar intervertebral disc degeneration in ovariectomized rats. Int Orthop. 2018;42(5):1183–90.

52. Kwon WK, Moon HJ, Kwon TH, Park YK, Kim JH. Influence of rabbit notochordal cells on symptomatic intervertebral disc degeneration: anti-angiogenic capacity on human endothelial cell proliferation under hypoxia. Osteoarthr Cartil. 2017;25(10):1738–46.

53. Ji B, Zhang Z, Guo W, Ma H, Xu B, Mu W, Amat A, Cao L. Isoliquiritigenin blunts osteoarthritis by inhibition of bone resorption and angiogenesis in subchondral bone. Sci Rep. 2018;8(1):1721.

4

Association between brain-derived neurotrophic factor gene polymorphisms and fibromyalgia in a Korean population: a multicenter study

Dong-Jin Park[1], Seong-Ho Kim[2], Seong-Su Nah[3], Ji Hyun Lee[4], Seong-Kyu Kim[5], Yeon-Ah Lee[6], Seung-Jae Hong[6], Hyun-Sook Kim[7], Hye-Soon Lee[8], Hyoun Ah Kim[9], Chung-Il Joung[10], Sang-Hyon Kim[11] and Shin-Seok Lee[1]*⊙

Abstract

Background: Several lines of evidence imply that brain-derived neurotrophic factor (BDNF) is involved in the pathophysiology of fibromyalgia (FM); in this regard, patients with FM have altered blood and cerebrospinal fluid levels of BDNF. In this study, we explored the association between *BDNF* gene polymorphisms and FM susceptibility and the severity of symptoms.

Methods: In total, 409 patients with FM and 423 healthy controls in 10 medical centers were enrolled from the Korean nationwide FM survey. The alleles and genotypes at 10 positions in the *BDNF* gene were genotyped.

Results: The allele and genotype frequencies of *BDNF* rs11030104 differed significantly between the patients with FM and the controls ($P = 0.031$). The GG genotype of rs11030104 had a protective effect against FM ($P = 0.016$), and the G allele of rs11030104 was negatively associated with the presence of FM compared with the A allele ($P = 0.013$). In comparison, although the allele and genotype frequencies of *BDNF* rs12273539 did not differ between the two groups, the TT genotype of *BDNF* rs12273539 was associated with susceptibility to FM ($P = 0.038$). Haplotype analyses implied that some *BDNF* haplotypes have a protective effect against FM. Finally, several genotypes and haplotypes of the *BDNF* gene contributed to specific symptoms of FM.

Conclusions: This study is the first to evaluate the associations between *BDNF* gene polymorphisms and FM. Our results imply that some *BDNF* single-nucleotide polymorphisms and haplotypes are associated with susceptibility to, and contribute to the symptoms of, FM.

Keywords: Fibromyalgia, Brain-derived neurotrophic factor, Genetics, Polymorphism

Background

Fibromyalgia (FM) is a common rheumatic syndrome characterized by chronic widespread pain, and is often accompanied by diverse symptoms including fatigue, sleep disorders, memory loss, joint stiffness, and affective distress [1]. The prevalence of FM in the general population is reportedly 1–5%, and it is more prevalent among women than men [2]. Although its pathogenesis is

unclear, FM is recognized as an outcome of the interactions of multiple genetic, psychological, neurobiological, and environmental factors [3].

The familial aggregation observed among patients with FM implies that genetic factors are important contributors to the etiology of FM [4]. Recent genetic studies have advanced our understanding of the pathogenesis of FM. These studies have shown that certain gene polymorphisms alter pain sensitivity and increase susceptibility to FM [5]. In particular, polymorphisms of genes involved in the pain transmission pathway, such as the serotoninergic, dopaminergic, and catecholaminergic systems, have received much attention as possible genetic factors in FM

* Correspondence: shinseok@chonnam.ac.kr
[1]Division of Rheumatology, Department of Internal Medicine, Chonnam National University Medical School and Hospital, 42 Jebong-ro, Dong-gu, Gwangju 61469, Republic of Korea
Full list of author information is available at the end of the article

[6, 7]. However, those genetic factors do not fully account for the pathophysiology and symptoms of FM. Therefore, efforts to identify other genetic factors that contribute to FM are ongoing.

Brain-derived neurotrophic factor (BDNF) is involved in neuronal survival, growth, and differentiation during development of the central and peripheral nervous systems [8]. BDNF is important in the transmission of physiologic or pathologic pain [9]. BDNF is responsible for modulation of nociceptive inputs and enhanced hyperalgesia by a N-methyl-D-aspartate (NMDA) receptor-mediated mechanism [10]. Moreover, dysregulation of BDNF in the dorsal root ganglion (DRG) and spinal cord contributes to chronic pain hypersensitivity [11]. In addition, several lines of evidence have converged to imply that BDNF is involved in the pathophysiology of FM. Indeed, patients with FM have been shown to have altered serum and plasma levels of BDNF compared to healthy controls [12–14].

However, whether polymorphisms of the *BDNF* gene are associated with FM remains an open question. The objective of this study was to evaluate the associations between *BDNF* gene polymorphisms and FM susceptibility and clinical symptoms, using a large population of ethnically homogenous Koreans.

Methods
Study design and population
We performed a multicenter, nationwide FM cohort study (the Korean Nationwide FM Survey) in the Korean population. In the Korean Nationwide FM Survey, we established a prospective cohort to evaluate the pathophysiology of FM, and the clinical manifestations and outcomes of Korean patients with FM. The study participants were recruited from the outpatient rheumatology clinics of 10 medical centers. In this study, a cross-sectional design was employed to evaluate the association between *BDNF* gene polymorphisms and susceptibility to, and symptom severity of, FM. As reported previously [15], we enrolled 409 patients with FM (382 women and 27 men) with a mean (SD) age of 48.1 (10.9) years. At the time of the initial diagnosis, patients with FM were diagnosed according to the classification criteria for FM proposed by the American College of Rheumatology (ACR) in 1990 [1]. The mean (SD) symptom duration before diagnosis was 8.5 (8.3) years, and the mean (SD) disease duration after initial diagnosis was 1.9 (3.0) years. Based on health surveys for chronic pain, we recruited 423 healthy controls (397 women, 25 men) with a mean (SD) age of 45.5 (12.5) years and no history of chronic pain, including FM. Healthy controls were recruited randomly, without matching for age or sex, among the individuals visiting the general health examination clinics at each medical center. This research complied with the Helsinki Declaration, and written informed consent was obtained from all participants at the time of recruitment. Exactly the same informed consult form (ICF) and study protocol were provided to the independent Institutional Review Board/Ethics Committee (IRB/EC) at each medical center, and each IRB/EC reviewed the appropriateness of the protocol and risks and benefits to the study participants. Ultimately, the IRB/EC at each medical center independently approved this study without revision of the ICF or study protocol.

Procedures
The patients with FM were interviewed at the time of enrollment to determine their demographics and clinical characteristics, including age, sex, body mass index, and symptom and disease duration. In addition, at enrollment, peripheral venous blood was sampled and then stored in an ethylenediaminetetraacetate (EDTA)-coated tube. Tender points were assessed by thumb palpation according to the standardized tender point survey protocol [16]. The number of tender points was assessed at 18 sites on the body. The intensity at each tender point was assessed by determining the tender point score as follows: 0, no tenderness; 1, light tenderness (confirming answer when asked); 2, moderate tenderness (spontaneous verbal response); and 3, severe tenderness (moving away). Therefore, the number of tender points ranged from 0 to 18, and the possible total scores of the tender points ranged from 0 to 54. Furthermore, extensive clinical assessments of patients with FM enrolled in the cohort were undertaken using a self-report questionnaire and semi-structured questionnaires. The Korean version of the Fibromyalgia Impact Questionnaire (FIQ) was used to assess the functional abilities and severity of FM [17], and the Brief Fatigue Inventory (BFI) and the Beck Depression Inventory (BDI) were used to evaluate the severity of fatigue and depression, respectively [18, 19]. The 36-item Medical Outcomes Study Short-Form Health Survey (SF-36) was used to access the quality of life of the patients with FM [20]. In addition, we also evaluated the severity of anxiety using the State-Trait Anxiety Inventory (STAI)-I and STAI-II [21].

The patients had been treated with standard medications for FM, based on the clinical judgment of their attending rheumatologist. Concomitant medications, used at the time of enrollment, included tricyclic antidepressants (TCA), selective serotonin reuptake inhibitors (SSRI), serotonin-norepinephrine reuptake inhibitors (SNRI), pregabalin, gabapentin, nonsteroidal anti-inflammatory drugs (NSAIDs), acetaminophen, benzodiazepine, tramadol, and muscle relaxants.

Genotyping of *BDNF* polymorphisms
The assay reagents for rs2883187(C > T), rs7103873 (G > C), rs7103411(C > T), rs10835210(C > A), rs11030104 (A > G), rs12273539(C > T), rs11030102(C > G), rs11030101(A > T), rs6265(G > A) and rs7124442(C > T) in the *BDNF* gene

were designed by Applied Biosystems (Applied Biosystems). The reagents consisted of TaqMan MGB probes (FAM and VIC dye-labeled). Each reaction (10 μL) comprised 0.125 μL of 40X reagents, 5 μL of 2X TaqMan Genotyping Master Mix (Applied Biosystems) and 2 μL of 50 ng genomic DNA. The PCR conditions were 1 cycle at 95 °C for 10 min, followed by 40 cycles at 95 °C for 15 s and 60 °C for 1 min. The PCR reactions were performed using an ABI plus instrument (Applied Biosystems). The samples were read and analyzed using ABI plus software (Applied Biosystems). The sequences of the primers used for TaqMan probe genotyping of the *BDNF* gene are summarized in Table 1.

Statistical analysis

Statistical analyses were performed using IBM SPSS statistics (SPSS version 21; IBM SPSS Inc., Chicago, IL, USA). *P* values <0.05 were considered to indicate statistical significance. Each *BDNF* gene polymorphism was tested for Hardy-Weinberg equilibrium. The genotype and haplotype frequencies of the *BDNF* single-nucleotide polymorphisms (SNPs) were compared between the patients with FM and controls by Fisher's exact test or Pearson's chi-squared test. The association between each *BDNF* genotype and haplotype and susceptibility to FM was defined by logistic regression analysis. Analysis of covariance

Table 1 Primer sequences used for TaqMan probe genotyping of *BDNF*

Regions	Primers	Primer sequence (5′ → 3′)
rs 2883187	Forward	GTGAGGCATCCGGCCCGGCTGGGGA
	Reverse	CGGAGCGCGGTCTCGGCAGCTCCCC
rs 7103873	Forward	AGGACCTTTTACCCCCAAATGTAGA
	Reverse	ACTAAATGAAAAACCATTCTTTAAA
rs 7103411	Forward	GGAGCGCACTGTAAAGATACTGATA
	Reverse	GAACACGAATGTGAGATCAATGTTG
rs 10835210	Forward	CTTAACTGTAAAGCACAGGAAAGTG
	Reverse	TCATTACTTGTAGCTTAATGCAGGA
rs 11030104	Forward	ATTAAAAAGCAGATAACACTACCAC
	Reverse	TACTAACTGTCCTACAATTTCCTGT
rs 12273539	Forward	ACTCAATGCTTCATCACTTCTGCTC
	Reverse	GATCAGGACAGAGTCCTTGGAGTGC
rs 11030102	Forward	CTACTTCTCAGTTCTGAGGCATGGA
	Reverse	TTACAAAAAGACACATACATGCAAT
rs 11030101	Forward	GATACTCTATTATAGCAAAGAAGAA
	Reverse	GATAATTTCATTGAGCCATCCTGTT
rs 6265	Forward	TCCTCATCCAACAGCTCTTCTATCA
	Reverse	GTGTTCGAAAGTGTCAGCCAATGAT
rs 7124442	Forward	AAGGAAGCTGCATAAAGTTGACATA
	Reverse	AGCAGATATTCCAAGCATTCCTTAC

BDNF brain-derived neurotrophic factor

(ANCOVA), adjusted for age and sex, was used to explore the differences in the clinical measurements of the patients with FM according to *BDNF* genotype and haplotype. Haplotype structures were constructed and their frequencies estimated by combined allele analysis using PHASE v2.1.1 software (Department of Statistics, University of Washington, Seattle, WA, USA). We carried out a permutation test for the null hypothesis that the patients with FM and the healthy controls are random draws from a common set of haplotype frequencies (number of permutations performed = 10,000).

Results
BDNF genotypes and alleles and their association with clinical measurements

The *BDNF* SNPs were successfully genotyped in all enrolled subjects, except for 5 controls with *BDNF* rs2883187, 1 patient and 16 controls with *BDNF* rs7103873, 2 controls with *BDNF* rs7103411, 1 patient and 10 controls with *BDNF* rs10835210, 2 patients and 3 controls with *BDNF* rs11030104, 1 control with *BDNF* rs12273539, 1 patient and 1 control with *BDNF* rs11030102, 1 patient and 3 controls with *BDNF* rs11030101, 1 patient and 4 controls with *BDNF* rs6265, and 2 patients and 2 controls with *BDNF* rs7124442. The genotype distributions of the *BDNF* SNPs were consistent with Hardy-Weinberg equilibrium in both the patients and controls.

Among the *BDNF* SNPs, the allele and genotype frequencies of *BDNF* SNP rs11030104 were significantly different between the patients with FM and controls. Furthermore, patients with the GG genotype of rs11030104 were found less frequently in patients with FM after adjusting for age and sex (OR 0.619; 95% confidence interval (CI) 0.419–0.0913; $P = 0.016$). In addition, the G allele was negatively associated with the presence of FM compared to the A allele (OR = 0.781, 95% CI 0.641–0.950, $P = 0.013$). In comparison, although the allele and genotype frequencies of the SNPs of *BDNF* rs12273539 were not significantly different between the patients with FM and controls, the TT genotype of rs12273539 was found more frequently in patients with FM in the age-adjusted and sex-adjusted model (OR 2.586; 95% CI 1.052–6.360; $P = 0.038$) (Table 2).

Within the FM cohort, patients with the CG genotype of *BDNF* rs11030102 had more severe fatigue symptoms (measured by the BFI) and anxiety symptoms (measured by the STAI-I) than did the other genotypes ($P = 0.001$ and $P = 0.032$, respectively). Furthermore, both rs11030101 and rs10835210 were associated with the trait of anxiety (measured by the STAI-II) in patients with FM ($P = 0.029$ and $P = 0.033$, respectively). No associations were observed between clinical measurements and the other *BDNF* SNPs (Table 3).

Table 2 Genotype and allele analyses of *BDNF* in patients with fibromyalgia and healthy controls[a]

Marker	Genotype/allele	Contol, n (%)	Fibromyalgia, n (%)	Exact p value[b]	OR (95% CI), p value[c]	OR (95% CI), p value, adjusted by age, sex[‡]
rs2883187	C/C	115 (27.5)	100 (24.4)	0.218	1	1
	C/T	220 (52.6)	208 (50.9)		1.087 (0.783–1.510), $p = 0.617$	1.044 (0.747–1.458), $p = 0.802$
	T/T	83 (19.9)	101 (24.7)		1.399 (0.943–2.078), $p = 0.096$	1.340 (0.897–2.002), $p = 0.152$
	C	450 (53.8)	408 (49.9)	0.119	1	1
	T	386 (46.2)	410 (50.1)		1.172 (0.966–1.421), $p = 0.108$	1.147 (0.943–1.395), $p = 0.171$
rs7103873	G/G	113 (27.8)	98 (24.0)	0.245	1	1
	C/G	210 (51.6)	208 (51.0)		1.142 (0.820–1.591), $p = 0.432$	1.110 (0.791–1.556), $p = 0.546$
	C/C	84 (20.6)	102 (25.0)		1.400 (0.943–2.080), $p = 0.095$	1.345 (0.899–2.010), $p = 0.149$
	G	436 (53.6)	404 (49.5)	0.112	1	1
	C	378 (46.4)	412 (50.5)		1.176 (0.968–1.429), $p = 0.102$	1.153 (0.946–1.405), $p = 0.158$
rs7103411	C/C	120 (28.5)	128 (31.3)	0.638	1	1
	C/T	208 (49.4)	198 (48.4)		0.892 (0.651–1.224), $p = 0.48$	0.884 (0.641–1.220), $p = 0.454$
	T/T	93 (22.1)	83 (20.3)		0.837 (0.568–1.232), $p = 0.366$	0.865 (0.584–1.280), $p = 0.468$
	C	448 (53.2)	454 (55.5)	0.374	1	1
	T	394 (46.8)	364 (44.5)		0.912 (0.751–1.106), $p = 0.348$	0.925 (0.76–1.125), $p = 0.435$
rs10835210	C/C	204 (49.4)	196 (48.0)	0.725	1	1
	A/C	175 (42.4)	172 (42.2)		1.023 (0.767–1.364), $p = 0.877$	0.991 (0.740–1.326), $p = 0.949$
	A/A	34 (8.2)	40 (9.8)		1.224 (0.745–2.014), $p = 0.425$	1.183 (0.714–1.957), $p = 0.514$
	C	583 (70.6)	564 (69.1)	0.554	1	1
	A	243 (29.4)	252 (30.9)		1.072 (0.868–1.324), $p = 0.518$	1.048 (0.846–1.297), $p = 0.671$
rs11030104	A/A	101 (24.0)	126 (31.0)	0.031	1	1
	A/G	205 (48.8)	196 (48.2)		0.766 (0.553–1.063), $p = 0.111$	0.758 (0.544–1.057), $p = 0.102$
	G/G	114 (27.1)	85 (20.9)		0.598 (0.407–0.877), $p = 0.009$	0.619 (0.419–0.913), $p = 0.016$
	A	407 (48.5)	448 (55.0)	0.009	1	1
	G	433 (51.5)	366 (45.0)		0.768 (0.633–0.932), $p = 0.007$	0.781 (0.641–0.95), $p = 0.013$
rs12273539	C/C	283 (67.1)	268 (65.4)	0.101	1	1
	C/T	132 (31.3)	125 (30.5)		1 (0.744–1.345), $p = 1$	1.009 (0.747–1.362), $p = 0.955$
	T/T	7 (1.7)	17 (4.1)		2.564 (1.047–6.282), $p = 0.039$	2.586 (1.052–6.36), $p = 0.038$
	C	698 (82.7)	661 (80.6)	0.299	1	1
	T	146 (17.3)	159 (19.4)		1.150 (0.897–1.475), $p = 0.27$	1.161 (0.902–1.493), $p = 0.246$
rs11030102	C/C	419 (99.3)	402 (98.5)	0.334	1	1
	C/G	3 (0.7)	6 (1.5)		2.085 (0.518–8.392), $p = 0.301$	2.129 (0.524–8.649), $p = 0.291$
	C	841 (99.6)	810 (99.3)	0.335	1	1
	G	3 (0.4)	6 (0.7)		2.077 (0.518–8.326), $p = 0.302$	2.12 (0.524–8.58), $p = 0.292$
rs11030101	A/A	208 (49.5)	197 (48.3)	0.752	1	1
	A/T	178 (42.4)	172 (42.2)		1.020 (0.766–1.358), $p = 0.891$	0.985 (0.737–1.317), $p = 0.92$
	T/T	34 (8.1)	39 (9.6)		1.211 (0.735–1.996), $p = 0.452$	1.152 (0.694–1.912), $p = 0.583$
	A	594 (70.7)	566 (69.4)	0.585	1	1
	T	246 (29.3)	250 (30.6)		1.067 (0.864–1.316), $p = 0.548$	1.036 (0.837–1.283), $p = 0.743$
rs6265	G/G	96 (22.9)	87 (21.3)	0.770	1	1
	A/G	204 (48.7)	197 (48.3)		1.066 (0.751–1.512), $p = 0.722$	1.017 (0.712–1.451), $p = 0.928$
	A/A	119 (28.4)	124 (30.4)		1.150 (0.783–1.688), $p = 0.476$	1.110 (0.752–1.638), $p = 0.599$
	G	396 (47.3)	371 (45.5)	0.496	1	

Table 2 Genotype and allele analyses of *BDNF* in patients with fibromyalgia and healthy controls[a] *(Continued)*

Marker	Genotype/allele	Contol, n (%)	Fibromyalgia, n (%)	Exact p value[b]	OR (95% CI), p value[c]	OR (95% CI), p value, adjusted by age, sex[‡]
	A	442 (52.7)	445 (54.5)		1.075 (0.886–1.304), p = 0.466	1.058 (0.869–1.287), p = 0.575
rs7124442	C/C	2 (0.5)	0 (0)	0.574	1	1
	C/T	51 (12.1)	47 (11.5)		718,117.521 (0-Inf), p = 0.972	683,123.831 (0-Inf), p = 0.972
	T/T	368 (87.4)	360 (88.5)		762,294.038 (0-Inf), p = 0.971	682,163.974 (0-Inf), p = 0.972
	C	55 (6.5)	47 (5.8)	0.590	1	
	T	787 (93.5)	767 (94.2)		1.140 (0.763–1.705), p = 0.521	1.078 (0.716–1.623), p = 0.72

BDNF brain-derived neurotrophic factor

[a] Missing data were excluded from the analyses: *BDNF* rs2883187 (5 controls), *BDNF* rs7103873 (1 patient and 16 controls), *BDNF* rs7103411 (2 controls), *BDNF* rs10835210 (1 patient and 10 controls), *BDNF* rs11030104 (2 patients and 3 controls), *BDNF* rs12273539 (1 control), *BDNF* rs11030102 (1 patient and 1 control), *BDNF* rs11030101 (1 patient and 3 controls), *BDNF* rs6265 (4 controls and 1 patient), and *BDNF* rs7124442 (2 patients and 2 controls)

[b] Value was determined by Fisher's exact test or χ^2 test

[c] Logistic regression analyses were used to calculate the OR (95% CI; confidence interval)

Haplotype frequencies and clinical measurements

Among the 39 haplotype structures included in the haplotype analysis of *BDNF* SNPs, seven frequent haplotypes (TGACCGCTGC, TATCCAACCT, TGACCACTGC, TAACTACCCT, TATCCGACCT, TAACTGCCCT, and CAACCACCGC) had a frequency of > 1% in the patients and controls. Although not shown in Table 4, the total frequency of the other haplotype structures was 30 (3.8%) for patients and 46 (6%) for controls. These haplotypes showed significantly different distributions between the patients with FM and the controls (P = 0.0001; Table 4).

Among the frequent haplotypes, the TGACCACTGC haplotype was found less frequently in the patients with FM after adjusting for age and sex (OR 0.004, 95% CI 0.0–0.026, P < 0.001; Table 5). Interestingly, the TATCCGACCT and TAACTGCCCT haplotypes were not detected in patients with FM (Table 5) (both P > 0.05). In the clinical measures, only anxiety, assessed using the STAI-II score, was significantly different among the patients according to *BDNF* haplotype (Table 6).

Discussion

To our knowledge, we were the first to investigate the association between *BDNF* SNPs and FM. We found that the allele and genotype frequencies of *BDNF* rs11030104 were significantly different between the patients with FM and the controls. In comparison, although the allele and genotype frequencies of *BDNF* rs12273539 were not significantly different between the patients with FM and the controls, the TT genotype of *BDNF* rs12273539 was associated with susceptibility to FM. In addition to the individual SNPs, certain *BDNF* haplotypes may be protective against FM or contribute to its symptoms. Therefore, our data imply that *BDNF* gene polymorphisms contribute to the development and symptom severity of FM in the Korean population.

Neurotrophic factors are a family of closely related proteins involved in neuronal survival, growth, and differentiation during development of the nervous system [9]. Neurotrophins comprise four structurally related factors: BDNF, nerve growth factor (NGF), neurotrophin 3 (NT-3), and neurotrophin 4/5 (NT-4/5). Neurotrophins play important roles in the transmission of physiologic and pathologic pain [22]. In particular, BDNF plays key roles in chronic pain conditions. BDNF is synthesized in the DRG, and is transported to the central terminals of the primary afferents in the spinal dorsal horn, where it is involved in the modulation of painful stimuli [9]. BDNF contributes to central sensitization by modulating nociceptive inputs and enhancing hyperalgesia through NMDA-receptor-mediated responses [23]. For these reasons, researchers have been interested in the role of BDNF in chronic pain disorders, including FM [24]. In addition, BDNF plays a role in depressive disorder, which is frequently comorbid with FM; indeed, the serum level of BDNF is altered in patients with depression [25, 26]. Moreover, it can be normalized by antidepressants such as milnacipran [26], which are frequently used in the treatment of FM.

Several clinical studies have evaluated the role of BDNF in the pathogenesis of FM. Patients with FM have increased levels of BDNF in blood [12, 14] and cerebrospinal fluid [27] compared to healthy controls, implying that BDNF is involved in the pathophysiology of FM. In particular, Zanette et al. reported that serum BDNF levels are inversely associated with the pressure-pain threshold in patients with FM [13]. Furthermore, increased serum BDNF mediates the disinhibition of motor cortex excitability and the function of the descending inhibitory pain modulation system in patients with FM [28]. In fact, recent studies have shown that disruptions in default mode network (DMN) connectivity may be associated with impaired pain modulation, leading to the chronic pain seen in FM [29, 30]. Furthermore, certain *BDNF* polymorphisms have an effect on specific aspects of brain function such as DMN connectivity, which is currently considered to be central in the pathogenesis of FM [31]. These findings could be a potential explanation that

Table 3 Least-squares means (95% CI) of responses in patients with fibromyalgia, according to genotype

Position	Genotype	Number[a]	Tender point number	Tender point count	FIQ	BFI	PCS	MCS	BDI	STAI-I	STAI-II
rs2883187	C/C	100	13.38 (12.21–14.56)	25.17 (21.2–29.14)	58.56 (53.23–63.9)	7.25 (5.28–9.22)	38.02 (35.88–40.16)	31.25 (27.83–34.67)	18.09 (15.05–21.12)	51.56 (48.06–55.06)	51.97 (48.73–55.21)
	C/T	208	13.80 (12.83–14.77)	25.70 (22.43–28.96)	610 (56.69–65.32)	6.27 (4.66–7.89)	37.29 (35.56–39.03)	32.62 (29.85–35.39)	18.57 (16.11–21.02)	49.73 (46.9–52.56)	50.2 (47.59–52.81)
	T/T	101	13.77 (12.54–15.0)	25.85 (21.68–30.03)	58.21 (52.66–63.77)	7.16 (5.11–9.22)	38.17 (35.94–40.41)	34.26 (30.69–37.83)	16.89 (13.7–20.08)	49.49 (45.82–53.15)	48.29 (44.9–51.68)
p value[†]			0.739	0.947	0.449	0.466	0.625	0.299	0.54	0.478	0.138
rs7103873	G/G	98	13.37 (12.18–14.55)	25.01 (21.01–29.01)	57.96 (52.56–63.35)	7.34 (5.35–9.32)	37.96 (35.8–40.12)	31.39 (27.93–34.85)	17.78 (14.71–20.85)	51.52 (47.98–55.06)	51.9 (48.63–55.18)
	G/C	208	13.84 (12.88–14.81)	25.97 (22.73–29.21)	60.89 (56.60–65.19)	6.25 (4.65–7.85)	37.34 (35.62–39.07)	32.83 (30.07–35.6)	18.45 (16.01–20.9)	49.51 (46.7–52.32)	50.08 (47.48–52.68)
	C/C	102	13.66 (12.42–14.9)	25.28 (21.08–29.49)	59.04 (53.43–64.64)	7.26 (5.19–9.33)	38.07 (35.82–40.32)	33.52 (29.92–37.13)	17.4 (14.18–20.62)	50.33 (46.64–54.02)	48.72 (45.31–52.13)
p value[b]			0.69	0.857	0.479	0.389	0.721	0.523	0.755	0.484	0.224
rs7103411	C/C	128	13.79 (12.68–14.9)	25.97 (22.21–29.72)	60.26 (55.22–65.3)	6.97 (5.11–8.83)	37.76 (35.73–39.79)	32.88 (29.64–36.12)	18.25 (15.37–21.14)	50.48 (47.17–53.8)	49.28 (46.21–52.35)
	C/T	198	13.74 (12.74–14.74)	25.65 (22.27–29.02)	60.54 (56.09–64.99)	6.07 (4.41–7.73)	37.5 (35.71–39.29)	33.0 (30.14–35.87)	18.32 (15.78–20.85)	49.55 (46.62–52.47)	50.44 (47.74–53.15)
	T/T	83	13.46 (12.23–14.68)	25.0 (20.87–29.14)	57.81 (52.24–63.38)	7.64 (5.59–9.68)	37.79 (35.55–40.02)	31.41 (27.84–34.98)	17.5 (14.33–20.67)	50.89 (47.22–54.55)	51.09 (47.69–54.48)
p value[b]			0.859	0.907	0.582	0.249	0.947	0.635	0.86	0.705	0.578
rs10835210	C/C	196	13.49 (12.50–14.47)	25.67 (22.37–28.97)	59.70 (55.30–64.10)	6.91 (5.27–8.55)	37.78 (36.02–39.55)	31.77 (28.96–34.58)	18.87 (16.37–21.36)	51.04 (48.18–53.9)	51.77 (49.13–54.41)
	C/A	172	13.87 (12.84–14.91)	25.51 (22.04–28.99)	60.15 (55.46–64.85)	6.66 (4.93–8.4)	37.3 (35.41–39.18)	33.19 (30.18–36.2)	17.17 (14.5–19.83)	48.42 (45.35–51.48)	48.63 (45.81–51.45)
	A/A	40	13.96 (12.18–15.74)	24.85 (18.87–30.83)	59.67 (51.64–67.7)	5.46 (2.52–8.4)	38.45 (35.22–41.67)	35.31 (30.17–40.45)	17.78 (13.17–22.4)	51.79 (46.49–57.08)	47.51 (42.62–52.4)
p value[b]			0.675	0.962	0.977	0.609	0.728	0.301	0.384	0.138	0.029
rs11030104	A/A	126	13.80 (12.68–14.92)	25.99 (22.22–29.75)	60.27 (55.2–65.35)	7.0 (5.13–8.87)	37.82 (35.77–39.86)	32.86 (29.6–36.12)	18.33 (15.43–21.23)	50.46 (47.13–53.79)	49.29 (46.2–52.37)
	A/G	196	13.79 (12.79–14.8)	25.67 (22.3–29.03)	60.66 (56.19–65.13)	6.09 (4.42–7.76)	37.4 (35.60–39.20)	32.9 (30.02–35.77)	18.41 (15.87–20.95)	49.69 (46.76–52.61)	50.53 (47.82–53.24)
	G/G	85	13.31 (12.08–14.53)	24.75 (20.64–28.86)	57.55 (51.98–63.12)	7.58 (5.53–9.62)	37.86 (35.63–40.1)	31.6 (28.03–35.16)	17.31 (14.15–20.47)	50.63 (46.99–54.28)	50.88 (47.49–54.27)
p value[b]			0.677	0.845	0.498	0.274	0.871	0.731	0.757	0.821	0.616
rs12273539	C/C	268	13.63 (12.7–14.55)	25.24 (22.11–28.37)	5903 (54.81–63.25)	6.51 (4.95–8.07)	37.67 (35.98–39.37)	33.14 (30.42–35.86)	17.45 (15.05–19.85)	49.9 (47.14–52.66)	49.52 (46.96–52.09)
	C/T	125	14.13 (13.01–15.24)	27.04 (23.26–30.81)	62.11 (57.15–67.08)	6.75 (4.89–8.61)	37.48 (35.48–39.47)	31.56 (28.36–34.76)	19.34 (16.5–22.18)	50.66 (47.4–53.92)	51.73 (48.7–54.75)
	T/T	17	11.90 (9.7–14.1)	21.96 (14.52–29.41)	57.64 (47.31–67.96)	8.92 (5.15–12.69)	38.13 (33.98–42.27)	31.82 (25.17–38.48)	20.22 (14.35–26.09)	49.54 (42.8–56.29)	50.87 (44.61–57.14)
p value[b]			0.131	0.319	0.349	0.432	0.945	0.533	0.26	0.862	0.271
rs11030102	C/C	402	13.67 (12.8–14.55)	25.57 (22.61–28.53)	59.83 (55.89–63.77)	6.62 (5.17–8.07)	37.66 (36.07–39.25)	32.67 (30.14–35.21)	18.06 (15.83–20.29)	50.02 (47.45–52.59)	50.16 (47.78–52.55)
	C/G	6	17.58 (13.01–22.15)	36.13 (20.73–51.54)	72.91 (51.53–94.29)	19.07 (11.35–26.79)	35.01 (26.4–43.63)	23.8 (10.04–37.56)	29.58 (17.47–41.69)	65.06 (51.13–78.99)	62.56 (49.62–75.51)
p value[b]			0.089	0.172	0.224	0.001	0.542	0.2	0.059	0.032	0.057
rs11030101	A/A	197	13.49 (12.51–14.47)	25.69 (22.38–29.01)	59.82 (55.43–64.22)	6.91 (5.27–8.55)	37.79 (36.02–39.55)	31.73 (28.92–34.54)	18.94 (16.45–21.43)	51.01 (48.15–53.87)	51.77 (49.13–54.42)
	A/T	172	13.84 (12.81–14.87)	25.38 (21.9–28.87)	60.26 (55.57–64.95)	6.69 (4.95–8.43)	37.34 (35.45–39.22)	33.14 (30.14–36.15)	17.1 (14.43–19.76)	48.41 (45.34–51.48)	48.57 (45.75–51.4)
	T/T	39	14.23 (12.45–16.01)	26.37 (20.36–32.37)	58.75 (50.73–66.77)	5.33 (2.39–8.27)	38.16 (34.93–41.39)	35.94 (30.8–41.08)	17.66 (13.12–22.21)	52.15 (46.94–57.37)	48.07 (43.25–52.89)
p value[b]			0.605	0.943	0.929	0.555	0.816	0.212	0.325	0.126	0.033
rs6265	G/G	87	13.29 (12.07–14.51)	24.66 (20.55–28.78)	57.67 (52.14–63.21)	7.55 (5.52–9.59)	37.83 (35.61–40.06)	31.56 (28.01–35.11)	17.44 (14.29–20.59)	50.62 (46.97–54.26)	50.94 (47.56–54.32)

Table 3 Least-squares means (95% CI) of responses in patients with fibromyalgia, according to genotype (Continued)

Position	Genotype	Number[a]	Tender point number	Tender point count	FIQ	BFI	PCS	MCS	BDI	STAI-I	STAI-II
	G/A	197	13.77 (12.77–14.77)	25.62 (22.26–28.99)	60.72 (56.27–65.18)	6.11 (4.44–7.77)	37.45 (35.65–39.24)	32.92 (30.05–35.79)	18.27 (15.74–20.81)	49.6 (46.67–52.52)	50.43 (47.71–53.14)
	A/A	124	13.88 (12.76–15)	26.34 (22.56–30.13)	60.17 (55.09–65.24)	6.98 (5.11–8.86)	37.83 (35.79–39.88)	32.91 (29.64–36.18)	18.37 (15.47–21.28)	50.58 (47.24–53.91)	49.37 (46.28–52.46)
p value[b]			0.634	0.746	0.513	0.293	0.898	0.702	0.829	0.766	0.657
rs7124442	C/T	47	13.57 (12.12–15.03)	26.18 (21.3–31.07)	62.15 (55.49–68.81)	5.60 (3.16–8.05)	37.37 (34.69–40.05)	30.74 (26.46–35.03)	19.98 (16.2–23.76)	50.67 (46.27–55.07)	51.35 (47.3–55.39)
	T/T	360	13.72 (12.81–14.62)	25.53 (22.48–28.57)	59.53 (55.49–63.57)	6.88 (5.37–8.39)	37.69 (36.06–39.32)	32.94 (30.34–35.54)	17.81 (15.51–20.1)	50.01 (47.36–52.66)	50.04 (47.58–52.5)
p value[b]			0.836	0.777	0.411	0.274	0.804	0.285	0.23	0.755	0.501

Abbreviations: CI confidence interval, *FIQ* Fibromyalgia Impact Questionnaire, *BFI* Brief Fatigue Inventory, *PCS* Physical Component Summary, *MCS* Mental Component Summary, *BDI* Beck Depression Inventory, *STAI-I* State-Trait Anxiety Inventory-I, *STAI-II* State-Trait Anxiety Inventory-II
[a]Missing data were excluded from the analyses: *BDNF* rs2883187 (5 controls), *BDNF* rs7103411 (2 controls), *BDNF* rs10835210 (1 patient and 10 controls), *BDNF* rs11030104 (2 patients and 3 controls), *BDNF* rs12273539 (1 control), *BDNF* rs11030102 (1 patient and 1 control), *BDNF* rs11030101 (1 patient and 3 controls), *BDNF* rs6265 (4 controls and 1 patient), and *BDNF* rs7124442 (2 patients and 2 controls)
[b]*p* values derived by analysis of covariance adjusted for age and sex

Table 4 Estimates of haplotype frequencies in patients with fibromyalgia ($n = 393$) and healthy controls ($n = 388$)[a]

Combined alleles[a]	All subjects	Controls	Fibromyalgia	p value[b]
TGACCGCTGC	29.6 ± 0.75	20.22 ± 0.9	38.87 ± 0.88	0.0001
TATCCAACCT	20.16 ± 0.44	12.94 ± 0.57	27.29 ± 0.52	
TGACCACTGC	14.8 ± 0.75	25.26 ± 0.89	4.47 ± 0.88	
TAACTACCCT	11.97 ± 0.42	6.99 ± 0.5	16.89 ± 0.53	
TATCCGACCT	8.94 ± 0.45	15.76 ± 0.59	2.21 ± 0.52	
TAACTGCCCT	5.74 ± 0.42	9.8 ± 0.5	1.72 ± 0.53	
CAACCACCGC	3.20 ± 0.17	2.06 ± 0.22	4.33 ± 0.24	

[a]Data are percentages ± SE
[a]Missing data were excluded ($n = 51$). Among 39 haplotype structures, 7 haplotypes with frequency of at least 1% in both the patients and controls are presented
[b]p values for permutation test of the null hypothesis that cases and controls are random draws from a common set of haplotype frequencies (number of permutations = 10,000)

supports the existence of a mechanistic link between *BDNF* polymorphisms and FM. However, although multiple lines of evidence imply a role for BDNF in the pathogenesis of FM, *BDNF* polymorphisms in these patients have not been investigated extensively.

In this study, we found that certain *BDNF* SNPs are associated with susceptibility to FM. The GG genotype and the G allele of *BDNF* rs11030104 exert a protective effect against FM. In contrast, although the allele and genotype frequencies of *BDNF* rs12273539 did not differ between the patients with FM and controls, the TT genotype of *BDNF* rs12273539 was associated with susceptibility to FM. To date, only one study has evaluated associations between *BDNF* gene polymorphisms and FM. Xiao et al. [32] evaluated whether the *BDNF* Val66Met polymorphism was associated with FM; their results implied that the *BDNF* Val66 Met SNP is associated with a subgroup of patients with FM with high-sensitivity C-reactive protein and high body mass index. Nevertheless, the relative distribution of the *BDNF* Val66Met SNP did not differ between the patients with FM and healthy controls. Similarly, in our study, *BDNF* Val66Val Met was not associated

with susceptibility to FM. However, our data demonstrate that other *BDNF* SNPs, such as rs11030104 and rs12273539, were associated with the risk of FM in a Korean population.

Furthermore, our data imply that certain *BDNF* haplotypes exert a protective effect against FM. A haplotype refers to a particular set of closely linked alleles that are inherited as a unit, and haplotype analysis can reveal the pattern of genetic variation associated with certain diseases [33]. Several haplotypes of certain genes are reportedly significantly associated with FM. Diatchenko et al. [34] reported that the ACCG haplotype, which consists of four SNPs (rs6269, rs4633, rs4818, and rs4680) of the catechol-O-methyltransferase (*COMT*) gene, is associated with both FM susceptibility and symptom severity [35, 36]. Similarly, we also suggested that a particular haplotype of *TRPV2* may be associated with susceptibility to FM [37]. In the current study, our findings imply that *BDNF* haplotypes may be involved in the pathophysiology of FM.

Notably, we failed to uncover a direct association between *BDNF* gene polymorphisms and pain-related symptom scales such as the tender point number and count. However, those polymorphisms were related to certain psychological symptoms in patients with FM. In particular, certain *BDNF* SNPs and haplotypes were associated with anxiety symptoms. Since patients with FM have a significantly higher prevalence of anxiety disorders (13–63.8%) [38], our findings imply that *BDNF* gene polymorphisms may indirectly affect FM through their effect on anxiety. However, diverse factors affect the development of FM, including psychological symptoms such as anxiety, so our results should be interpreted carefully.

This study had several limitations. First, it was of a case-control design. Because the purpose of this study was to evaluate the role of *BDNF* SNPs associated with susceptibility to FM, we adopted a target-gene-based approach. Therefore, like the majority of SNP studies, we selected candidate SNPs for a case-control analysis of their association with FM. Second, the multiple tests

Table 5 Combined allele frequencies and odds ratios in patients with fibromyalgia and healthy controls[a]

Combined alleles	Controls, n (%)	Fibromyalgia, n (%)	Crude OR (95% CI)	p value[b]	Age and sex adjusted OR (95% CI)	p value[b]
TGACCGCTGC	193 (26.6)	340 (45)	1.0 (reference)		1.0 (reference)	
TATCCAACCT	119 (16.4)	232 (30.7)	1.107 (0.834–1.469)	0.483	1.106 (0.833–1.47)	0.487
TGACCACTGC	160 (22)	1 (0.1)	0.004 (0–0.026)	< 0.001	0.004 (0.0–0.026)	< 0.001
TAACTACCCT	66 (9.1)	146 (19.3)	1.256 (0.894–1.765)	0.19	1.248 (0.887–1.756)	0.204
TATCCGACCT	103 (14.2)	0 (0)	0 (0-Inf)	0.963	0 (0-Inf)	0.963
TAACTGCCCT	65 (9)	0 (0)	0 (0-Inf)	0.971	0 (0-Inf)	0.97
CAACCACCGC	20 (2.8)	37 (4.9)	1.05 (0.593–1.861)	0.867	1.088 (0.612–1.934)	0.774

Abbreviations: OR odds ratio, CI confidence interval
[a]Missing data were excluded ($n = 51$). Among 39 haplotype structures, 7 haplotypes with a frequency of at least 1% in both the patients and controls are presented; the total frequency of the other haplotype structures was 46 (6%) for controls and 30 (3.8%) for patients. Logistic regression models were used to calculate ORs
[b]Computed for the estimated coefficient of each haplotype in the logistic regression

Table 6 Numbers of haplotypes and least-squares means (95% CI) of responses in patients with fibromyalgia

Combined alleles	Number[a]	Tender point number	Tender point count	FIQ	BFI	PCS	MCS	BDI	STAI-I	STAI-II
TGACCGCTGC	340	13.61 (12.89–14.33)	25.33 (22.93–27.73)	59.67 (56.48–62.87)	6.81 (5.6–8.01)	37.56 (36.25–38.87)	32.12 (30.06–34.18)	18.02 (16.22–19.83)	50.66 (48.56–52.76)	51.01 (49.07–52.95)
TATCCAACCT	232	13.91 (13.1–14.72)	25.29 (22.6–27.99)	59.88 (56.26–63.5)	6.35 (4.99–7.71)	37.49 (36–38.98)	33.88 (31.54–36.21)	17.25 (15.21–19.3)	49.31 (46.92–51.69)	48.26 (46.07–50.46)
TAACTACCCT	146	13.66 (12.75–14.58)	26.34 (23.29–29.38)	61.2 (57.17–65.23)	7.32 (5.8–8.85)	37.49 (35.84–39.15)	31.73 (29.13–34.33)	19.5 (17.21–21.78)	50.49 (47.83–53.14)	51.16 (48.71–53.6)
CAACCACCGC	37	13.53 (12.02–15.05)	25.96 (20.93–31)	63.17 (56.22–70.11)	5.67 (3.09–8.25)	37.78 (34.92–40.63)	30.7 (26.22–35.18)	20.06 (16.15–23.97)	52.65 (48.1–57.2)	52.74 (48.54–56.93)
p value[b]		0.874	0.902	0.696	0.527	0.998	0.271	0.221	0.459	0.027

Abbreviations: CI confidence interval, *FIQ* Fibromyalgia Impact Questionnaire, *BFI* Brief Fatigue Inventory, *PCS* Physical Component Summary, *MCS* Mental Component Summary, *BDI* Beck Depression Inventory, *STAI-I* State-Trait Anxiety Inventory-I, *STAI-II* State-Trait Anxiety Inventory-II
[a]Missing data were excluded from the analyses
[b]*p* values derived by analysis of covariance adjusted for age and sex

performed in this study may have increased the type I error. In genetics, controlling for multiple testing is important in estimating thresholds of significance accurately, particularly in genome-wide association studies (GWAS) [39]. However, in this target-gene-based SNP study, we did not consider the potential effects of multiple testing in the analyses. In fact, most published FM SNP case-control studies have not considered the potential effects of multiple testing. Third, we were unable to prospectively evaluate the associations between *BDNF* genetic variation and clinical outcomes. Therefore, further studies are needed to investigate the effect of those genetic polymorphisms on the long-term clinical outcomes of patients with FM. Finally, to overcome the insufficient statistical power, we conducted a large-scale study involving > 800 samples. However, our findings should be replicated in a larger population comprising multiple ethnicities.

Conclusions

In this study, we evaluated the association between *BDNF* polymorphisms and FM in a large sample of the Korean population. We found that *BDNF* gene polymorphisms influenced susceptibility to FM, and contributed to the severity of certain symptoms of FM. Further evidence from large prospective studies is needed to determine the generalizability of our findings to the broader population and their impact on the clinical outcomes of FM. Moreover, further work is needed to elucidate the biologic and epigenetic mechanisms underlying the complex role of the *BDNF* gene in FM.

Abbreviations

BDI: Beck Depression Inventory; BDNF: Brain-derived neurotrophic factor; BFI: Brief Fatigue Inventory; CI: Confidence interval; DRG: Dorsal root ganglion; FIQ: Fibromyalgia Impact Questionnaire; FM: Fibromyalgia; ICF: Informed consent form; MCS: Mental Component Summary; NMDA: N-methyl-D-aspartate; NSAIDs: Nonsteroidal anti-inflammatory drugs; PCS: Physical Component Summary; SF-36: 36-Item Medical Outcomes Study Short-Form Health Survey; SNP: Single-nucleotide polymorphism; SNRI: Serotonin-norepinephrine reuptake inhibitors; SSRI: Selective serotonin reuptake inhibitor; STAI-I: State-Trait Anxiety Inventory-I; STAI-II: State-Trait Anxiety Inventory-II; TCA: Tricyclic antidepressant

Acknowledgements
We would like to thank the patients and their families for participating in this study.

Funding
This study was supported by the Bio & Medical Technology Development Program of the NRF funded by the Korean government, MSIP (2017M3A9E8023014), and by a grant (CRI16015–1) from Chonnam National University Hospital Biomedical Research Institute.

Authors' contributions
D-J P and S-SL conceived and designed the study. S-HK, S-SN, JHL, S-KK, Y-AL, S-JH, H-SK, H-SL, HAK, C-IJ, and S-HK acquired data. D-J P and S-SL performed statistical analysis and drafted the manuscript. All authors critically revised the manuscript for important intellectual content. All authors read and approved the final manuscript.

Consent for publication
Not applicable.

Competing interests
The authors declare that they have no competing interests.

Author details
[1]Division of Rheumatology, Department of Internal Medicine, Chonnam National University Medical School and Hospital, 42 Jebong-ro, Dong-gu, Gwangju 61469, Republic of Korea. [2]Department of Internal Medicine, Inje University Haeundae Paik Hospital, Busan, Korea. [3]Department of Internal Medicine, Soonchunhyang University, College of Medicine, Cheonan, Korea. [4]Department of Internal Medicine, Maryknoll Medical Center, Busan, Korea. [5]Department of Internal Medicine, Catholic University of Daegu, School of Medicine, Daegu, Korea. [6]Department of Internal Medicine, School of Medicine, Kyung Hee University, Seoul, Korea. [7]Department of Internal Medicine, Soonchunhyang University Seoul Hospital, Seoul, Korea. [8]Hanyang University College of Medicine and the Hospital for Rheumatic Diseases, Seoul, Korea. [9]Department of Allergy and Rheumatology, Ajou University Hospital, Ajou University School of Medicine, Suwon, Korea. [10]Department of Internal Medicine, Konyang University Medical School, Daejeon, Korea. [11]Departments of Internal Medicine, School of Medicine, Keimyung University, Daegu, Korea.

References

1. Wolfe F, Smythe HA, Yunus MB, Bennett RM, Bombardier C, Goldenberg DL, et al. The American College of Rheumatology 1990 Criteria for the classification of fibromyalgia. report of the Multicenter Criteria Committee. Arthritis Rheum. 1990;33(2):160–72.
2. Jones GT, Atzeni F, Beasley M, Fluss E, Sarzi-Puttini P, Macfarlane GJ. The prevalence of fibromyalgia in the general population: a comparison of the American College of Rheumatology 1990, 2010, and modified 2010 classification criteria. Arthritis Rheumatol. 2015;67(2):568–75.
3. Maletic V, Raison CL. Neurobiology of depression, fibromyalgia and neuropathic pain. Front Biosci (Landmark Ed). 2009;14:5291–338.
4. Ablin JN, Buskila D. Update on the genetics of the fibromyalgia syndrome. Best Pract Res Clin Rheumatol. 2015;29(1):20–8.
5. Park DJ, Lee SS. New insights into the genetics of fibromyalgia. Korean J Intern Med. 2017;32(6):984–95.
6. Buskila D, Sarzi-Puttini P, Ablin JN. The genetics of fibromyalgia syndrome. Pharmacogenomics. 2007;8(1):67–74.
7. Park DJ, Kim SH, Nah SS, Lee JH, Kim SK, Lee YA, et al. Association between catechol-O-methyl transferase gene polymorphisms and fibromyalgia in a Korean population: a case-control study. Eur J Pain. 2016;20(7):1131–9.
8. Wu YJ, Kruttgen A, Moller JC, Shine D, Chan JR, Shooter EM, et al. Nerve growth factor, brain-derived neurotrophic factor, and neurotrophin-3 are sorted to dense-core vesicles and released via the regulated pathway in primary rat cortical neurons. J Neurosci Res. 2004;75(6):825–34.
9. Obata K, Noguchi K. BDNF in sensory neurons and chronic pain. Neurosci Res. 2006;55(1):1–10.
10. Wu K, Len GW, McAuliffe G, Ma C, Tai JP, Xu F, et al. Brain-derived neurotrophic factor acutely enhances tyrosine phosphorylation of the AMPA receptor subunit GluR1 via NMDA receptor-dependent mechanisms. Brain Res Mol Brain Res. 2004;130(1–2):178–86.
11. Yajima Y, Narita M, Usui A, Kaneko C, Miyatake M, Yamaguchi T, et al. Direct evidence for the involvement of brain-derived neurotrophic factor in the development of a neuropathic pain-like state in mice. J Neurochem. 2005; 93(3):584–94.
12. Laske C, Stransky E, Eschweiler GW, Klein R, Wittorf A, Leyhe T, et al. Increased BDNF serum concentration in fibromyalgia with or without depression or antidepressants. J Psychiatr Res. 2007;41(7):600–5.
13. Zanette SA, Dussan-Sarria JA, Souza A, Deitos A, Torres ILS, Caumo W. Higher serum S100B and BDNF levels are correlated with a lower pressure-pain threshold in fibromyalgia. Mol Pain. 2014;10:46.

14. Haas L, Portela LV, Bohmer AE, Oses JP, Lara DR. Increased plasma levels of brain derived neurotrophic factor (BDNF) in patients with fibromyalgia. Neurochem Res. 2010;35(5):830–4.

15. Kim SK, Kim SH, Nah SS, Lee JH, Hong SJ, Kim HS, et al. Association of guanosine triphosphate cyclohydrolase 1 gene polymorphisms with fibromyalgia syndrome in a Korean population. J Rheumatol. 2013;40(3):316–22.

16. Okifuji A, Turk DC, Sinclair JD, Starz TW, Marcus DA. A standardized manual tender point survey. I. Development and determination of a threshold point for the identification of positive tender points in fibromyalgia syndrome. J Rheumatol. 1997;24(2):377–83.

17. Kim YA, Lee SS, Park K. Validation of a Korean version of the Fibromyalgia Impact Questionnaire. J Korean Med Sci. 2002;17(2):220–4.

18. Mendoza TR, Wang XS, Cleeland CS, Morrissey H, Johnson BA, Wendt JK, et al. The rapid assessment of fatigue severity in cancer patients - use of the brief fatigue inventory. Cancer. 1999;85(5):1186–96.

19. Richter P, Werner J, Heerlein A, Kraus A, Sauer H. On the validity of the Beck Depression Inventory. Rev Psychopathol. 1998;31(3):160–8.

20. Ware JE Jr, Sherbourne CD. The MOS 36-item short-form health survey (SF-36). I Conceptual framework and item selection. Med Care. 1992;30(6):473–83.

21. Kim JT, Shin DK. A study based on the standardization of the STAI for Korea. New Med J. 1978;21(11):69–75.

22. Malik-Hall M, Dina OA, Levine JD. Primary afferent nociceptor mechanisms mediating NGF-induced mechanical hyperalgesia. Eur J Neurosci. 2005;21(12):3387–94.

23. Kerr BJ, Bradbury EJ, Bennett DLH, Trivedi PM, Dassan P, French J, et al. Brain-derived neurotrophic factor modulates nociceptive sensory inputs and NMDA-evoked responses in the rat spinal cord. J Neurosci. 1999;19(12):5138–48.

24. Siniscalco D, Giordano C, Rossi F, Maione S, de Novellis V. Role of neurotrophins in neuropathic pain. Curr Neuropharmacol. 2011;9(4):523–9.

25. Karege F, Perret G, Bondolfi G, Schwald M, Bertschy G, Aubry JM. Decreased serum brain-derived neurotrophic factor levels in major depressed patients. Psychiatry Res. 2002;109(2):143–8.

26. Yoshimura R, Mitoma M, Sugita A, Hori H, Okamoto T, Umene W, et al. Effects of paroxetine or milnacipran on serum brain-derived neurotrophic factor in depressed patients. Prog Neuro-Psychopharmacol Biol Psychiatry. 2007;31(5):1034–7.

27. Sarchielli P, Mancini ML, Floridi A, Coppola F, Rossi C, Nardi K, et al. Increased levels of neurotrophins are not specific for chronic migraine: evidence from primary fibromyalgia syndrome. J Pain. 2007;8(9):737–45.

28. Caumo W, Deitos A, Carvalho S, Leite J, Carvalho F, Dussan-Sarria JA, et al. Motor cortex excitability and BDNF levels in chronic musculoskeletal pain according to structural pathology. Front Hum Neurosci. 2016;10:357.

29. Fallon N, Chiu Y, Nurmikko T, Stancak A. Functional connectivity with the default mode network is altered in fibromyalgia patients. PLoS One. 2016;11(7):e0159198.

30. Hsiao FJ, Wang SJ, Lin YY, Fuh JL, Ko YC, Wang PN, et al. Altered insula-default mode network connectivity in fibromyalgia: a resting-state magnetoencephalographic study. J Headache Pain. 2017;18(1):89.

31. Jang JH, Yun JY, Jung WH, Shim G, Byun MS, Hwang JY, et al. The impact of genetic variation in comt and bdnf on resting-state functional connectivity. Int J Imaging Syst Technol. 2012;22(1):97–102.

32. Xiao Y, Russell IJ, Liu YG. A brain-derived neurotrophic factor polymorphism Val66Met identifies fibromyalgia syndrome subgroup with higher body mass index and C-reactive protein. Rheumatol Int. 2012;32(8):2479–85.

33. International HapMap C. A haplotype map of the human genome. Nature. 2005;437(7063):1299–320.

34. Diatchenko L, Nackley AG, Slade GD, Bhalang K, Belfer I, Max MB, et al. Catechol-O-methyltransferase gene polymorphisms are associated with multiple pain-evoking stimuli. Pain. 2006;125(3):216–24.

35. Martinez-Jauand M, Sitges C, Rodriguez V, Picornell A, Ramon M, Buskila D, et al. Pain sensitivity in fibromyalgia is associated with catechol-O-methyltransferase (COMT) gene. Eur J Pain. 2013;17(1):16–27.

36. Vargas-Alarcon G, Fragoso JM, Cruz-Robles D, Vargas A, Lao-Villadoniga JI, Garcia-Fructuoso F, et al. Catechol-O-methyltransferase gene haplotypes in Mexican and Spanish patients with fibromyalgia. Arthritis Res Ther. 2007;9(5):R110.

37. Park DJ, Kim SH, Nah SS, Lee JH, Kim SK, Lee YA, et al. Polymorphisms of the TRPV2 and TRPV3 genes associated with fibromyalgia in a Korean population. Rheumatology (Oxford). 2016;55(8):1518–27.

38. Arnold LM, Hudson JI, Keck PE, Auchenbach MB, Javaras KN, Hess EV. Comorbidity of fibromyalgia and psychiatric disorders. J Clin Psychiatry. 2006;67(8):1219–25.

39. Clarke GM, Anderson CA, Pettersson FH, Cardon LR, Morris AP, Zondervan KT. Basic statistical analysis in genetic case-control studies. Nat Protoc. 2011;6(2):121–33.

5

Low bone mineral density predicts the formation of new syndesmophytes in patients with axial spondyloarthritis

Hyoung Rae Kim[1], Yeon Sik Hong[1,2], Sung-Hwan Park[1], Ji Hyeon Ju[1] and Kwi Young Kang[1,2]*

Abstract

Background: This study aimed to investigate whether the presence of low bone mineral density (BMD) in patients with axial spondyloarthritis (axSpA) predicts formation of new syndesmophytes over 2 years.

Methods: One hundred and nineteen patients fulfilling the imaging arm of the Assessment of SpondyloArthritis International Society axSpA criteria were enrolled. All patients were under 50 years of age. The modified Stoke Ankylosing Spondylitis Spinal Score (mSASSS) was assessed by two trained readers blinded to the patients' data. BMD (lumbar spine, femoral neck or total hip) at baseline was assessed using dual-energy absorptiometry. Low BMD was defined as Z score ≤ -2.0. Spinal radiographic progression was defined as worsening of the mSASSS by ≥ 2 points over 2 years. Logistic regression analyses were performed to identify predictors associated with development of new syndesmophytes and spinal radiographic progression.

Results: At baseline, 19 (16%) patients had low BMD. New syndesmophytes had developed in 22 (21%) patients at 2-year follow-up. New syndesmophyte formation after 2 years occurred more in patients with low BMD than in those with normal BMD ($p = 0.047$). In the multivariable analysis, current smoking, existing syndesmophytes and low BMD at baseline were associated with spinal radiographic progression (OR (95% CI) 3.0 (1.1, 7.7), 4.6 (1.8, 11.8) and 3.6 (1.2, 11.2), respectively). The presence of syndesmophytes at baseline and low BMD were predictors of new syndesmophytes over the following 2 years (OR (95% CI) 5.5 (2.0, 15.2) and 3.6 (1.1, 11.8), respectively).

Conclusions: Low BMD and existing syndesmophytes at baseline were independently associated with the development of new syndesmophytes in young axSpA patients.

Keywords: Axial spondyloarthritis, Ankylosing spondylitis, Bone mineral density, Syndesmophyte

Background

Axial spondyloarthritis (axSpA) is a chronic inflammatory disease that predominantly affects the sacroiliac joints and the spine. axSpA includes the subtypes ankylosing spondylitis (AS) and non-radiographic axSpA (nr-axSpA). These separate entities are discriminated by the structural damage to the sacroiliac joints visible on conventional X-ray images [1].

For most patients with SpA, the burden of disease results from a combination of inflammation and structural bone damage [2]. Radiographic damage in the spine presents as syndesmophyte formation leading to bridging of the intervertebral spaces. Structural damage not only affects patients by causing disability and permanent loss of function, but also has secondary effects, with ankylosis changing the balance of loads and forces on the skeletal system, leading to muscle stiffness and accelerated degenerative spine disease [3]. As structural damage contributes to impairment of spinal mobility and function, the retardation of spinal radiographic progression should be an important treatment goal [4].

Spinal progression varies widely among axSpA patients, and previous studies examined predictors influencing the heterogeneous formation of syndesmophytes within these patients. The strongest predictor of radiographic spinal

* Correspondence: kykang@catholic.ac.kr
[1]Division of Rheumatology, Department of Internal Medicine, College of Medicine, The Catholic University of Korea, Seoul, South Korea
[2]Division of Rheumatology, Department of Internal Medicine, Incheon St. Mary's Hospital, College of Medicine, The Catholic University of Korea, #56, Dongsu-Ro, Bupyung-Gu, Incheon, South Korea

progression is the presence of syndesmophytes at baseline [5, 6]. Furthermore, increased levels of acute phase reactants and smoking are independent predictors of radiographic spinal progression in early axSpA patients [6].

In a recent study, persisting high disease activity according to the Ankylosing Spondylitis Disease Activity Score (ASDAS) was found to be associated with accelerated radiographic spinal progression in early axSpA patients [7]. This advocates the early use of anti-inflammatory treatment in patients with early and active disease, in the hope that decreasing the disease activity will also slow down the radiographic progression. Identification of the predictors of spinal progression at baseline is important for clinical decision-making on aggressive anti-inflammatory treatment.

Chronic inflammation of the spine leads not only to new bone formation in axial joints and vertebral spaces, but also to bone resorption leading to osteoporosis, which is increased in axSpA [8]. It has been established that the generalised bone loss may be due to systemic inflammation and disease activity [9], and as disease activity in AS contributes to the rate of bone loss, osteoporosis is considered to be a manifestation of the disease itself, rather than a comorbidity [10].

Low bone mass in axSpA is a result of increased bone resorption through differentiation and activation of osteoclasts caused by inflammation. Therefore, bone mass changes reflect the severity of persistent inflammation, rather than a time-specific inflammatory state. Trabecular bone loss has been clearly and repeatedly demonstrated in the spines of patients with axSpA [11]. In a recent study, trabecular bone microarchitecture was found to be associated with spinal structural damage, as well as systemic inflammatory markers [12]. Furthermore, inflammation on spinal MRI is related to low bone mass in patients with nr-axSpA [13]. These studies show the site-specific relationship between low bone mass and inflammation in the spine. Earlier studies also reported the association between low bone mass in AS and spinal structural damage [14–16]; however, despite the identification of this relationship, it is not yet known whether the presence of low bone mass can independently predict radiographic spinal progression in axSpA patients.

The aims of the present study were therefore to evaluate the association between low bone mass and the formation of new syndesmophytes, and to investigate whether low bone mass independently predicts radiographic progression in axSpA patients.

Methods

Study population

Between August 2013 and December 2015, consecutive axSpA patients from Incheon Saint Mary's Hospital (Incheon, Korea) were recruited to this study. All enrolled patients fulfilled the imaging arm of the Assessment of SpondyloArthritis International Society (ASAS) axSpA criteria [17]. To exclude the effects of age, patients aged 50 years or older were excluded. Further exclusion criteria included patients with thyroid or parathyroid disorders, the presence of chronic renal or liver disease, cancer, coeliac disease or concurrent rheumatoid arthritis and the use of corticosteroids.

Bone mineral density (BMD) using dual-energy absorptiometry (DXA) and lateral radiographs of the cervical and lumbar spine were assessed at the time of enrolment, and demographic data were collected at the time of BMD assessment. All participants provided written informed consent according to the Declaration of Helsinki, and the study was approved by the ethics committee at Incheon Saint Mary's Hospital (study number OC16OISI0138).

Clinical data

Disease-related data and disease activity scores were collected at baseline. Clinical data included the time after symptom onset, the presence of HLA B27, family history and peripheral arthritis. A 44-joint count has been proposed to measure peripheral joint involvement, with this including the sternoclavicular joints, acromioclavicular joints, shoulders, elbows, wrists, knees and ankles, and the MCP, MTP and PIP joints of the hands [18]. Measures of disease activity were collected using the Bath Ankylosing Spondylitis Disease Activity Index (BASDAI) [19]. The ASDAS was calculated as described in a previous study [20]. The Bath Ankylosing Spondylitis Functional Index (BASFI) [21] was also recorded, and the erythrocyte sedimentation rate (ESR) and C-reactive protein (CRP) were measured. The use of medications such as non-steroidal anti-inflammatory drugs (NSAIDs), sulfasalazine, tumour necrosis factor (TNF) inhibitors, calcium, bisphosphonate and vitamin D was recorded, with patients who had taken treatment agents for periods of 1 year or longer being considered sustained users.

Radiographic scoring

For all patients, conventional radiographs of the spine were obtained at baseline and at 2-year follow-up. Lateral views of the cervical and lumbar spine were scored according to the modified Stoke Ankylosing Spondylitis Spinal Score (mSASSS) [22]. The mSASSS was scored by two trained experts who were blinded to the patients' demographic and clinical data and orders. In the mSASSS, a lateral view of the anterior parts of the cervical and lumbar spine is scored for squaring and/or erosion and/or sclerosis (1 point), syndesmophytes (2 points) and bridging syndesmophytes (3 points). As determination of cervical spine squaring may be unreliable, this element was not scored on the radiographs [23]. The total scores ranged from 0 to 72. Significant 'spinal radiographic progression' was defined as an increase in the mSASSS of ≥ 2 units over 2 years [7]. In the present analysis, the formation of new syndesmophytes at individual vertebral levels was of interest. Therefore, a 'new syndesmophyte' was defined as the formation of a syndesmophyte (mSASSS 2 points) or a bridge (mSASSS 3 points) at a vertebral level that was previously uninvolved or with only signs of squaring, erosion or sclerosis at baseline (mSASSS 0 or 1 point).

Two investigators independently scored the baseline and 2-year follow-up radiographs for each patient. To quantify the reliability of the radiographic scoring, the intraclass correlation coefficients (ICCs) for status scores (one time point) and change scores were calculated. There were few discrepancies between the two independent trained readers, but when they did occur the two investigators reached a consensus.

BMD assessment

BMD of the lumbar spine and left hip was assessed using DXA (Lunar Prodigy densitometer, Madison, WI, USA) at the baseline enrolment. All measurements were taken by experienced operators using the same machine and standardised procedures for participant positioning. BMD was measured at the lumbar spine using an anteroposterior projection at L1–L4, and at the left hip from the femoral neck and total proximal femur, and was expressed as the number of grams of bone mineral per square centimetre (g/cm^2) and calculated as Z scores using the manufacturer's reference. For patients under 50 years of age, a Z score ≤ -2.0 standard deviations (SDs) relative to the age-matched mean is considered to be below the expected range [24]; therefore, low BMD was defined as Z score ≤ -2.0.

Statistical analysis

Continuous data are expressed as the mean $\pm$ SD, and categorical data are expressed as percentages. Clinical variables were compared using independent t tests, and the chi-squared test was used to compare categorical variables between axSpA patients with and without a new syndesmophyte. The numbers of syndesmophytes at baseline and 2-year follow-up were compared using a paired t test.

Between-reader agreement in the determination of numbers of syndesmophytes at baseline and 2-year follow-up was estimated by the ICC. Agreement between the two readers regarding the presence of syndesmophytes was very good both at baseline (ICC 0.967 (95% CI 0.953–0.977)) and at 2 years (ICC 0.970 (95% CI 0.957–0.979)). Agreement over the change in the number of syndesmophytes was also good (ICC 0.739 (95% CI 0.625–0.818)).

Univariable and multivariable logistic regression analyses were used to identify predictors associated with the formation of new syndesmophytes and spinal radiographic progression over the 2-year follow-up period. Odds ratios (ORs) with 95% CIs were calculated. Variables identified in the univariate analysis ($p < 0.05$) were entered into a backward stepwise multiple logistic regression model.

$p \leq 0.05$ was considered statistically significant. Statistical analysis was performed with IBM SPSS Statistics version 18.

Results

A total of 217 patients with axSpA were enrolled at baseline. All patients were aged between 20 and 50 years. For 126 of the 217 patients, radiographs in the spine were available at baseline and at 2-year follow-up. Four patients with total ankylosis in the cervical and lumbar spine at enrolment were excluded from the analysis. One patient with stomach cancer, one patient with concurrent rheumatoid arthritis and one patient with chronic hepatitis B were also excluded. Thus, 119 patients with definite axSpA were included in this analysis. Baseline characteristics of the total group, as well as for the groups stratified according to the formation of new syndesmophytes, are presented in Table 1. In total, 34 (29%) patients had syndesmophytes at baseline. Ninety (76%) patients had radiographic sacroiliitis fulfilling the modified New York criteria for the classification of AS [25], and 19 (16%) patients had low BMD.

New syndesmophytes had developed in 22 (21%) patients at the 2-year follow-up. The patient group with new syndesmophytes had a higher percentage of current smokers at baseline and patients with a longer symptom duration than the patient group without new syndesmophytes ($p = 0.038$ and $p = 0.035$, respectively). Patients with new syndesmophytes had a higher frequency of syndesmophytes at baseline and a higher baseline mSASSS score than those who did not develop new syndesmophytes ($p = 0.001$ and $p = 0.015$, respectively). Low BMD in any site (lumbar spine, femoral neck or total hip) at baseline was more frequent in patients with new syndesmophytes ($p = 0.047$). There were no significant differences in disease activity scores, inflammatory markers and treatment agents.

Patients with low BMD at baseline showed higher levels of ESR and CRP ($p = 0.019$ and $p = 0.022$, respectively), as presented in Table 2. Patients with low BMD received more calcium agent and vitamin D treatments.

Table 3 presents the mean number of syndesmophytes at baseline and 2-year follow-up for the total group and the groups with or without low BMD at baseline. The number of syndesmophytes significantly increased in the period from baseline to 2 years in the total patient group (0.4 over 2 years) and both subgroups dichotomised according to low BMD. In the group of patients without

Table 1 Baseline patient characteristics

Variable	Total patients (n = 119)	New syndesmophytes at 2 years		p value
		No (n = 97)	Yes (n = 22)	
Age (years)	35 ± 9	34 ± 10	38 ± 8	0.075
Male sex	91 (77)	74 (76)	17 (77)	1.000
BMI (kg/m^2)	23.2 ± 3.4	22.9 ± 3.2	24.4 ± 4.1	0.072
Current smoking	36 (30)	25 (26)	11 (50)	0.038
Alcohol ≥ 3 units/day	3 (3)	3 (3)	0 (0)	1.000
Symptom duration (years)	8.6 ± 7.6	7.9 ± 7.3	11.6 ± 8.0	0.035
Family history of axSpA	12 (10)	12 (12)	0 (0)	0.120
HLA B27-positive	110 (92)	90 (93)	20 (91)	0.671
Peripheral arthritis	27 (23)	22 (23)	5 (23)	1.000
Radiographic sacroiliitis	90 (76)	70 (72)	20 (91)	0.097
BASDAI score (range 0–10)	3.9 ± 2.1	3.9 ± 2.0	3.7 ± 2.7	0.683
BASFI score	1.7 ± 2.1	1.7 ± 2.2	1.8 ± 1.8	0.722
ESR (mm/h)	23 ± 20	23 ± 20	23 ± 19	0.960
CRP (mg/L)	9.1 ± 14.9	8.9 ± 15.2	10.2 ± 14.1	0.703
ASDAS-ESR	2.6 ± 1.1	2.6 ± 1.1	2.5 ± 1.3	0.707
ASDAS-CRP	2.2 ± 1.3	2.2 ± 1.2	2.2 ± 1.5	0.883
mSASSS	7.6 ± 14.3	5.7 ± 13.0	15.8 ± 17.1	0.015
Number of syndesmophytes	2.3 ± 4.8	1.6 ± 4.3	5.0 ± 6.0	0.021
Presence of syndesmophytes	34 (29)	21 (22)	13 (59)	0.001
Patients on NSAIDs	106 (89)	86 (89)	20 (91)	1.000
Patients on sulfasalazine	42 (35)	34 (35)	8 (36)	1.000
Patients on TNF inhibitors	36 (30)	27 (28)	9 (41)	0.303
Patients on bisphosphonate	2 (2)	2 (2)	0 (0)	1.000
Patients on calcium	17 (14)	11 (11)	6 (27)	0.085
Patients on vitamin D	18 (15)	12 (12)	6 (27)	0.099
BMD (g/cm^2)				
Lumbar spine	1.16 ± 0.17	1.17 ± 0.16	1.13 ± 0.22	0.949
Femoral neck	0.94 ± 0.14	0.94 ± 0.14	0.92 ± 0.16	0.401
Total hip	0.98 ± 0.15	0.99 ± 0.15	0.95 ± 0.15	0.338
Low BMD (Z score ≤ −2.0)				
Any site	19 (16)	12 (12)	7 (32)	0.047
Lumbar spine	15 (13)	10 (10)	5 (23)	0.150
Femoral neck	3 (3)	1 (1)	2 (12)	0.070
Total hip	5 (4)	3 (3)	2 (9)	0.233

Data presented as n (%) or mean ± standard deviation

BMI body mass index, *axSpA* axial spondyloarthritis, *BASDAI* Bath Ankylosing Spondylitis Disease Activity Index, *BASFI* Bath Ankylosing Spondylitis Functional Index, *ESR* erythrocyte sedimentation rate, *CRP* C-reactive protein, *ASDAS* Ankylosing Spondylitis Disease Activity Score, *mSASSS* Modified Stoke Ankylosing Spondylitis Spinal Score, *NSAID* non-steroidal anti-inflammatory drug, *TNF* tumour necrosis factor, *BMD* bone mineral density

low BMD at baseline, the mean increase was 0.3 over the 2 years, while in those with low BMD at baseline it was 1.2 (Fig. 1a). New syndesmophytes after 2 years occurred in 15% of patients without low BMD and in 37% of patients with low BMD (p = 0.047; Fig. 1b).

Among the total of 119 patients, 27% (32) showed spinal radiographic progression (change of mSASSS ≥ 2 points) over 2 years. In the univariable logistic regression analysis, age (OR 1.1), current smoking (OR 4.1), radiographic sacroiliitis (OR 4.1), presence of syndesmophytes (OR 5.7) and low BMD (OR 3.0) at baseline were associated with spinal radiographic progression (Table 4). In the multivariable analysis, current smoking, presence of syndesmophytes and low BMD at baseline were independently

Table 2 Baseline patient characteristics in relation to low BMD at baseline

Variable	Low BMD at baseline		p value
	No (n = 100)	Yes (n = 19)	
Age (years)	35 ± 9	32 ± 11	0.245
Male sex	75 (75)	16 (84)	0.558
BMI (kg/m^2)	23.1 ± 3.2	23.5 ± 4.2	0.671
Current smoking	30 (30)	6 (32)	1.000
Alcohol ≥ 3 units/day	3 (3)	0 (0)	1.000
Symptom duration (years)	8 ± 7	9 ± 8	0.615
Family history of axSpA	10 (10)	2 (11)	1.000
HLA B27-positive	92 (92)	18 (95)	1.000
Peripheral arthritis	24 (24)	3 (16)	0.559
Radiographic sacroiliitis	73 (73)	17 (90)	0.154
BASDAI score (range, 0–10)	3.9 ± 2.2	3.8 ± 2.0	0.849
BASFI score	1.7 ± 2.1	1.9 ± 2.0	0.672
ESR (mm/h)	21 ± 20	32 ± 18	0.019
CRP (mg/L)	7.4 ± 13.4	18.0 ± 19.2	0.032
ASDAS-ESR	2.5 ± 1.2	2.9 ± 1.0	0.169
ASDAS-CRP	2.1 ± 1.3	2.7 ± 1.2	0.051
mSASSS	7 ± 14	11 ± 16	0.215
Number of syndesmophytes	2.1 ± 4.7	3.1 ± 5.6	0.430
Presence of syndesmophytes	28 (28)	6 (32)	0.785
Patients on NSAIDs	88 (88)	18 (95)	0.690
Patients on sulfasalazine	33 (33)	9 (47)	0.296
Patients on TNF inhibitors	28 (28)	8 (42)	0.227
Patients on bisphosphonate	0 (0)	2 (11)	0.024
Patients on calcium	10 (10)	7 (37)	0.006
Patients on vitamin D	10 (10)	8 (42)	0.002

Data presented as n (%) or mean ± standard deviation
BMD bone mineral density, BMI body mass index, axSpA axial spondyloarthritis, BASDAI Bath Ankylosing Spondylitis Disease Activity Index, BASFI Bath Ankylosing Spondylitis Functional Index, ESR erythrocyte sedimentation rate, CRP C-reactive protein, ASDAS Ankylosing Spondylitis Disease Activity Score, mSASSS modified Stoke Ankylosing Spondylitis Spinal Score, NSAID nonsteroidal anti-inflammatory drug, TNF tumour necrosis factor

associated with significant spinal progression (OR 3.0 (95% CI 1.1–7.7), OR 4.6 (95% CI 1.8–11.9) and OR 3.6 (95% CI 1.2–11.2), respectively). In the univariable logistic regression analysis to identify predictors of the formation of new syndesmophytes over 2 years (Table 5), symptom duration (OR 1.1), current smoking (OR 2.9), presence of syndesmophytes (OR 5.2) and low BMD (OR 3.3) at baseline were statistically significant factors and were included in the subsequent multivariable logistic regression analysis. This identified the presence of baseline syndesmophytes and low BMD at any site (OR 5.5 (95% CI 2.0–15.2) and OR 3.6 (95% CI 1.1–11.8), respectively) as significant predictors of new syndesmophytes.

Discussion

In this longitudinal observational study, we investigated the formation of new syndesmophytes in the spines of patients with axSpA over a period of 2 years, and identified predictors of new syndesmophyte formation and spinal radiographic progression. About 20% of the patients developed a new syndesmophyte over 2 years. The presence of a syndesmophyte at baseline and low BMD were predictors of the formation of new syndesmophytes and significant mSASSS progression.

Abnormal bone metabolism in axSpA is characterised by pathological new bone formation in the cortical zone of the vertebrae and the loss of trabecular bone from the centres of the vertebral bodies. Osteoproliferation leads to syndesmophytes, while the loss of trabecular bone leads to low BMD [26].

This study is the first to demonstrate that low BMD predicts radiographic progression in axSpA. The main determinants of low BMD in axSpA patients are systemic inflammation and bone-specific inflammation [27]. The inflammatory process is associated with altered systemic bone remodelling, increased bone resorption and impaired bone formation resulting from the effects of inflammatory mediators on the differentiation and activity of osteoclasts and osteoblasts. Proinflammatory cytokines can influence osteoclastogenesis and osteoblastic activity [28]. Thus, the presence of low BMD in axSpA is considered to be a result of altered bone remodelling caused by persistent inflammation. In the present study, serum levels of ESR correlated with BMD values of the lumbar spine, femoral neck and total hip, and Z scores of the femoral neck and total hip. Additionally, CRP levels correlated with the Z score at the lumbar spine and femoral neck (data not shown).

Table 3 Number of syndesmophytes at baseline and after 2 years for the total group and groups stratified for the presence or absence of low BMD

Group	Baseline syndesmophytes	2-year syndesmophytes	p value
Total patients (n = 119)	2.3 ± 4.8	2.7 ± 5.4	< 0.001
Normal BMD (n = 100)	2.1 ± 4.7	2.4 ± 5.0	< 0.001
Low BMD (n = 19)	3.0 ± 5.6	4.2 ± 7.4	< 0.001

Values presented as mean ± standard deviation
BMD bone mineral density

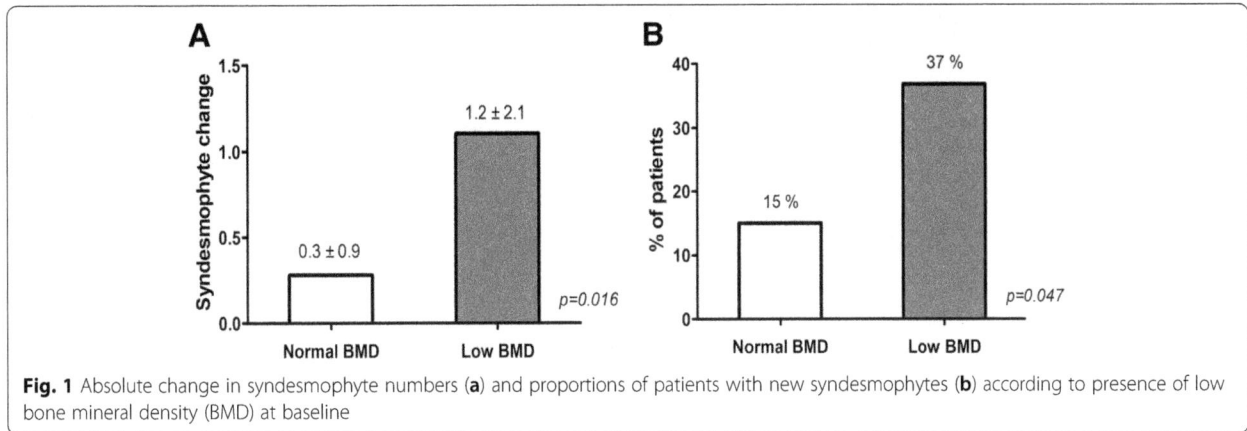

Fig. 1 Absolute change in syndesmophyte numbers (**a**) and proportions of patients with new syndesmophytes (**b**) according to presence of low bone mineral density (BMD) at baseline

Table 4 Univariable and multivariable analysis of significant progression of mSASSS over 2 years

Variable	Univariable analysis			Multivariable analysis[a]		
	OR	95% CI	p value	OR	95% CI	p value
Male sex	0.5	0.2–1.5	0.223			
Age (years)	1.1	1.0–1.1	0.019			
Symptom duration (years)	1.1	1.0–1.1	0.064			
BMI (kg/m^2)			0.817			
< 18.5	1.0	0.2–5.3	0.964			
18.5–22.9	1.0 (reference)					
23.0–24.9	1.4	0.5–4.0	0.487			
≥ 25.0	1.5	0.6–4.2	0.408			
Current smoking	4.1	1.7–9.6	0.001	3.0	1.1–7.7	0.025
HLA B27-positive	1.3	0.3–6.7	0.743			
Peripheral arthritis	0.5	0.2–1.6	0.269			
Radiographic sacroiliitis	4.1	1.2–14.7	0.029			
Presence of syndesmophytes	5.7	2.4–13.8	< 0.001	4.6	1.8–11.9	0.002
BASFI score, per 1 point	1.0	0.8–1.2	0.678			
BASDAI score ≥ 4	0.9	0.7–1.1	0.328			
ASDAS-CRP			0.313			
Low (< 1.3)	1.0 (Reference)					
Moderate (< 2.1)	1.2	0.4–3.6	0.769			
High (≤ 3.5)	0.3	0.2–1.3	0.135			
Very high (> 3.5)	0.9	0.2–3.2	0.839			
Increased ESR (≥ 20 mm/h)	1.1	0.5–2.4	0.842			
Increased CRP (≥ 5 mg/L)	1.4	0.6–3.3	0.431			
Patients on NSAIDs	0.7	0.2–3.1	0.716			
Patients on sulfasalazine	0.7	0.3–1.9	0.530			
Patients on TNF inhibitors	1.6	0.7–3.7	0.298			
Patients on calcium	3.0	0.8–11.3	0.097			
Patients on vitamin D	2.1	0.4–10.1	0.336			
Low BMD, any site (Z score ≤ − 2.0)	3.0	1.1–8.3	0.033	3.6	1.2–11.2	0.028

mSASSS Modified Stoke Ankylosing Spondylitis Spinal Score, *OR* odds ratio, *CI* confidence interval, *BMI* body mass index, *BASFI* Bath Ankylosing Spondylitis Functional Index, *BASDAI* Bath Ankylosing Spondylitis Disease Activity Index, *ASDAS* Ankylosing Spondylitis Disease Activity Score, *CRP* C-reactive protein, *ESR* erythrocyte sedimentation rate, *NSAID* non-steroidal anti-inflammatory drug, *TNF* tumour necrosis factor, *BMD* bone mineral density
[a]Adjusted for age, smoking, radiographic sacroiliitis, presence of syndesmophytes and presence of low BMD at any site at baseline

Table 5 Univariable and multivariable analysis of the formation of new syndesmophytes over 2 years

Variable	Univariable analysis			Multivariable analysis[a]		
	OR	95% CI	p value	OR	95% CI	p value
Male sex	1.0	0.3–2.9	0.922			
Age (years)	1.0	1.0–1.1	0.078			
Symptom duration (years)	1.1	1.0–1.1	0.040			
BMI (kg/m^2)			0.838			
< 18.5	1.7	0.3–9.8	0.567			
18.5–22.9	1.0 (reference)					
23.0–24.9	1.5	0.4–4.9	0.534			
≥ 25.0	1.6	0.5–5.2	0.403			
Current smoking	2.9	1.1–7.5	0.029			
HLA B27-positive	0.8	0.2–4.0	0.765			
Peripheral arthritis	1.0	0.3–3.0	0.996			
Radiographic sacroiliitis	3.9	0.8–17.6	0.082			
Presence of syndesmophytes	5.2	2.0–13.9	0.001	5.5	2.0–15.2	0.001
BASFI score, per 1 point	1.0	0.8–1.3	0.720			
BASDAI score ≥ 4	1.0	0.4–2.6	0.965			
ASDAS-CRP			0.632			
Low (< 1.3)	1.0 (reference)					
Moderate (< 2.1)	1.1	0.3–3.8	0.900			
High (≤ 3.5)	0.5	0.2–1.7	0.278			
Very high (> 3.5)	0.3	0.2–3.3	0.688			
Increased ESR (≥ 20 mm/h)	1.3	0.5–3.2	0.630			
Increased CRP (≥ 5 mg/L)	1.6	0.6–4.2	0.320			
Patients on NSAIDs	1.3	0.3–6.2	0.761			
Patients on sulfasalazine	1.1	0.4–2.8	0.907			
Patients on TNF inhibitors	1.8	0.7–4.7	0.232			
Patients on calcium	2.9	0.9–9.0	0.062			
Patients on vitamin D	2.7	0.9–8.1	0.086			
Low BMD, any site (Z score ≤ −2.0)	3.3	1.1–9.8	0.030	3.6	1.1–11.8	0.031

OR odds ratio, *CI* confidence interval, *BMI* body mass index, *BASFI* Bath Ankylosing Spondylitis Functional Index, *BASDAI* Bath Ankylosing Spondylitis Disease Activity Index, *ASDAS* Ankylosing Spondylitis Disease Activity Score, *CRP* C-reactive protein, *ESR* erythrocyte sedimentation rate, *NSAID* non-steroidal anti-inflammatory drug, *TNF* tumour necrosis factor, *BMD* bone mineral density
[a]Adjusted for symptom duration, presence of syndesmophytes, smoking and presence of low BMD at any site at baseline

Bone loss resulting from chronic inflammation and the associated changes in bone microarchitecture have been proposed as a potential driving mechanism for the ankylosing process [29]. The inflammatory process induces bone loss, which affects the microarchitecture in the trabecular bone, thereby leading to instability. Reduced bone strength triggers a stabilising anabolic effort that results in bone formation. Trabecular and cortical compartments appear to have different reactions to inflammation; in axSpA, inflammation has a direct effect on the trabecular bone of the vertebrae, but not on the cortical bone [8]. As persistent inflammation in the trabecular bone of the vertebral bodies may prevent the anabolic response from correcting the instability, new

bone formation in the cortical bone of the vertebrae may be increased [30]. This would result in the formation of syndesmophytes: compensatory stability for the spine but with a loss of normal mobility [31].

Another explanation is that low BMD may represent the presence of a repairing area that was affected by active inflammation in the past. There is increasing evidence that new bone formation in axSpA is the consequence of previous inflammation in the subchondral bone marrow, with the appearance of granulated repair tissue occurring as a mandatory intermediate step, with this then being followed by new bone formation. It has been proposed that the best current treatment for the prevention of bone formation is the early and effective suppression of bony inflammation [32]. Additionally, if it is possible to detect the presence of repair tissue, the risk of new syndesmophyte formation could also be predicted. The presence of a low BMD means that the repair process may become apparent, to compensate for bone loss resulting from the inflammatory process. Therefore, the presence of low BMD may represent areas with ongoing repair affected by inflammation, such as fatty lesions on MRI.

In the current study, the presence of baseline syndesmophytes in axSpA was found to be the strongest predictor for the formation of new syndesmophytes. This finding is consistent with those of earlier studies. Similar results with respect to spinal radiographic progression have been found in early axSpA patients, as well as in AS patients [5, 33, 34]. However, a substantial proportion of patients with baseline syndesmophytes do not show progression over 2 years. Furthermore, it is arguable whether the presence of baseline syndesmophytes should be considered a true predictor, because the patients already exhibited the features that the model was designed to predict [5].

Smoking is reported to be associated with spinal radiographic progression in early axSpA [6] and the radiographic severity of AS [35], although the exact mechanisms for the influence of smoking on radiographic progression are not known. In the present study, smoking was associated with new syndesmophyte formation only in the univariable analysis, whereas it was independently associated with significant mSASSS progression over 2 years after adjustment for confounding factors. Only the status of smoking at baseline was included in the analysis, and the relatively small number of patients may have influenced the inconsistent results with respect to smoking. The influence of smoking on new syndesmophyte formation should be studied in a larger cohort.

The presence of radiographic sacroiliitis was significantly associated with spinal radiographic progression over 2 years, but this significant association was not present in the multivariable analysis. This finding is consistent with a previous result in early axSpA patients [6]. In the present study, 90% of patients with low BMD had radiographic sacroiliitis. This high proportion of radiographic sacroiliitis in the patients with low BMD could have affected the result. The exact effect of radiographic sacroiliitis on spinal progression should be clarified in a large patient cohort including non-radiographic axSpA patients with low BMD.

Although we did not observe a significant result in this study, systemic inflammatory markers were reported as predictors of radiographic progression in patients with early axSpA in the German Spondyloarthritis Inception Cohort (GESPIC) [6]. This previous study included early axSpA patients with short symptom duration (mean 4.2 years) and low mSASSS (mean 4.25) [6]. In this study, the mean symptom duration and mSASSS were 8.6 years and 7.6 points. These differences suggest that our study patients had more severe and longstanding symptoms and were advanced patients. In a prospective observation of a cohort with longstanding AS, inflammatory markers did not emerge as independent predictors, as per the results of the present study [5]. These discordant results could possibly be explained by the differences in disease duration and structural damage severity. Furthermore, we only analysed the associations between baseline ESR and CRP measurements and new syndesmophyte formation, not time-averaged inflammatory markers. Baseline inflammatory markers may be less reflective of the status of persistent systemic inflammation than time-averaged values. Therefore, our results for the predictive role of systemic inflammation should be interpreted with caution.

Inflammation plays a key role in bone loss in axSpA, and anti-inflammatory drugs are expected to have a beneficial effect on bone through both the increased mobility related to pain relief and the direct effects on bone [28]. The best treatment for the prevention of bone formation/progression is currently the early and effective suppression of bony inflammation [32]. Our results suggest that successful anti-inflammatory treatment reduces inflammation and allows the bone metabolism to normalise, thereby taking away the compensatory anabolic response that leads to new bone formation in the cortical bone of the spine. Although we did not find a beneficial effect of NSAIDs or TNF inhibitors in this 2-year follow-up study, recent long-term follow-up data show that TNF inhibitors suppress radiographic spinal progression [36, 37]. Thus, if patients are treated for a longer time with a TNF inhibitor (preventing new occurrences of the sequence of inflammation, repair and new bone formation), or if they are treated early in the course of their disease, such a treatment seems to be effective in retarding the process of new bone formation [32]. Taken together, active anti-inflammatory treatment is crucial for the prevention of spinal ankylosis in young axSpA patients, especially those with low BMD.

This study has some limitations. First, the number of axSpA patients was relatively small; therefore, the regression analysis could be underpowered. In our patients, those with low BMD received more calcium agents and vitamin D treatments, and these agents could have affected the bone metabolism. Although calcium and vitamin D intake were not significant in the regression analysis, their effects on spinal progression need to be clarified in a large cohort including more patients with low BMD. The BMD in axSpA can be affected by the presence of syndesmophytes or other structural lesions such as an ankylosed posterior arch and periosteal bone formation. Therefore, the BMD of the lumbar spine in patients with syndesmophytes could have been overestimated. Lastly, it is known that there is an association between serum levels of sex hormones and BMD in AS [38], but these were not measured in this study.

Conclusions

The presence of low BMD and syndesmophytes at baseline were independently associated with the formation of new syndesmophytes in young axSpA patients. Current smoking, syndesmophytes and low BMD at baseline were also associated with significant mSASSS progression. Effective anti-inflammatory treatment may modify radiographic spinal progression in young axSpA patients with low BMD. Our findings require confirmation in other large cohorts of axSpA patients.

Abbreviations

AS: Ankylosing spondylitis; ASAS: Assessment of SpondyloArthritis International Society; ASDAS: Ankylosing Spondylitis Disease Activity Score; axSpA: Axial spondyloarthritis; BASDAI: Bath Ankylosing Spondylitis Disease Activity Index; BASFI: Bath Ankylosing Spondylitis Functional Index; BMD: Bone mineral density; CRP: C-reactive protein; DXA: Dual-energy absorptiometry; ESR: Erythrocyte sedimentation rate; ICC: Intraclass correlation coefficient; mSASSS: Modified Stoke Ankylosing Spondylitis Spinal Score; nr-axSpA: Non-radiographic axSpA; NSAID: Non-steroidal anti-inflammatory drug; OR: Odds ratio; SD: Standard deviation; TNF: Tumour necrosis factor

Funding

No specific funding was received from any bodies in the public, commercial or not-for-profit sectors to carry out the work described in this manuscript.

Authors' contributions

HRK contributed to conception, design, acquisition of data and drafting of the article. JHJ contributed to conception, design and acquisition of data, and helped to draft the manuscript. YSH and S-HP contributed to design, acquisition of data and analysis and interpretation of data. KYK contributed to statistical analysis and interpretation of data. All authors read and approved the final manuscript.

Competing interests

The authors declare that they have no competing interests.

References

1. Sieper J, van der Heijde D. Review: Nonradiographic axial spondyloarthritis: new definition of an old disease? Arthritis Rheum. 2013;65:543–51.
2. Machado P, Landewe R, Braun J, Hermann KG, Baker D, van der Heijde D. Both structural damage and inflammation of the spine contribute to impairment of spinal mobility in patients with ankylosing spondylitis. Ann Rheum Dis. 2010;69:1465–70.
3. Lories RJ, Schett G. Pathophysiology of new bone formation and ankylosis in spondyloarthritis. Rheum Dis Clin N Am. 2012;38:555–67.
4. Poddubnyy D, Sieper J. Radiographic progression in ankylosing spondylitis/axial spondyloarthritis: how fast and how clinically meaningful? Curr Opin Rheumatol. 2012;24:363–9.
5. van Tubergen A, Ramiro S, van der Heijde D, Dougados M, Mielants H, Landewe R. Development of new syndesmophytes and bridges in ankylosing spondylitis and their predictors: a longitudinal study. Ann Rheum Dis. 2012;71:518–23.
6. Poddubnyy D, Haibel H, Listing J, Marker-Hermann E, Zeidler H, Braun J, et al. Baseline radiographic damage, elevated acute-phase reactant levels, and cigarette smoking status predict spinal radiographic progression in early axial spondylarthritis. Arthritis Rheum. 2012;64:1388–98.

7. Poddubnyy D, Protopopov M, Haibel H, Braun J, Rudwaleit M, Sieper J. High disease activity according to the Ankylosing Spondylitis Disease Activity Score is associated with accelerated radiographic spinal progression in patients with early axial spondyloarthritis: results from the GErman SPondyloarthritis Inception Cohort. Ann Rheum Dis. 2016;75:2114–8.
8. Schett G. Structural bone changes in spondyloarthritis: mechanisms, clinical impact and therapeutic considerations. Am J Med Sci. 2011;341:269–71.
9. Szentpetery A, Horvath A, Gulyas K, Petho Z, Bhattoa HP, Szanto S, et al. Effects of targeted therapies on the bone in arthritides. Autoimmun Rev. 2017;16:313–20.
10. Rosenbaum J, Chandran V. Management of comorbidities in ankylosing spondylitis. Am J Med Sci. 2012;343:364–6.
11. Carter S, Lories RJ. Osteoporosis: a paradox in ankylosing spondylitis. Curr Osteoporos Rep. 2011;9:112–5.
12. Kang KY, Goo HY, Park SH, Hong YS. Trabecular bone score as an assessment tool to identify the risk of osteoporosis in axial spondyloarthritis: a case-control study. Rheumatology (Oxford). 2018;57:462–9.
13. Akgol G, Kamanli A, Ozgocmen S. Evidence for inflammation-induced bone loss in non-radiographic axial spondyloarthritis. Rheumatology (Oxford). 2014;53:497–501.
14. Klingberg E, Lorentzon M, Gothlin J, Mellstrom D, Geijer M, Ohlsson C, et al. Bone microarchitecture in ankylosing spondylitis and the association with bone mineral density, fractures, and syndesmophytes. Arthritis Res Ther. 2013;15:R179.
15. Klingberg E, Lorentzon M, Mellstrom D, Geijer M, Gothlin J, Hilme E, et al. Osteoporosis in ankylosing spondylitis—prevalence, risk factors and methods of assessment. Arthritis Res Ther. 2012;14:R108.
16. Klingberg E, Nurkkala M, Carlsten H, Forsblad-d'Elia H. Biomarkers of bone metabolism in ankylosing spondylitis in relation to osteoproliferation and osteoporosis. J Rheumatol. 2014;41:1349–56.
17. Rudwaleit M, Landewe R, van der Heijde D, Listing J, Brandt J, Braun J, et al. The development of Assessment of SpondyloArthritis international Society classification criteria for axial spondyloarthritis (part I): classification of paper patients by expert opinion including uncertainty appraisal. Ann Rheum Dis. 2009;68:770–6.
18. Zochling J, Braun J. Assessments in ankylosing spondylitis. Best Pract Res Clin Rheumatol. 2007;21:699–712.
19. Garrett S, Jenkinson T, Kennedy LG, Whitelock H, Gaisford P, Calin A. A new approach to defining disease status in ankylosing spondylitis: the Bath Ankylosing Spondylitis Disease Activity Index. J Rheumatol. 1994;21:2286–91.
20. van der Heijde D, Lie E, Kvien TK, Sieper J, Van den Bosch F, Listing J, et al. ASDAS, a highly discriminatory ASAS-endorsed disease activity score in patients with ankylosing spondylitis. Ann Rheum Dis. 2009;68:1811–8.
21. Calin A, Garrett S, Whitelock H, Kennedy LG, O'Hea J, Mallorie P, et al. A new approach to defining functional ability in ankylosing spondylitis: the development of the Bath Ankylosing Spondylitis Functional Index. J Rheumatol. 1994;21:2281–5.
22. Wanders AJ, Landewe RB, Spoorenberg A, Dougados M, van der Linden S, Mielants H, et al. What is the most appropriate radiologic scoring method for ankylosing spondylitis? A comparison of the available methods based on the Outcome Measures in Rheumatology Clinical Trials filter. Arthritis Rheum. 2004;50:2622–32.
23. Ward MM, Learch TJ, Weisman MH. Cervical vertebral squaring in patients without spondyloarthritis. J Rheumatol. 2012;39:1900.
24. Baim S, Leonard MB, Bianchi ML, Hans DB, Kalkwarf HJ, Langman CB, et al. Official Positions of the International Society for Clinical Densitometry and executive summary of the 2007 ISCD Pediatric Position Development Conference. J Clin Densitom. 2008;11:6–21.
25. van der Linden S, Valkenburg HA, Cats A. Evaluation of diagnostic criteria for ankylosing spondylitis. A proposal for modification of the New York criteria. Arthritis Rheum. 1984;27:361–8.
26. Hinze AM, Louie GH. Osteoporosis management in ankylosing spondylitis. Curr Treatm Opt Rheumatol. 2016;2:271–82.
27. Briot K, Durnez A, Paternotte S, Miceli-Richard C, Dougados M, Roux C. Bone oedema on MRI is highly associated with low bone mineral density in patients with early inflammatory back pain: results from the DESIR cohort. Ann Rheum Dis. 2013;72:1914–9.
28. Briot K, Geusens P, Em Bultink I, Lems WF, Roux C. Inflammatory diseases and bone fragility. Osteoporos Int. 2017;28:3301–14.

29. Van Mechelen M, Lories RJ. Microtrauma: no longer to be ignored in spondyloarthritis? Curr Opin Rheumatol. 2016;28:176–80.

30. Neerinckx B, Lories RJ. Structural disease progression in axial spondyloarthritis: still a cause for concern? Curr Rheumatol Rep. 2017;19:14.

31. Neerinckx B, Lories R. Mechanisms, impact and prevention of pathological bone regeneration in spondyloarthritis. Curr Opin Rheumatol. 2017;29:287–92.

32. Poddubnyy D, Sieper J. Mechanism of new bone formation in axial spondyloarthritis. Curr Rheumatol Rep. 2017;19:55.

33. Baraliakos X, Listing J, Rudwaleit M, Haibel H, Brandt J, Sieper J, et al. Progression of radiographic damage in patients with ankylosing spondylitis: defining the central role of syndesmophytes. Ann Rheum Dis. 2007;66:910–5.

34. Baraliakos X, Listing J, von der Recke A, Braun J. The natural course of radiographic progression in ankylosing spondylitis—evidence for major individual variations in a large proportion of patients. J Rheumatol. 2009;36: 997–1002.

35. Ward MM, Hendrey MR, Malley JD, Learch TJ, Davis JC Jr, Reveille JD, et al. Clinical and immunogenetic prognostic factors for radiographic severity in ankylosing spondylitis. Arthritis Rheum. 2009;61:859–66.

36. Maas F, Arends S, Brouwer E, Essers I, van der Veer E, Efde M, et al. Reduction in spinal radiographic progression in ankylosing spondylitis patients receiving prolonged treatment with tumor necrosis factor inhibitors. Arthritis Care Res (Hoboken). 2017;69:1011–9.

37. Haroon N, Inman RD, Learch TJ, Weisman MH, Lee M, Rahbar MH, et al. The impact of tumor necrosis factor alpha inhibitors on radiographic progression in ankylosing spondylitis. Arthritis Rheum. 2013;65:2645–54.

38. Aydin T, Karacan I, Demir SE, Sahin Z. Bone loss in males with ankylosing spondylitis: its relation to sex hormone levels. Clin Endocrinol. 2005;63:467–9.

6

Role of the mTOR pathway in minor salivary gland changes in Sjogren's syndrome and systemic sclerosis

Zeki Soypaçacı[1*], Zeynep Zehra Gümüş[2], Fulya Çakaloğlu[3], Mustafa Özmen[4], Dilek Solmaz[4], Sercan Gücenmez[4], Önay Gercik[4] and Servet Akar[4]

Abstract

Background: To examine the activity of the mammalian target of rapamycin (mTOR) pathway and its regulators, transforming growth factor (TGF)-β1 and phosphatase and tensin homolog (PTEN), in minor salivary gland biopsies of Sjogren's syndrome (SS) and systemic sclerosis (SSc) patients.

Methods: We retrospectively evaluated SS, SSc, and SS-SSc overlap patients admitted to our outpatient rheumatology clinic between January 2007 and December 2015 who underwent a minor salivary gland biopsy. Patient demographics and some clinical features were obtained from hospital records. Immunohistochemistry was used to analyze total mTOR, total PTEN, and TGF-β1 expression in the biopsied tissues. The biopsy specimens were also examined for the presence and degree of fibrosis.

Results: Minor salivary gland biopsies of 58 SS, 14 SSc, and 23 SS-SSc overlap patients were included in the study. There was no significant difference in mTOR expression between these groups ($P = 0.622$). PTEN protein was expressed in 87.2% of patients with SS, 57.9% with overlap syndrome, and 100% of the SSC patients, and these differences were statistically different ($P = 0.023$). Although ductal epithelial TGF-β1 expression was similar between the groups ($P = 0.345$), acinar cell expression was found to be more frequent in the SSc (72.7%) and overlap patients (85.7%) in comparison with the SS cases (58.2%; $P = 0.004$).

Conclusion: mTOR may be one of the common pathways in the pathology of both SS and SSc. Hence, there may be a role for mTOR inhibitors in the treatment of both diseases. Additionally, PTEN and TGF-β1 expression may be a distinctive feature of SSc.

Keywords: Target of rapamycin proteins, mTOR pathway, Sjogren's syndrome, Systemic sclerosis, PTEN protein, Human, Transforming growth factor beta

Background

Sjogren's syndrome (SS) is a chronic, systemic, inflammatory disease [1]. The characteristic pathologic findings for this disorder are lymphocytic infiltration of the exocrine glands leading to autoantibody production and tissue destruction [1, 2]. Consistent with its pathogenesis, the first symptoms of SS are generally xerostomia and keratoconjunctivitis sicca [2]. SS can occur as an isolated primary condition or secondary to another connective tissue disease. At the beginning of SS onset, CD4-positive T helper cells play a pathogenic role whereas, in late-term SS, B cells play a predominant role. Recent studies have indicated that epithelial cells are central to autoimmune pathways where they produce human leukocyte antigen (HLA), adhesion and costimulatory molecules, and cytokines and chemokines [2]. The term 'autoimmune epitheliitis' has thus been suggested to describe the etiology of SS.

Systemic sclerosis (SSc) is a chronic autoimmune disease characterized by increased fibrosis and slightly enlightened pathogenesis [3, 4]. The most frequent skin sign of SSc is dermal infiltration by myofibroblasts that

* Correspondence: soypacaci@yahoo.com
[1]Department of Internal Medicine, Division of Nephrology, İzmir Katip Celebi University School of Medicine, Karabağlar, 35360 İzmir, Turkey
Full list of author information is available at the end of the article

synthesize type I collagen and alpha smooth muscle actin (α-SMA) [4]. Increased profibrotic mediators, such as transforming growth factor (TGF)-β, and increased mammalian target of rapamycin (mTOR) activity have also been reported in dermal fibroblasts of SSc patients [4, 5]. mTOR is a serine kinase that plays a role in the regulation of cell growth and proliferation. The mTOR complex includes two multiprotein complexes, mTOR complex 1 (mTORC1) and mTOR complex 2 (mTORC2) [6]. mTORC1 activates S6 kinase 1 (S6K1) and eukaryotic translation initiation factor 4E (eIF4E) which are responsible for mRNA translation [5]. mTOR also regulates cell survival and is stimulated by growth factors, nutrients, stress signals, phosphoinositol-3-kinase (PI3K), mitogen-activated protein kinase (MAPK), adenosine monophosphate (AMP), and adenosine monophosphate-activated protein kinase (AMPK). mTORC2 regulates the actin cytoskeleton and activates protein kinase C (PKC)-α and Akt (protein kinase B, or PKB) [6]. mTOR multiprotein complexes have a positive effect on fibrotic interleukins (ILs). Liang et al. reported previously that IL-4, IL-6, IL-17, and TGF-β are downregulated after mTOR inhibition with rapamycin [5]. Phosphatase and tensin homolog (PTEN) is also involved in the regulation of mTOR activity and usually inhibits mTOR via the inhibition of Akt [7]. Decreased intracellular levels of PTEN cause PI3K/Akt/mTOR pathway activation and increase cell proliferation, survival, adhesion, migration, and angiogenesis [7]. Another mTOR regulator molecule, TGF-β, activates intracellular signaling pathways such as PI3K/Akt/mTOR and SMAD [8, 9]. TGF-β can also both enhance and suppress PTEN, an effect that depends on Ras/ERK pathway activation [7].

Multiple signaling pathways such as MAPK, Akt, NF-κB, Bcl-2, and JAK/STAT are found to be activated in systemic diseases in which the mTOR pathway is also an attractive therapeutic target [10]. The relationship between mTOR and increased skin fibrosis in SSc has previously been investigated both in vivo and in vitro. The role of rapamycin, an mTOR inhibitor, was investigated previously in only a murine model of SS, the results of which suggested that it has therapeutic potential [11]. We therefore aimed, in our current study, to investigate the role of the mTOR pathway in the pathologic changes observed in minor salivary gland biopsies (MSGBs) from SS, SSc, and SS/SSc overlap syndrome patients.

Methods

Patients and data collection

Patients admitted to the outpatient rheumatology clinic in our tertiary hospital between January 2007 and December 2015 were retrospectively reviewed. These patients were divided into SSc, SS, and SSc/SS overlap subgroups. Demographic (age, gender), clinical (duration of disease, presence of sicca symptoms, Schirmer's and tear breakup time (BUT) test results), and serum autoantibody data for these cases were collected using their medical records. Patients who answered positively to at least one of the questions regarding keratoconjunctivitis sicca and xerostomia were considered positive for sicca symptoms. A BUT test result < 10 s and a Schirmer's test finding ≤ 5 mm/5 min were also considered positive indicators of sicca symptoms.

SS and SSc patients aged ≥ 18 years who fulfilled the American-European Consensus Group (AECG) classification criteria for Sjogren's syndrome [12] and the ACR/EULAR 2013 criteria for systemic sclerosis [13], respectively, and who underwent MSGB were screened for inclusion in the study cohort. All of the SSc patients who underwent MSGB had at least one sicca symptom or had a positive autoantibody related to sicca symptoms. We excluded patients who had received any previous treatment with mTOR inhibitors. We also excluded any secondary SS or SSc patients other than overlap cases. We did not use an informed consent form since this was a retrospective study.

Histopathological evaluation

The MSGBs were fixed with 10% buffered formalin for at least 6 h and then monitored with a closed-loop tissue monitoring machine overnight. Serial sections of 4–5 μm thickness were obtained from a single paraffin-embedded block for each patient, stained with hematoxylin and eosin (H&E), and examined under a light microscope by a single expert pathologist (FC). The specimens were evaluated for the presence and number of lymphocytic foci, the presence and grade of fibrosis, and lobular or acinar atrophy. Focal lymphocytic sialadenitis with a score of ≥ 1 foci/4 mm^2 was accepted as diagnostic for SS [14]. The extent of fibrosis in the MSGB specimens was assessed semiquantitatively and graded as mild (less than 25% of the surface area), moderate (between 25 and 50%), or severe (> 50%).

Immunohistochemical staining

The MSGB specimens were evaluated by immunohistochemical (IHC) staining with antibodies for total PTEN (Spring Bioscience Rabbit Anti-Human PTEN Rabbit Monoclonal, Clone SP170), total mTOR (Spring Bioscience Rabbit Anti-Human mTOR Polyclonal Antibody), and TGF-β1 (Spring Bioscience Rabbit Anti-Human Transforming Growth Factor 1β Polyclonal Antibody) by a single expert pathologist (FC). IHC staining slides were evaluated via light microscopy. The positive controls used in this study were prostate adenocarcinoma tissue for PTEN, placenta for TGF-β1, and breast cancer tissue for mTOR.

Immunohistochemical evaluation

IHC staining of mTOR was semiquantitatively assessed as mild (1+) (Fig. 1a), moderate (2+), or strong (3+) (Fig. 1b) positivity [15]. IHC staining of PTEN was graded as negative (Fig. 1c), or as mild (1+) or strong (2+) positivity (Fig. 1d) [16]. IHC staining of TGF-β1 was semiquantitatively assessed and graded between 0 and 4 according to the level of staining [17] (Fig. 1e, f).

Statistical analysis

Unless otherwise stated, results are presented as a mean and standard deviation (SD) or percentage as appropriate. Comparisons of categorical data between groups were made using the chi-square test. The Spearman's rank correlation test was performed for bivariate correlations between variables. All tests were two-tailed and a P value of < 0.05 was considered statistically significant for all measurements. All statistical analyses were made

using the Statistical Package of Social Science (SPSS) version 16.0 software (Chicago, IL).

Results

Patient demographic and baseline features

Demographic and baseline features of the patients are presented in Table 1. Formalin-fixed MSGB sections from 58 patients with SS, 16 with SSc, and 23 with SSc/SS overlap syndrome were initially included in the study samples. However, two female SSc samples had to be excluded to due to difficulties with IHC staining. As expected, the frequency of sicca symptoms was higher in the SS patients (90%) than in the SSc (77%) or overlap syndrome cases (70%). BUT test positivity was determined as 60% in the SS patients, 36% in the SSc patients, and 74% in the overlap syndrome patients. Schirmer test positivity was found to be 58% in the SS patients, 50% in the SSc patients, and 58% in the overlap

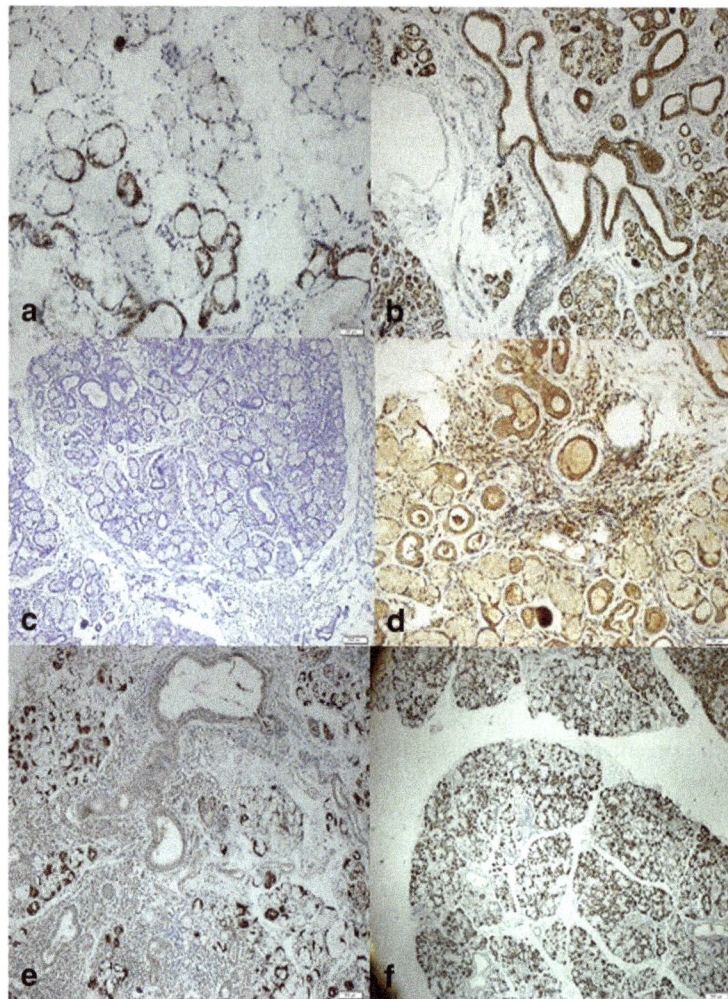

Fig. 1 Immunohistochemical staining of mTOR, PTEN, and TGF-β1 in minor salivary gland biopsies. Representative samples showing mild (**a**) and strong (**b**) positivity for mTOR, negative (**c**) and strong positivity for PTEN (**d**), and mild (**e**) and strong positivity for TGF-β staining (**f**). Positive staining for TGF-β was mainly observed in the acinar regions of the salivary glands

Table 1 Demographic and baseline features of the patients

	Sjogren's syndrome ($n = 58$)	Systemic sclerosis ($n = 14$)	Overlap syndrome ($n = 23$)
Age, years (mean ± SD)	52.6 ± 13.1	53.9 ± 14.2	48.0 ± 9.3
Duration of disease, months (mean ± SD)	58.3 ± 23.4	43.0 ± 23.9	56.8 ± 35.4
Sicca symptom positivity, %	90	77	70
Schirmer test positivity, %	58	50	58
Breakup time test positivity, %	60	36	74
Anti-Ro (SSA) or La (SSB) positivity, %	96	55	71

syndrome patients. Anti-Ro (SSA) or anti-La (SSB) positivity was higher in the SS patients (96%) than SSc (55%) and overlap syndrome (71%) patients. Examination of the biopsy specimens revealed a focus score of ≥ 1 foci/4 mm^2 in 52 out of the 58 (90%) SS patients, 22 out of the 23 (96%) overlap patients, and none of the SSc patients.

mTOR, PTEN, and TGF-β1 expressions

mTOR expression was evident in 94% of the SS group, 100% of the overlap cases, and 91% of the SSc patients (Table 2). There were no significant differences in the presence ($P = 0.462$) or degree ($P = 0.622$) of mTOR expression between these groups. PTEN protein expression was detected in 87% of the SS patients, 58% of the overlap cases, and 100% of the SSc patients (Table 2) with significant differences in the presence ($P = 0.004$) and intensity ($P = 0.023$) of staining. Although the ductal epithelial TGF-β1 expression was similar between the groups ($P = 0.345$), acinar cell expression (Table 2) was more frequent in the SSc (73%) and overlap patients (86%) in comparison with the SS (58%) cases with borderline significance ($P = 0.05$). Additionally, more of the acinar TGF-β1 staining was strongly positive in SSC patients (46% vs 19% and 4%; $P = 0.004$).

Fibrosis features

In general, fibrosis was evident in all of our patient groups but we did not observe severe fibrosis in any

MSGB sections. There was also no significant difference found between the study groups in terms of the presence of fibrosis ($P = 0.833$). Correlation analysis between the immunohistochemical staining results, presence of fibrosis, and the demographic, clinical characteristics, and autoantibodies of the SS patients showed only a negative correlation between PTEN and TGF-β1 positivity ($r = -0.306$, $P = 0.041$). However, because of the small number of patients in the SSc and overlap syndrome groups, correlation analyses were not performed for these patients.

Discussion

Sicca symptoms were more frequent in our current SSc patients (77%) than has been reported previously [18]. It should be noted, however, that all SSc patients examined in our present study had undergone MSGB as they had either sicca symptoms or autoantibody positivity suggesting an accompanying SS.

Our current findings suggest that the mTOR pathway might play an active role in the pathology of SS, SSc, and overlap syndrome. We did not find any statistically significant differences in the mTOR expression profile among our study groups indicating a common role of this pathway in these diseases. It may be appropriate, therefore, to use mTOR inhibitors more frequently in rheumatology practice.

We are not aware of any prior human study that has evaluated mTOR inhibitors in SS patients. Shah

Table 2 Immunohistochemical staining results in the three patient groups (mTOR, PTEN, and TGF-β1 in acinus)

		Negative	Mild positivity	Moderate positivity	Strong positivity
mTOR	SS	3 (6)	25 (46)	20 (37)	6 (11)
	Overlap syndrome	0	11 (55)	9 (45)	0
	SSc	1 (9)	4 (36)	5 (46)	1 (9)
PTEN	SS	6 (13)	23 (49)	–	18 (38)
	Overlap syndrome	8 (42)	5 (26)	–	6 (32)
	SSc	0	7 (58)	–	5 (42)
TGF-β1	SS	23 (42)	20 (36)	10 (18)	2 (4)
	Overlap syndrome	3 (14)	10 (48)	4 (19)	4 (19)
	SSc	3 (27)	2 (18)	1 (9)	5 (46)

All values are shown as n (%)

mTOR mammalian target of rapamycin, *PTEN* phosphatase and tensin homolog, *SS* Sjogren's syndrome, *SSc* systemic sclerosis, *TGF* transforming growth factor

and colleagues have previously reported in a mouse model of SS that the mTOR inhibitor sirolimus may suppress the lymphocytic infiltration of lacrimal glands [11]. Our present observations may encourage other investigators to test mTOR inhibitors as potential new SS therapeutics.

Forestier et al. recently showed an altered B cell homeostasis in SSc patients compared with healthy controls [19]. This altered B cell homeostasis was found to be related to the mTOR pathway. However, the most important limitation of this study is the lack of a control group. Thus, further studies with healthy control groups may shed light on the pathogenesis of SSc and SS and may help us to understand the role of the mTOR pathway in the rheumatologic diseases.

We found a statistically significant difference between the acinar TGF-β1 expression levels in our study groups. As expected, strong TGF-β1 expression, a well-known fibrosis indicator, was found most frequently in the SSc patients. In addition, PTEN expression was similar in SS and SSc patients and this was significantly different from the overlap patients. These data suggest that epithelopathogenesis follows a different pathway in overlap syndrome than in SS or SSc. Although PTEN is known as an endogenous mTOR inhibitor, it has also previously been shown that increased mTOR activity is accompanied by increased PTEN levels and it was hypothesized that this might be due an autoimmune-related impairment in the PTEN pathway [7]. However, further studies are needed to investigate the effects of PTEN and PTEN-related molecules on autoimmune diseases.

Our correlation analysis in the SS group did not reveal any association between mTOR, PTEN, or TGF-β1 expression. This might indicate that PTEN and TGF-β1 operate independently of the mTOR pathway in SS pathogenesis. We also found a negative association between TGF-β1 and PTEN expression in our SS samples. Under normal physiological conditions in the cell, TGF-β1 may have both enhancing and reducing effects on PTEN. When the Ras/ERK pathway is activated, TGF-β suppresses PTEN by the SMAD4-independent signal pathway [7]. However, when the Ras/ERK pathway is inactivated, TGF-β upregulates the classic SMAD-dependent PTEN molecule [7]. The negative correlation between TGF-β1 and PTEN in SS suggests that the Ras/ERK pathway is active in this disease, but no precise information is yet available because other pathway members have yet to be identified. In addition, some notable limitations of our present study include the small number of SSc and overlap syndrome patients, the lack of sicca controls, and other reasons and technical difficulties with analyzing some of the biopsy materials.

Conclusions

In conclusion, mTOR may be one of the common pathways leading to the pathology/inflammation observed in both SS and SSc and may provide a new alternative for the development of new treatments for both diseases. Additionally, higher PTEN and TGF-β1 expression, in particular a higher acinar TGF-β1 level, may be a distinctive feature of SSc.

Key messages

- The mTOR pathway appears to be similarly active in minor salivary gland biopsies of SS and SSc patients.
- PTEN and TGF-β1 expression may be a distinctive feature of salivary gland pathology in SSc.

Abbreviations

α-SMA: Alpha smooth muscle actin; ACR: American College of Rheumatology; AECG: American-European Consensus Group; Akt: Protein kinase B; AMP: Adenosine monophosphate; AMPK: Adenosine monophosphate-activated protein kinase; Bcl-2: B-cell lymphoma 2; BUT: Breakup time; CD4: Cluster of differentiation; eIF4E: Eukaryotic translation initiation factor 4E; ERK: Extracellular signal-regulated kinases; EULAR: European League Against Rheumatism; H&E: Hematoxylin and eosin; HLA: Human leukocyte antigen; IHC: Immunohistochemical; IL: Interleukin; JAK: Janus activated kinase; MAPK: Mitogen-activated protein kinase; mRNA: Messenger ribonucleic acid; MSGB: Minor salivary gland biopsy; mTOR: Mammalian target of rapamycin; mTORC1: Mammalian target of rapamycin complex 1; mTORC2: Mammalian target of rapamycin complex 2; NF-κB: Nuclear factor kappa B; PI3K: Phosphoinositol-3-kinase; PKB: Protein kinase B; PKC: Protein kinase C; PTEN: Phosphatase and tensin homolog; S6K1: S6 kinase 1; SD: Standard deviation; SMAD: Small mothers against decapentaplegic; SPSS: Statistical Package of Social Science; SS: Sjogren's syndrome; SSc: Systemic sclerosis; STAT: Signal transducer and activator of transcription; TGF: Transforming growth factor

Funding

This study was supported by the Izmir Katip Celebi University Science Research Project Coordinator.

Authors' contributions

SA designed the research and revised the manuscript. ZS analyzed data and wrote the manuscript. ZZG collected data, analyzed data, and wrote the manuscript. FÇ helped with pathology diagnosis. MÖ and DS participated in case and data collection. SG and ÖG helped optimize the research and proofread the paper. All authors read and approved the final manuscript.

Consent for publication

We did not use an informed consent form since this was a retrospective study.

Competing interests

The authors declare that they have no competing interests.

Author details

[1]Department of Internal Medicine, Division of Nephrology, Izmir Katip Celebi University School of Medicine, Karabağlar, 35360 İzmir, Turkey. [2]Dogubeyazit Public Hospital, Internal Medicine, Agri, Turkey. [3]Department of Pathology, Izmir Katip Celebi University, Izmir, Turkey. [4]Department of Internal Medicine, Division of Rheumatology, Izmir Katip Celebi University, Izmir, Turkey.

References

1. Kassan SS, Moutsopoulos HM. Clinical manifestations and early diagnosis of Sjögren syndrome. Arch Intern Med. 2004;164(12):1275–84. https://doi.org/10.1001/archinte.164.12.1275.

2. Moriyama M, Tanaka A, Maehara T, Furukawa S, Nakashima H, Nakamura S. T helper subsets in Sjögren's syndrome and IgG4-related dacryoadenitis and sialoadenitis: a critical review. J Autoimmun. 2014; https://doi.org/10.1016/j.jaut.2013.07.007.

3. Manno R, Boin F. Immunotherapy of systemic sclerosis. Immunotherapy. 2010;2(6):863–78. https://doi.org/10.2217/imt.10.69.

4. Gilbane AJ, Denton CP, Holmes AM. Scleroderma pathogenesis: a pivotal role for fibroblasts as effector cells. Arthritis Res Ther. 2013;15(3):215. https://doi.org/10.1186/ar4230.

5. Liang M, Lv J, Chu H, Wang J, Chen X, Zhu X, et al. Vertical inhibition of PI3K/Akt/mTOR signaling demonstrates in vitro and in vivo anti-fibrotic activity. J Dermatol Sci. 2014;76(2):104–11. https://doi.org/10.1016/j.jdermsci.2014.08.002.

6. Populo H, Lopes JM, Soares P. The mTOR signalling pathway in human cancer. Int J Mol Sci. 2012;13(2):1886–918. https://doi.org/10.3390/ijms13021886.

7. Assinder SJ, Dong Q, Kovacevic Z, Richardson DR. The TGF-beta, PI3K/Akt and PTEN pathways: established and proposed biochemical integration in prostate cancer. Biochem J. 2009;417(2):411–21. https://doi.org/10.1042/BJ20081610.

8. Xu J, Lamouille S, Derynck R. TGF-beta-induced epithelial to mesenchymal transition. Cell Res. 2009;19(2):156–72. https://doi.org/10.1038/cr.2009.

9. Lamouille S, Connolly E, Smyth JW, Akhurst RJ, Derynck R. TGF-β-induced activation of mTOR complex 2 drives epithelial-mesenchymal transition and cell invasion. J Cell Sci. 2012; https://doi.org/10.1242/jcs.095299.

10. Wu T, Mohan C. The AKT axis as a therapeutic target in autoimmune diseases. Endocrine, Metab immune Disord -drug Targets. 2009;9(2):145–50.

11. Shah M, Edman MC, Janga SR, Shi P, Dhandhukia J, Liu S, et al. A rapamycin-binding protein polymer nanoparticle shows potent therapeutic activity in suppressing autoimmune dacryoadenitis in a mouse model of Sjogren's syndrome. J Control Release. 2013;171(3):269–79. https://doi.org/10.1016/j.jconrel.2013.07.016.

12. Vitali C, Bombardieri S, Jonsson R, Moutsopoulos HM, Alexander EL, Carsons SE, et al. Classification criteria for Sjögren's syndrome: a revised version of the European criteria proposed by the American-European consensus group. Ann Rheum Dis. 2002;61(6):554–8.

13. van den Hoogen F, Khanna D, Fransen J, Johnson SR, Baron M, Tyndall A, et al. 2013 classification criteria for systemic sclerosis: an American College of Rheumatology/European league against rheumatism collaborative initiative. Ann Rheum Dis. 2013;72(11):1747–55. https://doi.org/10.1136/annrheumdis-2013-204424.

14. Chisholm DM, Mason DK. Labial salivary gland biopsy in Sjögren's disease. J Clin Pathol. 1968;21(5):656–60.

15. Mutee AF, Kaur G, Kumar G, Muhammad TST, Khalid IA, Tan ML. Immunohistochemical evaluation of mTOR and Beclin-1 protein expression in human breast cancer and adjacent normal tissues, a study in Malaysian patients. Open Pathol J. 2009;3:111–7. https://doi.org/10.2174/1874375700903010111.

16. Sakr RA, Barbashina V, Morrogh M, Chandarlapaty S, Andrade VP, Arroyo CD, et al. Protocol for PTEN expression by immunohistochemistry in formalin-fixed paraffin-embedded human breast carcinoma. Appl Immunohistochem Mol Morphol. 2010;18(4):371–4. https://doi.org/10.1097/PAI.0b013e3181d50bd5.

17. Xie S, Macedo P, Hew M, Nassenstein C, Lee KY, Chung KF. Expression of transforming growth factor-β in idiopathic cough. Respir Res 2009; doi: https://doi.org/10.1186/1465-9921-10-40.

18. Hunzelmann N, Genth E, Krieg T, Lehmacher W, Malchers I, Meurer M, et al. The registry of the German network for systemic scleroderma: frequency of disease subsets and patterns of organ involvement. Rheumatology (Oxford). 2008;47(8):1185–92. https://doi.org/10.1093/rheumatology/ken179.

19. Forestier A, Guerrier T, Jouvray M, Giovannelli J, Lefèvre G, Sobanski V, et al. Altered B lymphocyte homeostasis and functions in systemic sclerosis. Autoimmun Rev. 2018;17(3):244–55. https://doi.org/10.1016/j.autrev.2017.10.015.

7

Relevance of interferon-gamma in pathogenesis of life-threatening rapidly progressive interstitial lung disease in patients with dermatomyositis

Yuichi Ishikawa[1], Shigeru Iwata[1], Kentaro Hanami[1], Aya Nawata[1,2], Mingzeng Zhang[1], Kaoru Yamagata[1], Shintaro Hirata[1,3], Kei Sakata[1,4], Yasuyuki Todoroki[1], Kazuhisa Nakano[1], Shingo Nakayamada[1], Minoru Satoh[5] and Yoshiya Tanaka[1*]

Abstract

Background: Dermatomyositis (DM) with rapidly progressive interstitial lung disease (DM RP-ILD) is a life-threatening condition. Serum cytokine levels are potentially suitable biomarkers for DM RP-ILD. However, the relationships among cytokine levels, lung imaging findings, and lung pathology have not been investigated. The aim of the present retrospective study was to determine the association between hypercytokinemia and lung inflammation in patients with DM RP-ILD.

Methods: The study subjects were nine patients with life-threatening DM RP-ILD and severe hypoxemia (partial arterial oxygen pressure (PaO_2)/fraction of inspired oxygen (FiO_2) ratio ≤ 200) before receiving intensive care management, who were admitted to our hospital between 2006 and 2015. The controls included 10 patients with DM without RP-ILD and 19 healthy subjects. We assessed the association between serum cytokine levels and computed tomography (CT) scores of the lung (ground glass opacity-score, G-score; fibrosis-score, F-score). Lung, hilar lymph nodes, and spleen from two autopsies were examined by hematoxylin-eosin (H&E) staining and immunostaining.

Results: Serum interferon (IFN)-γ, interleukin (IL)-1β and IL-12 levels were significantly higher in patients with DM RP-ILD than in the other two groups, whereas serum IL-6 levels were elevated in the two patient groups but not in the healthy subjects. Serum levels of IL-2, IL-4, IL-8, IL-10, IFN-α, and TNF (tumor necrosis factor)-α were not characteristically elevated in the DM RP-ILD group. Serum IFN-γ levels correlated with G-scores in patients with DM RP-ILD, while IL-1β was negatively correlation with F-scores. Immunohistochemical staining showed infiltration of numerous IFN-γ-positive histiocytes in the lung and hilar lymph nodes; but not in the spleen. Serum IL-6 levels did not correlate with the CT scores. Numerous IL-6-positive plasma cells were found in hilar lymph nodes, but not in the lungs or spleen.

Conclusions: Our results suggest strong IFN-γ-related immune reaction in the lungs and hilar lymph nodes of patients with life-threatening DM RP-ILD, and potential IFN-γ involvement in the pathogenesis of DM, specifically in the pulmonary lesions of RP-ILD.

Keywords: Rapidly progressive interstitial lung disease, Dermatomyositis, IFN-γ

* Correspondence: tanaka@med.uoeh-u.ac.jp
[1]The First Department of Internal Medicine, School of Medicine, University of Occupational and Environmental Health, Japan, 1-1 Iseigaoka, Yahatanishi-ku, Kitakyushu City 807-8555, Japan
Full list of author information is available at the end of the article

Background

The rate of interstitial lung disease (ILD) in patients with dermatomyositis (DM) is approximately 30% [1, 2]. While most patients exhibit slow progression of ILD, some exhibit rapidly progressive ILD (RP-ILD), in which the respiratory status deteriorates rapidly within 2–3 months from the onset of ILD [3–5]. In particular, a high incidence of RP-ILD has been reported in patients with clinically amyopathic dermatomyositis (cADM) who are positive for anti-melanoma differentiation-associated gene 5 (MDA5) antibodies (Abs) [6, 7]. RP-ILD in cADM is extremely difficult to treat and associated with a high mortality rate. Kameda et al. [8] reported the efficacy of intensive therapy with high-dose glucocorticoids (GC), intravenous cyclophosphamide (IVCY), and cyclosporine-A (CsA) in patients with DM complicated with RP-ILD (DM RP-ILD). Nakashima et al. [9] also reported marked improvement in prognosis of anti-MDA5 Abs-positive patients with DM using the same regimen, from the early stages of RP-ILD, with 75% survival rate by intensive immunosuppressive regimen versus only about 29% by conventional step-up therapy. Despite these encouraging reports, poor prognosis has been reported even in patients on intensive therapy, such as those with anti-MDA5 Abs-positive cADM, with a mortality rate after 6 months of treatment of as high as 25% [8]. In a retrospective analysis of 56 patients (including 49 patients with RP-ILD) treated in the intensive care unit (ICU) for exacerbation of DM/polymyositis (PM), Peng et al. [10] reported an overall survival rate of 14% (n = 8 out of 56), though the survival rate after 28 days was 0% in patients with cADM. Thus, the prognosis of anti-MDA5 Abs-positive cADM patients with RP-ILD is poor, as is the prognosis of patients with DM who develop RP-ILD during the course of treatment. Although it has been reported that treatment with tacrolimus (TAC), a calcineurin inhibitor, similar to CsA, and rituximab (RTX), is effective for life-threatening DM RP-ILD refractory to the above intensive therapy [11–13], this outcome remains to be confirmed.

Almost all anti-MDA5 Abs-positive patients have cADM with a high incidence of acute or subacute ILD [6, 14]. In a retrospective analysis of 13 patients with anti-MDA5 Abs-positive cADM, Takada et al. [15] reported that mortality was associated with high levels of anti-MDA5 Abs, suggesting that the levels of anti-MDA5 Abs could be useful in predicting prognosis. Since a strong association between DM RP-ILD and anti-MDA5 Abs has been confirmed previously in several studies, research on the pathophysiology of DM RP-ILD has been conducted mainly in anti-MDA5 Abs-positive patients [16]. High serum levels of ferritin and several types of inflammatory cytokines have been described in patients with DM RP-ILD [17–21], suggesting their involvement in the pathogenesis of RP-ILD. The pathophysiology of DM RP-ILD could be similar to that of macrophage activation syndrome (MAS), in which a variety of cytokines (e.g., interleukin (IL)-1, IL-6, tumor necrosis factor (TNF)-α) are involved [22]. However, despite studies suggesting that serum cytokines levels could be useful biomarkers for monitoring disease activity and to predict the prognosis of DM RP-ILD, the associations among serum cytokine levels, pulmonary image findings (e.g., computed tomography (CT) score) and lung pathology, have not been investigated thoroughly. The present study was designed to determine the relationships among serum cytokine levels, CT scores of the lung, and the histopathologic assessment of lung tissue.

Methods

Study design and patients

This study included nine Japanese patients with DM, aged ≥ 20 years, who had life-threatening RP-ILD and were admitted to our department between 2006 and 2015 and treated at the in-patient intensive care management unit. The term RP-ILD is not well-established and is used mainly by rheumatologists but not by pneumologists. Since we understand that the lack of standardization of the term RP-ILD can cause clinical bias and confusion, we defined RP-ILD with reference to the definition of acute respiratory distress syndrome (ARDS) in this study [23, 24]. Life-threatening RP-ILD was defined based on previous reports [7, 23, 24] as "a critical condition characterized by severe hypoxemia (PaO_2/FiO_2 ratio ≤200) that progressed within 3 months before initiation of treatment or intensification". The control groups included 10 patients with DM with ILD (that did not meet the definition of RP-ILD) who underwent high-dose GC therapy (equivalent to prednisolone (PSL) of > 1 mg/kg/day) and 19 healthy individuals. Age-matched patients with DM without RP-ILD were randomly selected from the cohort of patients with DM/PM who were admitted to our department (n = 38) between 2014 and 2015. Thus, the total number of subjects in this study was 38. With regard to evaluation of serum cytokines, the major cytokines (IL-1β, IL-2, IL-4, IL-6, IL-8, IL-10, IL-12, interferon (IFN)-γ, IFN-α, TNF-α) involved in DM RP-ILD and MAS were selected based on the literature [17–22]. Cytokine levels were measured in all disease groups before the initiation or intensification of the treatment.

For patients with DM RP-ILD, the CT scores of the lung (ground glass opacity (GGO) score (G-score), fibrosis score (F-score)) and their association with serum cytokine levels were analyzed. This study was approved by the institutional review board of our university (#H28–033).

Diagnostic criteria

The diagnosis of DM was based on the Bohan and Peter criteria for PM/DM while that of cADM was

based on the diagnostic criteria of Euwer and Sontheimer [25–28].

Exclusion criteria

Patients with pulmonary lesions due to bacterial
pneumonia, fungal pneumonia, or pneumocystis pneumonia (PCP) and those with sepsis were excluded.
Bacterial pneumonia was diagnosed based on positive
sputum culture and detection of bacteria phagocy-
tosed by leukocytes. Fungal pneumonia was diagnosed
based on positive sputum or bronchoalveolar lavage
fluid (BALF) culture for fungi, high serum β-D-glucan
levels, positivity for antigens of Candida, Aspergillus
or Cryptococcus, and chest CT findings consistent
with fungal pneumonia. PCP was diagnosed based on
positive polymerase chain reaction (PCR) of the sputum or BALF for *Pneumocystis jirovecii*, and chest CT
findings consistent with PCP. Sepsis was diagnosed
based on The Third International Consensus Definitions for Sepsis and Septic Shock [29].

RP-ILD assessment by CT scores

Lung CT was evaluated semi-quantitatively using two-types
of CT score; the G-score, which reflects changes in the acute
and active phases, and the F-score, which reflects changes
mainly in the chronic phase. Images were scored by two
rheumatologists with at least 15 years of clinical experience,
who were blinded to the demographic and clinical information. The left and right lung fields were divided into three regions and total of six lung zones were scored separately:
upper (aortic arch zone), middle (tracheal bifurcation zone),
and lower (supradiaphragmatic zone). The G-score and
F-score of each zone were scored on a scale of 0–3 (maximum score = 3 points). The final CT score used for the analysis was the mean score of the six zones assessed by the two
rheumatologists. The criteria used for the G-score were as
follows: 1 point for predominantly subpleural partial GGO
(Fig. 1A-a), 2 points for more pronounced GGO relative to
that of G-score 1 point (Fig. 1A-b), and 3 points for
diffuse GGO extending over a wide area (Fig. 1A-c).
On the other hand, the criteria used for the F-score
were as follows: 1 point for thickening and fibrosis of
parts of the interlobular septa, mainly in the subpleural area (Fig. 1B-a), 2 points for more pronounced fibrosis and bronchiectasis compared with
that for 1 point (Fig. 1B-b), and 3 points for diffuse
and widespread fibrosis, honeycomb lung, and bronchiectasis (Fig. 1B-c) [30–32].

Endpoints and clinical assessment

The primary endpoint was elucidation of the significance
of the elevated cytokines in DM RP-ILD. The secondary
endpoint was the correlation between serum cytokines
and CT scores in DM RP-ILD.

Measurements of serum cytokine levels

We measured the serum concentrations of various cytokines (IL-1β, IL-2, IL-4, IL-6, IL-8, IL-10, IL-12, IFN-α,
IFN-γ, TNF-α) at the time of admission. Serum samples
were isolated and stored at − 80 °C until analysis. The
concentrations of these cytokines were measured by cytometric bead array (Becton Dickinson, Franklin Lakes,
NJ, USA) using a FACSVerse flow cytometer (Becton
Dickinson). Data were analyzed using the FCAP Array
software (Becton Dickinson).

Immunohistochemical analysis

Immunohistochemical analysis was performed as described previously [33]. Antigen retrieval was performed
by soaking the specimen on slides in 5 M sodium citrate
solution in phosphate-buffered saline containing 0.05%
(v/v) Tween 20 (PBST) (pH 6.0). The slides were subsequently blocked with serum-free protein block (Dako,
2016–08) for 30 min at room temperature and incubated
at 4 °C overnight optimally with rabbit polyclonal antibodies to IFN-γ (ab25101, Abcam Inc., Boston, MA,
USA) or IL-6 (21865–1-AP, Proteintech Inc., Rosemont,
IL, USA) diluted 1:200 in DAKO antibody diluent. After
washing three times with PBST, the slides were incubated with anti-rabbit IgG secondary antibody conjugated with horseradish peroxidase-labeled polymer
(DakoCytomation, Glostrup, Denmark) and subsequently visualized by treatment with 3,3′ diaminobenzi-
dine (DAB) Chromogen (DakoCytomation, #K3465)
according to the instructions provided by the manufacturer. Nuclei were visualized using Mayer's hematoxylin
(MERCK, 1:1000 dilution in PBST). For mounting, the
sections were rinsed with water, dehydrated in graded
ethanol (90% ethanol for 30 s × 3 and 100% ethanol for
30 s × 3), cleared in xylene (for 30 s × 2), and sealed
using multi-mount 480 (Matsunami, FM48001). Images
were acquired and processed digitally.

Measurement of myositis-specific autoantibodies (MSAs)

We tested all serum samples by immunoprecipitation and
enzyme-linked immunosorbent assay (ELISA) using recombinant proteins for anti-MDA5, anti-Jo-1, centromere
protein A (CENP-A), CENP-B, Ro-52, and Ro-60 Abs. In
addition, in patients positive for anti-aminoacyl-transfer
ribonucleic acid synthetase (anti-ARS) Abs, the levels of
anti-glycyl-tRNA synthetase (anti-EJ), anti-threonyl-tRNA
synthetase (PL-7), anti-PL12, and anti-KS Abs were analyzed by ELISA.

Immunoprecipitation

Myositis-specific autoantibodies in serum were analyzed
by immunoprecipitation of K562 cell extracts radiola-
beled with ^{35}S-methionine as described previously [34];
the specificities of the autoantibodies were determined

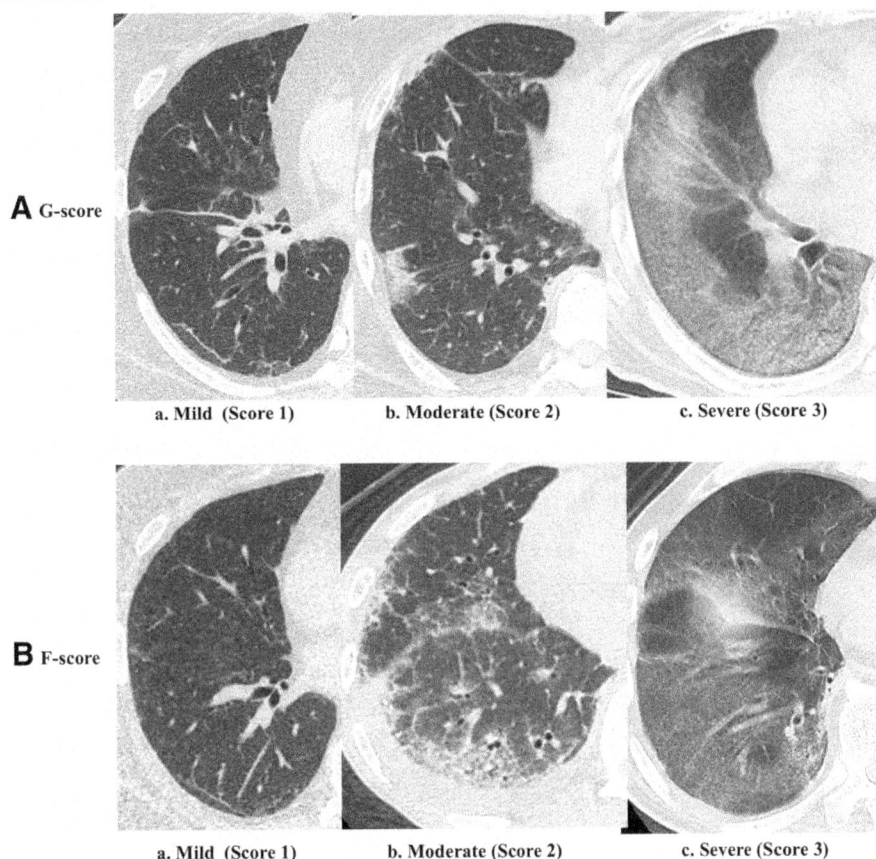

Fig. 1 Assessment of rapidly progressive interstitial lung disease (RP-ILD) by computed tomography (CT) scores. **A** Assessment of RP-ILD by CT ground glass opacity (GGO) scores (G-scores): (**a**) thin-section CT scan shows small areas with GGO compared with normal parenchyma at the right lower lobe (mild GGO = 1); (**b**) CT scan shows extensive GGO that could be easily identified when compared with the normal parenchyma at the right lower lobe (moderate GGO = 2); (**c**) thin-section CT scan shows areas with diffuse GGO at the right lower lobe (severe GGO = 3). **B** Assessment of RP-ILD by CT fibrosis scores (F-scores): (**a**) thin-section CT scan shows areas with thickened interlobular septum or predominant peripheral fibrosis (mild fibrosis = 1). (**b**) CT scan shows extensive fibrosis that could be easily identified when compared with normal parenchyma at the right lower lobe (moderate fibrosis = 2), moderate fibrosis and bronchiolectasis. (**c**) thin-section CT scan shows areas with diffuse fibrosis at the right lower lobe (severe fibrosis = 3). Note honeycombing, bronchiectasis, peribronchovascular thickening, and subpleural cysts

using specific reference serum. Analysis of RNA components of the immunoprecipitates was also performed when necessary.

Anti-MDA5 and Jo-1 ELISA

Anti-MDA5 and Jo-1 Abs were tested by enzyme-linked immunosorbent assay, using recombinant proteins (0.5 µg/ml; Diarect AG, Freiburg, Germany) and 1:250 diluted serum, as described previously [34, 35]. The optical density was measured and converted into units using a standard curve created by a prototype-positive serum. The specificity of ELISA-positive serum was confirmed by immunoprecipitation.

Statistical analysis

Continuous variables were reported as mean plus or minus standard deviation or median (interquartile range). Differences between two groups were compared using the Mann-Whitney U test. Differences among multiple groups were compared using the Kruskal-Wallis test, followed by post-hoc Dunn's multiple comparison test. Multiple group tests using the median test were also performed to determine the median values; the Wilcoxon test was used as the post-hoc test. The correlation between serum cytokine levels and CT scores was calculated using Spearman's correlation coefficient. Statistical significance was set at $p < 0.05$. Statistical analyses were performed using the JMP version 9.0 (SAS Institute Inc., Cary, NC, USA).

Results

Demographic data of patients

The demographic data of patients in the DM RP-ILD groups are summarized in Table 1. The disease duration

Table 1 Clinical characteristics of patients

	DM with RP-ILD	DM without RP-ILD	p value
n	9	10	
Age, years	69.3 ± 3.9	63.9 ± 14.2	0.68
Female (n, %)	8, 88.9	6, 60.0	0.31
Disease duration (months)	18.1 ± 39.8	7.6 ± 8.7	0.40
Smokers (current and past) (%)	11.1	30.0	0.31
Number of GC pulses	2.2 ± 1.1	N/A	
PaO$_2$/FiO$_2$ ratio	160 ± 90	N/A	
Leukocyte count (/μL)	9438 ± 5751	7620 ± 5458	0.35
LDH (U/L)	549 ± 357	376 ± 168	0.27
KL-6 (U/mL)	1087 ± 584	1419 ± 1756	0.46
IgG (mg/dL)	1225 ± 398	1452 ± 454	0.27
Positivity for anti-CADM140/MDA5 Ab (%)	66.7	50.0	0.76
CT score (G)	2.1 ± 0.7	N/A	
CT score (F)	1.2 ± 0.6	N/A	

Data are mean ± SD or number of patients (percentage)
DM dermatomyositis, *RP-ILD* rapidly progressive-interstitial lung disease, *GC* glucocorticoid, *PaO₂/FiO₂* partial arterial pressure of oxygen/fraction of inspired oxygen, *KL-6* Kerbs von Lungren 6 antigen, *CT* computed tomograpghy, *G* ground glass opacity, *F* fibrosis

of DM with and without RP-ILD was 18.1 ± 39.8 and 7.6 ± 8.7 months, respectively (Table 1). Among the 19 patients, 11 were considered to have new-onset untreated anti-MDA5 Abs-positive DM. All six anti-MDA5 antibody-positive patients with DM with RP-ILD had hypoxemia (partial arterial pressure of oxygen (PaO$_2$)/fraction of inspired oxygen (FiO$_2$) ratio ≤ 200) before starting intensive therapy and their disease duration was 1.2 ± 0.4 months. On the other hand, none of the five anti-MDA5 antibody-positive patients with DM who were free of RP-ILD were hypoxemic before the start of treatment, and their disease duration was 5.5 ± 4.3 months.

The DM RP-ILD group included two patients positive for anti-PL-7 Ab (Additional file 1: Table S1), who developed RP-ILD during the course of remission maintenance therapy and thus, had long disease duration (35 and 120 months). One patient was treated with 7.5 mg/day PSL and the other with 3 mg/day TAC. The disease duration was long in the DM with RP-ILD group because this group not only included anti-MDA5 Abs-positive patients but also two anti-PL-7 antibody-positive patients.

High serum IFN-γ, IL-1β, and IL-12 levels in patients with DM RP-ILD

Figure 2 and Additional file 2: Table S2 compare serum cytokine levels among the DM RP-ILD, DM without

RP-ILD, and HD groups, while Additional file 1: Table S1 shows antibody profiles and serum cytokine profiles in the same three groups. Serum levels of IFN-γ, IL-1β, and IL-12 were significantly higher in the DM RP-ILD group compared with the other two groups (IFN-γ, $p < 0.01$ vs DM without RP-ILD, and $p < 0.01$ vs healthy donors (HD); IL-1β, $p = 0.03$ vs DM without RP-ILD, and $p < 0.01$ vs HD; IL-12, $p < 0.01$ vs DM without RP-ILD and $p < 0.01$ vs HD). Furthermore, serum levels of IL-6, IL-10, and IFN-α were significantly higher in the DM RP-ILD group compared with the healthy donors, but were not significantly different from those in the DM without RP-ILD group. Interestingly, the serum levels of IL-2, IL-4, IL-8, and TNF-α levels were within the normal ranges in the DM RP-ILD group (Fig. 2). These results suggest that high serum levels of IFN-γ, IL-1β, and IL-12 are characteristic of DM RP-ILD. Unlike previous studies [17, 20, 21], our results showed no characteristic rises in IL-6, IL-8, IL-10, IFN-α, and TNF-α in DM RP-ILD.

Serum IFN-γ levels correlate significantly with G-score in patients with DM RP-ILD

In addition to the high serum levels of IFN-γ (Fig. 2), in the DM RP-ILD group there was positive correlation between serum IFN-γ levels and the G-scores (ρ = 0.69, $p = 0.04$, Table 2). Although serum IL-1β also correlated significantly with the F-scores, the correlation was negative (ρ = − 0.68, $p = 0.045$, Table 2). None of the other cytokines were significantly correlated with the CT scores. These results demonstrate characteristically high serum IFN-γ in patients with DM RP-ILD, and significant correlation between IFN-γ and the G-score, which is a marker of the acute phase and disease activity in ILD. Moreover, the results suggest that IFN-γ plays a major role in the pathophysiology of DM RP-ILD.

Accumulation of IFN-γ-positive histiocytes in lungs and hilar lymph nodes, and IL-6-positive plasma cells in hilar lymph nodes in patients with DM RP-ILD

Serum IFN-γ was characteristically high and correlated with the G-scores in the DM RP-ILD group, whereas serum IL-6 was not elevated characteristically and did not correlate with the CT scores (Fig. 2 and Table 2), although IL-6 is reported to be important in DM RP-ILD [17, 19, 36, 37]. In the next step, we examined the roles of IFN-γ and IL-6 in the pulmonary pathophysiology of DM RP-ILD by immunostaining and hematoxylin-eosin (H&E) staining of lung tissues, hilar lymph nodes, and spleen tissues from two patients from whom specimens were obtained on autopsy (Fig. 3).

The first patient (Case 1) was a 70-year-old man with anti-MDA5 antibody-positive cADM. The patient was treated with four courses of GC pulse therapy, TAC,

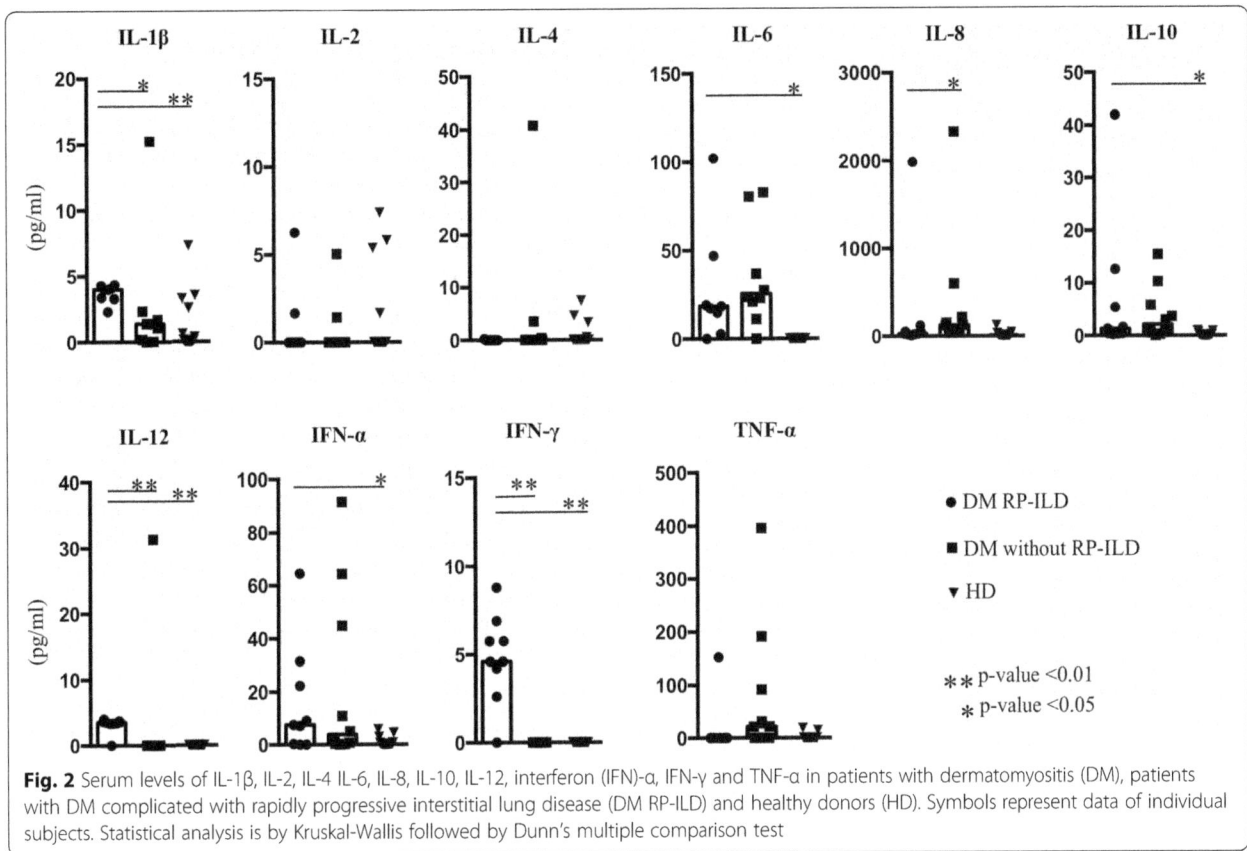

Fig. 2 Serum levels of IL-1β, IL-2, IL-4 IL-6, IL-8, IL-10, IL-12, interferon (IFN)-α, IFN-γ and TNF-α in patients with dermatomyositis (DM), patients with DM complicated with rapidly progressive interstitial lung disease (DM RP-ILD) and healthy donors (HD). Symbols represent data of individual subjects. Statistical analysis is by Kruskal-Wallis followed by Dunn's multiple comparison test

CsA, IVCY, and RTX (Fig. 3a). H&E staining showed diffuse hyaline membrane formation in the alveolar spaces. Fibroblast proliferation and incorporation of this hyaline membrane were observed in some parts, suggesting diffuse alveolar damage (DAD) extending from the exudative phase to the organizing phase (Fig. 3a (1)). Further analysis showed extravasation of erythrocytes and infiltration and aggregation of histiocytes in the alveolar spaces (Fig. 3a (2)). In these same tissues, IFN-γ-stained histiocytes had abundant cytoplasm and eccentrically distributed large nuclei (Fig. 3a (3, 4), red arrows). Marked infiltration of histiocytes was also noted into the lymph sinus of the hilar lymph nodes, with disappearance of nearly all lymphoid follicles (Fig. 3a (5, 6)). In addition to the lung tissue, IFN-γ-stained histiocytes were also found in the hilar lymph nodes (Fig. 3a (7, 8), histiocytes marked by red arrows). However, H&E staining of the spleen showed no marked histopathological changes other than splenic white pulp atrophy (Fig. 3a (9, 10)), with no infiltration of IFN-γ-positive histiocytes (Fig. 3a (11, 12)). The results of IL-6 staining are shown in Fig. 3a (13, 14, 15, 16, 17, 18). In the lung and spleen tissues, a few IL-6-positive histiocytes were observed, but cytoplasmic immunostaining was relatively weak

(Fig. 3a (13, 14, 17, 18), histiocytes marked by the red arrow). Numerous IL-6-positive plasma cells were observed in hilar lymph nodes (Fig. 3a (15, 16), plasma cells marked by blue arrows). A small number of IL-6-positive histiocytes and plasma cells were also found in the spleen (Fig. 3a (17, 18), histiocytes and plasma cells are marked by the red and blue arrows).

The other autopsy specimen was from a 65-year-old woman with anti-PL-7 antibody-positive DM treated with one course of GC pulse therapy and IVCY (Fig. 3b). At the onset of RP-ILD, she was treated with 7.5 mg/day PSL, followed by a course of GC pulse therapy, TAC, and IVCY. The histopathological findings were similar to those of the first patient, despite different treatment histories and types of MSA. These results suggest that the pathophysiology of DM RP-ILD seems to be characterized by local appearance of IFN-γ-positive histiocytes in the lung tissues and related lymphoid tissues and the appearance of IL-6-positive plasma cells in hilar lymph nodes, regardless of the treatment history and type of MSA.

Discussion

The present study demonstrated the presence of characteristically high serum IFN-γ in patients with life-threatening

Table 2 Association between CT scores and cytokines in patients with DM RP-ILD

	ρ	p value
CT scores (F)		
IFN-γ	0.10	0.80
IL-1β	− 0.68	0.05
IL-6	0.35	0.36
IL-12	− 0.14	0.71
TNF-α	− 0.43	0.25
IL-2	− 0.17	0.67
IL-4	− 0.07	0.85
IL-8	− 0.56	0.12
IL-10	−0.49	0.18
IFN-α	− 0.15	0.70
CT scores (G)		
IFN-γ	0.69	0.04
IL-1β	0.14	0.72
IL-6	0.24	0.53
IL-12	0.10	0.80
TNF-α	− 0.21	0.59
IL-2	− 0.45	0.22
IL-4	0.07	0.86
IL-8	− 0.12	0.76
IL-10	− 0.53	0.14
IFN-α	− 0.35	0.35

DM dermatomyositis, *RP-ILD* rapidly progressive-interstitial lung disease, *CT* computed tomography, *G* ground glass opacity, *F* fibrosis, *IFN* interferon, *IL* interleukin, *TNF* tumor necrosis factor

DM RP-ILD and that such levels correlated significantly with CT scores and histopathologic findings of pulmonary lesions. While high serum IL-6 reported in previous studies was also observed in patients with DM without RP-ILD, this finding might not be a characteristic of DM RP-ILD. Our results also showed significant correlation between serum IFN-γ levels and CT scores/G-scores, and infiltration of IFN-γ-positive histiocytes into the lung and hilar lymph node tissues, but not in the spleen, in patients with high disease activity. Numerous IL-6-positive plasma cells were also observed in the hilar lymph nodes but not in the lung. In the DM RP-ILD group, serum IFN-γ was elevated even in anti-MDA5 antibody-negative cases, whereas in the DM without RP-ILD group, serum IFN-γ was not elevated even in the majority of anti-MDA5 antibody-positive cases (Additional file 1: Table S1 and Additional file 2: Table S2). These results suggest that high serum IFN-γ is associated with the onset of RP-ILD, regardless of the presence of anti-MDA5 antibodies in patients with DM. Gono et al. [19] reported that anti-MDA5 antibody-positive ILD

patients with high disease activity and poor prognosis tend to have a low IL-4/IFN-γ ratio, relative to patients with anti-ARS antibody-positive DM complicated with ILD. Considered together, these findings highlight the potential role of IFN-γ in the pathophysiology of anti-MDA5 antibody-positive DM.

No common pathophysiological processes between MAS and DM RP-ILD have previously been described. MAS is a secondary hemophagocytic syndrome (HPS) or hemophagocytic lymphohistiocytosis (i.e., autoimmune-associated HPS), in which various vital organs are damaged due to abnormal production of pro-inflammatory cytokines, such as IFN-γ [38]. It has been reported that hyperferritinemia, which reflects macrophage activation, is observed in 82% of patients with MAS [39, 40]. Moreover, cytopenia and liver dysfunction were often observed in patients with MAS [39, 41]. On the other hand, serum ferritin levels correlated with disease activity in patients with anti-MDA5 antibody-positive DM complicated with RP-ILD [6], who often have liver dysfunction and cytopenia [6, 42, 43]. We identified high serum IFN-γ and the presence of IFN-γ-positive histiocytes in the lung in patients with DM RP-ILD. These results suggest that in addition to its importance in MAS, IFN-γ seems to have a pathological influence in DM RP-ILD by activating macrophages and accelerating inflammation. This is the first study to report the characteristic presence of high serum IFN-γ in DM RP-ILD and that these levels correlate with the severity of pulmonary lesions assessed by CT scores/G-scores and histopathological examination.

In DM, serum IL-6 levels correlate with disease activity [44], and the use of tocilizumab (TCZ) is effective in patients with refractory DM [45]. However, there is no information on whether TCZ is effective against DM complicated with ILD or DM RP-ILD. Our study showed that (1) serum IL-6 was not specifically high only in DM RP-ILD but also in patients with DM without RP-ILD; (2) unlike IFN-γ, high serum IL-6 did not correlate with CT scores; and (3) numerous IL-6-positive plasma cells were found in hilar lymph nodes but not in the lungs. These results suggest that while IL-6 is important in the pathogenesis of DM RP-ILD, it is unlikely to be involved in local lung injury. Although serum IL-1β levels also correlated significantly with F-scores, the correlation was negative. Correlation between serum IL-1β levels and disease activity and pulmonary lesions was examined in previous studies, but no significant correlation was detected [17]. Our results also showed no significant correlation among other cytokines and CT scores in DM RP-ILD.

We expected to find systemic autoimmune inflammation, particularly in secondary lymphoid tissues, such as the spleen, in patients with DM RP-ILD.

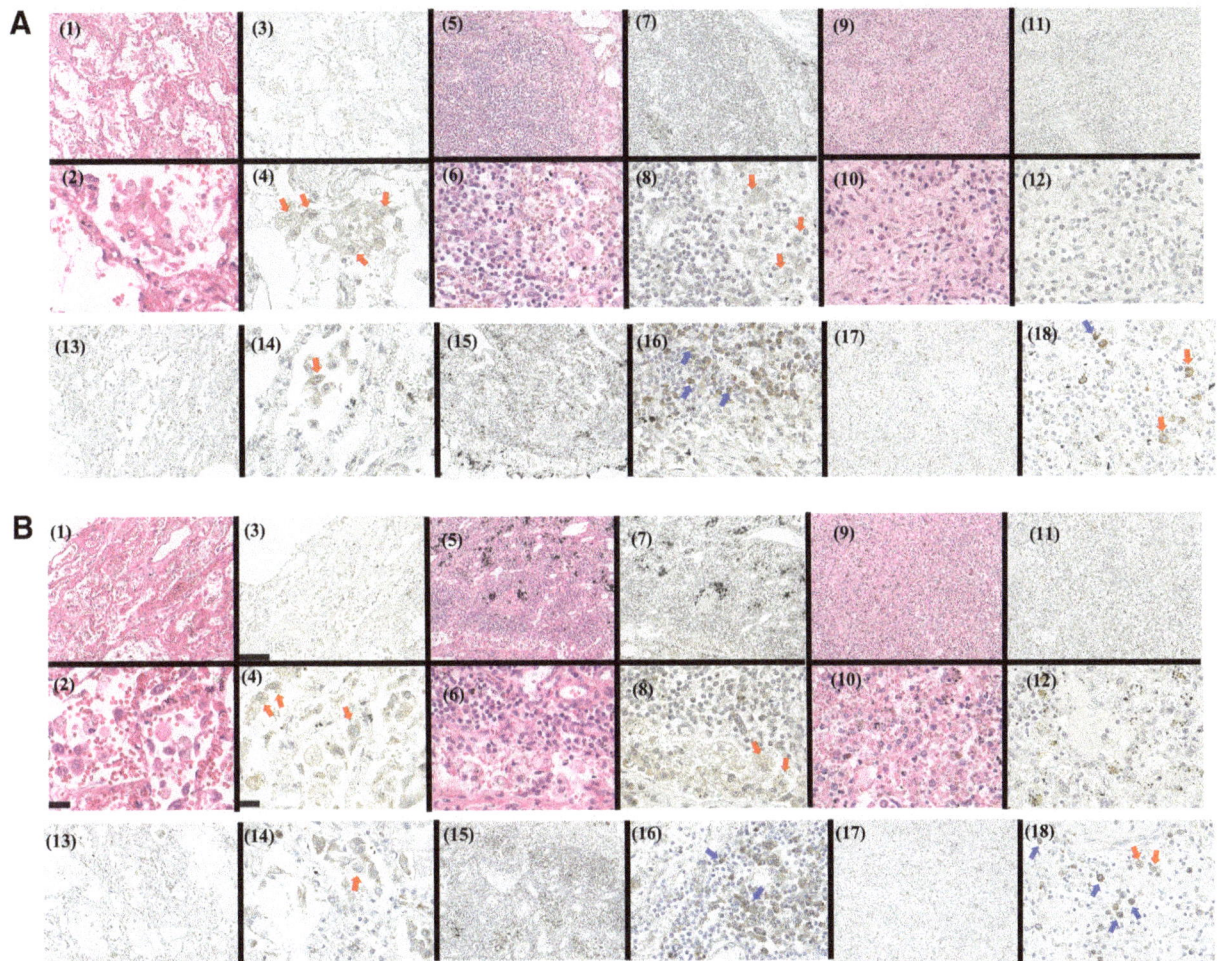

Fig. 3 Histopathological findings from two autopsies. **a** Case 1: (1, 2) lung; hematoxylin-eosin (H&E) staining; (3, 4) lung, immunostaining for interferon (IFN)-γ; (5, 6) hilar lymph nodes, H&E staining; (7, 8) hilar lymph nodes, immunostaining for IFN-γ; (9, 10) spleen, H&E staining; (11, 12) spleen immunostaining for IFN-γ; (13, 14) lung, immunostaining for interleukin (IL)-6; (15, 16) hilar lymph nodes, immunostaining for IL-6; (17, 18) spleen, immunostaining for IL-6. **b** Case 2: (1, 2) lung, H&E staining; (3, 4) lung, immunostaining for IFN-γ; (5, 6) hilar lymph nodes, H&E staining; (7, 8) hilar lymph nodes, immunostaining for IFN-γ; (9, 10) spleen, H&E staining; (11, 12) spleen, immunostaining for IFN-γ; (13, 14) lung, immunostaining for IL-6; (15, 16) hilar lymph nodes, immunostaining for IL-6; (17, 18) spleen, immunostaining for IL-6. Red arrows show histiocytes, blue arrows show plasma cells

However, contrary to our expectation, the presence of IFN-γ-positive histiocytes was limited to local regions of the lungs and pulmonary hilar lymph nodes showing diffuse DAD. Neither infiltration of IFN-γ-positive histiocytes nor histopathological changes suggestive of inflammation were observed in the spleen. Inflammation limited to localized regions of the lungs may be a significant finding that could influence the selection of the drug administration route in the future.

The present study has certain limitations. First, the number of enrolled patients was relatively small because RP-ILD is an uncommon disease. Thus, our findings need to be confirmed in larger cohort studies. Second, it is possible that immunosuppressive therapy itself altered serum cytokine levels in the present study.

Conclusions

IFN-γ was characteristically high in patients with DM RP-ILD after the onset of life-threatening RP-ILD. Furthermore, serum IFN-γ levels correlated with GGO, as evaluated by CT. Our results also suggested that inflammation might occur in localized regions of the lungs. Considered together, the results suggest the high potential of IFN-γ involvement in the pathophysiology of DM, specifically in the formation of pulmonary lesions seen in RP-ILD. Further prospective studies in large numbers of patients are needed.

Abbreviations

Abs: Antibodies; ARDS: Acute respiratory distress syndrome; ARS: Aminoacyl-transfer ribonucleic acid synthetase; BALF: Bronchoalveolar lavage fluid; cADM: Clinically amyopathic dermatomyositis; CsA: Cyclosporine-A; CT: Computed tomography; DAD: Diffuse alveolar damage; DM RP-ILD: Dermatomyositis with rapidly progressive interstitial lung disease; DM: Dermatomyositis; ELISA: Enzyme-linked immunosorbent assay; FiO$_2$: Fraction of inspired oxygen; F-score: Fibrosis score; GC: Glucocorticoid; GGO: Ground glass opacity; G-score: Ground glass opacity score; H&E: Hematoxylin-eosin; HD: Healthy donors; ICU: Intensive care unit; IFN-α: Interferon alpha; IFN-γ: Interferon gamma; IL: Interleukin; IL-1β: Interleukin-1beta; ILD: Interstitial lung disease; IVCY: Intravenous cyclophosphamide; MAS: Macrophage activation syndrome; MDA5: Melanoma differentiation-associated gene 5; MSA: Myositis-specific antibody; PaO$_2$: Partial pressure of arterial oxygen; PCP: Pneumocystis pneumonia; PM: Polymyositis; PSL: Prednisolone; RNA: Ribonucleic acid; RP-ILD: Rapidly progressive interstitial lung disease; RTX: Rituximab; TAC: Tacrolimus; TNF-α: Tumor necrosis factor-alpha

Acknowledgements

The authors acknowledge the technical assistance and expertise of Ms Narumi Sakaguchi, Ms Kahoru Noda, Ms Tomoko Hasegawa, and Dr Shin Tanaka (University of Occupational and Environmental Health, Kitakyushu, Japan).

Funding

This work was supported in part by a Grant-In-Aid for Scientific Research from the Ministry of Education, Culture, Sports, Science, and Technology of Japan (#22249025, #16 K09928, #15 K08790), the Ministry of Health, Labor, and Welfare of Japan (#H26–008), and Japan Agency for Medical Research and Development (#16ek0410016h0003).

Authors' contributions

YI, SI, KH, SN, KN, and YT conceived the design of the study. YI and YT acquired the clinical data. SI, KH, and SH evaluated the CT scores. KH and SI performed statistical analyses. YI, SI, and KH interpreted the data. KS and MZ measured serum cytokines. MS tested MSA. AN and KY performed histopathological examination. YI drafted the manuscript. All authors revised the manuscript for intellectual content and approved the final version.

Competing interests

Kei Sakata is an employee of Mitsubishi Tanabe Pharma. Shingo Nakayamada has received speaking fees from Bristol-Myers, Sanofi, AbbVie, Eisai, Eli Lilly, Chugai, Pfizer, Takeda (less than US $10,000 each), and research grants from Mitsubishi-Tanabe, Novartis and MSD. Dr Tanaka has received consulting fees, speaking fees, and/or honoraria from Mitsubishi Tanabe Pharma, Eisai, Pfizer, Abbott Immunology, Janssen, Takeda Industrial Pharma, Santen, AstraZeneca, Astellas, Asahi Kasei, UCB, and GlaxoSmithKline (less than US $10,000 each) and from AbbVie and Chugai (more than US $10,000 each) and research grants from Bristol-Myers Squibb, Mitsubishi Tanabe, MSD, Takeda Industrial Pharma, Astellas, Eisai, Chugai, Pfizer, and Daiichi-Sankyo. All other authors declare no conflict of interest.

Author details

The First Department of Internal Medicine, School of Medicine, University of Occupational and Environmental Health, Japan, 1-1 Iseigaoka, Yahatanishi-ku, Kitakyushu City 807-8555, Japan. [2]Department of Pathology and Cell Biology, School of Medicine, University of Occupational and Environmental Health, Japan, Kitakyushu City, Japan. [3]Department of Clinical Immunology and Rheumatology, Hiroshima University Hospital, Hiroshima, Japan. [4]Mitsubishi Tanabe Pharma Corporation, Yokohama, Japan. [5]Department of Clinical Nursing, School of Health Sciences, University of Occupational and Environmental Health, Japan, Kitakyushu City, Japan.

References

1. Ikezoe J, Johkoh T, Kohno N, Takeuchi N, Ichikado K, Nakamura H. High-resolution CT findings of lung disease in patients with polymyositis and dermatomyositis. J Thorac Imaging. 1996;11(4):250–9.
2. Fathi M, Vikgren J, Boijsen M, Tylen U, Jorfeldt L, Tornling G, et al. Interstitial lung disease in polymyositis and dermatomyositis: longitudinal evaluation by pulmonary function and radiology. Arthritis Rheum. 2008;59(5):677–85.
3. Fathi M, Lundberg IE. Interstitial lung disease in polymyositis and dermatomyositis. Curr Opin Rheumatol. 2005;17(6):701–6.
4. Bouros D, Nicholson AC, Polychronopoulos V, du Bois RM. Acute interstitial pneumonia. Eur Respir J. 2000;15(2):412–8.
5. Al-Hameed FM, Sharma S. Outcome of patients admitted to the intensive care unit for acute exacerbation of idiopathic pulmonary fibrosis. Can Respir J. 2004;11(2):117–22.
6. Nakashima R, Imura Y, Kobayashi S, Yukawa N, Yoshifuji H, Nojima T, et al. The RIG-I-like receptor IFIH1/MDA5 is a dermatomyositis-specific autoantigen identified by the anti-CADM-140 antibody. Rheumatology (Oxford). 2010;49(3):433–40.
7. Sato S, Hirakata M, Kuwana M, Suwa A, Inada S, Mimori T, et al. Autoantibodies to a 140-kd polypeptide, CADM-140, in Japanese patients with clinically amyopathic dermatomyositis. Arthritis Rheum. 2005;52(5):1571–6.
8. Kameda H, Nagasawa H, Ogawa H, Sekiguchi N, Takei H, Tokuhira M, et al. Combination therapy with corticosteroids, cyclosporin A, and intravenous pulse cyclophosphamide for acute/subacute interstitial pneumonia in patients with dermatomyositis. J Rheumatol. 2005;32(9):1719–26.
9. Nakashima R, Hosono Y, Mimori T. Clinical significance and new detection system of autoantibodies in myositis with interstitial lung disease. Lupus. 2016;25(8):925–33.
10. Peng JM, Du B, Wang Q, Weng L, Hu XY, Wu CY, et al. Dermatomyositis and polymyositis in the intensive care unit: a single-center retrospective cohort study of 102 patients. PLoS One. 2016;11(4):e0154441.
11. Kurita T, Yasuda S, Amengual O, Atsumi T. The efficacy of calcineurin inhibitors for the treatment of interstitial lung disease associated with polymyositis/dermatomyositis. Lupus. 2015;24(1):3–9.
12. Watanabe R, Ishii T, Araki K, Ishizuka M, Kamogawa Y, Fujita Y, et al. Successful multi-target therapy using corticosteroid, tacrolimus, cyclophosphamide, and rituximab for rapidly progressive interstitial lung disease in a patient with clinically amyopathic dermatomyositis. Mod Rheumatol. 2016;26(3):465–6.
13. Kurita T, Yasuda S, Oba K, Odani T, Kono M, Otomo K, et al. The efficacy of tacrolimus in patients with interstitial lung diseases complicated with polymyositis or dermatomyositis. Rheumatology (Oxford). 2015;54(1):39–44.
14. Sato S, Hoshino K, Satoh T, Fujita T, Kawakami Y, Kuwana M. RNA helicase encoded by melanoma differentiation-associated gene 5 is a major autoantigen in patients with clinically amyopathic dermatomyositis: association with rapidly progressive interstitial lung disease. Arthritis Rheum. 2009;60(7):2193–200.
15. Takada T, Aoki A, Asakawa K, Sakagami T, Moriyama H, Narita I, et al. Serum cytokine profiles of patients with interstitial lung disease associated with anti-CADM-140/MDA5 antibody positive amyopathic dermatomyositis. Respir Med. 2015;109(9):1174–80.
16. Abe Y, Matsushita M, Tada K, Yamaji K, Takasaki Y, Tamura N. Clinical characteristics and change in the antibody titres of patients with anti-MDA5 antibody-positive inflammatory myositis. Rheumatology (Oxford). 2017;56(9):1492–7.
17. Kawasumi H, Gono T, Kawaguchi Y, Kaneko H, Katsumata Y, Hanaoka M, et al. IL-6, IL-8, and IL-10 are associated with hyperferritinemia in rapidly progressive interstitial lung disease with polymyositis/dermatomyositis. Biomed Res Int. 2014;2014(8):15245.
18. Gono T, Sato S, Kawaguchi Y, Kuwana M, Hanaoka M, Katsumata Y, et al. Anti-MDA5 antibody, ferritin and IL-18 are useful for the evaluation of response to treatment in interstitial lung disease with anti-MDA5 antibody-positive dermatomyositis. Rheumatology (Oxford). 2012;51(9):1563–70.
19. Gono T, Kawaguchi Y, Hara M, Masuda I, Katsumata Y, Shinozaki M, et al. Increased ferritin predicts development and severity of acute interstitial lung disease as a complication of dermatomyositis. Rheumatology (Oxford). 2010;49(7):1354–60.
20. Gono T, Kaneko H, Kawaguchi Y, Hanaoka M, Kataoka S, Kuwana M, et al. Cytokine profiles in polymyositis and dermatomyositis complicated by rapidly progressive or chronic interstitial lung disease. Rheumatology (Oxford). 2014;53(12):2196–203.
21. Horai Y, Koga T, Fujikawa K, Takatani A, Nishino A, Nakashima Y, et al. Serum interferon-α is a useful biomarker in patients with anti-melanoma differentiation-associated gene 5 (MDA5) antibody-positive dermatomyositis. Mod Rheumatol. 2015;25(1):85–9.
22. Schulert GS, Grom AA. Macrophage activation syndrome and cytokine-directed therapies. Best Pract Res Clin Rheumatol. 2014;28(2):277–92.
23. Ranieri VM, Rubenfeld GD, Thompson BT, Ferguson ND, Caldwell E, Fan E, et al. Acute respiratory distress syndrome: the Berlin Definition. JAMA. 2012; 307(23):2526–33.

24. Fan E, Brodie D, Slutsky AS. Acute respiratory distress syndrome: advances in diagnosis and treatment. JAMA. 2018;319(7):698–710.

25. Bohan A, Peter JB. Polymyositis and dermatomyositis (first of two parts). N Engl J Med. 1975;292(7):344–7.

26. Bohan A, Peter JB. Polymyositis and dermatomyositis (second of two parts). N Engl J Med. 1975;292(8):403–7.

27. Euwer RL, Sontheimer RD. Amyopathic dermatomyositis: a review. J Invest Dermatol. 1993;100(1):124S–7S.

28. Sontheimer RD. Would a new name hasten the acceptance of amyopathic dermatomyositis (dermatomyositis siné myositis) as a distinctive subset within the idiopathic inflammatory dermatomyopathies spectrum of clinical illness? J Am Acad Dermatol. 2002;46(4):626–36.

29. Singer M, Deutschman CS, Seymour CW, Shankar-Hari M, Annane D, Bauer M, et al. The third international consensus definitions for sepsis and septic shock (Sepsis-3). JAMA. 2016;315(8):801–10.

30. Brantly M, Avila NA, Shotelersuk V, Lucero C, Huizing M, Gahl WA. Pulmonary function and high-resolution CT findings in patients with an inherited form of pulmonary fibrosis, Hermansky-Pudlak syndrome, due to mutations in HPS-1. Chest. 2000;117(1):129–36.

31. Terriff BA, Kwan SY, Chan-Yeung MM, Müller NL. Fibrosing alveolitis: chest radiography and CT as predictors of clinical and functional impairment at follow-up in 26 patients. Radiology. 1992;184(2):445–9.

32. Ichikado K, Suga M, Muranaka H, Gushima Y, Miyakawa H, Tsubamoto M, et al. Prediction of prognosis for acute respiratory distress syndrome with thin-section CT: validation in 44 cases. Radiology. 2006;238(1):321–9.

33. Yamagata K, Li X, Ikegaki S, Oneyama C, Okada M, Nishita M, et al. Dissection of Wnt5a-Ror2 signaling leading to matrix metalloproteinase (MMP-13) expression. J Biol Chem. 2012;287(2):1588–99.

34. Satoh M, A C MH, EKL C. Immunodiagnosis of autoimmune myopathies. In: B D RGH, JL S, editors. Manual of molecular and clinical laboratory immunology, eighth edition. 8th ed. Washington, D. C: ASM Press; 2016. p. 878–87.

35. Ceribelli A, Fredi M, Taraborelli M, Cavazzana I, Tincani A, Selmi C, et al. Prevalence and clinical significance of anti-MDA5 antibodies in European patients with polymyositis/dermatomyositis. Clin Exp Rheumatol. 2014;32(6):891–7.

36. Nara M, Komatsuda A, Omokawa A, Togashi M, Okuyama S, Sawada K, et al. Serum interleukin 6 levels as a useful prognostic predictor of clinically amyopathic dermatomyositis with rapidly progressive interstitial lung disease. Mod Rheumatol. 2014;24(4):633–6.

37. Yasuda H, Ikeda T, Hamaguchi Y, Furukawa F. Clinically amyopathic dermatomyositis with rapidly progressive interstitial pneumonia: the relation between the disease activity and the serum interleukin-6 level. J Dermatol. 2017;44(10):1164–7.

38. Grom AA, Mellins ED. Macrophage activation syndrome: advances towards understanding pathogenesis. Curr Opin Rheumatol. 2010;22(5):561–6.

39. Kumakura S, Ishikura H, Kondo M, Murakawa Y, Masuda J, Kobayashi S. Autoimmune-associated hemophagocytic syndrome. Mod Rheumatol. 2004; 14(3):205–15.

40. Bracaglia C, de Graaf K, Pires Marafon D, Guilhot F, Ferlin W, Prencipe G, et al. Elevated circulating levels of interferon-γ and interferon-γ-induced chemokines characterise patients with macrophage activation syndrome complicating systemic juvenile idiopathic arthritis. Ann Rheum Dis. 2017; 76(1):166–72.

41. Kumakura S, Murakawa Y. Clinical characteristics and treatment outcomes of autoimmune-associated hemophagocytic syndrome in adults. Arthritis Rheumatol. 2014;66(8):2297–307.

42. Gono T, Kawaguchi Y, Ozeki E, Ota Y, Satoh T, Kuwana M, et al. Serum ferritin correlates with activity of anti-MDA5 antibody-associated acute interstitial lung disease as a complication of dermatomyositis. Mod Rheumatol. 2011;21(2):223–7.

43. Hoshino K, Muro Y, Sugiura K, Tomita Y, Nakashima R, Mimori T. Anti-MDA5 and anti-TIF1-gamma antibodies have clinical significance for patients with dermatomyositis. Rheumatology (Oxford). 2010;49(9):1726–33.

44. Bilgic H, Ytterberg SR, Amin S, McNallan KT, Wilson JC, Koeuth T, et al. Interleukin-6 and type I interferon-regulated genes and chemokines mark disease activity in dermatomyositis. Arthritis Rheum. 2009;60(11):3436–46.

45. Narazaki M, Hagihara K, Shima Y, Ogata A, Kishimoto T, Tanaka T. Therapeutic effect of tocilizumab on two patients with polymyositis. Rheumatology (Oxford). 2011;50(7):1344–6.

8

Baseline metabolic profiles of early rheumatoid arthritis patients achieving sustained drug-free remission after initiating treat-to-target tocilizumab, methotrexate, or the combination: insights from systems biology

Xavier M Teitsma[1][*][†], Wei Yang[2][†], Johannes W G Jacobs[1], Attila Pethö-Schramm[4], Michelle E A Borm[5], Amy C Harms[2,3], Thomas Hankemeier[2,3], Jacob M van Laar[1], Johannes W J Bijlsma[1] and Floris P J G Lafeber[1]

Abstract

Background: We previously identified, in newly diagnosed rheumatoid arthritis (RA) patients, networks of co-expressed genes and proteomic biomarkers associated with achieving sustained drug-free remission (sDFR) after treatment with tocilizumab- or methotrexate-based strategies. The aim of this study was to identify, within the same patients, metabolic pathways important for achieving sDFR and to subsequently study the complex interactions between different components of the biological system and how these interactions might affect the therapeutic response in early RA.

Methods: Serum samples were analyzed of 60 patients who participated in the U-Act-Early trial (ClinicalTrials.gov number NCT01034137) and initiated treatment with methotrexate, tocilizumab, or the combination and who were thereafter able to achieve sDFR ($n = 37$); as controls, patients were selected who never achieved a drug-free status ($n = 23$). Metabolomic measurements were performed using mass spectrometry on oxidative stress, amine, and oxylipin platforms covering various compounds. Partial least square discriminant analyses (PLSDA) were performed to identify, per strategy arm, relevant metabolites of which the biological pathways were studied. In addition, integrative analyses were performed correlating the previously identified transcripts and proteins with the relevant metabolites.

Results: In the tocilizumab plus methotrexate, tocilizumab, and methotrexate strategy, respectively, 19, 13, and 12 relevant metabolites were found, which were subsequently used for pathway analyses. The most significant pathway in the tocilizumab plus methotrexate strategy was "histidine metabolism" ($p < 0.001$); in the tocilizumab strategy it was "arachidonic acid metabolism" ($p = 0.018$); and in the methotrexate strategy it was "arginine and proline metabolism" ($p = 0.022$). These pathways have treatment-specific drug interactions with metabolites affecting either the signaling of interleukin-6, which is inhibited by tocilizumab, or affecting protein synthesis from amino acids, which is inhibited by methotrexate.

(Continued on next page)

* Correspondence: x.m.teitsma@umcutrecht.nl
†Xavier M Teitsma and Wei Yang contributed equally to this work.
[1]Department of Rheumatology & Clinical Immunology, University Medical Center Utrecht, Heidelberglaan 100, 3584 CX Utrecht, Netherlands
Full list of author information is available at the end of the article

(Continued from previous page)

Conclusion: In early RA patients treated-to-target with a tocilizumab- or methotrexate-based strategy, several metabolites were found to be associated with achieving sDFR. In line with our previous observations, by analyzing relevant transcripts and proteins within the same patients, the metabolic profiles were found to be different between the strategy arms. Our metabolic analysis further supports the hypothesis that achieving sDFR is not only dependent on predisposing biomarkers, but also on the specific treatment that has been initiated.

Keywords: Rheumatoid arthritis, Tocilizumab, Methotrexate, Drug-free remission, Metabolomics

Background

Rheumatoid arthritis (RA) is a systemic disease characterized by inflammation and damage of the affected joints; although the cause is not known, both genetic as well as environmental factors are reported to be associated with the condition [1–4]. Initiating treatment, aiming for sustained remission or low disease activity early in the course of the disease, is important to preserve physical function and improve long-term prognosis [5–7]. Biological disease-modifying anti-rheumatic drugs (DMARDs) are to date mainly used as the second line of therapy in the management of early RA, although several studies showed their superior efficacy over traditional DMARDs in reducing disease activity and halting joint damage [8, 9]. Starting biological therapy in newly diagnosed RA patients as standard care, however, still remains highly controversial considering costs and unnecessary exposure to adverse events as a proportion of patients will be over-treated when using such an approach. Therefore, predictors are not only needed for treatment response to the currently recommended conventional DMARDs, but also for identifying patients for whom it would be favorable to initiate, as first therapy, a step-down biological-based strategy (i.e. tapering and finally discontinuing treatment) as achieving remission in the early stage of the disease improves the long-term clinical outcome.

Recent developments in "omics" technologies—such as genomics, transcriptomics, proteomics, and metabolomics—made it feasible to measure a broader spectrum of disease biomarkers for prediction of disease progression and development of personalized treatment strategies in RA [10]. Metabolomics is the non-targeted study of small-molecule metabolites and has become of increased interest in recent years due to the development and accessibility of new high-throughput technologies, including nuclear magnetic resonance spectroscopy and mass spectrometry (MS) [11]. Metabolites provide, under a given set of conditions, detailed information on cellular processes that are indicative for the disease state and are considered as the final downstream product of gene expression [12]. Especially in RA, metabolites are of particular interest as widespread cytokine-mediated inflammatory processes alter the cellular metabolism, when macrophages

and lymphocytes become activated [13]. The role of these compounds in biomarker discovery has also been demonstrated previously, suggesting that metabolic analysis is potentially valuable in identifying markers for treatment response in patients with RA [14–17].

The aim of this study was to identify relevant metabolites and important metabolomic pathways associated with achieving sustained drug-free remission (sDFR) after a treat-to-target tocilizumab- or methotrexate-based strategy initiated in DMARD-naïve early RA patients. We previously identified, within the same patients, networks of co-expressed genes [18] and several inflammatory proteins [19] associated with sDFR and now, in the present study, by revealing metabolic biomarkers, exploring the systems biology of these patients in more detail by also integrating the findings of our previous studies.

Methods

Patient selection

From the U-Act-Early strategy trial, patients were selected who achieved sDFR, defined as being drug-free for ≥ 3 months until end of the study, after initiating tocilizumab, step-up methotrexate, or tocilizumab plus methotrexate therapy. As controls, we selected patients who never achieved a drug-free status at any time point during the study. A detailed description of the study design has been reported previously [20]. Briefly, DMARD-naïve patients with early RA were randomized (1:1:1) to one of the three strategy arms and treated to the target of sustained remission, defined as disease activity score assessing 28 joints (DAS28) < 2.6 with ≤ 4 swollen joints for ≥ 24 weeks. Tocilizumab was administered intravenously every four weeks at a dose of 8 mg/kg with a maximum of 800 mg. Methotrexate (oral) was given every week with a starting dose of 10 mg and was increased to 30 mg (or maximum tolerable dose) with steps of 5 mg every four weeks until remission was reached. If the treatment target was achieved, medication was tapered stepwise and finally discontinued, if remission persisted.

Metabolomic platforms

Baseline serum samples were measured on oxidative stress, amines, and oxylipins MS platforms, which have been applied previously and are validated [21–23]. The oxidative stress platform covers various isoprostane classes, signaling lipids from the sphingosine and sphinganine classes and their phosphorylated forms, as well as three classes of lysophosphatidic acids: lysophosphatidic acids, alkyl-lysophosphatidic acids, and cyclic-lysophosphatidic acids (all in the chain length species range of C14–C22). The amine platform covers amino acids and biogenic amines and the oxylipin platform covers classical and non-classical eicosanoids from different polyunsaturated fatty acids. In total, 263 metabolites were measured for each sample on the different platforms: 57 signaling lipid mediators, 128 oxylipins, and 78 amines. Serum samples were thawed on ice and vortexed before preparation procedures following inner standard protocols [22, 23]; extra samples were pooled for internal quality control (QC). For each platform, QC samples were added and the relative standard deviation (RSD) per metabolite was calculated. Only those metabolites that complied with the acceptance criteria (RSD < 15% for amines; RSD < 30% for oxidative stress and oxylipins) were selected for further data analysis. Additional information about the metabolite profiling on the different platforms is provided in Additional file 1. All metabolite analyses were performed by the Biomedical Metabolomics Facility Leiden department at Leiden University.

Data pre-processing

For peak determination and integration, signaling lipid mediators profiled by the oxidative stress platform were pre-processed by LabSolutions (Shimadzu, Version 5.65); peak-picking of oxylipins was performed with Agilent MassHunter Quantitative Analysis software (Agilent, Version B.05.01) and amines with MultiQuant Software for Quantitative Analysis (AB SCIEX, Version 3.0.2). For all metabolites, raw data correction was accomplished using selected internal standards by calculating the ratio of peak area of the target compound to the peak area of assigned internal standard from which a response ratio for each analyte was obtained. QC samples were used for evaluating the quality of the targeted compounds according to the in-house written protocol and the data were hereafter ready to be used for statistical analyses.

Statistical analyses

Baseline clinical characteristics are described as mean (standard deviation [SD]), median (interquartile range [IQR]) or as proportions (%); between-group differences (sDFR versus controls) were tested within each strategy arm using independent t test, Mann–Whitney U test, or Pearson χ^2 test, respectively. A linear mixed model with a random intercept and baseline DAS28, week of visit, and group (sDFR versus controls) as fixed effects was built to evaluate, within the strategy arms, differences in

disease activity over time. As metabolite concentrations are influenced by a variety of factors, we performed principal component analyses (PCA) to identify possible confounders. The following parameters were considered: age; body mass index, gender, ethnicity, disease duration, smoking, alcohol consumption, seropositivity for rheumatoid factor (RF) or cyclic citrullinated peptide (CCP), erythrocyte sedimentation rate (ESR), and C-reactive protein (CRP). Thereafter, supervised partial least square discriminant analyses (PLSDA) were performed for each class (lipids, amines, and oxylipins) to identify relevant metabolites within each strategy arm. Several multivariate discrimination techniques currently exist but the main advantage of PLSDA is the handling of collinearity and noisy data (i.e. more observations than samples), both common in metabolomics experiments [24]. Data were first normalized (natural log-transformed) and then standardized (z-score) to ensure that all metabolite scores are comparable by giving them equal weight. The variable importance on projection (VIP) was used for metabolite selection; this measure accumulates the importance of each variable, whereas a higher VIP score shows that it is more relevant to predict the outcome [25]. Metabolites with VIP > 1 in the first component were considered important as the squared sum of all VIP values is equal to "1", i.e. the average VIP. Thereafter, the Mann–Whitney U test (sDFR versus controls) was performed within these selected metabolites to identify those who are most relevant ($p < 0.10$) within each strategy arm (not corrected for multiple testing), which were subsequently used for pathway analysis in the Kyoto Encyclopedia of Genes and Genomes (KEGG) databases. Pathways were considered relevant when $p \leq 0.05$. In addition, integrative analyses between the previously identified transcripts [18] and proteins [19] and relevant metabolites were performed by calculating statistically significant ($p \leq 0.05$) transcript–protein and protein–metabolite correlations (Pearson correlation coefficients [PCC]). These network analyses were visualized using VisANT 5.0 software [26, 27]. All other analyses were performed using the web-based tool MetaboAnalyst version 4.0 [28] and R version 3.4.3 (R Foundation for Statistical Computing, Vienna, Austria).

Results

Serum samples were analyzed for 60 patients (tocilizumab plus methotrexate arm: $n = 14$ sDFR, $n = 5$ controls; tocilizumab arm: $n = 13$ sDFR, $n = 11$ controls; methotrexate arm: $n = 10$ sDFR, $n = 7$ controls) and their baseline characteristics are summarized in Table 1. The mean (SD) age of all patients was 53 (14) years with a median (IQR) symptom duration of 23 (18–40) days; the majority was seropositive for rheumatoid factor (60%) or cyclic citrullinated peptide (60%). At baseline, the mean (SD) DAS28 of these patients was 4.9 (1.1) with a median

Table 1 Baseline characteristics of the patients included in the analyses

	Tocilizumab plus methotrexate		Tocilizumab		Methotrexate	
	sDFR (n = 14)	Controls (n = 5)	sDFR (n = 13)	Controls (n = 11)	sDFR (n = 10)	Controls (n = 7)
Female gender, n (%)	6 (43)	4 (80)	9 (69)	8 (73)	8 (80)	6 (86)
Age (years)	53 (16)	64 (10)	58 (14)	51 (13)	50 (14)	46 (17)
BMI (kg/m^2)	25 (4)	27 (4)	25 (2)	25 (5)	29 (4)	26 (3)
Caucasian, n (%)	13 (93)	4 (80)	13 (100)	10 (91)	10 (100)	7 (100)
Current smokers, n (%)	3 (21)	1 (20)	2 (15)	3 (27)	1 (10)	1 (14)
Symptom duration (days), median (IQR)	22 (21–40)	19 (14–55)	24 (18–39)	21 (16–25)	30 (13–40)	31 (20–45)
RF positive, n (%)	5 (34)	3 (60)	8 (62)	6 (55)	9 (90)	5 (71)
Anti-CCP positive, n (%)	5 (34)	3 (60)	8 (62)	7 (64)	7 (70)	6 (86)
CRP (mg/L), median (IQR)	5 (2–13)	5 (4–9)	15 (4–27)	14 (4–30)	11 (5–18)	5 (4–12)
ESR (mm/h), median (IQR)	18 (12–39)	25 (23–29)	26 (14–28)	20 (9–39)	25 (13–47)	16 (13–25)
DAS28 (range 0–9.4, 9.4 = maximum)	4.7 (1.2)	5.1 (0.9)	5.0 (1.1)	5.3 (1.3)	4.6 (1.2)	4.8 (0.9)
HAQ (range 0–3, 3 = worst function)	0.8 (0.5)	1.5 (0.9)	1.0 (0.6)	1.4 (0.7)	0.9 (0.6)	1.0 (0.5)
Sharp/van der Heijde score, median (IQR)	0 (0–0)	0 (0–0)	0 (0–3)	0 (0–2)	0 (0–1)	0 (0–0)

Continuous data presented as mean (SD) unless otherwise indicated

SD standard deviation, *IQR* interquartile range, *sDFR* sustained drug-free remission, *BMI* body mass index, *RF* rheumatoid factor, *CCP* cyclic citrullinated peptide, *CRP* C-reactive protein, *ESR* erythrocyte sedimentation rate, *DAS28* disease activity score assessing 28 joints, *HAQ* health assessment questionnaire

(IQR) ESR of 20 (11–32) mm/1thh and median (IQR) CRP of 9 (3–18) mg/L. No significant differences were noted in clinical characteristics at baseline between the groups (sDFR versus controls) within the strategy arms ($p \geq 0.07$). The mean (standard error) DAS28 scores over time of the sDFR and control groups are shown in Fig. 1. In the longitudinal analysis, significant lower DAS28 scores were found in the sDFR group within the tocilizumab plus methotrexate (mean − 1.18, 95% confidence interval [CI] − 0.87, − 1.50; $p < 0.001$), tocilizumab (mean − 0.87, 95% CI − 0.62, − 1.12; $p < 0.001$), and methotrexate (mean − 0.43, 95% CI -0.16, − 0.69; $p = 0.009$) arms, when compared to the control group.

Metabolite biomarkers for sDFR

PCA revealed no clear confounders (data not shown) and therefore metabolite concentrations were not corrected for clinical characteristics in further analyses. PLSDA identified 35 metabolites (15 signaling lipid mediators, 14 oxylipins, 6 amines) in the tocilizumab plus

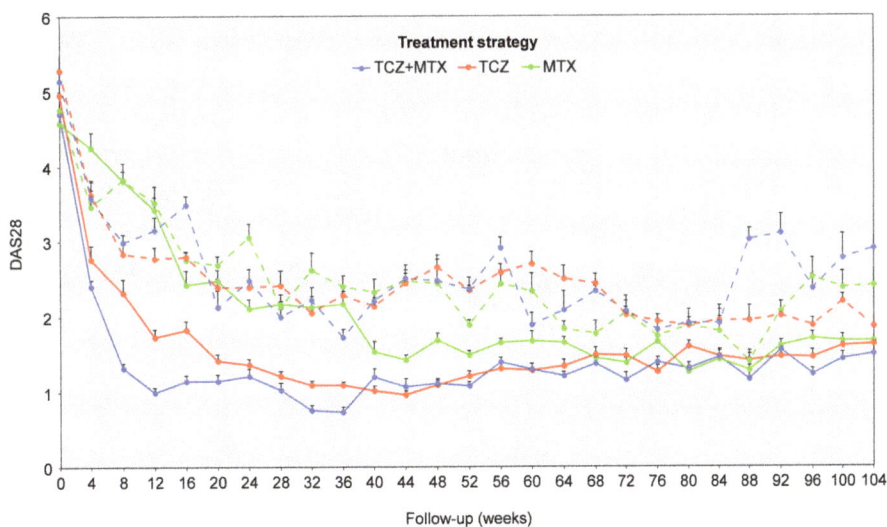

Fig. 1 Mean (SE) DAS28-ESR over time in those achieving sDFR (*continuous line*) vs controls (*dotted line*) within the three strategy arms. DAS28 disease activity score assessing 28 joints, ESR erythrocyte sedimentation rate, MTX methotrexate, sDFR sustained drug-free remission, SE standard error, TCZ tocilizumab

methotrexate arm, 33 metabolites (9 signaling lipid mediators, 15 oxylipins, 9 amines) in the tocilizumab arm, and 33 metabolites (11 signaling lipid mediators, 13 oxylipins, 9 amines) in the methotrexate arm. Of these metabolites, 19, 13, and 12, respectively, were subsequently selected for further pathway analyses (Table 2). When comparing the metabolites between the strategy arms, one (LPA c16:1) showed overlap in the tocilizumab plus methotrexate and tocilizumab arm; two (12,13-DiHODE and LPA c16:0) in the tocilizumab plus methotrexate and methotrexate strategy, and one (3-Methylhistidine) in the tocilizumab and methotrexate strategy.

Pathway analyses

Pathway overviews for each strategy arm are shown in Additional file 2. The three most relevant KEGG pathways in the tocilizumab plus methotrexate arm were "histidine metabolism" ($p < 0.001$), "sphingolipid metabolism" ($p = 0.004$), and "arachidonic acid metabolism" ($p = 0.037$). Within the "histidine metabolism" pathway, a significant lower concentration of histamine ($p = 0.002$) was found in the sDFR group when compared to controls (Fig. 2). In the "arachidonic acid metabolism" pathway, production of PGD2 and 12,13-DiHODE, 9,10,13-TriHOME, and 9,12,13-TriHOME through lipoxygenase was higher in those who achieved sDFR. Within the "sphingolipid metabolism" pathway, significantly lower levels of sphinganine (Spha c18:0, $p = 0.007$) and sphingosine (Sph c18:1, $p = 0.012$) were found in the sDFR (versus controls) group, which are both related to ceramide generation. In the tocilizumab arm, three most relevant pathways were identified: "arachidonic acid metabolism" ($p = 0.018$); "lysine degradation" ($p = 0.023$); and "cysteine and methionine metabolism" ($p = 0.030$, Fig. 2). In the "arachidonic acid metabolism" pathway, higher concentrations of prostaglandin E2 (PGE2), 8-isoprostaglandin E2 (8-iso-PGE2), prostaglandin A2 (PGA2), 8-isoprostaglandin A2 (8-iso-PGA2), 8,9-DiHETrE, and 5,6-DiHETrE ($p \le 0.08$) were found in the sDFR group, compared to controls, implying a more active role of prostaglandins and isoprostanes, which are critical signaling molecules in various inflammatory disease including RA [29–31]. Furthermore, in the "lysine degradation" pathway, significantly higher concentrations were found in the sDFR group (versus controls) of L-pipecolic acid ($p = 0.026$) and in the "cysteine and methionine metabolism" pathway, slightly but not statistically significantly lower concentrations were found in the sDFR group for cystathionine ($p = 0.052$) and homocysteine ($p = 0.09$). Most metabolites in

Table 2 Identified metabolites associated with achieving sustained drug-free remission in the three strategy arms

Tocilizumab plus methotrexate	SMD	p value	Tocilizumab	SMD	p value	Methotrexate	SMD	p value
Histamine ▼	− 1.75	0.002	PGE2 ▲	0.93	0.019	L-Lysine ▲	0.95	0.032
9,12,13-TriHOME ▲	0.52	0.002	L-Pipecolic acid ▲	0.42	0.026	L-Proline ▲	0.98	0.040
Spha c18:0 ▼	− 1.34	0.007	8,9-DiHETrE ▲	0.81	0.026	3-Methylhistidine ▼	− 1.05	0.06
9,10,13-TriHOME ▲	1.05	0.010	5,6-DiHETrE ▲	0.79	0.034	Anserine ▲	0.73	0.06
LPA c20:3 ▼	− 1.29	0.012	8-iso-PGE2 ▲	0.89	0.034	19,20-DiHDPA ▼	− 1.03	0.06
Sph c18:1 ▼	− 0.83	0.012	20-carboxy-LTB4 ▲	0.50	0.035	5-Hydroxy-L-tryptophan ▼	− 0.40	0.08
LPA c18:1 ▼	− 0.93	0.033	Cystathionine ▼	− 0.96	0.052	L-Arginine ▲	0.98	0.08
L-Methionine sulfoxide ▲	1.01	0.033	Norepinephrine ▼	− 0.39	0.052	LPA c18:3 (w3/w6) ▲	0.80	0.08
8,9-DiHETrE ▼	− 0.94	0.042	3-Methylhistidine ▼	− 0.61	0.07	12,13-DiHODE ▼	− 0.60	0.10
LPA c16:0 ▼	− 0.81	0.052	TXB2 ▲	0.82	0.08	14,15-DiHETE ▼	− 0.96	0.10
NO2-OA ▼	− 0.98	0.052	8-iso-PGA2 ▲	0.58	0.08	cLPA c16:0 ▲	0.71	0.10
L-Kynurenine ▼	− 1.03	0.06	aLPA c16:1 ▼	− 0.24	0.08	PAF c16:0 ▲	0.87	0.10
LPA c22:4 ▼	− 1.03	0.06	Homocysteine ▼	− 0.78	0.09			
LPA c20:4 ▼	− 0.97	0.06						
Methyldopa ▼	− 0.88	0.08						
PGD2 ▲	0.02	0.08						
LPA c16:1 ▼	− 0.84	0.08						
Hydroxylysine ▲	0.66	0.10						
PGF3a ▲	0.07	0.10						
12,13-DiHODE ▲	0.85	0.10						

▲On average, higher concentration in the sDFR group *vs* controls; ▼on average, lower concentration in the sDFR group *vs* controls. *sDFR* sustained drug-free remission, *SDM* standardized mean difference

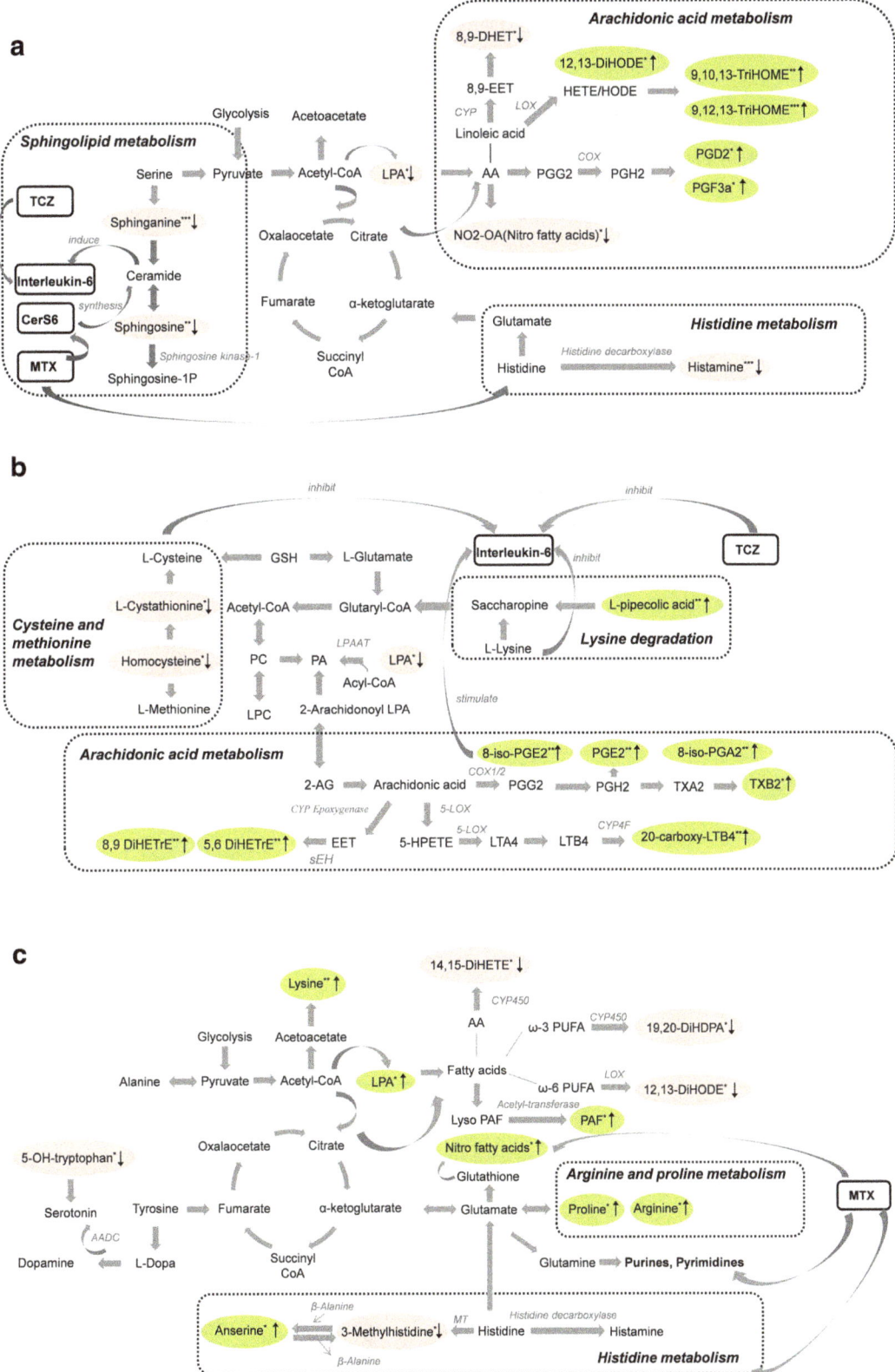

Fig. 2 (See legend on next page.)

(See figure on previous page.)

Fig. 2 Pathway analysis within the identified metabolites in the (**a**) tocilizumab plus methotrexate, (**b**) tocilizumab, and (**c**) methotrexate strategy arms. Metabolites depicted in *red* nodes have, on average, lower concentration in the sDFR group compared to controls; those depicted in *green* nodes have a higher concentration. *$p \leq 0.10$, **$p \leq 0.05$, ***$p \leq 0.01$. Metabolites not included in the top three most relevant pathways are not displayed

the methotrexate arm were associated with the "arginine and proline" and "histidine metabolism" pathways ($p = 0.022$ and $p = 0.025$, respectively). When compared to controls, lower oxylipin levels of 14,15-DiHETE, 19,20-DiHDPA, and 12,13-DiHODE were found in the sDFR group ($p \leq 0.10$), which indicates fewer active cytochromes P450 (CYP450) and lipoxygenase-based fatty acids metabolism, while the observed increased L-proline ($p = 0.040$) and L-arginine ($p = 0.08$) levels suggest a more active role of this pathway (Fig. 2). In the "histidine metabolism" pathway, decreased levels of 3-methylhistidine ($p = 0.06$) and higher levels of anserine ($p = 0.06$) were observed in the sDFR group (versus controls). Other changes of amine levels included

higher concentrations of lysine ($p = 0.032$) and lower concentrations of 5-hydroxy-tryptophan ($p = 0.08$). Another significant pathway in the methotrexate arm was "aminoacyl-tRNA biosynthesis" ($p = 0.027$).

Systems biology: from transcripts to proteins and metabolites

Figure 3 shows significant transcript–protein and protein–metabolite correlations within the three strategy arms. The average PCC between the biomarkers in the tocilizumab plus methotrexate arm was 0.54; these were 0.48 and 0.57 in the tocilizumab and methotrexate arm, respectively. Biomarkers showing > 10 connections within the networks were considered most important (i.e.

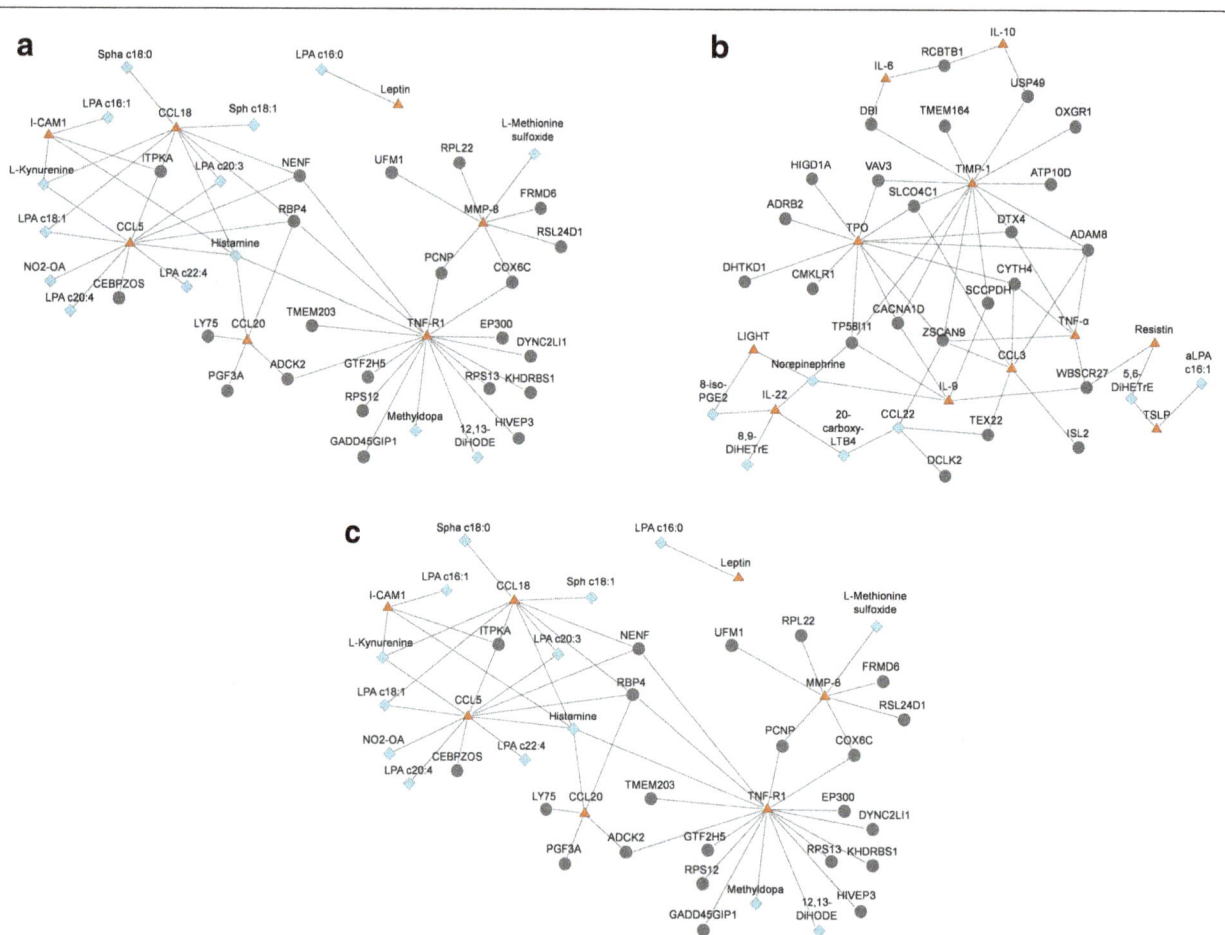

Fig. 3 Network correlation between transcriptomic (*gray* nodes), proteomic (*orange* nodes), and metabolomic (*blue* nodes) biomarkers in the (**a**) tocilizumab plus methotrexate, (**b**) tocilizumab, and (**c**) methotrexate strategy arms. Only significant transcriptomic–proteomic and proteomic–metabolomic correlations are displayed

signature biomarker) as they show the highest connectivity and therefore contribute most to the pathway analyses. The signature biomarkers in the tocilizumab plus methotrexate arm were the protein chemokine (C-C motif) ligand 5 (CCL5), as it was significantly correlated to seven metabolites and four transcripts, and the protein tumor necrosis factor receptor 1 (TNF-R1), being significantly correlated to three metabolites and 14 transcripts. In the tocilizumab arm, the proteins TIMP metallopeptidase inhibitor 1 (TIMP-1, 13 with transcripts) and thyroid peroxidase (TPO, 12 with transcripts) showed the highest number of correlations and in the methotrexate arm the protein granulocyte colony-stimulating factor (G-CSF, 4 with metabolites; 26 with transcripts).

Discussion

We identified several small-molecule metabolites, by using high-throughput MS, associated with achieving sDFR after treatment with tocilizumab- or methotrexate-based strategies in newly diagnosed RA patients. In line with our previous observations, by measuring transcripts and proteins within the same patients, different metabolic profiles were found between the treatment strategies, further supporting the hypothesis that achieving sDFR is likely dependent on pre-treatment concentrations of specific biomarkers as no differences in clinical characteristics could be found. Although we did find different metabolic pathways between the treatment strategies when using the identified metabolites, the pathways within each strategy arm were found to be specific for the respective treatment, which shows the possibility of selecting biomarkers for prediction of a good treatment-specific response.

An important metabolic pathway within the tocilizumab plus methotrexate strategy was "sphingolipid metabolism," in which ceramide synthases is closely associated with the consumption of both sphingosine, a lipid signaling molecule stimulating several cellular processes important in RA, such as cell growth, differentiation, and migration [32], and its derivative sphinganine [33]. These metabolites have been found to induce IL-6 production and may thus influence the treatment response to tocilizumab, a humanized monoclonal antibody against the IL-6 receptor. In the present analysis, lower baseline levels of sphingosine and sphinganine were found in the sDFR group of the tocilizumab plus methotrexate strategy arm when compared to controls although the opposite was expected (i.e. less inhibition resulting in higher disease activity); a possible explanation for these findings could be that patients with higher levels of IL-6 are more likely to respond to tocilizumab. To test this hypothesis, we evaluated within the same patients the absolute IL-6 concentrations in baseline (i.e. pre-treatment) serum, as was measured previously using Luminex® [19], but found no statistically significant difference between those who

would later achieve sDFR and the controls (mean 65 versus 70 pg/mL, respectively). This result confirms the findings of others showing that baseline levels of IL-6 are not predictive of clinical outcomes of tocilizumab treatment [34]. Further studies are required to elucidate on how metabolite levels are altered and how these pathophysiological changes eventually affect the response to specific therapies. Ceramide synthase 6 (CerS6), an enzyme also important in sphingolipid biosynthesis, is mediated by methotrexate [35], which might indicate a role of sphingolipids in the treatment response to a tocilizumab plus methotrexate-based strategy in early RA.

In the tocilizumab strategy arm, several involved metabolic pathways were found to be associated with signaling of the IL-6 protein whereas increased levels of prostaglandins and isoprostanes were observed in the sDFR group when compared to controls. These metabolites are involved in the metabolism of arachidonic acid, a polyunsaturated fatty acid reported to be a key intermediate promoting inflammation. Prostaglandins are known to have a stimulating effect on IL-6 and could thus influence the response to tocilizumab therapy [36]. Other important metabolites involved in IL-6 signaling are L-pipecolic acid, which is produced during the degradation of lysine, and cysteine, which is synthesized from serine. Both lysine and serine are essential amino acids in humans as they are being used in the biosynthesis of proteins whereas lysine has been reported to downregulate the release of IL-6 [37].

In the methotrexate strategy, important metabolites were proline and arginine for which higher concentrations were observed in those achieving sDFR when compared to controls. Arginine, apart from its role in protein synthesis, serves as the precursor of proline and glutamate; glutamates are involved in the generation of glutamine, which stimulates purine and pyrimidine formation that is required for cell proliferation. These organic compounds thus seem to play a crucial role in the direct treatment response to methotrexate as this drug antagonizes folic acid [38], which is important for purine and pyrimidine formation, and inhibits via this pathway the synthesis of nucleic acids and subsequently protein synthesis [39]. One of the other important amino acids for protein synthesis is histidine, of which the post-translational modified product, 3-methylhistidine, was found to have a decreased metabolism in the present study in those achieving sDFR in the methotrexate strategy. Histidine is also involved in the local immune response as it is a precursor of histamine, a compound that induces permeability of capillaries allowing, for example, leukocytes and pro-inflammatory molecules to elicit an immune response. These amino acids thus might directly affect the treatment response to methotrexate therapy.

There are some limitations to this study. First, although not uncommon in metabolomic studies, the number of samples measured was relatively small, enhancing the likelihood of false-negative findings (i.e. type II error). To minimize this risk, we used for detecting relevant metabolites analyses suitable for handling such datasets consisting of more markers than samples. Second, before the samples were measured, serum was pre-processed according to usual guidelines, which differed for each platform, and compounds were, after analyses, corrected using internal standards. These variety of factors could potentially impair replicating or external validation of findings. Third, for defining remission, and thus tapering medication, we used DAS28 criteria which is highly dependent of acute phase response and might not always reflect an inflammation-free state of the patient. To minimize this risk, no more than four swollen joints were allowed during the remission period, enhancing the likelihood that patients were also clinically in remission. Nevertheless, American College of Rheumatology (ACR)/European League Against Rheumatism (EULAR) Boolean-based remission criteria might have been a more reliable tool for assessing disease activity as it is more stringent in assessing inflammation [40].

Conclusions

We have identified several relevant metabolites in baseline serum related to achieving sDFR after treatment with tocilizumab- or methotrexate-based strategies in DMARD-naïve RA patients. In line with our previous work on the analyses of transcripts and proteins, performed within the same patients, the identified metabolic pathways were shown to be specific for the treatment that was initiated. These results might provide further insight into the role of predisposing biomarkers for eventually achieving sDFR in early RA. Signature metabolite biomarkers have been identified which could potentially serve as key prognostic factors for developing personalized care but need to be validated in large replication studies. Further studies are also warranted to elucidate on the drug metabolism in those patients with refractory disease to, by initiating other therapies based on pharmacogenomics, achieve better treatment outcomes.

Additional files

Additional file 1: Additional information regarding the metabolite profiling on the three platforms.

Additional file 2: Overview of the pathway analysis in the (a) tocilizumab plus methotrexate, (b) tocilizumab, and (c) methotrexate strategy arms. The top three most relevant pathways in the tocilizumab plus methotrexate arm were (1) "histidine metabolism," (2) "sphingolipid metabolism," and (3) "arachidonic acid metabolism;" in the tocilizumab arm, these were (1) "arachidonic acid metabolism," (2) "lysine degradation," and (3) "cysteine and methionine metabolism;" in the

methotrexate arm, these were (1) "arginine and proline metabolism," (2) "histidine metabolism," and (3) "aminocyl-tRNA biosynthesis." KEGG Kyoto Encyclopedia of Genes and Genomes, tRNA transfer ribonucleic acid. The colors of the nodes, varying from *yellow* to *red*, indicates the level of significance with *red* being highly significant; the size of the nodes depicts the impact of the pathway with larger nodes illustrating a higher impact.

Abbreviations
8-iso-PGE2: 8-isoprostaglandin E2; ACR: American College of Rheumatology; CCL5: Chemokine (c-c motif) ligand 5; CCP: Cyclic citrullinated peptide; CerS6: Ceramide synthase 6; CI: Confidence interval; CRP: C-reactive protein; CYP450: Cytochromes P450; DAS28: Disease activity score assessing 28 joints; DMARDs: Disease-modifying anti-rheumatic drugs; ESR: Erythrocyte sedimentation rate; EULAR: European League Against Rheumatism; G-CSF: Granulocyte colony-stimulating factor; IL: Interleukin; IQR: Interquartile range; KEGG: Kyoto Encyclopedia of Genes and Genomes; MS: Mass spectrometry; PCA: Principal component analyses; PGA2: Prostaglandin A2; PGE2: Prostaglandin E2; PLSDA: Partial least square discriminant analyses; QC: Quality control; RA: Rheumatoid arthritis; RF: Rheumatoid factor; SD: Standard deviation; sDFR: Sustained drug-free remission; TIMP1: TIMP metallopeptidase inhibitor 1; TNF-R1: Tumour necrosis factor receptor 1; TPO: Thyroid peroxidase; VIP: Variable importance on projection

Acknowledgements
The authors thank all participating institutions and personnel who were involved in the study, particularly (research) nurses, physicians' assistants, and rheumatologists. Lastly, the authors thank the participating patients for their kind willingness to participate.

Funding
The U-Act-Early trial was funded by Roche Nederland BV.

Authors' contributions
XMT: study design, data collection, data interpretation, and writing. WY: study design, data collection, data interpretation, and writing. JWGJ: study design, data interpretation, and writing. AP-S: data interpretation and writing. MEAB: data interpretation and writing. ACH: study design, data interpretation, and writing. TH: study design, data interpretation, and writing. JMVL: data interpretation and writing. JWJB: study design, data interpretation, and writing. FPJGL: study design, data interpretation, and writing. All authors read and approved the manuscript.

Consent for publication
Not applicable.

Competing interests
The department of the authors who included patients (JWGJ and JWJB) in the U-Act-Early trial received reimbursements from Roche Nederland BV. JWJB reported grants and fees from Roche, AbbVie, Bristol-Myers Squibb, Merck Sharp & Dohme, Pfizer, and UCB. JMvL received fees from Arthrogen, MSD, Pfizer, Eli Lilly, and BMS and research grants from Astra Zeneca, Roche-Genentech. FPJGL reports grants from Roche. AP-S is an employee of F Hoffmann-La Roche and MEAB is an employee of Roche Nederland BV. XMT, WY, ACH, and TH declare no competing interests.

Author details
[1]Department of Rheumatology & Clinical Immunology, University Medical Center Utrecht, Heidelberglaan 100, 3584 CX Utrecht, Netherlands. [2]Leiden Academic Center for Drug Research, Leiden University, 2300 RA Leiden, Netherlands. [3]Netherlands Metabolomic Centre, Einsteinweg 55, 2333 CC Leiden, Netherlands. [4]F. Hoffmann-La Roche, Grenzacherstrasse 124, 4070 CH Basel, Switzerland. [5]Roche Nederland BV, Beneluxlaan 2a, 3446 GR Woerden, Netherlands.

References

1. Pedersen M, Jacobsen S, Klarlund M, Pedersen BV, Wiik A, Wohlfahrt J, Frisch M. Environmental risk factors differ between rheumatoid arthritis with and without auto-antibodies against cyclic citrullinated peptides. Arthritis Res Ther. 2006;8(4):R133.
2. Viatte S, Plant D, Raychaudhuri S. Genetics and epigenetics of rheumatoid arthritis. Nat Rev Rheumatol. 2013;9(3):141–53.
3. Stolt P, Bengtsson C, Nordmark B, Lindblad S, Lundberg I, Klareskog L, Alfredsson L, EIRA study group. Quantification of the influence of cigarette smoking on rheumatoid arthritis: results from a population based case-control study, using incident cases. Ann Rheum Dis. 2003;62(9):835–41.
4. Liao KP, Alfredsson L, Karlson EW. Environmental influences on risk for rheumatoid arthritis. Curr Opin Rheumatol. 2009;21(3):279–83.
5. van Nies JA, Tsonaka R, Gaujoux-Viala C, Fautrel B, van der Helm-van Mil AH. Evaluating relationships between symptom duration and persistence of rheumatoid arthritis: does a window of opportunity exist? Results on the Leiden early arthritis clinic and ESPOIR cohorts. Ann Rheum Dis. 2015; 74(5):806–12.
6. Smolen JS, Landewe R, Bijlsma J, Burmester G, Chatzidionysiou K, Dougados M, Nam J, Ramiro S, Voshaar M, van Vollenhoven R, et al. EULAR recommendations for the management of rheumatoid arthritis with synthetic and biological disease-modifying antirheumatic drugs: 2016 update. Ann Rheum Dis. 2017;76(6):960–77.
7. van der Linden MP, le Cessie S, Raza K, van der Woude D, Knevel R, Huizinga TW, van der Helm-van Mil AH. Long-term impact of delay in assessment of patients with early arthritis. Arthritis Rheum. 2010;62(12): 3537–46.
8. Alfonso-Cristancho R, Armstrong N, Arjunji R, Riemsma R, Worthy G, Ganguly R, Kleijnen J. Comparative effectiveness of biologics for the management of rheumatoid arthritis: systematic review and network meta-analysis. Clin Rheumatol. 2017;36(1):25–34.
9. Hazlewood GS, Barnabe C, Tomlinson G, Marshall D, Devoe DJ, Bombardier C. Methotrexate monotherapy and methotrexate combination therapy with traditional and biologic disease modifying anti-rheumatic drugs for rheumatoid arthritis: A network meta-analysis. Cochrane Database Syst Rev. 2016;8:CD010227.
10. Priori R, Scrivo R, Brandt J, Valerio M, Casadei L, Valesini G, Manetti C. Metabolomics in rheumatic diseases: the potential of an emerging methodology for improved patient diagnosis, prognosis, and treatment efficacy. Autoimmun Rev. 2013;12(10):1022–30.
11. Kang J, Zhu L, Lu J, Zhang X. Application of metabolomics in autoimmune diseases: insight into biomarkers and pathology. J Neuroimmunol. 2015;279:25–32.
12. Morgan RP, Louise KC. Omic technologies: genomics, transcriptomics, proteomics and metabolomics. Obstet Gynaecol. 2011;13(3):189–95.
13. Chimenti MS, Triggianese P, Conigliaro P, Candi E, Melino G, Perricone R. The interplay between inflammation and metabolism in rheumatoid arthritis. Cell Death Dis. 2015;6:e1887.
14. Cuppen BV, Fu J, van Wietmarschen HA, Harms AC, Koval S, Marijnissen AC, Peeters JJ, Bijlsma JW, Tekstra J, van Laar JM, et al. Exploring the inflammatory metabolomic profile to predict response to TNF-alpha inhibitors in rheumatoid arthritis. PLoS One. 2016;11(9):e0163087.
15. Priori R, Casadei L, Valerio M, Scrivo R, Valesini G, Manetti C. ^{1}H-NMR-based metabolomic study for identifying serum profiles associated with the response to etanercept in patients with rheumatoid arthritis. PLoS One. 2015;10(11):e0138537.
16. Chimenti MS, Tucci P, Candi E, Perricone R, Melino G, Willis AE. Metabolic profiling of human CD4+ cells following treatment with methotrexate and anti-TNF-alpha infliximab. Cell Cycle. 2013;12(18):3025–36.
17. Kapoor SR, Filer A, Fitzpatrick MA, Fisher BA, Taylor PC, Buckley CD, McInnes IB, Raza K, Young SP. Metabolic profiling predicts response to anti-tumor necrosis factor alpha therapy in patients with rheumatoid arthritis. Arthritis Rheum. 2013;65(6):1448–56.
18. Teitsma XM, Jacobs JWG, Mokry M, Borm MEA, Petho-Schramm A, van Laar JM, Bijlsma JWJ, Lafeber FPJ. Identification of differential co-expressed gene networks in early rheumatoid arthritis achieving sustained drug-free remission after treatment with a tocilizumab-based or methotrexate-based strategy. Arthritis Res Ther. 2017;19(1):170.
19. Teitsma XM, Jacobs JWG, Concepcion AN, Petho-Schramm A, Borm MEA, van Laar JM, Bijlsma JWJ, Lafeber F. Explorative analyses of protein biomarkers in patients with early rheumatoid arthritis achieving sustained drug-free remission after treatment with tocilizumab- or methotrexate-based strategies: from transcriptomics to proteomics. Clin Exp Rheumatol. 2018; [Epub ahead of print].
20. Bijlsma JW, Welsing PM, Woodworth TG, Middelink LM, Petho-Schramm A, Bernasconi C, Borm ME, Wortel CH, ter Borg EJ, Jahangier ZN, et al. Early rheumatoid arthritis treated with tocilizumab, methotrexate, or their combination (U-Act-Early): a multicentre, randomised, double-blind, double-dummy, strategy trial. Lancet. 2016;388(10042):343–55.
21. Schoeman JC, Harms AC, van Weeghel M, Berger R, Vreeken RJ, Hankemeier T. Development and application of a UHPLC-MS/MS metabolomics based comprehensive systemic and tissue-specific screening method for inflammatory, oxidative and nitrosative stress. Anal Bioanal Chem. 2018; 410(10):2551–68.
22. Strassburg K, Huijbrechts AM, Kortekaas KA, Lindeman JH, Pedersen TL, Dane A, Berger R, Brenkman A, Hankemeier T, van Duynhoven J, et al. Quantitative profiling of oxylipins through comprehensive LC-MS/MS analysis: application in cardiac surgery. Anal Bioanal Chem. 2012;404(5):1413–26.
23. Noga MJ, Dane A, Shi S, Attali A, van Aken H, Suidgeest E, Tuinstra T, Muilwijk B, Coulier L, Luider T, et al. Metabolomics of cerebrospinal fluid reveals changes in the central nervous system metabolism in a rat model of multiple sclerosis. Metabolomics. 2012;8(2):253–63.
24. Gromski PS, Muhamadali H, Ellis DI, Xu Y, Correa E, Turner ML, Goodacre R. A tutorial review: Metabolomics and partial least squares-discriminant analysis--a marriage of convenience or a shotgun wedding. Anal Chim Acta. 2015;879:10–23.
25. Mehmood T, Hovde Liland K, Snipen L, Saebo S. A review of variable selection methods in Partial Least Squares Regression. Chemom Intell Lab Syst. 2012;118:62–9.
26. Hu Z, Mellor J, Wu J, DeLisi C. VisANT: an online visualization and analysis tool for biological interaction data. BMC Bioinformatics. 2004;5:17.
27. Hu Z, Snitkin ES, DeLisi C. VisANT: an integrative framework for networks in systems biology. Brief Bioinform. 2008;9(4):317–25.
28. Chong J, Soufan O, Li C, Caraus I, Li S, Bourque G, Wishart DS, Xia J. MetaboAnalyst 4.0: towards more transparent and integrative metabolomics analysis. Nucleic Acids Res. 2018;46(W1):W486–94.
29. Basu S. Bioactive eicosanoids: role of prostaglandin F(2alpha) and F(2)-isoprostanes in inflammation and oxidative stress related pathology. Mol Cell. 2010;30(5):383–91.
30. Hata AN, Breyer RM. Pharmacology and signaling of prostaglandin receptors: multiple roles in inflammation and immune modulation. Pharmacol Ther. 2004;103(2):147–66.
31. Fattahi MJ, Mirshafiey A. Prostaglandins and rheumatoid arthritis. Arthritis. 2012;2012:239310.
32. Hu PF, Chen Y, Cai PF, Jiang LF, Wu LD. Sphingosine-1-phosphate: a potential therapeutic target for rheumatoid arthritis. Mol Biol Rep. 2011; 38(6):4225–30.
33. Mullen TD, Hannun YA, Obeid LM. Ceramide synthases at the centre of sphingolipid metabolism and biology. Biochem J. 2012;441(3):789–802.
34. Wang J, Devenport J, Low JM, Yu D, Hitraya E. Relationship between baseline and early changes in C-reactive protein and interleukin-6 levels and clinical response to tocilizumab in rheumatoid arthritis. Arthritis Care Res. 2016;68(6):882–5.
35. Fekry B, Esmaeilniakooshkghazi A, Krupenko SA, Krupenko NI. Ceramide synthase 6 is a novel target of methotrexate mediating its antiproliferative effect in a p53-dependent manner. PLoS One. 2016;11(1):e0146618.
36. Li P, Shan JX, Chen XH, Zhang D, Su LP, Huang XY, Yu BQ, Zhi QM, Li CL, Wang YQ, et al. Epigenetic silencing of microRNA-149 in cancer-associated fibroblasts mediates prostaglandin E2/interleukin-6 signaling in the tumor microenvironment. Cell Res. 2015;25(5):588–603.
37. Al-Malki AL. Suppression of acute pancreatitis by L-lysine in mice. BMC Complement Altern Med. 2015;15:193.
38. Wessels JA, Huizinga TW, Guchelaar HJ. Recent insights in the pharmacological actions of methotrexate in the treatment of rheumatoid arthritis. Rheumatology (Oxford). 2008;47(3):249–55.
39. Guma M, Tiziani S, Firestein GS. Metabolomics in rheumatic diseases: desperately seeking biomarkers. Nat Rev Rheumatol. 2016;12(5):269–81.
40. Bykerk VP, Massarotti EM. The new ACR/EULAR remission criteria: rationale for developing new criteria for remission. Rheumatology (Oxford). 2012; 51(Suppl 6):vi16–20.

9

Musculoskeletal manifestations occur predominantly in patients with later-onset familial Mediterranean fever: Data from a multicenter, prospective national cohort study in Japan

Yushiro Endo[1], Tomohiro Koga[1*] [iD], Midori Ishida[1], Yuya Fujita[1], Sosuke Tsuji[1], Ayuko Takatani[1], Toshimasa Shimizu[1], Remi Sumiyoshi[1], Takashi Igawa[1], Masataka Umeda[1], Shoichi Fukui[1], Ayako Nishino[1], Shin-ya Kawashiri[1], Naoki Iwamoto[1], Kunihiro Ichinose[1], Mami Tamai[1], Hideki Nakamura[1], Tomoki Origuchi[1], Kazunaga Agematsu[2], Akihiro Yachie[3], Junya Masumoto[4], Kiyoshi Migita[5] and Atsushi Kawakami[1]

Abstract

Background: We showed previously that Japanese individuals with familial Mediterranean fever (FMF) have a more atypical phenotype compared to endemic areas. The clinical differences between young-onset FMF (YOFMF), adult-onset FMF (AOFMF), and late-onset FMF (LOFMF) in Japan are unclear.

Methods: We enrolled 395 consecutive patients. We defined YOFMF, AOFMF, and LOFMF as the onset of FMF at < 20, 20–39, and ≥ 40 years of age, respectively. We compared clinical manifestations and *MEFV* mutations patterns among these groups.

Results: Median ages at onset were YOFMF 12.5 years ($n = 182$), AOFMF 28 years ($n = 115$), and LOFMF 51 years ($n = 90$). A family history, *MEFV* mutations in exon 10, and more than two *MEFV* mutations were significantly more frequent in the earlier-onset groups ($p < 0.01$, $p < 0.0001$, and $p < 0.001$, respectively). In the accompanying manifestations, thoracic and abdominal pain were significantly more frequent in the earlier-onset groups ($p < 0.01$ and $p < 0.0001$, respectively), whereas arthritis and myalgia were significantly more frequent in the later-onset groups ($p < 0.0001$ and $p < 0.01$, respectively). The multiple logistic regression analysis revealed that the presence of *MEFV* exon 10 mutations and earlier onset were significantly associated with serositis, whereas the absence of *MEFV* exon 10 mutations, later onset, and the presence of erysipelas-like erythema were significantly associated with musculoskeletal manifestations. There was no significant between-group difference in the responsiveness to colchicine.

Conclusions: Our results indicate that the later-onset FMF patients had a lower percentage of *MEFV* mutations in exon 10 and predominantly presented arthritis and myalgia. It is important to distinguish their FMF from other inflammatory diseases.

Keywords: Familial Mediterranean fever, *MEFV* gene, Young onset, Late onset, Musculoskeletal manifestations

* Correspondence: tkoga@nagasaki-u.ac.jp
[1]Department of Immunology and Rheumatology, Unit of Advanced Preventive Medical Sciences, Nagasaki University Graduate School of Biomedical Sciences, 1-7-1 Sakamoto, Nagasaki 852-8501, Japan
Full list of author information is available at the end of the article

Background

Familial Mediterranean fever (FMF) is an autoinflammatory disease caused by Mediterranean fever (*MEFV*) gene mutations located on the short arm of chromosome 16 (16 pm 13.3) [1, 2]. FMF is characterized by recurrent and self-limiting fever attacks in a short period accompanied by serositis manifestations including peritonitis and pleuritis, musculoskeletal manifestations including synovitis and myalgia, and skin manifestations including erysipelas-like skin lesions [3–6]. A patient's FMF can be classified as a typical or an atypical case based on clinical findings and genetic testing [7–9]. According to the Tel Hashomer criteria, a typical case is characterized by fever attacks of ≥ 38.0 °C and lasting 12–72 h accompanied by pleuritis, nonlocalized peritonitis, and monoarthritis of the hip, knee, or ankle [7], whereas an atypical case is characterized by fever attacks of < 38.0 °C, lasting only a short period (i.e., 6–12 h) or lasting a long period (72 h–7 days), abdominal pain without definitive peritonitis, localized peritonitis, or arthritis outside the typical sites (i.e., hip, knee, and ankle) [7].

FMF is most prevalent in individuals in the Mediterranean and Middle Eastern regions, especially in Turks, Arabs, Armenians, and non-Ashkenazi Jews [10, 11]. However, FMF cases have increasingly been reported in some countries outside these regions, such as Japan and the USA [12]. In particular, Japanese FMF cases with *MEFV* mutations were described for the first time in 2002 [13], and there is accumulating evidence showing the characteristics of FMF in Japan [9, 14–19]. The frequency of FMF cases with high-penetrance *MEFV* mutations such as exon 10 is lower in Japan than in Western countries, and FMF cases in Japan have been reported to more often be adult onset and to more often show atypical clinical symptoms [9]. Because of the misunderstanding that FMF is rare in Japan, or that there is a higher percentage of earlier onset in Japan, it is possible that the condition's diagnosis has been delayed [16].

The onset of FMF in an individual over 40 years of age has been considered rare. A survey of 470 cases showed that approximately 60% of the patients experienced the first attack before 10 years of age, 90% of those experienced the first attack before 20 years of age, and most of the rest of the patients experienced the first attack before 40 years of age [5]. Although there is no definition to classify later-onset FMF including adult-onset FMF (AOFMF) and late-onset FMF (LOFMF), previous studies defined AOFMF and LOFMF as the onset of FMF over 20 and 40 years of age, respectively [20, 21], and revealed that a subgroup of patients with AOFMF or LOFMF is characterized by different demographic, clinical, and probably genetic features [20–23]. However, characteristics of later-onset FMF have not yet been fully elucidated in Japan.

In the present study, using data from a nationwide, multicenter, prospective study in Japan, we compared the clinical characteristics and the distribution of *MEFV* mutations among AOFMF, LOFMF, and YOFMF patients and determined the factors that can distinguish these three groups.

Methods
Patients

This was a prospective cohort study registered with the University Hospital Medical Information Network Clinical Trials Registry (#UMIN000015881; http://www.umin.ac.jp/ctr/). The study population consisted of 395 Japanese patients with FMF who were recruited consecutively and prospectively between January 2009 and March 2017 from 106 related centers of Nagasaki University, Shinshu University, Kanazawa University, and Nagasaki Medical Center in Japan. Each of the FMF patients fulfilled the Tel Hashomer criteria [7]. All patients underwent a clinical assessment and provided a blood sample for *MEFV* mutation analyses.

On the basis of the Tel Hashomer criteria, we divided the study patients into two groups: those with typical FMF and those with atypical FMF. The typical FMF patients had suffered typical episodes of peritonitis, pleuritis, monoarthritis, or fever alone as specified in the Tel Hashomer criteria. The atypical FMF patients had suffered an "incomplete" attack. An attack was considered incomplete if it differed from the definition of a typical attack in only one or two of the four following features: temperature < 38 °C; attack duration longer or shorter than specified periods (12 h–3 days), but not shorter than 6 h or longer than 1 week; no signs of peritonitis during an abdominal attack, or signs were localized; and atypical distribution of arthritis.

We defined YOFMF, AOFMF, and LOFMF as the onset of FMF at < 20, 20–39, and ≥ 40 years of age, respectively. We compared clinical manifestations including the characteristics of febrile episodes (duration and frequency), presence of serositis (chest or abdominal pain), arthritis, myalgia, erysipelas-like rash, and response to colchicine. We also compared the three groups' laboratory findings obtained during an attack including white blood cell count (WBC), C-reactive protein (CRP) level, serum amyloid A (SAA) level, erythrocyte sedimentation (ESR), and IgD level. All patients gave their signed informed consent to be subjected to the protocol, which was approved by the Institutional Review Board of Nagasaki University and related centers (Approval No. 14092946).

Mutational analysis

We extracted genomic DNA using the Promega Wizard® Genomic DNA Purification Kit (Promega, Madison, WI, USA). We subsequently performed polymerase chain reaction (PCR) using the forward and reverse primers for each exon of the *MEFV* gene as described [9]. We purified PCR products with the reagent ExoSAP-IT™ (GE Healthcare Japan, Tokyo) and sequenced directly, using specific primers and BigDye Terminator v1.1 (Applied Biosystems, Tokyo, Japan).

Statistical analysis

The demographic, clinical, and genomic characteristics among the YOFMF, AOFMF and LOFMF patients were compared with Fisher's exact test for discrete variables, and with Wilcoxon's test for continuous variables. The Kruskal–Wallis test followed by Dunn's multiple comparisons test were used to compare the groups.

We performed a sensitivity analysis by removing patients with mutations in exon 10 or overlapping rheumatic disease, because mutations of exon 10 in the *MEFV* gene are associated with typical FMF [9] and overlapping rheumatic disease influences clinical symptoms. To determine the independent factors of the patients' serositis or musculoskeletal manifestations, we performed a multiple logistic regression analysis. We selected variables with $p < 0.05$ by univariate analyses as model 1 (continuous variables for age at onset) or model 2 (binary variables for age at onset). Statistical analyses were performed in JMP pro 13.0 software (SAS Institute, Cary, NC, USA). All reported p values are two-sided. $p < 0.05$ was considered significant.

Results

Patient characteristics, classification, and complications

A total of 395 patients were enrolled in the study. We excluded eight patients from the analyses due to a lack of age data. The demographic characteristics of the patients with YOFMF ($n = 182$), AOFMF ($n = 115$), and LOFMF ($n = 90$) are presented in Table 1. The median age at diagnosis in the YOFMF, AOFMF, and LOFMF groups was 19, 34, and 58 years, respectively. The groups' median period between the onset of symptoms and the disease diagnosis was 7, 4, and 2 years, respectively (YOFMF vs others, $p < 0.0001$; others vs LOFMF, $p < 0.0001$). There was no significant difference in gender among the groups. The family history suggestive of FMF was observed in 28%, 17%, and 12% of the YOFMF, AOFMF, and LOFMF groups, respectively, and a significantly higher frequency of family history was observed among the earlier-onset groups (YOFMF vs others, $p < 0.01$; others vs LOFMF, $p < 0.05$).

The numbers of patients with the typical FMF phenotype according to the Tel Hashomer criteria [7] in the YOFMF, AOFMF, and LOFMF groups were 111 (61%), 57 (50%), and 46 (51%), respectively. We found that the YOFMF group had a significantly higher percentage of patients with typical FMF (YOFMF vs others, $p < 0.05$;

others vs LOFMF, $p = 0.40$). In the YOFMF, AOFMF, and LOFMF groups, the rates of amyloidosis as a complication were 1%, 4%, and 3% and the rates of the complication of autoimmune or autoinflammatory diseases were 5%, 10%, and 24%, respectively. Autoimmune or autoinflammatory diseases mainly included diseases such as rheumatoid arthritis (RA), systemic lupus erythematosus (SLE), Sjögren's syndrome (SS), Behçet's disease (BD), and adult-onset Still's disease (AOSD). There was a significantly higher percentage of overlapping autoimmune or autoinflammatory diseases among the later-onset group compared to the other groups (YOFMF vs others, $p < 0.001$; others vs LOFMF, $p < 0.0001$).

Clinical and laboratory characteristics

The demographic clinical characteristics of the patients with YOFMF, AOFMF, and LOFMF are presented in Table 2. No significant differences were found in the attack frequency or the attack duration among the three groups. Although we found no significant differences in the presence of fever, pericarditis, headache, or erysipelas erythema during the attack, the serositis symptoms such as chest pain and abdominal pain were significantly fewer in the later-onset group: YOFMF vs others, $p < 0.01$; others vs LOFMF, $p < 0.01$; YOFMF vs others, $p = 0.0001$; and others vs LOFMF, $p < 0.0001$. In contrast, musculoskeletal symptoms such as joint pain and myalgia were significantly more frequent in the later-onset group: YOFMF vs others, $p < 0.0001$; others vs LOFMF, $p < 0.0001$; YOFMF vs others, $p < 0.01$; and others vs LOFMF, $p < 0.01$. We examined the efficacy of colchicine therapy in each group and found no significant difference in this parameter among the three groups.

We next evaluated laboratory characteristics and found that there were no significant between-group differences in WBC count, CRP level, SAA level, or IgD level during the attack. The median ESR values during the attack in the YOFMF, AOFMF, and LOFMF groups were 40, 41.5, and 56 mm/h, respectively (YOFMF vs others, $p = 0.07$; others vs LOFMF, $p < 0.05$). It is likely that this difference in ESR can be explained by the influence of age.

Mutational analysis

The results of our demographic mutational analysis of the YOFMF, AOFMF, and LOFMF groups are presented in Table 3. Mutations accompanied by amino acid substitutions of the *MEFV* gene in the YOFMF, AOFMF, and LOFMF patients were observed in 94%, 92%, and 87%, respectively (data not significant). When we compared mutations in the groups by the site of mutations, we found no significant difference in exon 2 or exon 3 in each group. In contrast, mutations in exon 1 in the YOFMF, AOFMF, and LOFMF patients were observed at

Table 1 Patient characteristics, classification, and complications in patients with YOFMF, AOFMF, and LOFMF (univariate analyses)

Variable	YOFMF (n = 182)	AOFMF (n = 115)	LOFMF (n = 90)	p value		
				YOFMF vs AOFMF vs LOFMF	YOFMF vs others	Others vs LOFMF
Age at onset (years)	12.5 (6–15, n = 182)	28 (22–33, n = 115)	51 (45–61, n = 90)	NA	NA	NA
Age at diagnosis (years)	19 (12–30, n = 182)	34 (29–39, n =115)	58 (48.5–68, n = 90)	NA	NA	NA
Interval between disease onset and diagnosis (years)	7 (2–15.5, n = 182)	4 (1–11, n = 115)	2 (0.5–8, n = 90)	< 0.0001	< 0.0001	< 0.0001
Male gender	67/181 (37%)	53/115 (46%)	37/88 (44%)	0.29	0.15	0.81
Family history	51/182 (28%)	20/115 (17%)	11/90 (12%)	0.0055	0.0026	0.018
Typical FMF	111/182 (61%)	57/115 (50%)	46/90 (51%)	0.10	0.041	0.40
AA amyloidosis	2/182 (1%)	5/115 (4%)	3/90 (3%)	0.20	0.11	0.70
Autoimmune or autoinflammatory diseases	9/182 (5%)	12/115(10%)	22/90 (24%)	< 0.0001	0.0003	< 0.0001
RA	0/182 (0%)	0/115 (0%)	9/90 (10%)	< 0.0001	0.0040	< 0.0001
SLE	1/182 (1%)	1/115 (1%)	2/90 (2%)	0.43	0.63	0.23
SS	1/182 (1%)	3/115 (3%)	0/90 (0%)	0.13	0.63	0.58
PM or DM	0/182 (0%)	2/115 (2%)	1/90 (1%)	0.23	0.25	0.55
BD	0/182 (0%)	3/115 (3%)	1/90 (1%)	0.10	0.13	1.00
AOSD	0/182 (0%)	2/115 (2%)	2/90 (2%)	0.16	0.13	0.23
Others (i.e., RS3PE syndrome, Basedow disease, UC, ITP, MS, PBC, and unknown)	7/182 (4%)	1/115 (1%)	7/90 (8%)	0.040	0.98	0.054

Median (interquartile range, number) or number (percentage) presented. p values established using Fisher's exact test or Mann–Whitney U test

YOFMF young-onset FMF, *AOFMF* adult-onset FMF, *LOFMF* late-onset FMF, *FMF* familial Mediterranean fever, *NA* not available, *AA* amyloid A, *RA* rheumatoid arthritis, *SLE* systemic lupus erythematosus, *SS* Sjögren's syndrome, *PM* polymyositis, *DM* dermatomyositis, *BD* Behçet's disease, *AOSD* adult-onset Still's disease, *RS3PE* remitting seronegative symmetrical synovitis with pitting edema, *UC* ulcerative colitis, *ITP* idiopathic thrombocytopenic purpura, *MS* multiple sclerosis, *PBC* primary biliary cholangitis

Table 2 Clinical and laboratory characteristics in patients with YOFMF, AOFMF, and LOFMF (univariate analyses)

Variable	YOFMF (n = 182)	AOFMF (n = 115)	LOFMF (n = 90)	p value		
				YOFMF vs AOFMF vs LOFMF	YOFMF vs others	Others vs LOFMF
Frequency of febrile attack (/month)[a]	1.0 (0.3–1.0, n = 157)	1.0 (0.4–1.0, n = 97)	0.5 (0.4–1.0, n = 74)	0.90	0.66	0.66
Duration of fever attack (days)[a]	2.5 (2–4, n = 165)	3 (2–4.8, n = 101)	2.5 (2–5, n = 71)	0.25	0.25	0.75
Headache	25/161 (16%)	18/91 (20%)	10/65 (15%)	0.65	0.65	0.85
Thoracic pain	82/182 (45%)	38/115 (33%)	22/90 (24%)	0.0025	0.0015	0.0060
Abdominal pain	117/182 (64%)	64/115 (56%)	27/90 (30%)	< 0.0001	0.0001	< 0.0001
Pericarditis	3/161 (2%)	3/91 (3%)	4/65 (6%)	0.25	0.21	0.13
Arthritis	58/182 (32%)	55/115 (48%)	56/90 (62%)	< 0.0001	< 0.0001	< 0.0001
Myalgia	13/161 (8%)	16/91 (18%)	17/65 (26%)	0.0014	0.0012	0.0051
Erysipelas-like erythema	18/182 (10%)	16/115 (14%)	17/90 (19%)	0.11	0.10	0.076
Good response to colchicine	124/126 (98%)	85/87 (98%)	69/71 (97%)	0.84	0.70	0.64
WBC ($\times 10^3$/µl)[a]	10 (7.2–13, n = 126)	9.1 (7.2–12.5, n = 64)	9.1 (7.4–12, n = 48)	0.84	0.65	0.94
CRP (mg/dl)[a]	7.1 (4.0–12.7, n = 132)	7.1 (2.1–11.1, n = 65)	9.4 (3.4–15, n = 50)	0.12	0.46	0.22
SAA (µg/ml)[a]	85 (206–1246, n = 43)	423 (55–1100, n = 13)	300 (105–702, n = 9)	0.23	0.10	0.18
ESR (mm/h)[a]	40 (24–51, n = 39)	41.5 (15.5–56, n = 10)	56 (35–90, n = 15)	0.063	0.075	0.019
IgD (mg/dl)[a]	4.2 (1.1–10.9, n = 17)	1.5 (1.0–2.3, n = 3)	10 (1.9–18, n = 2)	0.41	0.64	0.46

Median (interquartile range, number) or number (percentage) presented. p values established using Fisher's exact test or Mann–Whitney U test

YOFMF young-onset FMF, AOFMF adult-onset FMF, LOFMF late-onset FMF, FMF familial Mediterranean fever, WBC white blood cell count, CRP C-reactive protein, SAA serum amyloid A, ESR erythrocyte sedimentation, IgD immunoglobulin D

Table 3 Comparison of mutational analysis in patients with YOFMF, AOFMF, and LOFMF (univariate analyses)

Variable	YOFMF (n = 182)	AOFMF (n = 115)	LOFMF (n = 90)	p value		
				YOFMF vs AOFMF vs LOFMF	YOFMF vs others	Others vs LOFMF
MEFV mutations (+)	171/182 (94%)	106/115 (92%)	78/90 (87%)	0.12	0.14	0.078
Exon 1 mutations (+)	11/182 (6%)	6/115 (5%)	0/90 (0%)	0.064	0.15	0.016
Exon 2 mutations (+)	127/182 (70%)	83/115 (72%)	61/90 (68%)	0.79	1.00	0.60
Exon 3 mutations (+)	22/182 (12%)	14/115 (12%)	15/90 (17%)	0.54	0.65	0.29
Exon 10 mutations (+)	89/182 (49%)	35/115 (30%)	16/90 (18%)	< 0.0001	< 0.0001	< 0.0001
Heterozygote mutations (+)	22/182 (12%)	13/115 (11%)	5/90 (6%)	0.23	0.32	0.11
More than two *MEFV* mutations (+)	125/182 (69%)	65/115 (57%)	41/90 (46%)	0.0009	0.0009	0.0022

Number (percentage) presented. *p* values established using Fisher's exact test or Mann–Whitney *U* test

YOFMF young-onset FMF, *AOFMF* adult-onset FMF, *LOFMF* late-onset FMF, *FMF* familial Mediterranean fever, *MEFV* Mediterranean fever gene

6%, 5%, and 0%, respectively (YOFMF vs others, $p = 0.15$; others vs LOFMF, $p < 0.0001$), and mutations in exon 10 were observed in 49%, 30%, and 18%, respectively (YOFMF vs others, $p < 0.0001$; others vs LOFMF, $p < 0.0001$).

We analyzed the percentage of patients with two or more *MEFV* mutations among the three groups and found that the rate of having two or more mutations in the *MEFV* gene was higher in the earlier-onset groups: YOFMF vs others, $p < 0.001$; and others vs LOFMF, $p < 0.01$.

Sensitivity analysis

To conduct a sensitivity analysis, we excluded patients with exon 10 mutation in the *MEFV* gene and patients with rheumatic disease, and reanalyzed the clinical and genetic characteristics among the YOFMF, AOFMF and LOFMF patients. A flow chart of this sensitivity analysis is shown in Additional file 1: Figure S1. As presented in Table 4, we found no significant between-group differences in the proportion of typical FMF, a positive family history, two or more mutations, or chest pain.

Interestingly, the presence of mutation in exon 1 and abdominal pain during the attack were significantly more frequently observed in the earlier-onset group: YOFMF vs others, $p < 0.05$; others vs LOFMF, $p < 0.01$; YOFMF vs others, $p < 0.001$; and others vs LOFMF, $p < 0.0001$. In contrast, the later-onset group presented musculoskeletal manifestations more frequently than the earlier-onset group: YOFMF vs others, $p < 0.05$; others vs LOFMF, $p < 0.05$; YOFMF vs others, $p < 0.001$; and others vs LOFMF, $p < 0.05$.

Identification of independent factors associated with serositis manifestations

To determine which variables are associated with serositis manifestations among the three groups, we evaluated the 20 variables presented in Tables 1, 2, 3. We found that the following nine variables were significantly associated with serositis in the univariate analyses: age at onset, family history, typical FMF, duration of fever attack, arthritis, erysipelas-like erythema, autoimmune or autoinflammatory diseases, exon 3 mutation, and exon 10 mutation.

We selected these variables for a logistic regression analysis and identified three independent factors associated with serositis manifestations: age at onset (odds ratio (OR) 0.43, 95% confidence interval (CI) 0.24–0.78, $p = 0.0051$), autoimmune or autoinflammatory diseases (OR 0.21, 95% CI 0.09–0.55, $p = 0.0006$), and positive exon 10 mutations (OR 10.7, 95% CI 4.15–27.7, $p < 0.0001$) (model 2 in Table 5). Taking these results together, we determined that age at FMF onset, complication of autoimmune or autoinflammatory diseases, and exon 10 mutation in the *MEFV* gene are independent factors that are associated with serositis manifestation.

Identification of independent factors associated with musculoskeletal manifestations

We next sought to determine variables that are associated with musculoskeletal manifestations among the three groups. We found that the following six variables were significantly associated with musculoskeletal manifestations in the univariate analyses: age at onset, typical FMF, abdominal pain, erysipelas-like erythema, autoimmune or autoinflammatory diseases, and exon 10 mutation. By performing a logistic regression analysis, we identified three independent factors associated with musculoskeletal manifestations: age at onset (OR 1.84, 95% CI 1.12–2.99, $p = 0.0077$), erysipelas-like erythema (OR 4.30, 95% CI 2.04–9.05, $p < 0.0001$), and positive exon 10 mutations (OR 0.54, 95% CI 0.31–0.93, $p < 0.0027$) (model 2 in Table 6). Collectively, these results led us to conclude that age at FMF onset, erysipelas-like erythema, and exon 10 mutation in the *MEFV* gene are independent factors associated with musculoskeletal manifestation.

Discussion

Our findings clarified the differences in later-onset FMF including AOFMF and LOFMF. Our data showed that later-onset FMF patients have a shorter diagnostic delay, a lower frequency of family history, a lower frequency of typical cases, a higher frequency of complications of autoimmune or autoinflammatory diseases, and a lower frequency of *MEFV* mutations in exons 1 and 10. Importantly, our analyses revealed that later-onset FMF patients predominantly present musculoskeletal manifestations, which is independent of overlapping rheumatic diseases and the *MEFV* mutation in exon 10.

The manifestations of FMF are attributed mainly to the difference in the mutational pattern in the *MEFV* gene [3, 9, 18, 19]. FMF patients with low-penetrance mutations tend to present with milder disease phenotypes and to be diagnosed with atypical FMF [24–26]. In addition, the M694 V mutations in exon 10 mutations, which is high penetrance, are associated with earlier onset and severe phenotypes [27, 28], suggesting an association between high penetrance and earlier onset. Consistent with these observations, our present analyses demonstrated that the earlier-onset FMF patients had a higher frequency of MEFV exon 10 mutations with high penetrance. Interestingly, our analyses also showed that E84K in exon 1 mutations was significantly more frequent in patients with earlier onset. We confirmed these results by performing the sensitivity analysis excluding the FMF cases with MEFV exon 10 mutations.

The age at disease onset is variable in FMF. As noted in the Introduction, the survey of 470 FMF cases in the 1960s showed that approximately 90% of patients experienced their first attack before 20 years of age, and the

Table 4 Characteristics of the YOFMF, AOFMF, and LOFMF patients in a sensitivity analysis removing patients with mutations in exon 10 or overlapping rheumatic diseases (univariate analyses)

Variable	YOFMF (n = 91)	AOFMF (n = 74)	LOFMF (n = 61)	p value		
				YOFMF vs AOFMF vs LOFMF	YOFMF vs others	Others vs LOFMF
Typical FMF	33/91 (36%)	25/74 (34%)	25/61 (41%)	0.68	1.00	0.44
Family history	15/91 (16%)	9/74 (12%)	6/61 (10%)	0.47	0.32	0.51
Exon 1 mutations (+)	11/91 (12%)	6/74 (8%)	0/61 (0%)	0.021	0.041	0.0078
Exon 2 mutations (+)	62/91 (68%)	58/74 (78%)	40/61 (66%)	0.20	0.55	0.32
Exon 3 mutations (+)	22/91 (24%)	14/74 (19%)	12/61 (20%)	0.67	0.41	0.86
More than two *MEFV* mutations (+)	48/91 (53%)	39/74 (53%)	24/61 (39%)	0.20	0.42	0.10
Thoracic pain	17/91 (19%)	19/74 (26%)	17/61 (28%)	0.36	0.20	0.38
Abdominal pain	55/91 (60%)	34/74 (46%)	13/61 (21%)	< 0.0001	0.0002	< 0.0001
Arthritis	40/91 (44%)	39/74 (53%)	39/61 (64%)	0.053	0.043	0.036
Myalgia	4/76 (5%)	12/56 (21%)	12/42 (29%)	0.0018	0.0007	0.016

Number (percentage) presented. *p* values established using Fisher's exact test or Mann–Whitney *U* test

YOFMF young-onset FMF, *AOFMF* adult-onset FMF, *LOFMF* late-onset FMF, *FMF* familial Mediterranean fever, *MEFV* Mediterranean fever gene

Table 5 Comparison of selected variables for thoracic or abdominal pain in multiple logistic regression analysis (continuous and binary variables)

Variable	p value	OR (95% CI)
Model 1		
Age at onset	0.0081	0.979 (0.963–0.995)
Family history	0.4012	1.415 (0.624–3.209)
Typical FMF	0.0437	2.023 (1.018–4.021)
Duration of fever attack	0.7985	1.012 (0.924–1.108)
Arthritis	0.8003	0.926 (0.510–1.681)
Erysipelas-like erythema	0.2824	0.655 (0.302–1.418)
Autoimmune or autoinflammatory diseases	0.0007	0.218 (0.0858–0.557)
Exon 3 mutations (+)	0.7587	0.890 (4.018–26.716)
Exon 10 mutations (+)	< 0.0001	10.361 (4.018–26.716)
Model 2		
Age at onset ≥20 years	0.0051	0.431 (0.238–0.782)
Family history	0.3733	1.445 (0.636–3.284)
Typical FMF	0.0527	1.970 (0.991–3.920)
Duration of fever attack	0.8415	1.009 (0.920–1.107)
Arthritis	0.7936	0.924 (0.509–1.675)
Erysipelas-like erythema	0.1723	0.589 (0.275–1.262)
Autoimmune or autoinflammatory diseases	0.0006	0.216 (0.085–0.545)
Exon 3 mutations (+)	0.7174	0.872 (0.414–1.835)
Exon 10 mutations (+)	< 0.0001	10.718 (4.148–27.694)

Odds ratio (OR), 95% confidence interval (CI), and p value in model 1 or model 2 presented
FMF familial Mediterranean fever

Table 6 Comparison of selected variables for arthritis or myalgia in multiple logistic regression analysis (continuous and binary variables)

Variable	p value	OR (95% CI)
Model 1		
Age at onset	0.0006	0.978 (0.965–0.991)
Typical FMF	0.8131	0.940 (0.565–1.564)
Abdominal pain	0.4751	0.842 (0.526–1.348)
Erysipelas-like erythema	< 0.0001	4.153 (1.960–8.802)
Autoimmune or autoinflammatory diseases	0.1988	1.609 (0.773–3.349)
Exon 10 mutations (+)	0.0315	0.550 (0.318–0.950)
Model 2		
Age at onset ≥ 20 years	0.0077	1.840 (1.175–2.882)
Typical FMF	0.7933	0.935 (0.564–1.549)
Abdominal pain	0.2795	0.7745 (0.488–1.229)
Erysipelas-like erythema	< 0.0001	4.295 (2.039–9.050)
Autoimmune or autoinflammatory diseases	0.1224	1.752 (0.851–3.605)
Exon 10 mutations (+)	0.0272	0.541 (0.313–0.935)

Odds ratio (OR), 95% confidence interval (CI), and p value in model 1 or model 2 presented
FMF familial Mediterranean fever

onset of FMF at > 40 years of age was rare [5]. A survey in the 2000s, when FMF had gradually come to be recognized, showed that the proportions of FMF patients whose age at onset was over 20 years and over 40 years were 14% and 1.25%, respectively [20]. Thus, later-onset FMF has been considered rare worldwide.

In contrast, later-onset FMF is more common in Japan compared to Western countries. Two studies from Japan revealed that the mean ± SD age at onset is 24.2 ± 18.1 years [9] and 23.7 ± 13.6 years [17], respectively. The present study showed that age at onset > 20 years and > 40 years occurred in 52% (205/395) and 23% (90/395) of all FMF patients, and our results support the idea that adult-onset FMF is not rare in Japan. We speculate that the genetic characteristics of Japanese FMF patients (i.e., with a lower percentage of *MEFV* exon 10 mutations and a higher percentage of *MEFV* exon 2 mutations [9]) may explain the reason for the higher percentage of later-onset Japanese FMF.

A delay in the diagnosis of FMF often occurs, even in endemic areas [20, 22]. Because of self-limiting attacks that occur in a short period, FMF patients may not see a doctor or may not be referred to a specialized department, making it difficult to diagnose FMF correctly in the early course of the disease. Two studies from endemic areas revealed that the mean delay before diagnosis was 6.0 ± 6.6 years (adult onset) versus 12.1 ± 9.0 years (others) [20] and was 4.9 ± 5.8 years (late onset) versus 20 ± 13 years (others) [21], respectively. In line with these observations, our present findings indicate that the age at earlier disease onset caused a delay in diagnosis. This may be attributed to more attention being paid by adults to new manifestations and more effort being made to receive a final diagnosis [21, 22].

Most studies of childhood FMF demonstrated that FMF affects both sexes equally [5, 29–32]. It was also shown that the proportion of males was not significantly different between the young-onset and adult-onset groups [20]. However, other studies showed that later-onset FMF is characterized by male predominance [21, 22]. This is because women with later-onset FMF present a milder disease phenotype, resulting in a lesser likelihood of being diagnosed with FMF [21]. In the present study, although the proportion of males tended to be higher in the AOFMF group than in the YOFMF group, there was no significant difference between the two groups.

Our previous investigation demonstrated that the presence of *MEFV* exon 10 mutations was associated with typical FMF presentation and that typical FMF had a higher frequency of a family history of FMF [9]. Our present findings showed that earlier-onset FMF patients have significantly higher frequency of a family history as well as *MEFV* mutations in exon 10. We considered that

high-penetrance mutations such as exon 10 increase the frequency of a family history. We also observed that the YOFMF group had a significantly higher frequency of typical FMF cases, probably because YOFMF patients more frequently have *MEFV* mutations in exon 10.

Our study showed that earlier-onset FMF patients predominantly present serositis manifestations including peritonitis and pleuritis, while later-onset FMF patients predominantly present musculoskeletal manifestations including synovitis and myalgia. Conversely, earlier studies showed that arthritis and erysipelas-like erythema are less frequent in adult-onset FMF compared to young-onset FMF [20, 22], which differs from our observations. However, these earlier studies did not perform sufficient analyses of the genetic differences with age at onset. Similar to our observations, a recent study from a Western country showed that LOFMF patients presented a high frequency of arthritis without significant difference and significantly less frequent chest pain compared to patients with a disease onset before 40 years of age [33]. It may thus be important to distinguish later-onset FMF from other inflammatory diseases such as crystalline-induced arthropathies and infectious arthritis.

Our multiple logistic regression analysis revealed that the presence of *MEFV* exon 10 mutations and earlier onset were significantly associated with serositis during attacks. Although this differs from some previous reports [20, 22], our analyses also revealed that the absence of *MEFV* exon 10 mutations, later onset, and the presence of erysipelas-like erythema were significantly associated with musculoskeletal manifestations. Collectively, our data indicate that the *MEFV* mutations in exon 10 with high penetrance are associated with both a high frequency of serositis and a low frequency of musculoskeletal manifestations. Japanese FMF patients not only have a lower percentage of *MEFV* exon 10 mutations but also a lower percentage of *MEFV* homozygous mutations associated with high penetrance [9, 17]. In addition, no Japanese FMF patients have the M694 V mutations in exon 10 mutations, which is especially high penetrance [9, 17]. The discrepancy between our findings and those of previous studies may be explained by the genetic characteristics of Japanese FMF patients, who have a lower percentage of *MEFV* mutations with high penetrance, especially in later-onset FMF. In addition, the discrepancy may be associated with racial differences including genetic characteristics other than the *MEFV* gene. This study is the first to describe the characteristics of FMF patients with adult onset and late onset in a country (Japan) other than endemic areas, suggesting different characteristics of FMF patients with later onset between endemic areas and other areas. We await the further accumulation of reports from locations other than endemic areas. Interestingly, the presence of erysipelas-like erythema was the strongest factor determining the presence of musculoskeletal manifestations. It was reported that the proportions of arthritis and erysipelas-like erythema are correlated [20, 22, 34], thus suggesting that these manifestations may develop with similar pathological conditions.

Since colchicine is primarily effective as a prophylactic treatment for FMF attacks, colchicine is recommended in all FMF patients regardless of the frequency and intensity of attacks. Later-onset FMF patients were described as having a milder form of disease and more favorable responses even to low-dose colchicine [21–23]. Most of the FMF patients in the present study had a good response to colchicine and there was no significant difference in secondary amyloidosis suggesting a severe phenotype among the three groups. There is a report showing that FMF patients with high-penetrance M694 V mutation in exon 10 needed higher-dose colchicine to achieve a good response [28], and there is also a report showing these patients have a significantly lower frequency of complete response to colchicine compared to patients with other MEFV mutations [35], suggesting that there may be an association between high-penetrance mutations and good response to colchicine. We suspect that Japanese FMF patients have good response to colchicine irrespective of age at onset and that there is no significant difference among the present three patient groups because of the higher frequency of low-penetrance mutations.

There are some study limitations to acknowledge. First, it remains questionable whether the diagnosis of FMF was correct in all of our cases. The diagnosis of FMF should be made based on clinical findings, not on the presence of MEFV gene mutations [36]. We also diagnosed FMF based on clinical findings in the present study. However, other hereditary autoinflammatory diseases cannot be completely ruled out. In addition, a good response to colchicine itself is one of the diagnostic criteria [7], and thus it is possible that patients with a poor response to colchicine were diagnosed as non-FMF.

Second, although we concluded an association with musculoskeletal symptoms and older-onset FMF by a sensitivity analysis after excluding patients with rheumatic disease, a few cases in later-onset FMF may have presented musculoskeletal symptoms due to the presence of subclinical rheumatic diseases. It has been reported that the MEFV gene mutations can be a risk for rheumatic diseases such as AOSD [37] and BD [38], and can modify clinical phenotypes of rheumatic diseases such as RA [39] and SLE [40]. In addition, it is generally known that the incidence of autoimmune diseases increases in proportion to age, and it is possible that rheumatic diseases before onset may be included in the adult-onset group or the late-onset group. Although each rheumatologist examined other overlapping rheumatic diseases at the diagnosis of FMF, there was no detailed information available on the profiles of autoantibodies.

Finally, there are no established standard criteria to evaluate the disease activity of FMF and the effectiveness of colchicine, and we were thus unable to evaluate these parameters accurately in the present study. The International Severity Score for FMF (ISSF) was recently recommended as a new criterion for evaluating the disease activity of FMF [41], and the FMF 50 score [42] is also recommended as a new criterion for evaluating the effectiveness of treatments such as colchicine and the necessity of intensive treatment. In the future, it is necessary to prospectively compare the disease activity and good response rate to colchicine of patients with young-onset, adult-onset, and late-onset FMF.

Conclusions

This is the first study to describe the characteristics of Japanese FMF patients with adult onset and late onset. Our results indicate that the later-onset FMF patients had a lower percentage of mutations in exon 1 and exon 10 of the MEFV gene, and they presented a higher frequency of musculoskeletal manifestations and a lower frequency of serositis during their attacks. It is thus important to distinguish their FMF from other inflammatory diseases such as crystalline-induced arthropathies and infectious arthritis.

Abbreviations
AOFMF: Adult-onset FMF; AOSD: Adult-onset Still's disease; BD: Behçet's disease; CI: Confidence interval; CRP: C-reactive protein; ESR: Erythrocyte sedimentation; FMF: Familial Mediterranean fever; ISSF: International Severity Score for FMF; LOFMF: Late-onset FMF; OR: Odds ratio; PCR: Polymerase chain reaction; RA: Rheumatoid arthritis; SAA: Serum amyloid A; SLE: Systemic lupus erythematosus; SS: Sjögren's syndrome; WBC: White blood cell count; YOFMF: Young-onset FMF

Acknowledgements
The authors wish to thank the patients and medical staff for their contribution to the study, and the 106 related centers of Nagasaki University, Shinshu University, Kanazawa University, and Nagasaki Medical Center for their assistance with patients' data.

Funding
This work was supported by the Japan Agency for Medical Research and Development (Grant no. 15657398).

Authors' contributions
TK had full access to all of the data in the study and takes responsibility for the integrity of the data and the accuracy of the data analysis. YE and TK were responsible for study design. YE, TK, MI, YF, ST, AT, TS, RS, TI, MU, SF, AN, S-yK, NI, KI, MT, HN, TO, KA, AY, JM, KM, and AK were responsible for acquisition of data. YE, TK were responsible for analysis and interpretation of data, manuscript preparation, and statistical analysis. All authors read and approved the final manuscript.

Consent for publication
All authors consented to publication of this manuscript.

Competing interests

The authors declare that they have no competing interests.

Author details

[1]Department of Immunology and Rheumatology, Unit of Advanced Preventive Medical Sciences, Nagasaki University Graduate School of Biomedical Sciences, 1-7-1 Sakamoto, Nagasaki 852-8501, Japan. [2]Department of Infection and Host Defense, Graduate School of Medicine, Shinshu University, 3-1-1 Asahi, Matsumoto 390-8621, Japan. [3]Department of Pediatrics, School of Medicine, Kanazawa University, 13-1 Takaramachi, Kanazawa 920-8641, Japan. [4]Proteo-Science Center, Ehime University, 3 Bunkyo-cho, Matsuyama 790-8577, Japan. [5]Department of Rheumatology, Fukushima Medical University School of Medicine, 1 Hikariga-oka, Fukushima 960-1295, Japan.

References

1. Ancient missense mutations in a new member of the RoRet gene family are likely to cause familial Mediterranean fever. The International FMF Consortium. Cell 1997, 90(4):797–807.
2. French FMF Consortium. A candidate gene for familial Mediterranean fever. Nat Genet. 1997;17(1):25–31.
3. Samuels J, Aksentijevich I, Torosyan Y, Centola M, Deng Z, Sood R, Kastner DL. Familial Mediterranean fever at the millennium. Clinical spectrum, ancient mutations, and a survey of 100 American referrals to the National Institutes of Health. Medicine (Baltimore). 1998;77(4):268–97.
4. El-Shanti H, Majeed HA, El-Khateeb M. Familial mediterranean fever in Arabs. Lancet. 2006;367(9515):1016–24.
5. Sohar E, Gafni J, Pras M, Heller H. Familial Mediterranean fever. A survey of 470 cases and review of the literature. Am J Med. 1967;43(2):227–53.
6. Majeed HA, Al-Qudah AK, Qubain H, Shahin HM. The clinical patterns of myalgia in children with familial Mediterranean fever. Semin Arthritis Rheum. 2000;30(2):138–43.
7. Livneh A, Langevitz P, Zemer D, Zaks N, Kees S, Lidar T, Migdal A, Padeh S, Pras M. Criteria for the diagnosis of familial Mediterranean fever. Arthritis Rheum. 1997;40(10):1879–85.
8. Marek-Yagel D, Berkun Y, Padeh S, Abu A, Reznik-Wolf H, Livneh A, Pras M, Pras E. Clinical disease among patients heterozygous for familial Mediterranean fever. Arthritis Rheum. 2009;60(6):1862–6.
9. Migita K, Agematsu K, Yazaki M, Nonaka F, Nakamura A, Toma T, Kishida D, Uehara R, Nakamura Y, Jiuchi Y, et al. Familial Mediterranean fever: genotype-phenotype correlations in Japanese patients. Medicine (Baltimore). 2014;93(3):158–64.
10. Ben-Chetrit E, Ben-Chetrit A. Familial Mediterranean fever and menstruation. BJOG. 2001;108(4):403–7.
11. Berkun Y, Eisenstein EM. Diagnostic criteria of familial Mediterranean fever. Autoimmun Rev. 2014;13(4–5):388–90.
12. Ben-Chetrit E, Touitou I. Familial mediterranean Fever in the world. Arthritis Rheum. 2009;61(10):1447–53.
13. Shinozaki K, Agematsu K, Yasui K, Nagumo H, Naitoh H, Naganuma K, Komiyama A. Familial Mediterranean fever in 2 Japanese families. J Rheumatol. 2002;29(6):1324–5.
14. Tomiyama N, Higashiuesato Y, Oda T, Baba E, Harada M, Azuma M, Yamashita T, Uehara K, Miyazato A, Hatta K, et al. MEFV mutation analysis of familial Mediterranean fever in Japan. Clin Exp Rheumatol. 2008;26(1):13–7.
15. Tsuchiya-Suzuki A, Yazaki M, Nakamura A, Yamazaki K, Agematsu K, Matsuda M, Ikeda S. Clinical and genetic features of familial Mediterranean fever in Japan. J Rheumatol. 2009;36(8):1671–6.
16. Migita K, Izumi Y, Jiuchi Y, Iwanaga N, Kawahara C, Agematsu K, Yachie A, Masumoto J, Fujikawa K, Yamasaki S, et al. Familial Mediterranean fever is no longer a rare disease in Japan. Arthritis Res Ther. 2016;18:175.
17. Kishida D, Nakamura A, Yazaki M, Tsuchiya-Suzuki A, Matsuda M, Ikeda S. Genotype-phenotype correlation in Japanese patients with familial Mediterranean fever: differences in genotype and clinical features between Japanese and Mediterranean populations. Arthritis Res Ther. 2014;16(5):439.
18. Migita K, Uehara R, Nakamura Y, Yasunami M, Tsuchiya-Suzuki A, Yazaki M, Nakamura A, Masumoto J, Yachie A, Furukawa H, et al. Familial Mediterranean fever in Japan. Medicine (Baltimore). 2012;91(6):337–43.
19. Migita K, Ida H, Moriuchi H, Agematsu K. Clinical relevance of MEFV gene mutations in Japanese patients with unexplained fever. J Rheumatol. 2012; 39(4):875–7.
20. Sayarlioglu M, Cefle A, Inanc M, Kamali S, Dalkilic E, Gul A, Ocal L, Aral O, Konice M. Characteristics of patients with adult-onset familial Mediterranean fever in Turkey: analysis of 401 cases. Int J Clin Pract. 2005;59(2):202–5.
21. Tamir N, Langevitz P, Zemer D, Pras E, Shinar Y, Padeh S, Zaks N, Pras M, Livneh A. Late-onset familial Mediterranean fever (FMF): a subset with distinct clinical, demographic, and molecular genetic characteristics. Am J Med Genet. 1999;87(1):30–5.
22. Nobakht H, Zamani F, Ajdarkosh H, Mohamadzadeh Z, Fereshtehnejad S, Nassaji M. Adult-onset familial Mediterranean fever in northwestern Iran; clinical feature and treatment outcome. Middle East J Dig Dis. 2011;3(1):50–5.
23. Rozenbaum M, Rosner I. The clinical features of Familial Mediterranean Fever of elderly onset. Clin Exp Rheumatol. 1994;12(3):347–8.
24. Ben-Chetrit E, Peleg H, Aamar S, Heyman SN. The spectrum of MEFV clinical presentations—is it familial Mediterranean fever only? Rheumatology (Oxford). 2009;48(11):1455–9.
25. Ryan JG, Masters SL, Booty MG, Habal N, Alexander JD, Barham BK, Remmers EF, Barron KS, Kastner DL, Aksentijevich I. Clinical features and functional significance of the P369S/R408Q variant in pyrin, the familial Mediterranean fever protein. Ann Rheum Dis. 2010;69(7):1383–8.
26. Soriano A, Manna R. Familial Mediterranean fever: new phenotypes. Autoimmun Rev. 2012;12(1):31–7.
27. Lidar M, Yonath H, Shechter N, Sikron F, Sadetzki S, Langevitz P, Livneh A, Pras E. Incomplete response to colchicine in M694V homozygote FMF patients. Autoimmun Rev. 2012;12(1):72–6.
28. Shinar Y, Livneh A, Langevitz P, Zaks N, Aksentijevich I, Koziol DE, Kastner DL, Pras M, Pras E. Genotype-phenotype assessment of common genotypes among patients with familial Mediterranean fever. J Rheumatol. 2000;27(7): 1703–7.
29. Gedalia A, Adar A, Gorodischer R. Familial Mediterranean fever in children. J Rheumatol Suppl. 1992;35:1–9.
30. Saatci U, Bakkaloglu A, Ozen S, Besbas N. Familial Mediterranean fever and amyloidosis in children. Acta Paediatr. 1993;82(8):705–6.
31. Schwabe AD, Peters RS. Familial Mediterranean Fever in Armenians. Analysis of 100 cases. Medicine (Baltimore). 1974;53(6):453–62.
32. Zemer D, Livneh A, Danon YL, Pras M, Sohar E. Long-term colchicine treatment in children with familial Mediterranean fever. Arthritis Rheum. 1991;34(8):973–7.
33. Kriegshauser G, Enko D, Hayrapetyan H, Atoyan S, Oberkanins C, 687 Sarkisian T. Clinical and genetic heterogeneity in a large cohort of 688 Armenian patients with late-onset familial Mediterranean fever. Genet 689 Med. Mar 15. https://doi.org/10.1038/gim.2018.46.
34. Tunca M, Akar S, Onen F, Ozdogan H, Kasapcopur O, Yalcinkaya F, Tutar E, Ozen S, Topaloglu R, Yilmaz E, et al. Familial Mediterranean fever (FMF) in Turkey: results of a nationwide multicenter study. Medicine (Baltimore). 2005;84(1):1–11.
35. Soylemezoglu O, Arga M, Fidan K, Gonen S, Emeksiz HC, Hasanoglu E, Buyan N. Unresponsiveness to colchicine therapy in patients with familial Mediterranean fever homozygous for the M694V mutation. J Rheumatol. 2010;37(1):182–9.
36. Giancane G, Ter Haar NM, Wulffraat N, Vastert SJ, Barron K, Hentgen V, Kallinich T, Ozdogan H, Anton J, Brogan P, et al. Evidence-based recommendations for genetic diagnosis of familial Mediterranean fever. Ann Rheum Dis. 2015;74(4):635–41.
37. Cosan F, Emrence Z, Erbag G, Azakli H, Yilmazer B, Yazici A, Ekmekci SS, Abaci N, Ustek D, Cefle A: The association of TNFRSF1A gene and MEFV gene mutations with adult onset Still's disease. Rheumatol Int 2013, 33(7): 1675–1680.
38. Wu Z, Zhang S, Li J, Chen S, Li P, Sun F, Wen X, Zheng W, Zhang F, Li Y: Association between MEFV Mutations M694V and M680I and Behcet's Disease: A Meta-Analysis. PLoS One. 2015;10(7):e0132704.
39. Rabinovich E, Livneh A, Langevitz P, Brezniak N, Shinar E, Pras M, Shinar Y: Severe disease in patients with rheumatoid arthritis carrying a mutation in the Mediterranean fever gene. Ann Rheum Dis 2005;64(7):1009–1014.
40. Deniz R, Ozen G, Yilmaz-Oner S, Alibaz-Oner F, Erzik C, Aydin SZ, Inanc N, Eren F, Bayalan F, Direskeneli H et al: Familial Mediterranean fever gene (MEFV) mutations and disease severity in systemic lupus erythematosus (SLE): implications for the role of the E148Q MEFV allele in inflammation. Lupus 2015;24(7):705–711.
41. Demirkaya E, Acikel C, Hashkes P, Gattorno M, Gul A, Ozdogan H, Turker T, Karadag O, Livneh A, Ben-Chetrit E et al: Development and initial validation of international severity scoring system for familial Mediterranean fever (ISSF). Ann Rheum Dis 2016, 75(6):1051–1056.

10

Cytokine production by activated plasmacytoid dendritic cells and natural killer cells is suppressed by an IRAK4 inhibitor

Karin Hjorton[1]* ⓘ, Niklas Hagberg[1], Elisabeth Israelsson[2], Lisa Jinton[2], Olof Berggren[1], Johanna K. Sandling[1], Kristofer Thörn[2], John Mo[2], The DISSECT consortium, Maija-Leena Eloranta[1] and Lars Rönnblom[1]

Abstract

Background: In systemic lupus erythematosus (SLE), immune complexes (ICs) containing self-derived nucleic acids trigger the synthesis of proinflammatory cytokines by immune cells. We asked how an interleukin (IL)-1 receptor-associated kinase 4 small molecule inhibitor (IRAK4i) affects RNA-IC-induced cytokine production compared with hydroxychloroquine (HCQ).

Methods: Plasmacytoid dendritic cells (pDCs) and natural killer (NK) cells were isolated from peripheral blood mononuclear cells (PBMCs) of healthy individuals. PBMCs from SLE patients and healthy individuals were depleted of monocytes. Cells were stimulated with RNA-containing IC (RNA-IC) in the presence or absence of IRAK4i I92 or HCQ, and cytokines were measured by immunoassay or flow cytometry. Transcriptome sequencing was performed on RNA-IC-stimulated pDCs from healthy individuals to assess the effect of IRAK4i and HCQ.

Results: In healthy individuals, RNA-IC induced interferon (IFN)-α, tumor necrosis factor (TNF)-α, IL-6, IL-8, IFN-γ, macrophage inflammatory protein (MIP)1-α, and MIP1-β production in pDC and NK cell cocultures. IFN-α production was selective for pDCs, whereas both pDCs and NK cells produced TNF-α. IRAK4i reduced the pDC and NK cell-derived cytokine production by 74–95%. HCQ interfered with cytokine production in pDCs but not in NK cells. In monocyte-depleted PBMCs, IRAK4i blocked cytokine production more efficiently than HCQ. Following RNA-IC activation of pDCs, 975 differentially expressed genes were observed (false discovery rate (FDR) < 0.05), with many connected to cytokine pathways, cell regulation, and apoptosis. IRAK4i altered the expression of a larger number of RNA-IC-induced genes than did HCQ (492 versus 65 genes).

Conclusions: The IRAK4i I92 exhibits a broader inhibitory effect than HCQ on proinflammatory pathways triggered by RNA-IC, suggesting IRAK4 inhibition as a therapeutic option in SLE.

Keywords: SLE, pDC, NK, HCQ, IRAK4

* Correspondence: karin.hjorton@medsci.uu.se
[1]Department of Medical Sciences, Rheumatology, Science for Life Laboratory, Uppsala University, Rudbecklaboratoriet, Dag Hammarskjölds v 20, C11, 751 85 Uppsala, Sweden
Full list of author information is available at the end of the article

Background

Systemic lupus erythematosus (SLE) is characterized by circulating immune complexes (ICs), an activation of the type I interferon (IFN) system, and production of proinflammatory cytokines and chemokines which cause an autoimmune reaction with organ inflammation [1]. The cellular and molecular mechanisms behind the ongoing inflammatory process in SLE have been partially clarified, and a number of different disease-associated pathways identified [2]. One important event is the induction of type I IFN production by plasmacytoid dendritic cells (pDCs) in response to ICs consisting of autoantibodies and apoptotic or necrotic cell-derived nucleic acids [3]. Such interferogenic ICs are internalized in pDCs via fragment crystallizable receptor IIA (FcγRIIA) and directed to the endosomes, where RNA and DNA interact with Toll-like receptor (TLR)7 and 9, respectively [4]. Activation of TLR7/9 triggers a signaling cascade, involving myeloid differentiation primary response protein 88 (MyD88), interleukin (IL)-1 receptor-associated kinase (IRAK)1, and IRAK4, that eventually leads to transcription of type I IFN genes. In addition to type I IFN production, MyD88 and IRAK4 signaling triggers the production of other proinflammatory cytokines, such as tumor necrosis factor (TNF)-α and IL-6, via activation of nuclear factor kappa-light-chain-enhancer of activated B cells (NFκB) or IFN regulatory factor (IRF) 5 [5]. Besides the pDCs, interferogenic ICs will also activate several other immune cells, such as natural killer (NK) cells, which contribute to enhanced cytokine production [6]. The final outcome in SLE is a complex inflammatory response that is difficult to bring into complete remission.

Current therapies in SLE aim to downregulate the autoimmune reaction. Treatment with antimalarials, such as hydroxychloroquine (HCQ), is considered the standard of care [7, 8]. The presumed central mechanism of action of HCQ is a reduction in the IFN-α production by inhibition of endosomal TLR signaling [9]. Studies have also shown that SLE patients treated with HCQ have a decreased type I IFN production after stimulation of pDCs with TLR ligands [10]. However, despite continuous HCQ treatment, few patients with SLE experience complete remission and flares still occur. A possible reason could be the limited number of disease-associated pathways affected by HCQ. Consequently, targeting a broader repertoire of inflammatory cytokines in SLE, yet avoiding severe infections, is needed. A potential therapeutic target in SLE is IRAK4 due to its essential role in MyD88 signaling [11]. IRAK4-deficient children are susceptible to life-threatening pyogenic infections that are reported to cease in adolescence, making IRAK4 inhibition an attractive therapeutic possibility [12].

In this study, we compared the effect of HCQ and the IRAK4 inhibitor (IRAK4i) I92 on the RNA-IC-induced cytokine production by pDCs and NK cells from healthy individuals and monocyte-depleted peripheral blood mononuclear cells (PBMCs) from SLE patients and healthy controls. Gene expression profiles of RNA-IC-stimulated pDCs treated with IRAK4i or HCQ were compared with nontreated cells to clarify the inflammatory response modulated by the drugs.

Methods

Patients and controls

All SLE patients ($n = 15$) fulfilled ≥ 4 of the American College of Rheumatology criteria for SLE [13]. Patients were a median 52 (range 32–81) years old with a disease duration of 15 (1–46) years (Additional file 1). Healthy age- and gender-matched controls ($n = 12$) were 53 (32–68) years old. The local ethics committee at Uppsala University approved the study and informed consent was obtained from all patients and controls.

Cell isolation and culture conditions

PBMCs were prepared from healthy donor buffy coats by Ficoll density-gradient centrifugation. pDCs (25×10^3/well) and NK cells (50×10^3/well) were isolated and cultivated as previously described [6, 14]. Cell purity was > 95% for pDC (blood dendritic cell antigen (BDCA)2⁺) and NK cells (cluster of differentiation (CD)56⁺) as determined by flow cytometry. Cell viability as measured by flow cytometry after 20 h was approximately 90%.

Interferon inducers

Necrotic material from U937 cell line and U1snRNP particles were prepared as previously described [3, 15]. Immunoglobulin (Ig)G was isolated from two Smith nuclear antigen (Sm) and ribonucleoprotein (RNP) antibody-containing SLE patient sera [14]. U1snRNP particles and SLE IgG were used at final concentrations of 2.5 μg/ml and 1 mg/ml, respectively.

Drugs

The small molecule drug IRAK4i I92 (ND-2158, Nimbus Discovery) [16] and HCQ (Sigma-Aldrich) were pretrated and used at final concentrations of 10 μM and 5.8 μM (pDCs and NK cells) or 7.8 μM (monocyte-depleted PBMCs) (Additional files 2, 3 and 4). The cells were preincubated with I92 or HCQ for 30 min at 5% CO_2 and 37 °C before adding IFN inducers.

Flow cytometry

pDCs and NK cells were cultivated for 5 or 9 h, with the final 4 h with brefeldin A. After gating live cells, singlets, and lymphocytes (Additional file 5), the cells were identified with anti-CD56-phycoerythrin (PE)Cy7 (NCAM 16.2, BD Biosciences) and BDCA-2-fluorescein isothiocyanate (FITC) (AC144, Miltenyi Biotech) monoclonal antibodies (mAbs). Intracellular cytokines were detected with anti-TNF-α-allophycocyanin (APC) (Mab11, BD Pharmingen) and anti-IFN-α-PE mAbs (LT27:295, Miltenyi Biotech). Isotype-matched irrelevant mAbs were used as controls. Live/dead Fixable Near-InfraRed Dead Cell Stain (Invitrogen) was used to distinguish live cells. Data were acquired with a FACS CantoII instrument and analyzed with Diva 6.1.3 software (BD Biosciences).

Immunoassays

TNF-α, IL-6, IL-8, IFN-γ, macrophage inflammatory protein (MIP)1-α, and MIP1-β were measured after 20 h by multiplex immunoassays (Milliplex Human Cytokine/ Chemokine (Millipore) or Luminex Screening Assay (R&D systems)). Lower limits of quantification (LLoQ) of cytokines were: TNF-α, 3.8 pg/ml; IL-6, 5.2 pg/ml; IL-8, 1.4 pg/ml; IFN-γ, 1.6 pg/ml; MIP1-α, 54.8; and MIP1-β, 162.2 pg/ml. IFN-α was measured by dissociation-enhanced lanthanide fluorescence immunoassay (DELFIA; LLoQ, 2 U/ml) [17].

RNA sequencing

pDCs from four healthy individuals were stimulated with RNA-IC for 6 h. RNA (RNA integrity number (RIN) ≥ 8) was extracted by the RNeasy 96 plus kit (Qiagen). RNA libraries were prepared with the TruSeq Stranded mRNA kit and sequenced by NextSeq500 (Illumina). RNAseq fastq files were processed using bcbio-nextgen (v.0.9.7) and mapped to the human genome GRCh38.79 [18]. Gene-level quantifications were generated with feature-Counts software (v.1.4.4) [19] and Sailfish (version 0.9.0) [20]. Pheatmap and ggplot2 (v.2.2.1, http://ggplot2.org/) were used for visualizations [21].

Statistical analysis

Statistical analysis was performed using GraphPad Prism software 7.0. Differences were analyzed with Friedman's test, and p values ≤ 0.05 were considered significant. For transcriptome analysis, a false discovery rate (FDR) < 0.05 was considered significant. Analyses were performed using R (version 3.3.3). Differential gene expression was assessed with DESeq2 (v.1.14.1) [22] using raw counts as input. Pathway enrichments were obtained from Pathway Studio® (Elsevier). A one-sided Mann-Whitney U test was performed to calculate the significance of the differences in distribution between the background (from the differential gene expression analysis) and the gene subnetworks (upstream regulators) or the gene sets (pathways).

Results

RNA-containing ICs induce TNF-α production more rapidly in NK cells than in pDCs

TNF-α and IFN-α are important drivers of inflammation in SLE and large amounts are produced in RNA-IC-stimulated

cocultures of pDCs and NK cells [6]. However, the cellular source and quantity produced by each cell type have not been determined. Therefore, we initially analyzed the frequency of TNF-α- and IFN-α-producing pDCs and NK cells in cocultures at 5 and 9 h, due to expected differences regarding peak cytokine production by the different cell types. A minority (< 20%) of both pDCs and NK cells produced TNF-α in response to RNA-IC (Fig. 1a, b; left panels). Furthermore, the TNF-α production was prominent in NK cells at 5 h, but occurred later in pDCs when the NK cell response had decreased.

Only pDCs produced IFN-α in response to RNA-IC (Fig. 1a, b; left panels), and synthesis of both TNF-α and IFN-α was most prominent at 9 h (Fig. 1b). Nearly all IFN-α-producing cells expressed TNF-α, whereas a fraction of the pDCs produced TNF-α only (Fig. 1b, left panel; Additional file 6). Almost no IFN-α-containing pDCs were detected at 5 h.

Therefore, RNA-containing ICs trigger the production of TNF-α in a fraction of pDCs and NK cells at different time points.

IRAK4i I92 inhibits TNF-α production by activated pDCs and NK cells, while HCQ affects TNF-α production by pDCs only

Next, we asked if HCQ inhibits the RNA-IC-induced TNF-α production in pDC/NK cell cocultures. As shown in Fig. 1a, b (right panels), HCQ completely blocked TNF-α production in pDCs but not in NK cells at 9 h. At 20 h, HCQ significantly reduced TNF-α production in cultures of pDCs and pDC/NK cells, but not in NK cells (Fig. 1e). In contrast, IFN-α production was completely blocked by HCQ. Subsequently, we investigated if IRAK4i I92 could inhibit the cytokine response in the cell cultures. As shown in Fig. 1c, d (right panels), intracellular IFN-α and TNF-α production by pDCs was effectively blocked by I92. The drug reduced the early (5-h) TNF-α response by approximately 75% in NK cells, whereas the inhibitory effect at a later time point (9 h) was less prominent. At 20 h, I92 reduced the TNF-α production by 70–95% in all cell cultures (Fig. 1e). In addition, the IFN-α levels in RNA-IC-stimulated pDC and pDC-NK cell cocultures were reduced by > 90% (Fig. 1f). No IFN-α was produced by NK cells. Thus, HCQ blocked TNF-α and IFN-α production by pDCs, whereas I92 reduced TNF-α production in both pDCs and NK cells, as well as the IFN-α production by pDCs.

IRAK4 inhibition reduces proinflammatory cytokine production by activated pDCs and NK cells more extensively than HCQ

To investigate whether IRAK4 inhibition affects production of other proinflammatory cytokines, levels of IL-6,

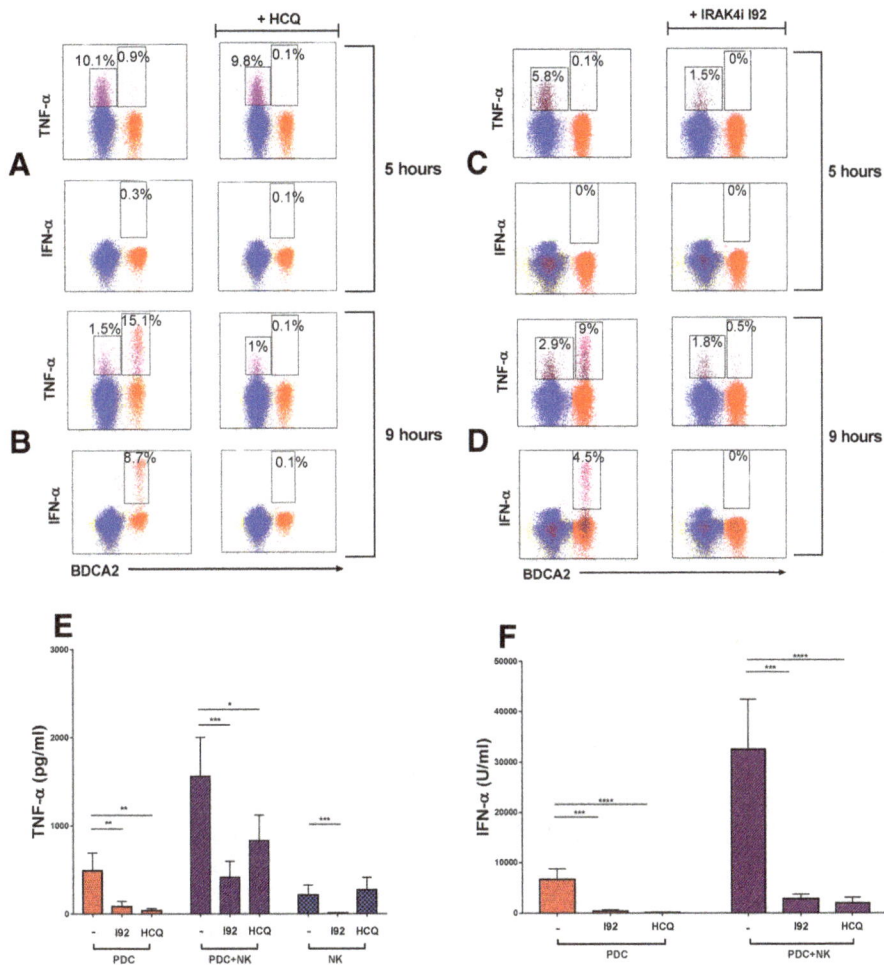

Fig. 1 Regulatory effect of hydroxychloroquine (HCQ) and the interleukin-1 receptor associated kinase 4 inhibitor (IRAK4i) I92 on tumor necrosis factor (TNF)-α and interferon (IFN)-α production. **a–d** Cocultures of plasmacytoid dendritic cells (pDC) and natural killer (NK) cells from healthy donors were stimulated with RNA-containing immune complexes (RNA-IC) for 5 h (**a,b**) or 9 h (**c,d**) in the absence or presence of HCQ or I92. The frequencies of TNF-α- and IFN-α-producing NK cells (blue) and pDCs (red) were determined by flow cytometry. The dot plots represent one representative individual donor from two (HCQ) and four (IRAK4i) donors analyzed. **e,f** pDCs or NK cells were cultivated separately or in coculture in the presence of RNA-IC with or without I92 or HCQ. Cytokine levels were measured by immunoassays after 20 h. No IFN-α is produced by NK cells (data not shown). No cytokines were detected in the cell cultures in the absence of RNA-IC. Bars represent the mean with standard error of the mean (SEM) of nine donors from at least three independent experiments. Friedman's test, uncorrected Dunn's test; $*p < 0.05$, $**p < 0.01$, $***p < 0.001$, $****p < 0.0001$. BDCA blood dendritic cell antigen

IL-8, IFN-γ, MIP1-α, and MIP1-β were measured in RNA-IC-stimulated cultures with pDCs, NK cells, or pDC/NK cell cocultures in the presence or absence of I92 or HCQ (Fig. 2). In pDC cultures and pDC/NK cocultures, both I92 and HCQ blocked IL-6, IL-8, and MIP1-α, whereas I92 also blocked IFN-γ and MIP1-β production. In NK cell cultures, I92 significantly reduced IL-6, IFN-γ, MIP1-α, and MIP1-β levels, whereas IL-8 was unaffected. HCQ did not inhibit cytokine production by NK cells. Hence, I92 showed a broader inhibitory effect than HCQ on proinflammatory cytokines produced by RNA-IC-stimulated pDCs and NK cells.

IRAK4 inhibition blocks production of proinflammatory cytokines by PBMCs from SLE patients

As healthy individuals and SLE patients may respond differently, we investigated if cytokine production in cells from patients with SLE also could be targeted with an IRAK4i. PBMCs from patients with SLE or healthy controls were stimulated after depletion of monocytes, due to their suppressive effect on the IFN-α response [14]. I92 inhibited TNF-α and IFN-α production by 80% and 97%, respectively, whereas HCQ interfered significantly only with IFN-α production (99%) (Fig. 3a, b). Furthermore, IL-6, IFN-γ,

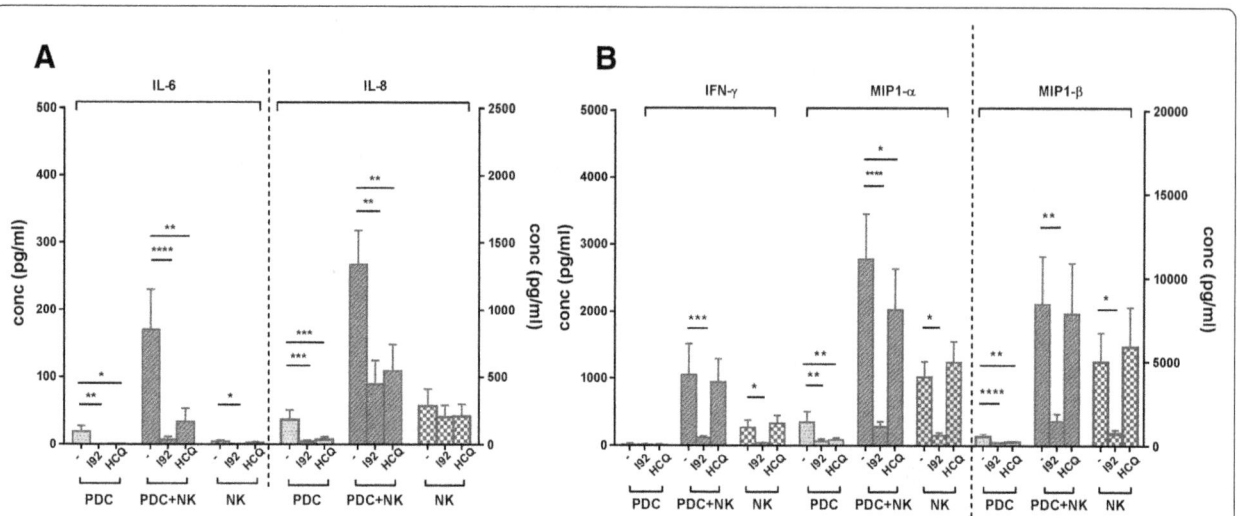

Fig. 2 The interleukin-1 receptor associated kinase 4 inhibitor (IRAK4i) I92 displays a more prominent inhibitory effect than hydroxychloroquine (HCQ) on the production of proinflammatory cytokines in plasmacytoid dendritic cells (pDC) and natural killer (NK) cell cocultures and in NK cells alone. pDCs and NK cells from healthy donors were cultivated separately or in coculture in the presence of RNA-containing immune complexes (RNA-IC), with or without I92 or HCQ. The levels of **a** interleukin (IL)-6 and IL-8, and **b** interferon (IFN)-γ, macrophage inflammatory protein (MIP)1-α, and MIP1-β were measured by immunoassays after 20 h. Bars represent the mean with standard error of the mean (SEM) of nine donors from at least three independent experiments. Friedman's test, uncorrected Dunn's test; *$p < 0.05$, **$p < 0.01$, ***$p < 0.001$, ****$p < 0.0001$

MIP1-α, and MIP1-β production was inhibited by I92, whereas only IL-6 and MIP1-β were significantly inhibited by HCQ (Fig. 4a, b). HCQ and I92 displayed the same inhibitory profile in monocyte-depleted PBMCs from healthy individuals. In summary, I92 reduced cytokine production in SLE patients and demonstrated a more extensive inhibitory profile on proinflammatory cytokines than did HCQ.

Gene expression changes in RNA-IC-stimulated pDCs are reversed by both IRAK4 inhibition and HCQ

To clarify the pathways affected by I92 and HCQ, we performed transcriptome sequencing (RNA-seq) of RNA-IC-stimulated pDCs. An RNA-IC activation signature was identified consisting of 975 differentially expressed genes (DEGs) compared with unstimulated pDCs (RNA-IC-DEGs, FDR < 0.05; Fig. 5, Additional file 7). A majority of

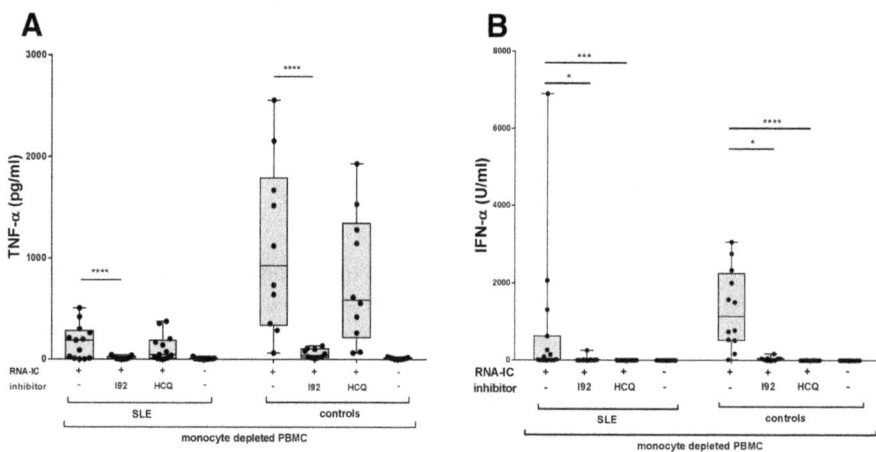

Fig. 3 The interleukin-1 receptor associated kinase 4 inhibitor (IRAK4i) I92 reduces both **a** tumor necrosis factor (TNF)-α and **b** interferon (IFN)-α production by monocyte-depleted peripheral blood mononuclear cells (PBMCs) from systemic lupus erythematosus (SLE) patients and healthy controls. The cells were stimulated with RNA-containing immune complexes (RNA-IC) in the presence or absence of I92 or hydroxychloroquine (HCQ), or were mock stimulated. TNF-α and IFN-α production in cell cultures was measured after 20 h by immunoassays. Box plots show median with interquartile range, based on 10–15 donors, in at least 10 independent experiments. Friedman's test, uncorrected Dunn's test; *$p < 0.05$, **$p < 0.01$, ***$p < 0.001$, ****$p < 0.0001$

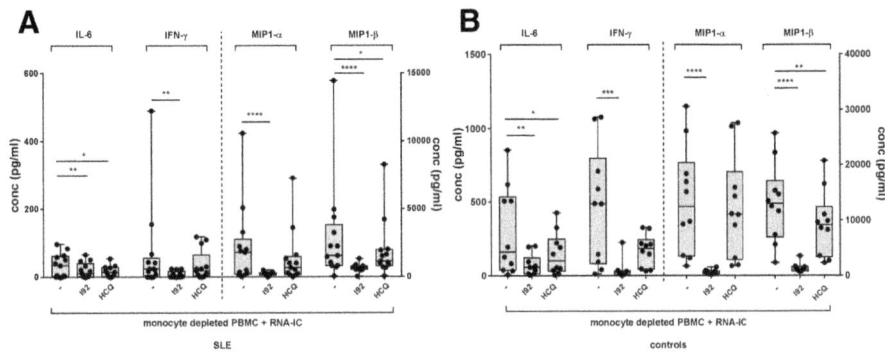

Fig. 4 The interleukin-1 receptor associated kinase 4 inhibitor (IRAK4i) I92 exhibits a broader inhibitory effect than hydroxychloroquine (HCQ) on cytokine production by monocyte-depleted peripheral blood mononuclear cells (PBMCs) from **a** systemic lupus erythematosus (SLE) patients and **b** healthy controls. Monocyte-depleted PBMCs were stimulated with RNA-containing immune complexes (RNA-IC) in the presence or absence of I92 or HCQ. Levels of interleukin (IL)-6, interferon (IFN)-γ, macrophage inflammatory protein (MIP)1-α, and MIP1-β in the cell cultures were measured after 20 h by immunoassays. Box plots show median with interquartile range, based on 10–13 donors from 10 independent experiments. Friedman's test, uncorrected Dunn's test; *$p < 0.05$, **$p < 0.01$, ***$p < 0.001$, ****$p < 0.0001$

the responding genes showed an upregulation after RNA-IC stimulation ($n = 670$), with 48 genes increased at least fourfold (Fig. 6a, Additional file 7). Among the 48 top RNA-IC-DEGs were genes mapping to the type I IFN signaling pathway (*IFNA2, IFIT1–3, GBP1*, and *OASL*), clearance of apoptotic material (*BCL2A1, CDKN1A*, and *TNFSF10*), and chemokine genes (*CXCL2, CXCL9, CXCL10*, and *CCL4*). Several regulators of inflammation and activation (e.g., *IRF1, IRF3, STAT1, STAT3, NFκB, RELA/B*, and *SP1*) were predicted to drive the RNA-IC-DEGs (Additional file 8).

I92 significantly altered the expression of almost 4000 genes (FDR < 0.05) in RNA-IC-activated pDCs, of which 492 overlapped with the RNA-IC-DEGs. In contrast, HCQ significantly altered only 73 genes, with 65 overlapping with the RNA-IC-DEGs (FDR < 0.05) (Fig. 5, Additional file 9). More RNA-IC-DEGs were strongly downregulated (log2 fold change > 2) by I92 ($n = 73$) than by HCQ ($n = 15$) (Fig. 6b, c). The expression of several top upregulated genes in the RNA-IC-DEGs was reversed by both I92 and HCQ, including *IFNA2, IFIT2–3, OASL, CXCL10, CD274, TNFSF10*, and *APOL6*.

Between HCQ- and I92-treated, RNA-IC-stimulated pDCs, 125 genes were differentially expressed. The greatest relative difference in expression was observed for *DKK4, LAD1*, and *EAF2* (Fig. 6d), which were more strongly downregulated by I92 than by HCQ. These genes have mainly been studied in the context of tumorigenesis [23–25]. The top enriched biological function pathway for these genes was macroautophagy decline, represented by *ATG14, AMBRA1*, and *BECN1*, contributing to the regulation of autophagy, autophagosomal maturation, endocytosis, and apoptosis (Additional file 10). Several STAT-related signaling pathways were more suppressed by I92 than by HCQ (Additional file 11). The expression of cytokine genes *TNF, IFNA2, CXCL8, CCL3*, and *CCL4* was significantly

suppressed by I92, compared with only *TNF* and *IFNA2* being suppressed by HCQ (Additional file 12). In conclusion, both I92 and HCQ reversed the effects of RNA-IC stimulation on the pDC gene expression profile, but I92 more extensively affected gene expression and modulated more cellular pathways than HCQ.

Discussion

This study demonstrates that the cytokine production by RNA-IC-stimulated pDCs and NK cells can be suppressed by HCQ and, more profoundly, by an IRAK4 inhibitor. The strong TNF-α induction by RNA-IC is interesting since TNF-α plays a critical role in several SLE disease manifestations, such as nephritis, skin lesions, and arthritis, all characterized by tissue deposition of ICs [26–28]. Increased IC formation precedes SLE flares and our findings may therefore partly explain the observed association between increased serum TNF-α levels and disease activity in SLE [29]. The difference in the TNF-α production rate between pDCs and NK cells indicates that RNA-ICs activate different induction pathways for TNF-α synthesis in these two cell types. Supporting this conjecture is the observed difference between pDCs and NK cells in response to HCQ. pDCs are mainly activated by ligation of endosomal TLRs [2] and this pathway is inhibited by HCQ [7]. TNF-α production by NK cells, on the other hand, can be induced by a number of different receptors, including TLR7 [30–32]. However, RNA-IC-induced production of cytokines and chemokines from NK cells was not dependent on endosomal TLR signaling since HCQ had no inhibitory effect. Consistent with a TLR7-independent activation of NK cells, heat-aggregated IgG was as efficient as RNA-IC in inducing TNF-α from purified NK cells, and a synthetic TLR7 agonist (DSR6434) did not induce TNF-α in NK cells (Additional file 13). Although no studies were performed

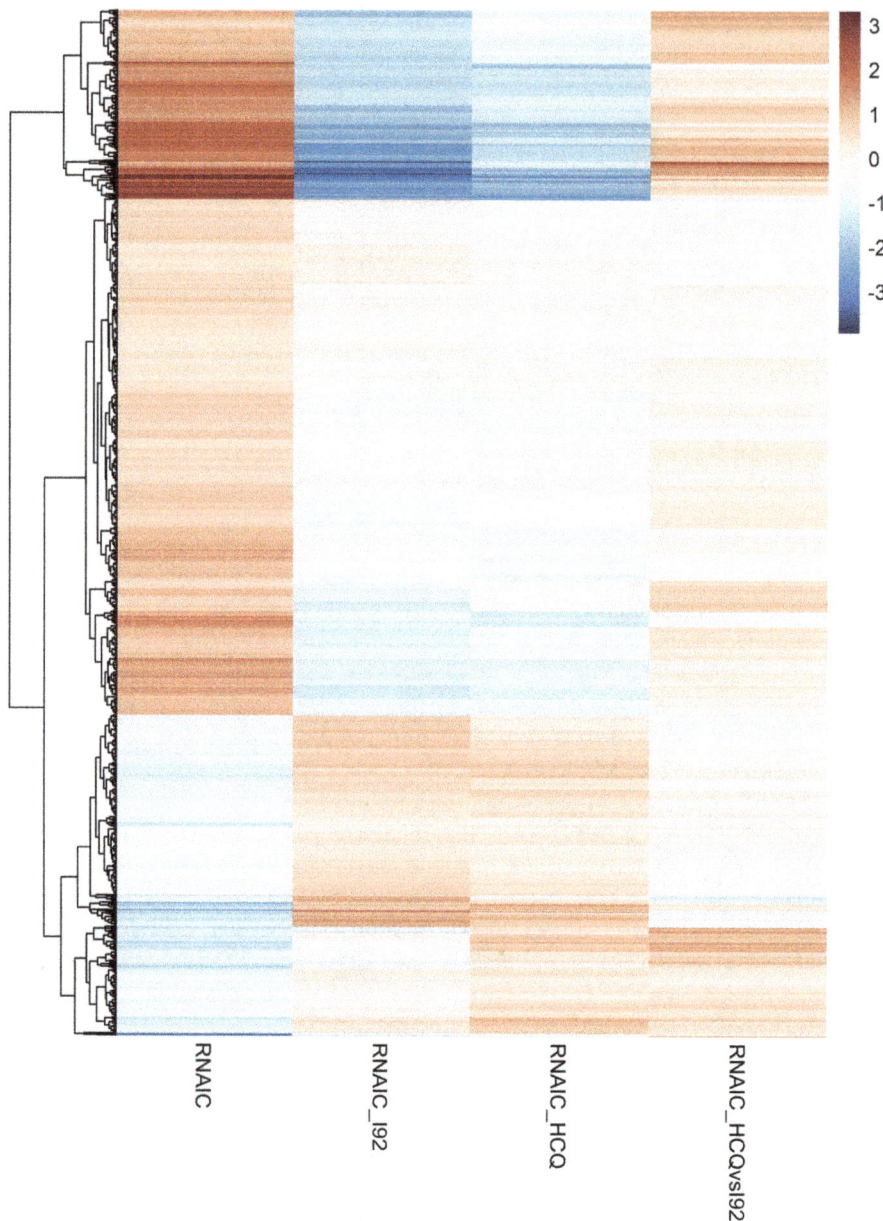

Fig. 5 Differential effects on gene expression in RNA-containing immune complex (RNA-IC)-stimulated plasmacytoid dendritic cells (pDCs) by the interleukin-1 receptor associated kinase 4 inhibitor (IRAK4i) I92 and hydroxychloroquine (HCQ). RNA-sequencing analysis was performed on RNA-IC-stimulated pDCs from healthy donors ($n = 4$), cultivated for 6 h in the presence or absence of I92 or HCQ. The heat map showing the mean log2 fold change values for the 975 activation signature genes from RNA-IC versus mock-stimulated cells (left), RNA-IC I92 versus RNA-IC (middle left), RNA-IC HCQ versus RNA-IC (middle right), and the difference between the two compounds RNA-IC I92 versus RNA-IC HCQ treated cultures (right)

regarding specific RNA-IC-responding NK cell receptors, the fact that TNF-α production was observed only in the CD56^{dim}, CD16-expressing NK cell population (Additional file 14) suggests NK cell activation by RNA-IC via CD16. The prominent effect of the IRAK4 inhibitor I92 on the TNF-α production by NK cells implies that NFκB-mediated and/or mitogen-activated protein kinase activation was involved in the NK cell response [33]. However, we cannot exclude that other

protein kinases were also affected by I92, despite the previously demonstrated high selectivity for IRAK4 by this drug [16].

When investigating the effect of HCQ and IRAK4 inhibitor I92 on other RNA-IC-induced cytokines, we noted that HCQ almost completely blocked the production of all investigated cytokines by pDCs. This was in stark contrast to the lack of effect on the cytokine response in NK cells. Conversely, HCQ markedly reduced

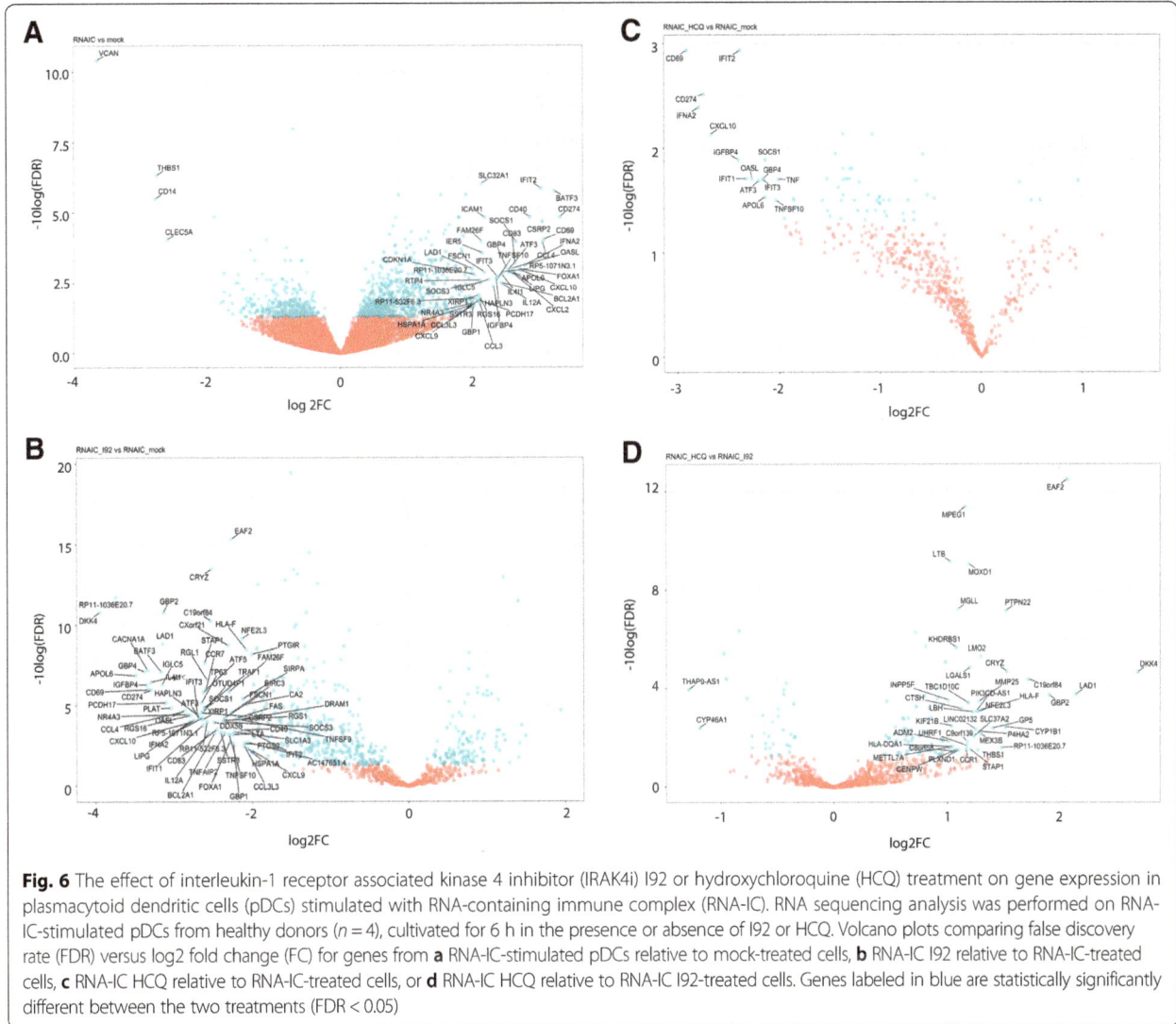

Fig. 6 The effect of interleukin-1 receptor associated kinase 4 inhibitor (IRAK4i) I92 or hydroxychloroquine (HCQ) treatment on gene expression in plasmacytoid dendritic cells (pDCs) stimulated with RNA-containing immune complex (RNA-IC). RNA sequencing analysis was performed on RNA-IC-stimulated pDCs from healthy donors (n = 4), cultivated for 6 h in the presence or absence of I92 or HCQ. Volcano plots comparing false discovery rate (FDR) versus log2 fold change (FC) for genes from **a** RNA-IC-stimulated pDCs relative to mock-treated cells, **b** RNA-IC I92 relative to RNA-IC-treated cells, **c** RNA-IC HCQ relative to RNA-IC-treated cells, or **d** RNA-IC HCQ relative to RNA-IC I92-treated cells. Genes labeled in blue are statistically significantly different between the two treatments (FDR < 0.05)

the production of most cytokines in the pDC/NK cell cocultures. The reason for this is unclear, but an optimal cytokine production in cell cocultures depends on both cell types since RNA-IC-activated pDC and NK cells promote the function of each other [6]. Consequently, inhibition of the pDC function in pDC/NK cell cocultures will also reduce the NK cell cytokine-producing capacity. However, in pDC/NK cocultures the production of IFN-γ and MIP-1β was not affected by HCQ, suggesting a pDC-independent production by NK cells, although the exact cellular source of these cytokines was not investigated. Nevertheless, this observation indicates the need for a therapeutic agent with broader effects than HCQ to achieve better control of IC-driven inflammatory processes.

The IRAK4 inhibitor I92 blocked the NK cell production of all cytokines in healthy individuals, except for IL-8. This could imply yet another induction mechanism

for IL-8 production in NK cells. In fact, IL-8 production was also remarkably high in monocyte-depleted PBMC cultures from SLE patients (Additional file 15) but, due to a shortage of patient material, the effects of I92 and HCQ on the IL-8 production could not be clarified. Studies have shown that patients with SLE have increased serum levels of IL-8 despite continuous standard treatment and being in remission [34]. An association between IL-8 gene polymorphisms and SLE further supports a role for IL-8 in SLE [35]. Additional studies are needed to determine the regulation of IL-8 production in patients with SLE, and some are now in progress. Notably, I92 inhibited all other investigated cytokines produced by RNA-IC-stimulated cells from SLE patients, whereas HCQ only reduced IL-6 and MIP1-β production significantly.

The RNA-IC activation signature in pDCs revealed an enrichment of pathways with connection to the IFN signaling system, antigen presentation, and apoptosis. This demonstrates that nucleic acid containing ICs elicit a powerful inflammatory response, but also trigger other cellular processes of importance in SLE. Both I92 and HCQ largely reversed the RNA-IC activation in pDCs, although some differences were observed. I92 increased the expression of genes involved in protein degradation and the autophagy process, in contrast to HCQ which downregulated these genes. The most strongly downregulated genes by I92 compared with HCQ were *DKK4*, *LAD1*, and *EAF2*, and suppression of these genes could have several effects on the SLE disease process. DKK4 is an inhibitor of the canonical Wnt signaling pathway, which has been suggested to contribute to disrupted T effector cell differentiation and the immune dysfunction in SLE [36, 37]. Ladinin 1, encoded by *LAD1*, modulates the EGF to ERK pathway and increased ERK activation is associated with organ damage in SLE [24, 38]. EAF2, on the other hand, is selectively upregulated in germinal center B cells and promotes their apoptosis [39]. Possibly, inhibition of EAF2 could therefore increase autoantibody production. The increased activation of the autophagy pathway by I92 might be beneficial in SLE since autophagy is reduced in SLE regulatory T cells and enhanced autophagy has been shown to improve both murine and human SLE [40]. On the other hand, activation of autophagy favors plasmablast development, enabling expansion of self-reactive B cells in SLE, as well as type I IFN production by facilitating intracellular IC transport [41, 42]. These observations merit further studies of the effects of I92 on different cell types, not least considering that IRAK4 inhibition ameliorates experimental murine lupus, suggesting a favorable effect also in human SLE [43]. Translating results of in-vitro studies of pharmaceutical compounds to potential drug effects in vivo has limitations. However, the approach to investigate drug candidates in cell cultures can be useful to determine the effects on central immune cells in the disease process [44]. Thus, we consider our system with IC-stimulated immune cells from SLE patients as one relevant model for an initial screening of potential drugs that target disease-associated pathways in SLE.

Conclusions

In conclusion, the IRAK4 inhibitor I92 reduced a number of proinflammatory cytokines triggered by RNA-IC that are involved in the immune pathogenesis of SLE equally, or more effectively, than HCQ. For the first time, we show the effects of an IRAK4 inhibitor on both transcription and protein synthesis in RNA-IC-activated pDCs, which demonstrates that IRAK4 inhibition affects many cellular pathways of importance in an autoimmune disease process.

Additional files

Additional file 1: Table S1. Patient clinical characteristics.

Additional file 2: Figure S1. Titration of IRAK4 inhibitor (I92) on cytokine production by cocultured plasmacytoid dendritic cells and NK cells.

Additional file 3: Figure S2. Titration of hydroxychloroquine in cocultured plasmacytoid dendritic cells and NK cells with regard to interferon-α production.

Additional file 4: Figure S3. Titration of hydroxychloroquine in cocultured plasmacytoid dendritic cells and NK cells.

Additional file 5: Figure S4. Flow cytometric gating strategy of stimulated plasmacytoid dendritic cells and NK cells.

Additional file 6: Figure S5. Flow cytometry showing total proportion of cytokine-producing cells in RNA-IC-stimulated pDC and NK cells.

Additional file 7: Table S2. Gene list of 975 differentially expressed genes.

Additional file 8: Table S3. Upstream regulators. (PDF 291 kb)

Additional file 9: Figure S6. Overlap of differentially expressed genes in plasmacytoid dendritic cells.

Additional file 10: Table S4. Enriched biological function pathways.

Additional file 11: Table S5. Enriched signal processing pathways.

Additional file 12: Figure S7. RNA-seq analysis of cytokine expression in plasmacytoid dendritic cells stimulated for 6 h in the presence of IRAK4 inhibitor or hydroxychloroquine.

Additional file 13: Figure S8. TNF-α production in NK cell cultures and NK cell/pDC cocultures.

Additional file 14: Figure S9. Flow cytometric analysis of TNF-α in NK cells. (PDF 165 kb)

Additional file 15: Figure S10. Interleukin-8 production by stimulated blood cells from SLE patients.

Additional file 16: Table S6. Gene expression in plasmacytoid dendritic cells (pDCs) from healthy donors.

Abbreviations

AMBRA1: Autophagy and beclin 1 regulator 1; APC: Allophycocyanin; *APOL6*: Apolipoprotein L6; *ATG14*: Autophagy related 14; *BCL2A1*: BCL2 related protein A1; BDCA: Blood dendritic cell antigen; *BECN1*: Beclin 1; *CCL*: C-C motif chemokine ligand; CD: Cluster of differentiation; *CD274*: CD274 molecule; *CDKN1A* : Cyclin dependent kinase inhibitor 1A; *CXCL*: C-X-C motif chemokine ligand; DEG: Differentially expressed gene; DELFIA: Dissociation-enhanced lanthanide fluorescence immunoassay; *DKK4*: Dickkopf WNT signaling pathway inhibitor 4; *EAF2*: ELL associated factor 2; FcγRIIA: Fragment crystallizable receptor IIA; FDR: False discovery rate; FITC: Fluorescein isothiocyanate; HCQ: Hydroxychloroquine; IC: Immune complex; *IFIT*: Interferon induced protein with tetratricopeptide repeats; IFN: Interferon; *IFNA2*: Interferon alpha 2; Ig: Immunoglobulin; IL: Interleukin; IRAK: Interleukin-1 receptor-associated kinase; IRAK4i: Interleukin-1 receptor-associated kinase 4 inhibitor; IRF: Interferon regulatory factor; *LAD1*: Ladinin 1; LLoQ: Lower limits of quantification; mAb: Monoclonal antibody; MIP: Macrophage inflammatory protein; MyD88: Myeloid differentiation primary response protein 88; NFκB: Nuclear factor kappa-light-chain-enhancer of activated B cells; NK: Natural killer; *OASL*: 2'-5'-Oligoadenylate synthetase like protein; PBMC: Peripheral blood mononuclear cell; pDC: Plasmacytoid dendritic cell; PE: Phycoerythrin; *RELA*: RELA proto-oncogene, NF-κB subunit; *RELB*: RELB proto-oncogene, NF-κB subunit; RIN: RNA integrity number; RNA-IC: Ribonucleic acid containing immune complex; RNP: Ribonucleoprotein; SLE: Systemic lupus erythematosus; Sm: Smith nuclear antigen; snRNP: Small nuclear ribonucleoprotein; *SP1*: Specificity protein 1 transcription factor; *STAT*: Signal transducer and activator of transcription; TLR: Toll-like receptor; TNF: Tumor necrosis factor; *TNFSF10*: TNF superfamily member 10

Acknowledgements
We thank Lisbeth Fuxler for excellent technical assistance, Rezvan Kiani Dehkordi for collecting the patient blood samples, and Dr. Gert Weber, Ernst-Moritz-Arndt University of Greifswald, for kindly providing the U1snRNP particles.

Funding
The study was supported by The Swedish Rheumatism Association, King Gustaf V's 80-years Foundation, Agnes and Mac Rudberg's Foundation, AstraZeneca Science for Life Research Collaboration grant (DISSECT), The Swedish Research Council, and the Swedish Society of Medicine (the Ingegerd Johansson donation). The funding bodies had no role in any aspect of study design, analysis, interpretation, or manuscript writing.

Authors' contributions
Study design: KH, JM, MLE, LR. Laboratory data acquisition: KH, NH, LJ, OB, KT, MLE. Data analysis and interpretation: KH, NH, EI, JKS, KT, JM, MLE. Draft writing: KH, NH, EI, MLE, LR. Final revision: KH, NH, EI, LJ, OB, JKS, KT, JM, MLE, LR. All authors read and approved the final manuscript.

Consent for publication
Not applicable.

Competing interests
EI, LJ, KT, and JM are employees of AstraZeneca. LR received a research grant from AstraZeneca. The remaining authors declare that they have no competing interests.

Author details
[1]Department of Medical Sciences, Rheumatology, Science for Life Laboratory, Uppsala University, Rudbecklaboratoriet, Dag Hammarskjölds v 20, C11, 751 85 Uppsala, Sweden. [2]Respiratory, Inflammation and Autoimmunity, IMED Biotech Unit, AstraZeneca, Gothenburg, Sweden.

References
1. Bengtsson AA, Ronnblom L. Systemic lupus erythematosus: still a challenge for physicians. J Intern Med. 2017;281:52–64.
2. Tsokos GC, Lo MS, Reis PC, Sullivan KE. New insights into the immunopathogenesis of systemic lupus erythematosus. Nat Rev Rheumatol. 2016;12:716–30.
3. Lovgren T, Eloranta ML, Bave U, Alm GV, Ronnblom L. Induction of interferon-alpha production in plasmacytoid dendritic cells by immune complexes containing nucleic acid released by necrotic or late apoptotic cells and lupus IgG. Arthritis Rheum. 2004;50:1861–72.
4. Eloranta ML, Alm GV, Rönnblom L. Disease mechanisms in rheumatology—tools and pathways: plasmacytoid dendritic cells and their role in autoimmune rheumatic diseases. Arthritis Rheum. 2013;65:853–63.
5. Takeuchi O, Akira S. Pattern recognition receptors and inflammation. Cell. 2010;140:805–20.
6. Hagberg N, Berggren O, Leonard D, Weber G, Bryceson YT, Alm GV, Eloranta ML, Ronnblom L. IFN-alpha production by plasmacytoid dendritic cells stimulated with RNA-containing immune complexes is promoted by NK cells via MIP-1beta and LFA-1. J Immunol. 2011;186:5085–94.
7. Wallace DJ, Gudsoorkar VS, Weisman MH, Venuturupalli SR. New insights into mechanisms of therapeutic effects of antimalarial agents in SLE. Nat Rev Rheumatol. 2012;8:522–33.
8. Ruiz-Irastorza G, Ramos-Casals M, Brito-Zeron P, Khamashta MA. Clinical efficacy and side effects of antimalarials in systemic lupus erythematosus: a systematic review. Ann Rheum Dis. 2010;69:20–8.
9. Rainsford KD, Parke AL, Clifford-Rashotte M, Kean WF. Therapy and pharmacological properties of hydroxychloroquine and chloroquine in treatment of systemic lupus erythematosus, rheumatoid arthritis and related diseases. Inflammopharmacology. 2015;23:231–69.
10. Sacre K, Criswell LA, McCune JM. Hydroxychloroquine is associated with impaired interferon-alpha and tumor necrosis factor-alpha production by plasmacytoid dendritic cells in systemic lupus erythematosus. Arthritis Res Ther. 2012;14:R155.
11. Ferrao R, Zhou H, Shan Y, Liu Q, Li Q, Shaw DE, Li X, Wu H. IRAK4 dimerization and trans-autophosphorylation are induced by Myddosome assembly. Mol Cell. 2014;55:891–903.
12. Picard C, von Bernuth H, Ghandil P, Chrabieh M, Levy O, Arkwright PD, McDonald D, Geha RS, Takada H, Krause JC, et al. Clinical features and outcome of patients with IRAK-4 and MyD88 deficiency. Medicine (Baltimore). 2010;89:403–25.
13. Tan EM, Cohen AS, Fries JF, Masi AT, McShane DJ, Rothfield NF, Schaller JG, Talal N, Winchester RJ. The 1982 revised criteria for the classification of systemic lupus erythematosus. Arthritis Rheum. 1982;25:1271–7.
14. Eloranta ML, Lövgren T, Finke D, Mathsson L, Rönnelid J, Kastner B, Alm GV, Rönnblom L. Regulation of the interferon-alpha production induced by RNA-containing immune complexes in plasmacytoid dendritic cells. Arthritis Rheum. 2009;60:2418–27.
15. Weber G, Trowitzsch S, Kastner B, Luhrmann R, Wahl MC. Functional organization of the Sm core in the crystal structure of human U1 snRNP. EMBO J. 2010;29:4172–84.
16. Kelly PN, Romero DL, Yang Y, Shaffer AL 3rd, Chaudhary D, Robinson S, Miao W, Rui L, Westlin WF, Kapeller R, et al. Selective interleukin-1 receptor-associated kinase 4 inhibitors for the treatment of autoimmune disorders and lymphoid malignancy. J Exp Med. 2015;212:2189–201.
17. Cederblad B, Blomberg S, Vallin H, Perers A, Alm GV, Ronnblom L. Patients with systemic lupus erythematosus have reduced numbers of circulating natural interferon-alpha- producing cells. J Autoimmun. 1998;11:465–70.
18. Kim D, Langmead B, Salzberg SL. HISAT: a fast spliced aligner with low memory requirements. Nat Methods. 2015;12:357–60.
19. Liao Y, Smyth GK, Shi W. featureCounts: an efficient general purpose program for assigning sequence reads to genomic features. Bioinformatics. 2014;30:923–30.
20. Patro R, Mount SM, Kingsford C. Sailfish enables alignment-free isoform quantification from RNA-seq reads using lightweight algorithms. Nat Biotechnol. 2014;32:462–4.
21. Wickham H. ggplot2: elegant graphics for data analysis. New York: Springer Verlag; 2009.
22. Love MI, Huber W, Anders S. Moderated estimation of fold change and dispersion for RNA-seq data with DESeq2. Genome Biol. 2014;15:550.
23. Pendas-Franco N, Aguilera O, Pereira F, Gonzalez-Sancho JM, Munoz A. Vitamin D and Wnt/beta-catenin pathway in colon cancer: role and regulation of DICKKOPF genes. Anticancer Res. 2008;28:2613–23.
24. Roth L, Srivastava S, Lindzen M, Sas-Chen A, Sheffer M, Lauriola M, Enuka Y, Noronha A, Mancini M, Lavi S, et al. SILAC identifies LAD1 as a filamin-binding regulator of actin dynamics in response to EGF and a marker of aggressive breast tumors. Sci Signal. 2018;11(Issue 515):14. https://doi.org/10.1126/scisignal.aan0949.
25. Ai J, Pascal LE, Wei L, Zang Y, Zhou Y, Yu X, Gong Y, Nakajima S, Nelson JB, Levine AS, et al. EAF2 regulates DNA repair through Ku70/Ku80 in the prostate. Oncogene. 2017;36:2054–65.
26. Postal M, Appenzeller S. The role of tumor necrosis factor-alpha (TNF-α) in the pathogenesis of systemic lupus erythematosus. Cytokine. 2011;56:537–43.
27. Aringer M, Smolen JS. The role of tumor necrosis factor-alpha in systemic lupus erythematosus. Arthritis Res Ther. 2008;10:202.
28. Cortes-Hernandez J, Egri N, Vilardell-Tarres M, Ordi-Ros J. Etanercept in refractory lupus arthritis: an observational study. Semin Arthritis Rheum. 2015;44:672–9.
29. Studnicka-Benke A, Steiner G, Petera P, Smolen JS. Tumour necrosis factor alpha and its soluble receptors parallel clinical disease and autoimmune activity in systemic lupus erythematosus. Br J Rheumatol. 1996;35:1067–74.
30. Fauriat C, Long EO, Ljunggren HG, Bryceson YT. Regulation of human NK-cell cytokine and chemokine production by target cell recognition. Blood. 2010;115:2167–76.
31. Qiu F, Maniar A, Diaz MQ, Chapoval AI, Medvedev AE. Activation of cytokine-producing and antitumor activities of natural killer cells and macrophages by engagement of toll-like and NOD-like receptors. Innate Immun. 2011;17:375–87.
32. Adib-Conquy M, Scott-Algara D, Cavaillon JM, Souza-Fonseca-Guimaraes F. TLR-mediated activation of NK cells and their role in bacterial/viral immune responses in mammals. Immunol Cell Biol. 2014;92:256–62.

33. Wang Z, Wesche H, Stevens T, Walker N, Yeh WC. IRAK-4 inhibitors for inflammation. Curr Top Med Chem. 2009;9:724–37.

34. Vega L, Barbado J, Almansa R, Gonzalez-Gallego R, Rico L, Jimeno A, Nocito M, Ortiz de Lejarazu R, Bermejo-Martin JF. Prolonged standard treatment for systemic lupus erythematosus fails to normalize the secretion of innate immunity-related chemokines. Eur Cytokine Netw. 2010;21:71–6.

35. Sandling J, Garnier S, Sigurdsson S, Wang C, Nordmark G, Gunnarsson I, Svenungsson E, Padyukov L, Sturfelt G, Jönsen A, et al. A candidate gene study of the type I interferon pathway implicates IKBKE and IL8 as risk loci for SLE. Eur J Hum Genet. 2011;19:479–84.

36. Niehrs C. Function and biological roles of the Dickkopf family of Wnt modulators. Oncogene. 2006;25:7469–81.

37. Olferiev M, Jacek E, Kirou KA, Crow MK. Novel molecular signatures in mononuclear cell populations from patients with systemic lupus erythematosus. Clin Immunol. 2016;172:34–43.

38. Bloch O, Amit-Vazina M, Yona E, Molad Y, Rapoport MJ. Increased ERK and JNK activation and decreased ERK/JNK ratio are associated with long-term organ damage in patients with systemic lupus erythematosus. Rheumatology (Oxford). 2014;53:1034–42.

39. Li Y, Takahashi Y, Fujii S, Zhou Y, Hong R, Suzuki A, Tsubata T, Hase K, Wang JY. EAF2 mediates germinal centre B-cell apoptosis to suppress excessive immune responses and prevent autoimmunity. Nat Commun. 2016;7:10836.

40. Kato H, Perl A. Blockade of Treg Cell differentiation and function by the Interleukin-21-Mechanistic Target of Rapamycin Axis Via Suppression of Autophagy in Patients With Systemic Lupus Erythematosus. Arthritis Rheumatol. 2018;70:427-38.

41. Clarke AJ, Ellinghaus U, Cortini A, Stranks A, Simon AK, Botto M, Vyse TJ. Autophagy is activated in systemic lupus erythematosus and required for plasmablast development. Ann Rheum Dis. 2015;74:912–20.

42. Gros F, Muller S. Pharmacological regulators of autophagy and their link with modulators of lupus disease. Br J Pharmacol. 2014;171:4337–59.

43. Dudhgaonkar S, Ranade S, Nagar J, Subramani S, Prasad DS, Karunanithi P, Srivastava R, Venkatesh K, Selvam S, Krishnamurthy P, et al. Selective IRAK4 inhibition attenuates disease in murine lupus models and demonstrates steroid sparing activity. J Immunol. 2017;198:1308–19.

44. Roy A. Early probe and drug discovery in Academia. A Minireview. High Throughput. 2018. p. 7. https://doi.org/10.3390/ht7010004.

11

Effects of CTLA4-Ig treatment on circulating fibrocytes and skin fibroblasts from the same systemic sclerosis patients: an in vitro assay

Maurizio Cutolo[1*], Stefano Soldano[1], Paola Montagna[1], Amelia Chiara Trombetta[1], Paola Contini[2], Barbara Ruaro[1], Alberto Sulli[1], Stefano Scabini[3], Emanuela Stratta[3], Sabrina Paolino[1], Carmen Pizzorni[1], Vanessa Smith[4] and Renata Brizzolara[1]

Abstract

Background: Systemic sclerosis (SSc) is characterized by vasculopathy and progressive fibrosis. CTLA4-Ig (abatacept) is able to interact with the cell surface costimulatory molecule CD86 and downregulate the target cell. The aim of this study was to evaluate the in-vitro effects of CTLA4-Ig treatment on circulating fibrocytes and skin fibroblasts isolated from the same SSc patient.

Methods: Circulating fibrocytes and skin fibroblasts were obtained from eight SSc patients with "limited" cutaneous involvement and from four healthy subjects (HSs). Samples were analyzed by fluorescence-activated cell sorter analysis (FACS) at baseline (T0) and after 8 days of culture (T8) for CD45, collagen type I (COL I), CXCR4, CD14, CD86, and HLA-DRII expression. Circulating fibrocytes were treated for 3 h and skin fibroblasts for 24/48 h with CTLA4-Ig (10, 50, 100, 500 μg/ml). Quantitative real-time polymerase chain reaction (qRT-PCR) was performed for CD86, COL I, FN, TGFβ, αSMA, S100A4, CXCR2, CXCR4, CD11a, and Western blotting was performed for COL I and FN.

Results: Using qRT-PCR, the T8-cultured SSc circulating fibrocytes which had not been treated with CTLA4-Ig showed higher gene expression for CD86, αSMA, S100A4, TGFβ, and COL I compared with HS circulating fibrocytes. Interestingly, αSMA/COL I gene expression was significantly lower only in the SSc circulating fibrocytes treated with CTLA4-Ig for 3 h ($p < 0.01$, $p < 0.05$). On the contrary, no effects were observed for either SSc or HS skin fibroblasts after CTLA4-Ig treatment. COL I and FN protein expression was unchanged in both SSc and HS skin fibroblasts by Western blot.

Conclusions: Circulating fibrocytes seem to be more responsive to CTLA4-Ig treatment than skin fibroblasts from the same SSc patient, likely due to their higher expression of CD86. CTLA4-Ig treatment might downregulate the fibrotic process in SSc patients by downregulating the fibrocytes, circulating progenitor cells.

Keywords: Fibrocytes, Skin fibroblasts, CTLA4-Ig, Systemic sclerosis, Connective tissue disease

* Correspondence: mcutolo@unige.it
[1]Research Laboratory and Academic Division of Clinical Rheumatology,
Department of Internal Medicine, University of Genoa, IRCCS San Martino
Polyclinic Hospital, Viale Benedetto XV, 616132 Genoa, Italy
Full list of author information is available at the end of the article

Key messages

Circulating fibrocytes seem to be more responsive to CTLA4-Ig (abatacept) treatment than skin fibroblasts isolated from the same SSc patients affected by limited or diffuse cutaneous involvement.

The described effetct exerted by abatacept may represent a new approach for early intervention in SSc, therefore acting on progenitor cells (fibrocytes) before their final homing and differentiation into active myofibroblasts.

A new therapeutic option for abatacept in SSc treatment should be taken into consideration based on its possible antifibrotic effect.

Background

Systemic sclerosis (SSc) is a systemic autoimmune connective tissue disease of complex etiology, characterized by microvasculopathy and progressive fibrosis [1, 2].

Activation of the immune response through autoantibody production, together with the recruitment and transition of endothelial cells and pericytes into active myofibroblasts, seems to play an important role in the progression of fibrosis in almost all organs. Therefore, although the pathogenesis of SSc remains unclear, myofibroblast activation is believed to be the final step following microvascular damage [3, 4]. Myofibroblasts are characterized by a higher expression of specific phenotype markers and profibrotic molecules, primarily α-smooth muscle actin (αSMA) and fibroblast-specific protein-1 (S100A4), as well as by the overproduction of extracellular matrix (ECM) proteins such as fibronectin (FN) and fibrillar collagens (type I and III) [5–7].

Various cell types, including endothelial cells, circulating mesenchymal cells, and even fibrocytes, may differentiate into myofibroblasts [8].

Fibrocytes are circulating progenitor cells derived from the bone marrow that express specific markers of both hematopoietic cells (CD34, CD43, CD45, LSP-1, and MHC class II) and stromal cells (collagen I and III), together with the chemokine receptors CCR2, CCR7, and CXCR4, which regulate their migration into inflammatory lesions [9–13]. Circulating fibrocytes are recruited through CXCR4/CXCL12 interaction into injured tissues where they differentiate into fibroblasts/myofibroblasts, thereby regulating the healing process (by producing cytokines, chemokines, and growth factors), secreting essential ECM proteins, and promoting angiogenesis [14–16].

Moreover, although fibrocytes are involved in physiological wound repair to local tissue injury, in chronic fibroproliferative disorders they may be the cause of excess deposition of ECM molecules [17].

In vitro, fibrocytes appear to differentiate from circulating CD14$^+$ monocytes into spindle-shaped, fibroblast-like cells and seem to have an antigen-presenting capability,

expressing class II major histocompatibility complex molecules (HLA-DP, -DQ, and -DR), the CD86 (B7.2) costimulatory molecule, and the CD11a, CD54 (ICAM-1: intracellular adhesion molecule-1), and CD58 adhesion molecules [9, 18–20]. When cultured in the presence of a specific antigen, human fibrocytes induce antigen-presenting cell (APC)-dependent T-cell proliferation which is significantly higher than that induced by monocytes and nearly as high as the proliferation of purified dendritic cells [20].

The costimulatory molecule CD86 is expressed on APCs, including macrophages, and the CTLA4-Ig fusion protein induces a significant downregulation of both proinflammatory cytokines (interleukin (IL)-6, tumor necrosis factor (TNF)α, and IL-1β) and transforming growth factor (TGF)β in cultured human macrophages [21]. Of note, these anti-inflammatory effects induced by the binding between CTLA4-Ig and CD86 on the macrophage surface are evident both in the presence and in the absence of T cells, indicating a direct action of CTLA4-Ig on APCs [21–23].

In addition, CTLA4-Ig interacts with the costimulatory molecule CD86 on human endothelial cells, masking its expression and modulating the expression of vascular endothelial growth factor receptor (VEGFR)-2 and ICAM-1, two important molecules involved in inflammatory and angiogenic processes that characterize several autoimmune diseases, including SSc [24].

Current treatment for SSc includes vasodilators, disease-modifying antirheumatic drugs (DMARDs), and immunosuppressive drugs, but with limited success. New approaches for the treatment of SSc and its fibrotizing processes are under investigation, including the use of CTLA4-Ig (abatacept) [25–27].

Since human fibrocytes seem to have an antigen-presenting capability, and would appear to be an important source of fibroblasts/myofibroblasts in the physiological and pathological tissue remodeling that characterizes SSc, the aim of this study was to isolate and culture human circulating fibrocytes and skin fibroblasts from the same SSc patients as well as from healthy subjects (HSs) to investigate the possible effects exerted in vitro by CTLA4-Ig treatment.

Methods

SSc patients and healthy subjects

Eight SSc patients (seven females and one male, mean age 65 ± 7 years) with "limited" cutaneous involvement (lSSc) and an "active" nailfold videocapillaroscopic (NVC) pattern of microvascular damage were recruited from the Division of Rheumatology at the University of Genova. Four age-matched HSs (three females, one male) were enrolled from the Department of Surgery of the IRCCS San Martino Hospital in Genoa during routine diagnostic procedures.

All enrolled SSc patients fulfilled the 2013 European League Against Rheumatism/American College of Rheumatology (EULAR/ACR) criteria for the diagnosis of SSc [28]. No evident clinical SSc complications were present at the time of skin sampling, and the patients were receiving treatment with vasodilators alone (mainly cyclic prostanoids). At the site of skin biopsy (forearm), the local average value of the modified Rodnan skin score (mRSS) was found to be equal to 1 [29].

All SSc patients and HSs provided informed consent and the study was approved by the local ethics committee (protocol number 273-REG-2015).

Cell culture and treatments

Fibrocytes were isolated from the peripheral blood mononuclear cells (PBMCs) by centrifugation over Ficoll-Paque (Sigma-Aldrich) according to the manufacturer's instructions. The cells were cultured at baseline (T0) on fibronectin-coated plates in Dulbecco's modified Eagle's medium (DMEM) with 20% fetal bovine serum (FBS), 1% penicillin-streptomycin, and 1% L-glutamine (Sigma-Aldrich) at 37 °C and 5% of CO_2. After overnight culture, the nonadherent cells were removed by a single gentle aspiration, while adherent fibrocytes were cultured for a further 8 days (T8) [30].

Fibrocytes at T8 were cultured for 3 h with or without CTLA4-Ig at various concentrations (10, 50, 100, and 500 μg/ml) in accordance with previous in-vitro studies [21, 22, 24].

Skin fibroblasts were isolated from the full thickness biopsies that had been carried out on the involved skin at one-third of the distal forearm of SSc patients and of HSs, in accordance with the EUSTAR protocol and the Declaration of Helsinki [31].

After fibroblast expansion, skin fragments were removed to allow cell growth. Fibroblasts that were collected between the third and fifth culture passage were cultured for 24 and 48 h in the absence or in the presence of various concentrations of CTLA4-Ig (10, 50, 100, and 500 μg/ml).

Fluorescence-activated cell sorter (FACS) analysis

After 8 days of culture (T8), adherent fibrocytes were lifted by incubation in ice-cold 0.05% EDTA in phosphate-buffered saline (PBS), and cell viability was determined by the trypan blue exclusion test.

Characterization and identification of fibrocytes was performed at T0 and T8 by FACS (Beckman Coulter Company) using anti-CD45 (anti-CD45-krome orange, Beckman Coulter Company), anti-COL I (anti-COL I-FITC, Milli-Mark, Millipore), anti-CXCR4 (anti-CXCR4-PE, Beckman Coulter Company), anti-CD14, anti-CD86, and anti-HLA-DRII monoclonal antibodies (anti-CD14-alexa Fluor 750, anti-CD86-PC7, and anti-HLA-DRII-PC5.5, Beckman Coulter Company) [30].

Relevant isotype controls for each monoclonal antibody were used in the initial setup and frequently between tests.

Quantitative real-time polymerase chain reaction (qRT-PCR)

Fibrocytes were cultured for 8 days whereas skin fibroblasts were cultured up to 80% confluency prior to treatment with CTLA4-Ig, as described in the "Cell culture and treatments" section above.

Total RNA was extracted with NucleoSpin RNA/protein (Macherey-Nagel) and quantified by NanoDrop (Thermo Scientific), which also evaluates RNA integrity, in accordance with the manufacturer's instructions. For each experimental condition, first-strand cDNA was synthesized from 1 μg total RNA using the QuantiTect Reverse Transcription Kit (Qiagen).

qRT-PCR was performed on an Eppendorf Realplex 4 Mastercycler using the Real MasterMix SYBR Green detection system (Eppendorf) in a total volume of 10 μl loaded in triplicate. Primers for CD86 (NM_175862.4), COL I (NM_000088), FN (NM_002026), TGFβ (NM_000660), αSMA (NM_001613), S100A4 (NM_002961), CXCR2 (NM_0 0116829), CXCR4 (NM_00100854), CD11a (NM_001 11438), and β-actin (NM_001101, housekeeping gene) were supplied by Primerdesign.

Gene expression values were calculated using the comparative $\Delta\Delta CT$ method and they corresponded to the expression level (fold-increase) of the target gene compared with the calibrator sample (untreated cells) taken as the unit value by definition [32]. In each qRT-PCR assay, the melting curve was performed to confirm the specificity of the SYBR green assay.

Western blotting

Skin fibroblasts were cultured to 80% confluency and treated as described in the "Cell culture and treatments" section above. At the end of treatment (24 and 48 h), cells were lysed with NucleoSpin RNA/protein (Macherey-Nagel). Protein quantification was performed by the Bradford method. For each experimental condition, 20 μg protein was separated by electrophoresis on Tris-Glycine gel and transferred onto Hybond-C-nitrocellulose membranes (Life Technologies Ltd.).

After 1 h in blocking solution (PBS 1× 0.1% triton-X, and 5% nonfat powdered milk) membranes were incubated overnight at 4 °C with the following primary antibodies: anti-human COL I (dilution 1:400, Vinci-Biochem) and FN (dilution 1:1000, Sigma-Aldrich). Membranes were also incubated with primary horseradish peroxidase (HRP)-conjugated antibody to human actin (dilution 1:10,

000, Santa-Cruz Biotechnology) to confirm similar loading of protein samples onto the gels and the efficiency of the electrophoretic transfer.

Membranes were subsequently incubated with the following secondary antibodies: anti-rabbit IgG for COL I (dilution 1:2000, Cell Signaling Technology) and anti-mouse IgG for FN (dilution 1:1000, Cell Signaling Technology). Protein synthesis was detected using the enhanced chemiluminescence system (Luminata Crescendo, Millipore). Densitometric analysis was performed by UVITEC Analysis Software (UVITEC Cambridge).

For each experimental condition, the values of collagen type I (COL I) and FN synthesis were normalized to those of the corresponding actin. The resulting values of each treatment were compared with those of the untreated cells (CNT; taken as the unit value by definition) to obtain the level of protein synthesis.

Statistical analysis

Statistical analysis was carried out by the nonparametric Mann-Whitney U test to compare unpaired treatment group data. Any p value below 0.05 was considered statistically significant. The final results of FACS, qRT-PCR, and Western blotting were the mean of the results obtained from the independent experiments performed on in-vitro cultures of fibrocytes and skin fibroblasts isolated from each SSc patient and HS. The results are reported as mean ± standard deviation (SD).

Results

FACS analysis

FACS analysis showed that at T0 the percentage of fibrocytes, identified as CD45$^+$COL I$^+$CXCR4$^+$ cells, was 1.0 ± 1.2% in SSc patients and 0.5 ± 0.2% in HSs (50% less) (Fig. 1a). Moreover, in this fibrocyte population, the percentage of HLA-DR$^+$ cells was very low (22.1 ± 21.1%

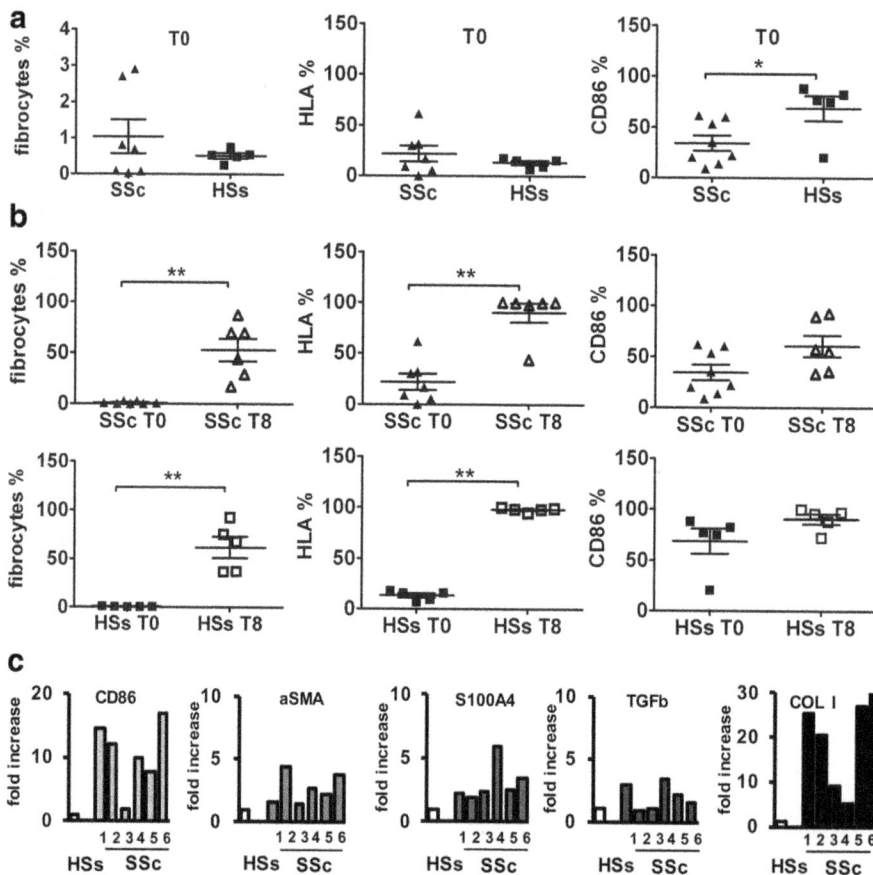

Fig. 1 Characterization of systemic sclerosis (SSc) and healthy subject (HS) fibrocytes at basal time (T0) and at 8 days of culture (T8). **a** FACS analysis of SSc and HS fibrocytes, identified among the CD45$^+$ cells, as CD45$^+$, COL I$^+$, CXCR4$^+$, and relative HLA-DR and CD86 expression at T0; **b** FACS analysis of SSc and HS fibrocytes, identified among the CD45$^+$ cells, as CD45$^+$, COL I$^+$, CXCR4$^+$, and relative HLA-DR and CD86 expression at T0 and T8. **c** Quantitative RT-PCR analysis for CD86, αSMA, S100A4, TGFβ, and COL I gene expression of cultured SSc fibrocytes (T8), compared with HS fibrocytes (T8), taken as the calibrator

and $13.1 \pm 4.7\%$, respectively), whereas the percentage of CD86$^+$ cells was higher in both SSc patients and HSs at T0 ($34.4 \pm 21.4\%$ and $68.9 \pm 27.6\%$) (Fig. 1a).

At T8, fibrocytes showed an adherent spindle-shaped morphology, and FACS analysis demonstrated that the percentage of CD45$^+$COL I$^+$CXCR4$^+$ fibrocytes was significantly higher in both SSc patients and in HSs compared with T0 (up to $52.8 \pm 27.1\%$ vs. $1.0 \pm 1.2\%$ and up to $61.9 \pm 24.4\%$ vs. $0.5 \pm 0.2\%$, respectively) ($p < 0.01$) (Fig. 1b).

At the same time, in this fibrocyte population, the HLA-DR$^+$ cells were significantly increased in SSc patients and HSs compared with T0 ($90.1 \pm 22.7\%$ vs. $22.1 \pm 21.1\%$ and 97.9 ± 1.9 vs $13.1 \pm 4.7\%$, respectively) ($p < 0.01$) (Fig. 1b).

Similarly, the percentage of CD86$^+$ fibrocytes was higher in SSc patients and HSs compared with T0 ($60.4 \pm 25.6\%$ vs. $34.4 \pm 21.4\%$, and $90.7 \pm 10.9\%$ vs. $68.9 \pm 27.6\%$, respectively) with a greater increment in SSc fibrocytes (Fig. 1b).

Quantitative real-time PCR

SSc fibrocytes

At T8, in the absence of CTLA4-Ig, SSc fibrocytes showed higher gene expression levels of CD86, αSMA, S100A4, TGFβ, and COL I compared with HS fibrocytes (Fig. 1c).

The SSc fibrocytes treated for 3 h with various concentrations of CTLA4-Ig (10, 50, 100, and 500 μg/ml) did not show any significant variations in the gene expression levels of TGFβ, IL-1β, and CXCR2 compared

with CNT (Fig. 2a). In these cells, CD86 gene expression decreased (not significantly) after treatment with CTLA4-Ig 500 μg/ml (Fig. 2a).

Interestingly, the gene expression of COL I was significantly lower in SSc fibrocytes treated with CTLA4-Ig even at 10 μg/ml compared with CNT ($p < 0.05$) (Fig. 2a). Of note, αSMA gene expression also decreased after CTLA4-Ig treatment (significantly after CTLA4-Ig 10 μg/ml treatment, $p < 0.05$, and CTLA4-Ig 500 μg/ml treatment, $p < 0.01$), whereas S100A4 gene expression was significantly higher compared with CNT ($p < 0.01$) excluding at the concentration of 500 μg/ml (Fig. 2a).

Moreover, while treatment with CTLA4-Ig 500 μg/ml did not significantly reduce the gene expression of CXCR4, it did significantly reduce that of CD11a as compared with CNT ($p < 0.05$) (Fig. 2a).

HS fibrocytes

Unlike SSc fibrocytes, HS fibrocytes treated for 3 h with various concentrations of CTLA4-Ig (10, 50, 100, and 500 μg/ml) did not show any significant modulation in the gene expression levels of CD86 (Fig. 2b).

In addition, gene expression levels of TGFβ, CXCR2, COL I, CXCR4, and CD11a remained unchanged after CTLA4-Ig treatment compared with CNT, as did gene expression of αSMA and S100A4 (Fig. 2b).

SSc fibroblasts

Cultured SSc fibroblasts showed very low gene expression levels of CD86 compared with cultured macrophages obtained from the PBMCs of SSc patients, which

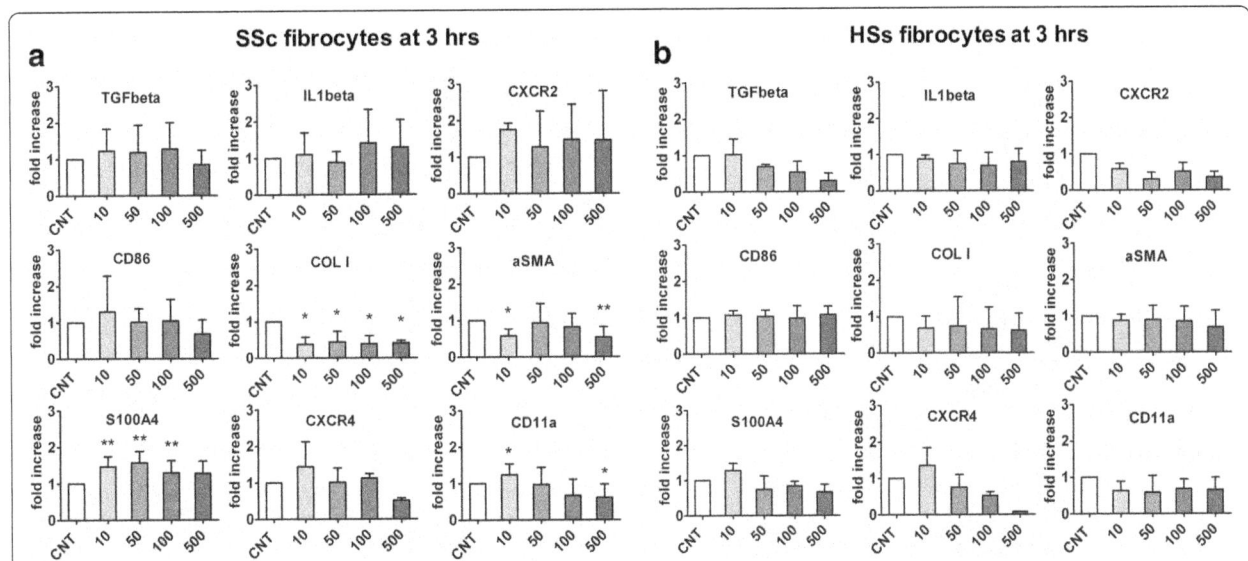

Fig. 2 Quantitative RT-PCR analysis for TGFβ, IL-1β, CXCR2, CD86, COL I, αSMA, S100A4, CXCR4, and CD11a gene expression in cultures of systemic sclerosis (SSc) and healthy subject (HS) fibrocytes after 3 h of CTLA4-Ig treatment. Quantitative RT-PCR analysis for TGFβ, IL-1β, CXCR2, CD86, COL I, αSMA, S100A4, CXCR4, and CD11a gene expression in cultures of SSc fibrocytes (**a**) and HS fibrocytes (**b**) either untreated (CNT) or treated for 3 h with CTLA4-Ig at various doses (10, 50, 100, and 500 μg/ml). *$p < 0.05$, **$p < 0.01$

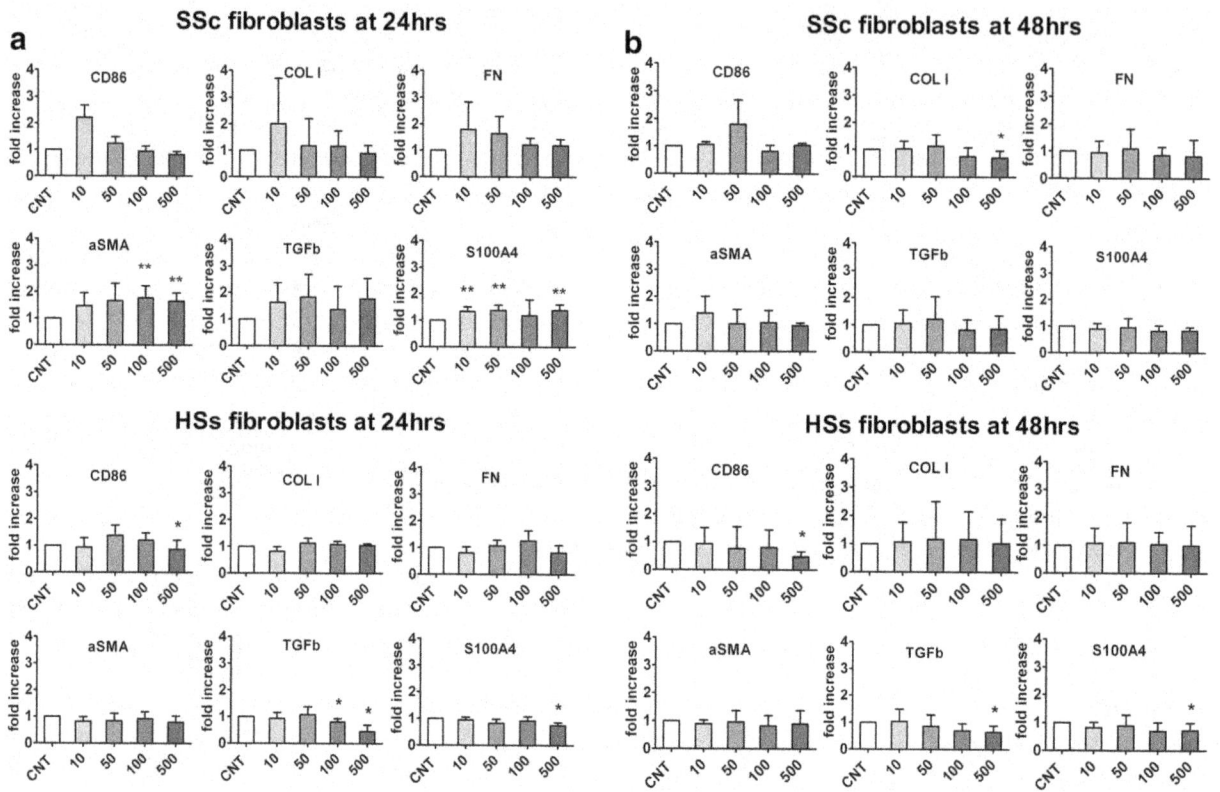

Fig. 3 Quantitative RT-PCR analysis for CD86, COL I, FN, αSMA, TGFβ, and S100A4 gene expression in cultured systemic sclerosis (SSc) and healthy subject (HS) fibroblasts after 24 and 48 h of CTLA4-Ig treatments. Quantitative RT-PCR analysis for CD86, COL I, FN, αSMA, TGFβ, and S100A4 gene expression in cultures of SSc and HS fibroblasts either untreated (CNT) or treated for 24 h (**a**) and 48 h (**b**) with CTLA4-Ig at various doses (10, 50, 100, and 500 μg/ml). *$p < 0.05$, **$p < 0.01$

were taken as positive controls for CD86 expression (Additional file 1).

Nevertheless, cultured SSc fibroblasts treated for 24 h with CTLA4-Ig (10, 50, 100, and 500 μg/ml) did not show any significant differences in gene expression levels of CD86 compared with CNT (a nonsignificant increase after treatment with CTLA4-Ig 10 μg/ml was observed) (Fig. 3a). At the same time, gene expression of COL I and FN was higher only in the cultured SSc fibroblasts which had been treated with the lowest concentration of CTLA4-Ig (10 μg/ml) (Fig. 3a).

In addition, in these cultured CTLA4-Ig-treated SSc cells, the gene expression levels of αSMA, TGFβ. and S100A4 were higher compared with CNT (significantly for αSMA and S100A4; $p < 0.01$) (Fig. 3a).

On the other hand, the cultured SSc fibroblasts treated for 48 h with CTLA4-Ig (10, 50, 100, and 500 μg/ml) did not show any significant modulation in the gene expression levels of CD86, FN, αSMA, TGFβ, and S100A4 compared with CNT, whereas the gene expression of COL I was significantly downregulated by the highest dose of CTLA4-Ig ($p < 0.05$) (Fig. 3b).

HS fibroblasts

Cultured HS fibroblasts treated with CTLA4-Ig for 24 h showed a significant decrease in the gene expression of CD86, although this was limited to the highest dose (500 μg/ml) compared with CNT ($p < 0.05$) (Fig. 3a).

Of note, the gene expression of TGFβ and S100A4 was significantly reduced by the higher doses of CTLA4-Ig ($p < 0.05$ after 100 and 500 μg/ml for TGFβ; $p < 0.05$ after 500 μg/ml for S100A4) (Fig. 3a).

Similar to the results obtained after 24 h of CTLA4-Ig treatment, cultured HS fibroblasts showed a significant decrease in the gene expression levels of CD86 compared with CNT after 48 h of treatment with CTLA4-Ig, though this was limited to the highest dose (500 μg/ml) ($p < 0.05$) (Fig. 3b).

After 48 h of treatment with the highest dose of CTLA4-Ig (500 μg/ml), gene expression of TGFβ and S100A4 was significantly reduced compared with CNT (both $p < 0.05$) (Fig. 3b).

Gene expression of COL I, FN, and αSMA was unchanged after both 24 and 48 h of CTLA4-Ig treatment in cultured HS fibroblasts (Fig. 3a, b).

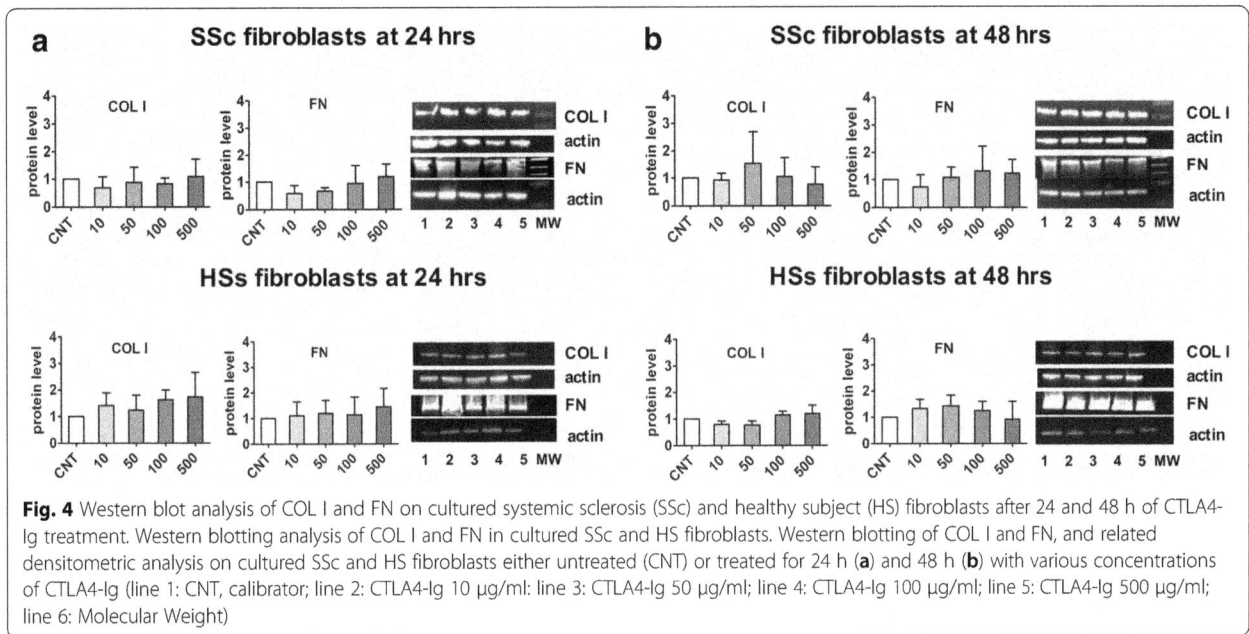

Fig. 4 Western blot analysis of COL I and FN on cultured systemic sclerosis (SSc) and healthy subject (HS) fibroblasts after 24 and 48 h of CTLA4-Ig treatment. Western blotting analysis of COL I and FN in cultured SSc and HS fibroblasts. Western blotting of COL I and FN, and related densitometric analysis on cultured SSc and HS fibroblasts either untreated (CNT) or treated for 24 h (**a**) and 48 h (**b**) with various concentrations of CTLA4-Ig (line 1: CNT, calibrator; line 2: CTLA4-Ig 10 μg/ml: line 3: CTLA4-Ig 50 μg/ml; line 4: CTLA4-Ig 100 μg/ml; line 5: CTLA4-Ig 500 μg/ml; line 6: Molecular Weight)

Western blotting

The protein expression of COL I and FN in cultured SSc and HS fibroblasts was unchanged even after treatment with CTLA4-Ig at both 24 and 48 h compared with CNT (Fig. 4).

Discussion

The present study reports for the first time that SSc circulating fibrocytes show an increased basal expression of αSMA and COL I compared with HS fibrocytes, suggesting their possible propensity for transition into activated myofibroblasts which are key cells involved in both tissue repair and fibrosis. Moreover, SSc circulating fibrocytes show a higher gene expression of CD86 and seem to be more responsive to treatment with the CTLA4-Ig fusion protein compared with the skin fibroblasts obtained from the same SSc patients.

This study also confirms that the percentage of circulating fibrocytes, characterized as CD45$^+$COL I$^+$CXCR4$^+$ cells, was at least twice as high in SSc patients compared with HSs, although these cells are a minor component of the circulating pool of cells [11, 16, 33].

On the basis of these characteristics, we observed that once circulating fibrocytes are cultured in vitro they become adherent, develop a spindle-shaped morphology, and maintain the expression of key fibrocyte phenotype markers (CD45, COL I, and CXCR4), with a further increase in CD86 and HLA-DRII expression.

The interaction between the CTLA4-Ig fusion molecule (abatacept) and CD86 expressed on circulating fibrocytes is believed to alter and interfere with the function of these cells under pathological conditions, such as SSc, and in

particular with their activation and differentiation into fibroblasts/myofibroblasts. The decrease in the gene expression of the main phenotypic markers of activated fibrocytes (COL I and CXCR4), together with the decreased gene expression of the myofibroblast phenotype marker αSMA induced by CTLA4-Ig treatment, suggests a possible downregulatory effect on the fibrocyte-myofibroblast transition process. It is interesting to note that these effects were evident in SSc circulating fibrocytes, but they were not observed in the HS circulating fibrocytes.

It is believed that, in response to injurious and inflammatory stimuli, human CD45$^+$COL I$^+$CXCR4$^+$ fibrocytes traffic through the bloodstream and may be recruited into, and activated within, the injured and inflamed tissues where the chemokine receptors CXCR4 and CCR7 are reported to be pivotal [10, 14]. Of note, the ability of CTLA4-Ig to trigger a decrease in the expression of CXCR4 and CD11a adhesion/migration molecules on SSc circulating fibrocytes may suggest its possible action in interfering with trafficking and migration of these cells into inflammatory/altered sites [10, 14].

Fibrocytes can also function as APCs for the activation of CD8$^+$ T cells by expressing major histocompatibility complex class I and II molecules and the costimulatory proteins CD80 and CD86 [20]. By binding to SSc circulating fibrocytes expressing CD86, CTLA4-Ig might interfere with their APC activity and could likely prevent the activation of T lymphocytes, as already demonstrated for other cellular targets (dendritic cells, B lymphocytes, macrophages, osteoclasts, endothelial cells) [21, 24, 34–37].

It is possible that, in SSc, circulating fibrocytes are already activated by the immune-inflammatory response associated with the disease, and that they are more responsive to other protein interactions, in particular to CTLA4-Ig, as compared with HS circulating fibrocytes.

A limitation of these in-vitro experiments relates to the small number of circulating fibrocytes that can be obtained from SSc patients and from HSs; therefore, larger samples are needed to confirm the obtained data. A further study evaluating SSc patients with diffuse skin involvement is already in progress. Very preliminary data obtained from in-vitro experiments on circulating fibrocytes isolated from only two patients, and treated with CTLA4-Ig, seem to show results similar to that described in our study.

Concerning fibroblasts, CD86 gene expression was found to be very low in cultured SSc fibroblasts, contrary to that found in circulating fibrocytes from the same patients, as already reported for murine fibroblasts [38]. As a possible consequence of the limited interaction with CD86, in the present short-term study (24 and 48 h) the CTLA4-Ig treatment did not induce a decrease in the ECM protein synthesis (COL I and FN) in cultured SSc fibroblasts or in HS fibroblasts.

A further study evaluating SSc patients with diffuse cutaneous involvement (dcSSc) is already in progress. Very preliminary data obtained from in-vitro experiments on circulating fibrocytes isolated from only two dcSSc patients, and treated with CTLA4-Ig, seem to show results similar to those described in lcSSc.

In addition, the histopathological literature in SSc attests that both the limited cutaneous as well as the diffuse cutaneous subset are characterized by the presence of myofibroblasts [39]. Hence, our study design should be equally applicable in limited cutaneous as well as diffuse cutaneous SSc.

Of note, the CTLA4-Ig treatment (at high doses) seems to induce a decrease in the TGFβ gene expression that can already be observed after 24 h of treatment; this, however, is limited to the cultured HS fibroblasts.

Conclusions

In conclusion, circulating fibrocytes seem to be more responsive to CTLA4-Ig treatment than skin fibroblasts isolated from the same SSc patients characterized by limited cutaneous involvement. Thus, a new therapeutic option for abatacept in SSc treatment should be taken into consideration based on its possible antifibrotic effect.

Therefore, as described for the first time in the present study, the higher efficacy exerted at the gene expression level by CTLA4-Ig in cultured circulating fibrocytes versus cultured skin fibroblasts/myofibroblasts isolated from the same SSc patients may represent a new approach for early intervention, acting on progenitor cells before their final homing and differentiation into active myofibroblasts.

Abbreviations
APC: Antigen-presenting cell; CNT: Untreated cells; COL I: Collagen type I; dcSSc: Diffuse cutaneous systemic sclerosis; DMARD: Disease-modifying antirheumatic drug; ECM: Extracellular matrix; EULAR/ACR: European League Against Rheumatism/American College of Rheumatology; FACS: Fluorescence-activated cell sorter; FN: Fibronectin; HS: Healthy subject; ICAM: Intracellular adhesion molecule; IL: Interleukin; lSSc: Limited systemic sclerosis; NVC: Nailfold videocapillaroscopy; PBMC: Peripheral blood mononuclear cell; PBS: Phosphate-buffered saline; qRT-PCR: Quantitative real-time polymerase chain reaction; S100A4: Fibroblast-specific protein-1; SMA: Smooth muscle actin; SSc: Systemic sclerosis; Tx: Day x; TGF: Transforming growth factor; TNF: Tumor necrosis factor; VEGFR: Vascular endothelial growth factor receptor

Acknowledgements
We thank Dr. Sara De Gregorio for the contribution to the figures.

Funding
Bristol Myers Squibb provided financial support (via a university research grant) and the CTLA4-Ig molecule for the in-vitro study.

Authors' contributions
MC made substantial contributions to the conception and design of the manuscript, revised it critically for important intellectual content, and gave final approval of the version to be published; SS participated in the conception and design of the study, participated in the interpretation of data, and revised the final version of the manuscript; PM performed the qRT-PCR analysis and made substantial contributions to the analysis and interpretation of data; ACT participated in the conception and design of the study and revised the final version of the manuscript; PC performed FACS analysis and made substantial contributions to the analysis of data; BR participated in the conception and design of the study and was clinically responsible for the selection and recruitment of SSc patients and healthy subjects; AS participated in the conception and design of the study and made substantial contributions to the analysis and interpretation of data; SS participated in the design of the study and performed the skin biopsies; ES performed the skin biopsies; SP participated in the recruitment of patients and healthy subjects; CP participated in the recruitment of patients and healthy subjects; VS revised the manuscript critically for important intellectual content and made substantial contributions to the analysis and interpretation of data; RB performed the in-vitro experiments and statistical analysis, made substantial contributions to the analysis and interpretation of data, and drafted the manuscript. All authors read and approved the final manuscript.

Competing interests
MC has obtained research funds from BMS, Actelion, Celgene, Boehringer. The remaining authors declare that they have no competing interests.

Author details
[1]Research Laboratory and Academic Division of Clinical Rheumatology, Department of Internal Medicine, University of Genoa, IRCCS San Martino Polyclinic Hospital, Viale Benedetto XV, 616132 Genoa, Italy. [2]Division of Clinical Immunology, Department of Internal Medicine, University of Genoa, Genoa, Italy. [3]Oncologic Surgery, Department of Surgery, IRCCS San Martino Polyclinic, Genoa, Italy. [4]Department of Rheumatology, Ghent University Hospital, Ghent University, Ghent, Belgium.

References
1. Allanore Y, Distler O. Systemic sclerosis in 2014: advances in cohort enrichment shape future of trial design. Nat Rev Rheumatol. 2015;11:72–4.
2. Balbir-Gurman A, Braun-Moscovici Y. Scleroderma: new aspects in pathogenesis and treatment. Best Pract Res Clin Rheumatol. 2012;26:13–24.
3. Bhattacharyya S, Wei J, Varga J. Understanding fibrosis in systemic sclerosis: shifting paradigms, emerging opportunities. Nat Rev Rheumatol. 2012;8:42–54.
4. Cutolo M, Montagna P, Brizzolara R, Smith V, Alessandri E, Villaggio B, et al. Effects of macitentan and its active metabolite on cultured human systemic sclerosis and control skin fibroblasts. J Rheumatol. 2015;42:456–63.
5. Tomcik M, Palumbo-Zerr K, Zerr P, Avouac J, Dees C, Sumova B, et al. S100A4 amplifies TGF-β-induced fibroblast activation in systemic sclerosis. Ann Rheum Dis. 2015;74:1748–55.

6. Eyden B. The myofibroblasts: phenotypic characterization as a prerequisite to understanding its functions in translational medicine. J Cell Mol Med. 2008;12:22–37.

7. Hinz B, Phan SH, Thannickal VJ, Galli A, Bothaton-Piallat ML, Gabbiani G. The myofibroblasts: one function, multiple origin. Am J Pathol. 2007;170:1807–16.

8. Brenner DA, Kisseleva T, Scholten D, Paik TH, Iwaisako K, Inokuchi S, et al. Origin of myofibroblasts in liver fibrosis. Fibrogenesis Tissue Repair. 2012;5(Suppl 1) https://doi.org/10.1186/1755-1536-5-S1-S17.

9. Bucala R. Fibrocytes at 20 years. Mol Med. 2015;21(Suppl 1):S3–5. https://doi.org/10.2119/molmed.2015.00043.

10. Grieb G, Bucala R. Fibrocytes in fibrotic diseases and wound healing. Adv Wound Care (New Rochelle). 2012;1:36–40.

11. Herzoga EL, Bucala R. Fibrocytes in health and disease. Exp Hematol. 2010;38:548–56.

12. Just SA, Lindegaard H, Hejbøl EK, Davidsen JR, Bjerring N, Hansen SWK, et al. Fibrocyte measurement in peripheral blood correlates with number of cultured mature fibrocytes in vitro and is a potential biomarker for interstitial lung disease in rheumatoid arthritis. Respir Res. 2017;18:141.

13. Strieter RM, Keeley EC, Hughes MA, Burdick MD, Mehrad B. The role of circulating mesenchymal progenitor cells (fibrocytes) in the pathogenesis of pulmonary fibrosis. J Leukoc Biol. 2009;86:1111–8.

14. Liu Y, Qingjuan S, Gao Z, Deng C, Wang Y, Guo C. Circulating fibrocytes are involved in inflammation and leukocyte trafficking in neonates with necrotizing enterocolitis. Medicine (Baltimore). 2017; https://doi.org/10.1097/MD.0000000000007400.

15. Dupin I, Allard B, Ozier A, Maurat E, Ousova O, Delbrel E, et al. Blood fibrocytes are recruited during acute exacerbations of chronic obstructive pulmonary disease through a CXCR4-dependent pathway. J Allergy Clin Immunol. 2016;137:1036–42.

16. Russo R, Medbury H, Guiffre A, Englert H, Manolios N. Lack of increased expression of cell surface markers for circulating fibrocyte progenitors in limited scleroderma. Clin Rheumatol. 2007;26:1136–41.

17. Keeleya EC, Mehradb B, Strieter RM. Fibrocytes: bringing new insights into mechanisms of inflammation and fibrosis. Int J Biochem Cell Biol. 2010;42:535–42.

18. Reilkoff RA, Bucala R, Herzog EL. Fibrocytes: emerging effector cells in chronic inflammation. Nat Rev Immunol. 2011;11:427–35.

19. Blakaj A, Bucala R. Fibrocytes in health and disease. Fibrogenesis Tissue Repair. 2012;5(Suppl 1):S6. https://doi.org/10.1186/1755-1536-5-S1-S6.

20. Chesney J, Bacher M, Bender A, Bucala R. The peripheral blood fibrocyte is a potent antigen presenting cell capable of priming naïve T cells in situ. Proc Natl Acad Sci. 1997;94:6307–12.

21. Cutolo M, Soldano S, Montagna P, Sulli A, Seriolo B, Villaggio B, et al. CTLA4-Ig interacts with cultured synovial macrophages from rheumatoid arthritis patients and downregulates cytokine production. Arthritis Res Ther. 2009;11:176–85.

22. Brizzolara R, Montagna P, Soldano S, Cutolo M. Rapid interaction between CTLA4-Ig (abatacept) and synovial macrophages from patients with rheumatoid arthritis. J Rheumatol. 2013;40:738–40.

23. Bonelli M, Ferner E, Göschl L, Blüml S, Hladik A, Karonitsch T, et al. Abatacept (CTLA-4IG) treatment reduces the migratory capacity of monocytes in patients with rheumatoid arthritis. Arthritis Rheum. 2013;65:599–607.

24. Cutolo M, Montagna P, Soldano S, Contini P, Paolino S, Pizzorni S, et al. CTLA4-IG/CD86 interaction in cultured human endothelial cells: effects on VEGFR-2 and ICAM1 expression. Clin Exp Rheumatol. 2015;33:250–4.

25. Ponsoye M, Frantz C, Ruzehaji N, Nicco C, Elhai M, Ruiz B, et al. Treatment with abatacept prevents experimental dermal fibrosis and induces regression of established inflammation-driven fibrosis. Ann Rheum Dis. 2016;75:2142–9.

26. Cutolo M. Disease modification in systemic sclerosis. Do integrated approaches offer new challenges? Z Rheumatol. 2013;72:326–8.

27. Gabrielli A, Avvedimento EV, Krieg T. Scleroderma. N Engl J Med. 2009;360:1989–2003.

28. van den Hoogen F, Khanna D, Fransen J, Johnson SR, Baron M, Tyndall A, et al. 2013 classification criteria for systemic sclerosis: an American College of Rheumatology/European League Against Rheumatism collaborative initiative. Arthritis Rheum. 2013;65:2737–47.

29. Czirják L, Nagy Z, Aringer M, Riemekasten G, Matucci-Cerinic M, Furst DE, EUSTAR. The EUSTAR model for teaching and implementing the modified Rodnan skin score in systemic sclerosis. Ann Rheum Dis. 2007;66:966–9.

30. Pilling D, Vakil V, Gomer RH. Improved serum-free culture conditions for the differentiation of human and murine fibrocytes. J Immunol Methods. 2009;351:62–70.

31. Beyer C, Distler JH, Allanore Y, Aringer M, Avouac J, Czirijak L, EUSTAR Biobanking Group, et al. EUSTAR biobanking: recommendations for the collection, storage and distribution of biospecimens in scleroderma research. Ann Rheum Dis. 2011;70:1178–82.

32. Livak KJ, Schmittgen TD. Analysis of relative gene expression data using real-time quantitative PCR and the 2(−Delta Delta C (T)) method. Methods. 2001;25:402–8.

33. Phillips RJ, Burdick MD, Hong K, Lutz MA, Murray LA, Xue YY, et al. Circulating fibrocytes traffic to the lungs in response to CXCL12 and mediate fibrosis. J Clin Invest. 2004;114:438–46.

34. Rau FC, Baumgarth N. CD86-1/2 (CD80/CD86) direct signaling to B cells enhances IgG secretion. J Immunol. 2009;183:7661–71.

35. Axnamm R, Herman S, Zaiss M, Franz S, Polzer K, Zwerina J, et al. CTLA-4 directly inhibit OC. Ann Rheum Dis. 2008;67:1603–9.

36. Vogt B, Warncke M, Micheel B, Sheriff A. Lentiviral gene transfer of CTLA4 generates B cells with reduced costimulatory properties. Autoimmunity. 2009;42:380–9.

37. Li H, Hong S, Qian J, Zheng Y, Yang J, Yi Q. Cross talk between the bone and immune systems: osteoclasts function as antigen-presenting cells and activate CD4+ and CD8+ T cells. Blood. 2010;116:210–7.

38. Pechhold K, Patterson NB, Craighead N, Lee KP, June CH, Harlan DM. Inflammatory cytokines IFN-gamma plus TNF-alpha induce regulated expression of CD80 (B7-1) but not CD86 (B7-2) on murine fibroblasts. J Immunol. 1997;158:4921–9.

39. Van Praet JT, Smith V, Haspeslagh M, Degryse N, Elewaut D, De Keyser F. Histopathological cutaneous alterations in systemic sclerosis: a clinicopathological study. Arthritis Res Ther. 2011;13(1):R35.

12

Disease-specific composite measures for psoriatic arthritis are highly responsive to a Janus kinase inhibitor treatment that targets multiple domains of disease

Philip Helliwell[1], Laura C. Coates[2], Oliver FitzGerald[3], Peter Nash[4], Enrique R. Soriano[5], M. Elaine Husni[6], Ming-Ann Hsu[7], Keith S. Kanik[7], Thijs Hendrikx[8], Joseph Wu[7] and Elizabeth Kudlacz[7*]

Abstract

Background: The multiple disease domains affected in psoriatic arthritis (PsA) may make composite endpoints appropriate for assessing changes in disease activity over time. Tofacitinib is an oral Janus kinase inhibitor for the treatment of PsA. Data from two phase 3 studies of patients with PsA were used to evaluate the effect of tofacitinib on composite endpoints.

Methods: Oral Psoriatic Arthritis triaL (OPAL) Broaden was a 12-month study of tumor necrosis factor inhibitor (TNFi)-naïve patients with an inadequate response to at least one conventional synthetic disease-modifying anti-rheumatic drug; OPAL Beyond was a 6-month study of patients with inadequate response to TNFi. Patients with active PsA received tofacitinib 5 or 10 mg doses twice daily (BID), adalimumab 40 mg subcutaneous injection once every 2 weeks (OPAL Broaden only), or placebo advancing at month 3 to tofacitinib 5 or 10 mg BID. The disease-specific composites were Psoriatic Arthritis Disease Activity Score (PASDAS), Disease Activity Index for Reactive Arthritis/Psoriatic Arthritis (DAPSA), and Composite Psoriatic Disease Activity Index (CPDAI). Change from baseline in composite endpoints was also assessed for minimal disease activity (MDA) responders versus non-responders.

Results: Overall, 422 patients from OPAL Broaden and 394 patients from OPAL Beyond were treated. The mean changes from baseline to month 3 for tofacitinib 5 mg BID, tofacitinib 10 mg BID (standard error; effect size) were OPAL Broaden: PASDAS, −2.0 (0.14; 1.73), −2.4 (0.14; 2.4); DAPSA, −20.2 (1.72; 0.9), −24.4 (1.73; 1.23); and CPDAI, −2.9 (0.34; 1.03), −4.2 (0.36; 1.53); OPAL Beyond: PASDAS, −1.9 (0.14; 1.53), −2.1 (0.14; 1.84); DAPSA, −22.5 (1.67; 0.81), −21.0 (1.70; 0.84); and CPDAI, −3.3 (0.31; 1.41), −3.4 (0.31; 1.45). Greater changes from baseline to month 3 ($P \leq 0.05$) were seen with both doses of tofacitinib versus placebo for all endpoints except CPDAI for tofacitinib 5 mg BID in OPAL Broaden. Effect sizes generally increased from 3 to 6 months. Mean changes from baseline were greater in MDA responders than MDA non-responders for all composite endpoints across all time points and treatments.

Conclusions: This analysis suggests that disease-specific composite measures are appropriate for evaluating treatment efficacy on multiple disease domains in PsA.

Keywords: Psoriatic arthritis, Assessment, PASDAS, DAPSA, CPDAI, DAS28–3(CRP)

* Correspondence: elizabeth.m.kudlacz@pfizer.com
[7]Pfizer Inc, 280 Shennecossett Rd, Groton, CT 06340, USA
Full list of author information is available at the end of the article

Background

Psoriatic arthritis (PsA) is a chronic, systemic, immune-mediated inflammatory disease with multiple disease manifestations, including peripheral arthritis, enthesitis, dactylitis, spondylitis, and psoriatic skin and nail disease [1–3]. Owing to the multiple diverse disease manifestations involved in PsA, the Group for Research and Assessment of Psoriasis and Psoriatic Arthritis (GRAPPA) bases its treatment recommendations on the domains affecting an individual [1]. Consequently, composite endpoints, which allow the assessment of multiple clinical outcomes in a single instrument, have been suggested to be particularly useful to assess changes in the multiple disease domains of PsA over time [3, 4]. Composite endpoints also have the potential to simplify statistical testing in clinical trials as a summary or total score is usually generated, thus requiring only a single hypothesis test, thereby avoiding issues with multiplicity and allowing for appropriate statistical power with relatively small numbers of patients [5].

A number of composite endpoints have been developed for PsA in order to assess multiple aspects of disease activity and identify patients who have achieved treatment targets of remission or minimal disease activity (MDA). Available instruments incorporate different types of assessments, including clinical (for example, tender and swollen joint counts [TJC and SJC]), laboratory (for example, C-reactive protein [CRP]), and patient-reported outcome (PRO) (for example, Health Assessment Questionnaire-Disability Index [HAQ-DI]) endpoints. Although there is no clear agreement on a standardized composite assessment approach that provides the optimal combination of individual variables [6], agreement has now been reached on a core domain set of variables that should be included [7].

Tofacitinib is an oral inhibitor of the Janus kinase (JAK) family for the treatment of PsA. Tofacitinib preferentially inhibits signaling via JAK3 or JAK1 (or both) with functional selectivity over JAK2 [8]. The efficacy and safety of tofacitinib 5 and 10 mg twice daily (BID) have been demonstrated in patients with PsA with an inadequate response to conventional synthetic disease-modifying anti-rheumatic drugs (csDMARDs) in Oral Psoriatic Arthritis triaL (OPAL) Broaden [9] and in patients with PsA who were tumor necrosis factor inhibitor (TNFi)-inadequate responders (IRs) in OPAL Beyond [10]. In both studies, tofacitinib had greater efficacy than placebo on the basis of the primary endpoints: a higher proportion of patients receiving tofacitinib than placebo achieved greater than or equal to 20% improvement according to the criteria of the American College of Rheumatology (ACR20 response) at month 3, and the mean change from baseline to month 3 in HAQ-DI score was greater in patients receiving tofacitinib versus placebo at month 3. In addition, between 21% and 26% of patients receiving tofacitinib and between 7% and 15% of patients receiving placebo had MDA responses at month 3 in OPAL Broaden and OPAL Beyond [9, 10]. This analysis evaluated the effect of tofacitinib on three disease-specific composite endpoints in patients with PsA by using data from the two placebo-controlled, double-blind, multicenter, global phase 3 studies of tofacitinib detailed above: OPAL Broaden and OPAL Beyond [9, 10].

Methods

Patients

Details of patient populations and study designs for both OPAL Broaden (A3921091; ClinicalTrials.gov Identifier: NCT01877668) and OPAL Beyond (A3921125; ClinicalTrials.gov Identifier: NCT01882439) have been published in detail [9, 10]. In brief, for inclusion in either OPAL Broaden or OPAL Beyond, patients were required to have active PsA with a duration of at least 6 months, to fulfill ClAShsification criteria for Psoriatic ARthritis (CASPAR) at screening, and to have evidence of active arthritis with both a TJC and SJC of three or higher. Patients in OPAL Broaden had an inadequate response to at least one csDMARD and were TNFi-naïve, whereas patients in OPAL Beyond had an inadequate response to at least one TNFi. The primary endpoints in both studies were ACR20 response rate and change from baseline in HAQ-DI score at month 3.

Study design

OPAL Broaden was a 12-month study in which patients were randomly assigned 2:2:2:1:1 to receive tofacitinib 5 mg BID, tofacitinib 10 mg BID, adalimumab 40 mg subcutaneous (SC) injection once every 2 weeks (Q2W), placebo advancing to tofacitinib 5 mg BID at month 3, or placebo advancing to tofacitinib 10 mg BID at month 3. OPAL Beyond was a 6-month study in which patients were randomly assigned 2:2:1:1 to receive tofacitinib 5 mg BID, tofacitinib 10 mg BID, placebo advancing to tofacitinib 5 mg BID at month 3, or placebo advancing to tofacitinib 10 mg BID at month 3. In both studies, patients also received one concomitant treatment with a stable dose of either methotrexate or another csDMARD (for example, sulfasalazine or leflunomide).

Assessments

Three disease-specific composite endpoints are discussed in this analysis. The Psoriatic Arthritis Disease Activity Score (PASDAS) (score range of 0–10) includes the following components: patient's global joint and skin assessment (visual analog scale; VAS [in millimeters]); physician's global assessment of PsA (VAS [in millimeters]); SJC (66 joints) and TJC (68 joints); Leeds Enthesitis Index

(LEI) score; tender dactylitic digit score; physical component summary (PCS) score of the 36-item short-form survey version 2 (SF-36v2 acute, norm-based scores); and CRP (in milligrams per liter) (Table 1) [11]. The Disease Activity Index for Reactive Arthritis/Psoriatic Arthritis (DAREA/DAPSA) (score range not defined; referred to as DAPSA herein) includes the components SJC (66 joints) and TJC (68 joints); patient's global assessment of arthritis and patient's pain assessment (both measured by VAS [in millimeters]); and CRP (in milligrams per liter) (Table 1) [6]. The Composite Psoriatic Disease Activity Index (CPDAI) (score range of 0–15) includes the components peripheral arthritis (SJC, TJC, and HAQ-DI); skin disease (Psoriasis Area and Severity Index [PASI] and Dermatology Life Quality Index [DLQI]); enthesitis (LEI score and HAQ-DI); dactylitis (number of digits and HAQ-DI); and spinal disease (Bath Ankylosing Spondylitis Disease Activity Index and Ankylosing Spondylitis Quality of Life [ASQoL]) (Table 1) [12]. For each of these composite endpoints, a higher score indicates higher disease activity. For comparison, a non-disease-specific composite outcome measure was also assessed: the three-component Disease Activity Score using 28 joints with CRP (DAS28–3 [CRP]; score range of 0–9.4, a higher score corresponds to worse symptoms) includes the components SJC (28 joints) and TJC (28 joints) and CRP (in milligrams per liter) (Table 1) [13].

Statistical analysis

The full analysis set (FAS) comprised all patients who were randomly assigned to the study and received at least one dose of study medication. Changes from baseline analyses were based on a repeated measures model, without imputation for missing values in the FAS, with the fixed effects of treatment, visit, treatment-by-visit interaction, geographic location, and baseline value; an unstructured covariance matrix was used. For results up to month 3, patients randomly assigned to the two placebo sequences were combined into a single placebo group. The repeated measures model included data from all visits up to month 3 for the treatment groups of tofacitinib 5 mg BID, tofacitinib 10 mg BID, adalimumab 40 mg SC Q2W (OPAL Broaden only), and placebo. For results beyond month 3 to the end of study, the two placebo

sequences were analyzed separately. The calculation of effect sizes and standardized response means for treatment groups of tofacitinib 5 mg BID, tofacitinib 10 mg BID, and adalimumab (OPAL Broaden only) at months 3, 6, and 12 (OPAL Broaden only at month 12) was based on patients with greater than or equal to 3% baseline psoriasis body surface area (BSA) in the FAS in order to permit comparison based on the same set of patients, with no missing values for any of the three disease-specific composite endpoints at baseline or months 3, 6, and 12 (OPAL Broaden only at month 12).

The effect size for a given composite endpoint at a time point was defined as (mean at baseline – mean at time point)/(standard deviation [SD] at baseline). The standardized response mean for a given composite endpoint at a time point was defined as (mean at baseline – mean at time point)/(SD of change from baseline at time point). Effect size and standardized response mean are unitless measures and are adjusted for the endpoints' variability, which allows comparisons to be made. For both effect sizes and standardized response means, levels of responsiveness have been proposed as small (≥ 0.20 to < 0.5), moderate (≥ 0.50 to < 0.8), and large (≥ 0.80), respectively [3, 14].

In order to investigate the relative strength of the composite endpoints in predicting MDA response at a given time point, multiple logistic regression was used to model MDA response as a dependent variable and the mean changes from baseline of the three disease-specific composite endpoints at the same time point as predictors. The estimated slope coefficient from this regression model is the change in log-odds of MDA response resulting from a 1-unit increase in change from baseline of the composite endpoint. It represents the strength of association between the composite endpoint and MDA response and is standardized (STB, range unbounded) to adjust for the variability of the composite endpoint to permit comparison of their associations with MDA response. In order to compare the correlations of the three disease-specific composite endpoints with MDA response, another standardized measure related to STB above, called logistic pseudo partial correlation (denoted as R, range of –1 to 1), was also calculated [15]. A value of R closer to 1 or –1 indicates strong correlation,

Table 1 Components of the composite endpoints PASDAS, DAPSA, CPDAI, and DAS28–3(CRP)

	Skin manifestations	Enthesitis	Dactylitis	Joints	Axial	PROs
PASDAS [11]	✓	✓	✓	✓		✓
DAPSA [6]				✓		✓
CPDAI [12]	✓	✓	✓	✓	✓	✓
DAS28–3(CRP) [13]				✓		

Abbreviations: *CPDAI* Composite Psoriatic Disease Activity Index, *DAPSA* Disease Activity Index for Psoriatic Arthritis, *DAS28–3(CRP)* 3-component Disease Activity Score using 28 joints with C-reactive protein, *PASDAS* Psoriatic Arthritis Disease Activity Score, *PRO* patient-reported outcomes

whereas a value of 0 indicates lack of correlation. This regression analysis was performed separately for months 3, 6, and 12 (OPAL Broaden only for month 12) and separately for tofacitinib 5 mg BID, 10 mg BID, and adalimumab 40 mg SC Q2W. These analyses included the same set of patients with baseline psoriasis BSA of greater than or equal to 3% in the FAS with no missing values for any of the three disease-specific composite endpoints and MDA at months 3, 6, and 12 (OPAL Broaden only at month 12). MDA was defined as any five of the following seven criteria being met: TJC ≤1, SJC ≤1, PASI score ≤1 or psoriasis BSA ≤3%, patient arthritis pain (VAS) ≤15 mm, patient's global assessment of arthritis (VAS) ≤20 mm, HAQ-DI ≤0.5, tender entheseal points (using LEI) ≤1 [16].

The PASDAS response rate was calculated at months 3, 6, and 12 (OPAL Broaden only for month 12) as the percentage of patients who had a good response (defined as a PASDAS score of less than or equal to 3.2 and a decrease from baseline in PASDAS score of greater than or equal to 1.6 at the relevant time point for patients with baseline PASDAS score of greater than 3.2 in FAS) [17]. Non-responder imputation was applied, and a missing response was treated as non-response.

The derivation of the composite endpoints was pre-specified in the original study protocols and statistical analysis plans; except for analysis using a repeated measures model, all analyses were performed post hoc. P values are reported for comparisons with placebo in repeated measures model analyses and for testing slope coefficients in multiple logistic regression analyses without adjustment for multiplicity. The significance level was set at two-sided, less than or equal to 0.05.

Results

Patients

The FAS comprised 422 patients from OPAL Broaden and 394 patients from OPAL Beyond (Table 2). Demographics and baseline disease characteristics have been published previously [9, 10]. Baseline values for composite endpoints were generally similar across treatment groups and studies (Table 2).

Composite endpoint outcomes

PASDAS

At baseline, mean PASDAS scores ranged from 5.92 to 6.43 across treatment groups in the OPAL Broaden and OPAL Beyond studies (Table 2). There were significantly greater improvements, as indicated by the least squares (LS) mean change from baseline in PASDAS score, with tofacitinib 5 and 10 mg BID versus placebo as early as month 1, continuing to month 3. Following advancement from placebo to tofacitinib treatments at month 3, patients showed similar improvements in disease activity at month 6 to those observed in patients receiving

tofacitinib 5 or 10 mg BID throughout (Additional file 1: Table S1 and Fig. 1a); this improvement was maintained until the end of the 12-month OPAL Broaden study (Table 2 and Fig. 1a) and was larger in patients in the placebo advancing to tofacitinib 10 mg BID group than the placebo advancing to tofacitinib 5 mg BID group. In OPAL Broaden, the mean absolute PASDAS scores decreased to 3.29 and 3.05 with tofacitinib 5 and 10 mg BID, respectively, at month 12, and in OPAL Beyond the mean PASDAS scores at month 6 were 3.87 and 3.97 with tofacitinib 5 and 10 mg BID, respectively (Table 2). In OPAL Broaden, decreases from baseline in PASDAS scores were also observed in patients receiving adalimumab 40 mg SC Q2W from month 1 and were maintained to month 12 (Additional file 1: Table S1 and Fig. 1a).

PASDAS response rates

The percentage of PASDAS responders increased with time on treatment in both studies and with both doses of tofacitinib (Fig. 2). A similar percentage of patients initially randomly assigned to receive placebo were PASDAS responders compared with those patients receiving tofacitinib throughout at month 6 in OPAL Beyond and month 12 in OPAL Broaden, following advancement from placebo to active treatment with tofacitinib at month 3 (Fig. 2).

DAPSA

At baseline, mean DAPSA scores in the two studies ranged from 38.52 to 51.54 across treatment groups (Table 2). In OPAL Broaden, significantly greater LS mean changes from baseline in the DAPSA score (indicating improvement) were observed versus placebo for tofacitinib 10 mg BID from week 2 and for tofacitinib 5 mg BID from month 2, and differences were maintained to month 3 for both doses (Fig. 1b). In OPAL Beyond, significantly greater improvements, as indicated by LS mean changes from baseline in the DAPSA score, were observed with both doses of tofacitinib versus placebo from week 2 throughout the placebo-controlled period (Fig. 1b). The LS mean changes from baseline in the DAPSA score showed further decreases to month 6 with tofacitinib treatment in both studies (Fig. 1b), and the improvement was maintained to month 12 in OPAL Broaden (Additional file 1: Table S1 and Fig. 1b). At month 12 in OPAL Broaden, the mean absolute DAPSA scores were 15.14 and 13.21 with tofacitinib 5 and 10 mg BID, respectively, whereas in OPAL Beyond they decreased to 20.69 and 28.30 at month 6 with tofacitinib 5 and 10 mg BID, respectively (Table 2). At month 6 in both studies and month 12 in OPAL Broaden, following advancement from placebo to tofacitinib at month 3, patients

Table 2 Composite endpoint scores in the OPAL Broaden and OPAL Beyond studies (FAS)

Mean composite endpoint scores (SD) [number of patients evaluable at time point]

	OPAL Broaden (N = 422)					OPAL Beyond (N = 394)			
	Tofacitinib 5 mg BID N = 107	Tofacitinib 10 mg BID N = 104	Adalimumab 40 mg SC Q2W N = 106	Placebo -> tofacitinib 5 mg BID N = 52[a]	Placebo -> tofacitinib 10 mg BID N = 53[a]	Tofacitinib 5 mg BID N = 131	Tofacitinib 10 mg BID N = 132	Placebo -> tofacitinib 5 mg BID N = 66[a]	Placebo -> tofacitinib 10 mg BID N = 65[a]
PASDAS									
Baseline	6.03 (1.15) [105]	6.01 (1.06) [102]	5.92 (1.25) [106]	6.03 (1.15) [103] (combined)		6.09 (1.22) [124]	6.43 (1.21) [128]	5.97 (1.26) [128] (combined)	
Month 3	4.17 (1.69) [98]	3.70 (1.43) [102]	3.89 (1.57) [98]	4.97 (1.41) [100] (combined)		4.26 (1.71) [122]	4.24 (1.78) [114]	5.07 (1.86) [117] (combined)	
Month 6	3.63 (1.61) [99]	3.43 (1.45) [98]	3.41 (1.47) [98]	4.00 (1.49) [48]	3.69 (1.46) [47]	3.87 (1.72) [117]	3.97 (1.75) [109]	3.81 (1.68) [55]	3.60 (1.71) [55]
Month 12	3.29 (1.37) [95]	3.05 (1.22) [95]	3.20 (1.56) [93]	3.50 (1.40) [44]	3.15 (1.21) [43]	—	—	—	—
DAPSA									
Baseline	45.55 (20.33) [107]	43.69 (19.51) [104]	38.52 (18.17) [105]	43.81 (22.46) [105] (combined)		45.53 (23.51) [130]	51.54 (27.80) [132]	42.64 (22.99) [131] (combined)	
Month 3	26.08 (23.53) [101]	20.29 (18.86) [103]	21.44 (20.43) [99]	31.64 (23.64) [101] (combined)		24.32 (20.53) [123]	29.14 (25.21) [117]	33.69 (27.69) [117] (combined)	
Month 6	21.42 (21.71) [100]	16.86 (17.99) [99]	16.34 (18.63) [99]	19.93 (18.14) [48]	19.42 (21.17) [48]	20.69 (17.55) [123]	28.30 (28.92) [113]	21.12 (20.75) [56]	20.28 (20.94) [55]
Month 12	15.14 (14.29) [95]	13.21 (13.87) [96]	13.84 (15.50) [93]	15.60 (18.07) [44]	14.83 (14.84) [44]	—	—	—	—
CPDAI[b]									
Baseline	9.9 (2.39) [81]	10.0 (2.76) [68]	9.7 (2.84) [77]	9.9 (2.65) [81] (combined)		10.1 (2.58) [79]	10.7 (2.56) [79]	9.6 (2.86) [85] (combined)	
Month 3	7.4 (3.57) [77]	6.0 (3.01) [68]	6.9 (3.19) [75]	8.0 (2.95) [78] (combined)		7.1 (3.23) [70]	7.1 (3.33) [74]	8.0 (3.80) [73] (combined)	
Month 6	6.2 (3.39) [76]	5.1 (2.87) [66]	5.6 (3.30) [74]	6.4 (3.45) [39]	6.4 (3.36) [34]	6.3 (3.42) [75]	6.5 (3.11) [69]	6.3 (3.43) [32]	6.1 (3.39) [35]
Month 12	5.1 (2.96) [73]	4.4 (2.71) [65]	5.0 (3.19) [71]	4.9 (3.17) [36]	5.1 (2.63) [32]	—	—	—	—
DAS28-3(CRP)									
Baseline	4.56 (0.92) [107]	4.48 (0.97) [104]	4.38 (1.02) [106]	4.50 (1.04) [105] (combined)		4.51 (1.04) [131]	4.67 (1.17) [132]	4.40 (1.03) [131] (combined)	
Month 3	3.25 (1.26) [101]	2.94 (1.15) [103]	2.96 (1.15) [99]	3.85 (1.30) [101] (combined)		3.18 (1.22) [123]	3.41 (1.39) [118]	3.77 (1.32) [117] (combined)	
Month 6	2.90 (1.25) [100]	2.60 (1.09) [99]	2.62 (1.08) [99]	2.99 (1.23) [48]	2.86 (1.23) [48]	2.98 (1.21) [123]	3.29 (1.36) [113]	2.87 (1.17) [56]	2.95 (1.35) [55]
Month 12	2.64 (1.11) [95]	2.43 (0.99) [96]	2.44 (1.04) [93]	2.60 (1.20) [44]	2.52 (1.05) [44]	—	—	—	—

[a]For baseline and month 3 visits, patients from the two placebo sequences were combined into a single placebo group

[b]Only patients with psoriasis body surface area (BSA) of greater than or equal to 3% were included

Abbreviations: BID twice daily, *CPDAI* Composite Psoriatic Disease Activity Index, *DAPSA* Disease Activity Index for Psoriatic Arthritis, *DAS28-3(CRP)* 3-component Disease Activity Score using 28 joints with C-reactive protein, *FAS* full analysis set, *N* number of patients in the full analysis set, *OPAL* Oral Psoriatic Arthritis trial, *PASDAS* Psoriatic Arthritis Disease Activity Score, *Q2W* once every 2 weeks, *SC* subcutaneous, *SD* standard deviation

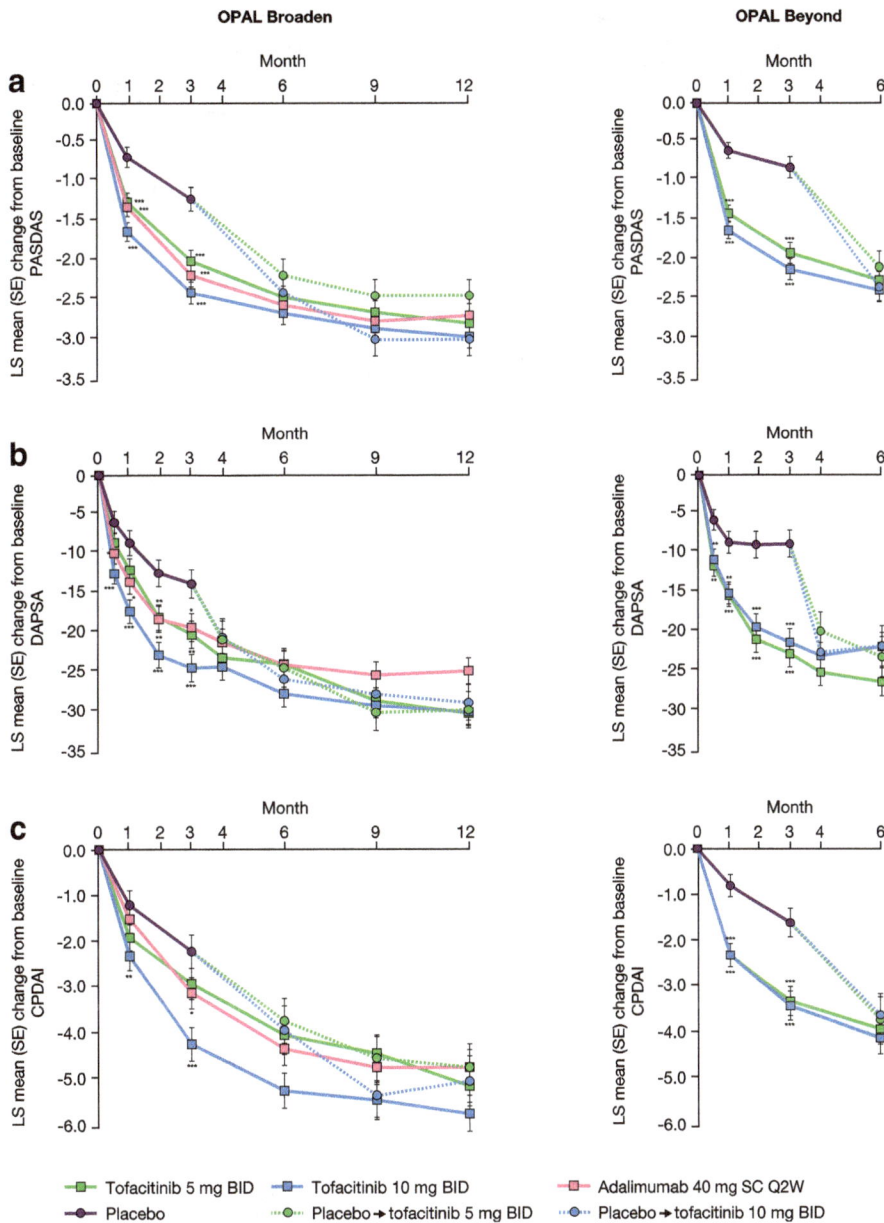

Fig. 1 LS mean change from baseline in (**a**) PASDAS, (**b**) DAPSA, and (**c**) CPDAI. For complete data, see Additional file 1: Table S1. *$P \leq 0.05$, **$P <0.01$, ***$P <0.001$ versus placebo. Abbreviations: *BID* twice daily, *CPDAI* Composite Psoriatic Disease Activity Index, *DAPSA* Disease Activity Index for Psoriatic Arthritis, *LS* least squares, *OPAL* Oral Psoriatic Arthritis triaL, *PASDAS* Psoriatic Arthritis Disease Activity Score, *Q2W* once every 2 weeks, *SC* subcutaneous, *SE* standard error

showed similar improvements in DAPSA scores to patients receiving tofacitinib throughout (Table 2 and Fig. 1b). Patients receiving adalimumab 40 mg SC Q2W showed decreases from baseline in DAPSA scores throughout both OPAL Broaden and OPAL Beyond (Table 2 and Fig. 1b).

CPDAI
At baseline, mean CPDAI scores ranged from 9.6 to 10.7 across studies and treatment groups (Table 2). For CPDAI, significant improvements in LS mean change from baseline were seen for tofacitinib 10 mg BID but not tofacitinib 5 mg BID versus placebo at months 1 and 3 in OPAL Broaden (Fig. 1c). Significant improvements in LS mean change from baseline in CPDAI score versus placebo at months 1 and 3 were reported for patients receiving tofacitinib 5 and 10 mg BID in OPAL Beyond (Fig. 1c). Decreases in LS mean change from baseline in CPDAI score with both doses of tofacitinib were maintained at months 6 and 12 (Fig. 1c). In OPAL Broaden,

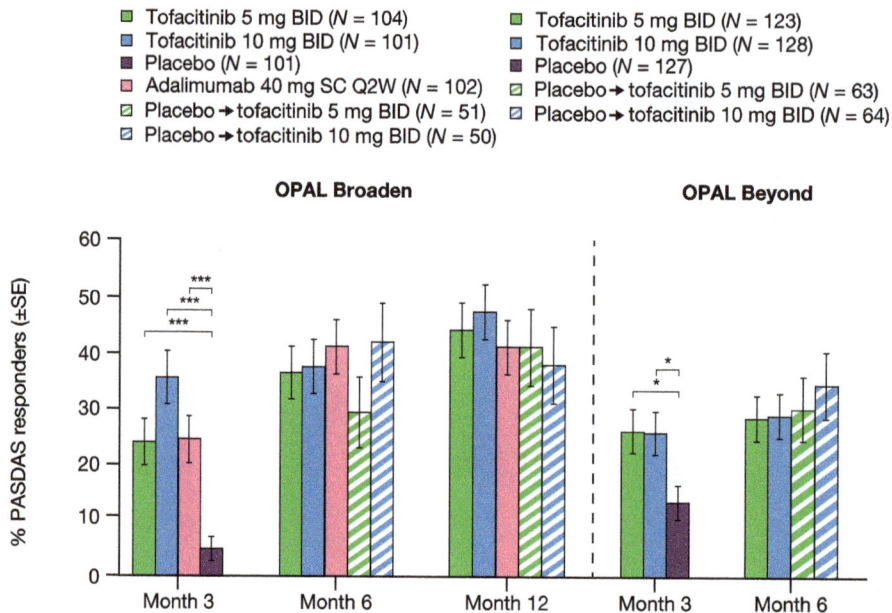

Fig. 2 PASDAS response rates for patients with baseline PASDAS >3.2 (FAS). *P≤0.05, ***P<0.001 versus placebo. PASDAS response was defined as the percentage of patients who had a PASDAS score ≤3.2 and a decrease from baseline in PASDAS score ≥1.6 at the relevant time point. A missing PASDAS response at a given time point was imputed as non-response. Abbreviations: *BID* twice daily, *FAS* full analysis set, *N* number of patients with baseline PASDAS >3.2 in the FAS, *OPAL* Oral Psoriatic Arthritis triaL, *PASDAS* Psoriatic Arthritis Disease Activity Score, *Q2W* once every 2 weeks, *SC* subcutaneous, *SE* standard error

the mean absolute CPDAI scores with tofacitinib 5 and 10 mg BID at month 12 were 5.1 and 4.4, respectively, and in OPAL Beyond they were 6.3 and 6.5, respectively, at month 6 (Table 2). Patients who advanced from placebo to tofacitinib treatments at month 3 showed similar improvements in CPDAI absolute scores and LS mean change from baseline in CPDAI at month 12 in OPAL Broaden and month 6 in OPAL Beyond to patients receiving tofacitinib 5 or 10 mg BID throughout (Table 2 and Fig. 1c). In OPAL Broaden, patients receiving adalimumab 40 mg SC Q2W showed improvements from baseline in CPDAI scores from month 1 to 12 (Table 2 and Fig. 1c).

DAS28–3(CRP)

For the non-disease-specific comparator included here, mean DAS28–3(CRP) at baseline was 4.38 to 4.67 across studies and treatment groups (Table 2). Patients receiving tofacitinib at either dose showed significant improvements from baseline in DAS28–3(CRP) versus placebo as early as week 2, which continued through the placebo-controlled period to month 3 in both studies (Additional file 1: Table S1). LS mean change from baseline in DAS28–3(CRP) continued to decrease with tofacitinib treatments through month 6 in both studies, and improvement was maintained until the end of the 12-month OPAL Broaden study (Additional file 1: Table S1). Patients who advanced from placebo to

tofacitinib treatments at month 3 showed improvements from baseline in DAS28–3(CRP) and LS mean change from baseline in DAS28–3(CRP) similar to patients receiving tofacitinib 5 or 10 mg BID throughout the studies at month 12 in OPAL Broaden and month 6 in OPAL Beyond (Additional file 1: Table S1).

Effect sizes and standardized response means

Based on the proposed levels of responsiveness, the effect sizes and standardized response means for all treatments across all composite endpoints were large (≥0.80). The effect size for the composite endpoints was highest for PASDAS across all treatment groups at months 3, 6, and 12 in OPAL Broaden and months 3 and 6 in OPAL Beyond and was lowest for DAPSA across treatments, studies, and time points, with the exception of the adalimumab group in OPAL Broaden at month 3, in which the effect size for both DAPSA and CPDAI was 1.05 (Table 3). Effect size increased with time on treatment across endpoints, studies, and treatment (Table 3). The effect size for all endpoints was higher in the OPAL Broaden study compared with OPAL Beyond at both months 3 and 6 with both tofacitinib doses, with the exception of CPDAI with tofacitinib 5 mg BID, which was lower (Table 3).

The highest standardized response mean was observed for PASDAS at months 3 and 6 in OPAL Beyond and at all time points with tofacitinib treatment at either dose in

Table 3 Effect sizes and standardized response means across studies

	Effect size					Standardized response mean				
	OPAL Broaden			OPAL Beyond		OPAL Broaden			OPAL Beyond	
	Tofacitinib 5 mg BID N = 68	Tofacitinib 10 mg BID N = 62	Adalimumab 40 mg SC Q2W N = 66	Tofacitinib 5 mg BID N = 64	Tofacitinib 10 mg BID N = 62	Tofacitinib 5 mg BID N = 68	Tofacitinib 10 mg BID N = 62	Adalimumab 40 mg SC Q2W N = 66	Tofacitinib 5 mg BID N = 64	Tofacitinib 10 mg BID N = 62
Month 3										
PASDAS	1.73	2.40	1.69	1.53	1.84	1.42	1.75	1.73	1.26	1.53
DAPSA	0.90	1.23	1.05	0.81	0.84	1.05	1.25	1.47	0.94	1.15
CPDAI	1.03	1.53	1.05	1.41	1.45	0.89	1.27	1.11	1.11	1.49
DAS28–3(CRP)	1.47	1.77	1.37	1.07	1.16	1.25	1.46	1.50	1.14	1.29
Month 6										
PASDAS	2.17	2.81	1.98	1.88	2.10	1.76	2.11	1.64	1.49	1.74
DAPSA	1.15	1.43	1.24	0.97	0.92	1.18	1.34	1.43	1.11	0.94
CPDAI	1.53	1.88	1.44	1.65	1.75	1.52	1.52	1.25	1.23	1.55
DAS28–3(CRP)	1.93	2.11	1.68	1.34	1.23	1.47	1.68	1.79	1.43	1.28
Month 12										
PASDAS	2.51	3.05	2.07	–	–	2.10	2.21	1.60	–	–
DAPSA	1.50	1.57	1.30	–	–	1.60	1.41	1.36	–	–
CPDAI	1.95	2.12	1.59	–	–	1.59	1.64	1.33	–	–
DAS28–3(CRP)	2.25	2.18	1.77	–	–	1.69	1.65	1.71	–	–

N = number of patients in the full analysis set with baseline psoriasis body surface area affected greater than or equal to 3% and with no missing values for any of the composite endpoints at baseline and months 3, 6, and 12 (OPAL Broaden only for month 12). This subset of patients was used for the calculation of effect sizes and standardized response means

Abbreviations: BID twice daily, *CPDAI* Composite Psoriatic Disease Activity Index, *DAPSA* Disease Activity Index for Psoriatic Arthritis, *DAS28–3(CRP)* 3-component Disease Activity Score using 28 joints with C-reactive protein, *OPAL* Oral Psoriatic Arthritis triaL, *PASDAS* Psoriatic Arthritis Disease Activity Score, *Q2W* once every 2 weeks, *SC* subcutaneous

OPAL Broaden (Table 3). In OPAL Broaden, with adalimumab treatment, the highest standardized response mean was observed for PASDAS at month 3 and for DAS28–3(CRP) at months 6 and 12 (Table 3). In both OPAL Broaden and OPAL Beyond, the standardized response mean increased with time on treatment in patients receiving tofacitinib 5 mg BID for all endpoints, and for patients receiving tofacitinib 10 mg BID, with the exception of DAS28–3(CRP) and DAPSA at month 6 in OPAL Beyond (Table 3). The standardized response mean for PASDAS, DAS28–3(CRP), and DAPSA was higher in the OPAL Broaden study compared with OPAL Beyond at both months 3 and 6 with both tofacitinib doses (Table 3). For CPDAI, the standardized response mean was lower at month 3 in OPAL Broaden versus OPAL Beyond with both tofacitinib doses; at month 6, the standardized response mean was higher with tofacitinib 5 mg BID and lower with tofacitinib 10 mg BID in OPAL Broaden versus OPAL Beyond (Table 3).

Outcomes stratified by MDA response and multiple regression analysis

Mean changes from baseline appeared greater in MDA responders than MDA non-responders for all composite endpoints across all time points and treatments;

however, no statistical comparison was made between these groups (Fig. 3 and Additional file 2: Table S2). Multiple logistic regression analysis of MDA response indicated that in both OPAL Broaden and OPAL Beyond there were statistically significant associations between change from baseline in PASDAS and MDA response at all time points in both studies for both doses of tofacitinib except month 3 for tofacitinib 10 mg BID (Table 4). For DAPSA, statistically significant associations were seen for tofacitinib 5 mg BID at 12 months in OPAL Broaden and at 6 months in OPAL Beyond. Significant associations were also observed for tofacitinib 10 mg BID at both 3 and 6 months in OPAL Beyond. In contrast, there were no statistically significant associations within CPDAI at any time point in either study. For comparison, statistically significant associations were noted for tofacitinib 10 mg BID at 6 and 12 months in OPAL Broaden and at 3 and 6 months in OPAL Beyond for DAS28–3(CRP).

Discussion

In the phase 3 studies OPAL Broaden and OPAL Beyond, patients with active PsA receiving tofacitinib 5 and 10 mg BID showed improvements versus placebo throughout the 3-month placebo-controlled period for

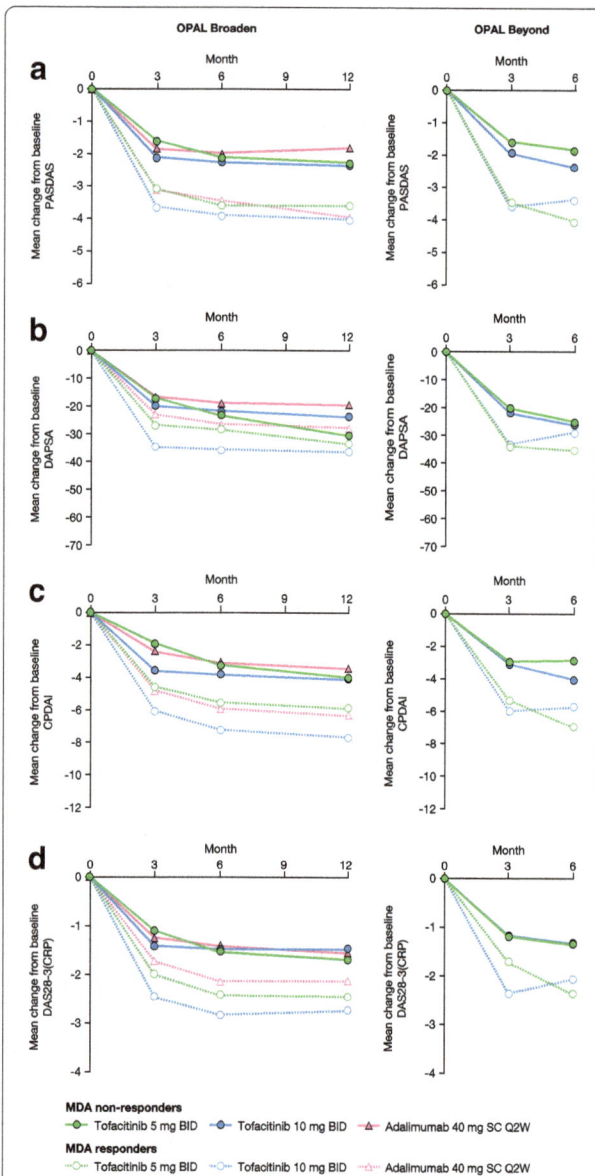

Fig. 3 Change from baseline in composite endpoint scores by MDA response status across studies, **a** PASDAS, **b** DAPSA, **c** CPDAI, **d** DAS28-3 (CRP). For complete data, see Additional file 2: Table S2. MDA response was defined as five of the following seven criteria being met: TJC ≤1, SJC ≤1, Psoriasis Area and Severity Index score ≤1 or psoriasis BSA ≤3%, patient arthritis pain (VAS) ≤15 mm, patient's global assessment of arthritis (VAS) ≤20 mm, HAQ-DI ≤0.5, tender entheseal points (using LEI) ≤1. Abbreviations: *BID* twice daily, *BSA* body surface area, *CPDAI* Composite Psoriatic Disease Activity Index, *DAPSA* Disease Activity Index for Psoriatic Arthritis, *DAS28–3(CRP)* 3-component Disease Activity Score using 28 joints with C-reactive protein, *FAS* full analysis set, *HAQ-DI* Health Assessment Questionnaire-Disability Index, *LEI* Leeds Enthesitis Index, *MDA* minimal disease activity, *OPAL* Oral Psoriatic Arthritis triaL, *PASDAS* Psoriatic Arthritis Disease Activity Score, *Q2W* once every 2 weeks, *SC* subcutaneous, *SJC* swollen joint count, *TJC* tender joint count, *VAS* visual analog scale

the composite endpoints assessed. These improvements were subsequently maintained to month 6 in OPAL Beyond and month 12 in OPAL Broaden. Adalimumab had comparable efficacy to tofacitinib across the composite endpoints in OPAL Broaden.

OPAL Broaden and OPAL Beyond involved two distinct populations of patients with PsA: csDMARD-IR/TNFi-naïve patients in OPAL Broaden and TNFi-IR patients in OPAL Beyond. Despite the difference in patient populations, baseline values for the composite endpoints were broadly similar across studies and treatments. Generally, LS mean changes from baseline were greater, and the effect size and standardized response mean were higher, in the OPAL Broaden study compared with OPAL Beyond. This suggests that the TNFi-naïve patients in OPAL Broaden showed more marked treatment responses than the TNFi-IR patients in OPAL Beyond, similar to previous reports for PsA treatment [18–20].

PASDAS baseline scores in OPAL Broaden were comparable with values reported in an equivalent study population [3]; however, along with the PASDAS baseline scores in OPAL Beyond, they were somewhat higher than those reported in a study of standard care [21] and patients in clinical practice [22]. In the GRACE (GRAPPA Composite Exercise) study, designed to develop composite disease activity and responder measures for PsA, a mean score of 5.30 for PASDAS was reported for patients changing treatment and this was taken as a surrogate for high disease activity [11]. The mean baseline PASDAS levels reported in this study were therefore suggestive of high disease activity in both OPAL Broaden and OPAL Beyond, and following 3 months of treatment, PASDAS levels dropped below this threshold. In addition, the GRACE study defined a good response as a PASDAS score of less than or equal to 3.2, following a decrease in score of greater than or equal to 1.6 from baseline [17]; in this study, this was achieved at month 12 in OPAL Broaden by 44.2% and 47.5% of patients receiving tofacitinib 5 and 10 mg BID, respectively, and at month 6 in OPAL Beyond by 28.5% and 28.9% of patients receiving tofacitinib 5 and 10 mg BID, respectively. Of note, a PASDAS score of less than or equal to 3.2 has been defined as low disease activity [17] and less than or equal to 1.9 as very low disease activity [23].

OPAL Broaden DAPSA baseline scores were slightly lower than baseline scores in an equivalent study population [3] but higher than reported in clinical practice [24]. In the GRACE study, patients changing treatment (considered to have high disease activity) had a mean DAPSA score of 41.91 [11], suggesting that patients in OPAL Broaden and OPAL Beyond had high levels of disease activity. Indeed, in a recent study analyzing data from 30 patients with PsA in an observational database, the cutoff for a

Table 4 Comparison of associations of composite endpoints with MDA response across time points and studies

| | OPAL Broaden | | | | | | OPAL Beyond | | | |
| | Tofacitinib 5 mg BID N = 68 | | Tofacitinib 10 mg BID N = 62 | | Adalimumab 40 mg SC Q2W N = 66 | | Tofacitinib 5 mg BID N = 64 | | Tofacitinib 10 mg BID N = 62 | |
	STB	R	STB	R	STB	R	STB	R	STB	R
Month 3										
PASDAS	−0.73*	−0.19	−0.71	−0.13	−0.70*	−0.20	−1.23**	−0.26	−0.53	0.00
DAPSA	0.64	0.10	0.09	0.00	0.35	0.00	0.38	0.00	0.87*	0.23
CPDAI	−0.07	0.00	0.15	0.00	−0.33	−0.02	0.17	0.00	−0.71	−0.16
DAS28–3(CRP)	−0.58	−0.06	−0.34	0.00	−0.11	0.00	−0.08	0.00	−0.75*	−0.22
Month 6										
PASDAS	−0.91*	−0.20	−0.83*	−0.17	−0.61	−0.12	−1.27*	−0.21	−0.77*	−0.16
DAPSA	0.78	0.15	0.83	0.15	0.47	0.04	0.82*	0.21	1.00**	0.26
CPDAI	0.08	0.00	−0.00	0.00	−0.17	0.00	−0.48	0.00	0.04	0.00
DAS28–3(CRP)	−0.53	−0.08	−1.23**	−0.26	−0.42	−0.11	−0.44	0.00	−0.69*	−0.20
Month 12										
PASDAS	−1.02**	−0.29	−0.87*	−0.18	−1.88***	−0.35	–	–	–	–
DAPSA	0.79**	0.24	0.51	0.04	0.86	0.11	–	–	–	–
CPDAI	0.08	0.00	−0.09	0.00	−0.00	0.00	–	–	–	–
DAS28–3(CRP)	−0.68*	−0.20	−0.75*	−0.19	−0.18	0.00	–	–	–	–

*$P \leq 0.05$, **$P < 0.01$, ***$P < 0.001$ testing the null hypothesis that the slope coefficient is equal to 0, based on the Wald statistic from the multiple logistic regression model

N = number of patients included in the multiple logistic regression model

For a given time point and treatment group, a multiple logistic regression was performed on MDA evaluated at this time point as a dependent variable and the changes from baseline in the composite endpoints measured at the same time point as predictors. The slope coefficient for a composite endpoint from this regression model is standardized (STB) to permit comparison of the associations of these composite endpoints with the MDA response. An additional statistic, logistic pseudo partial correlation (R, range − 1 to 1), was also computed as a measure of correlation between the composite endpoints and MDA response [15]

Abbreviations: BID twice daily, *CPDAI* Composite Psoriatic Disease Activity Index, *DAPSA* Disease Activity Index for Psoriatic Arthritis, *DAS28–3(CRP)* 3-component Disease Activity Score using 28 joints with C-reactive protein, *MDA* minimal disease activity, *OPAL* Oral Psoriatic Arthritis triaL, *PASDAS* Psoriatic Arthritis Disease Activity Score, *Q2W* once every 2 weeks, *SC* subcutaneous

DAPSA score indicating high disease activity was greater than 28 [25]. In this study, mean DAPSA scores were below the high disease activity score reported in the GRACE study after 3 months of active treatment in all groups [11].

In contrast to the findings with the other composite measures, the baseline CPDAI scores reported for OPAL Broaden and OPAL Beyond were somewhat lower than mean CPDAI score of 11.65 reported for patients changing treatment (surrogate for high disease activity) in the GRACE study [11]; thus, CPDAI scores did not appear to indicate patients with high baseline disease activity in these patient populations. However, another study has suggested a high disease activity threshold of greater than 7 for CPDAI [26]; mean CPDAI scores were below this threshold after 3 months of active treatment across all groups and both studies.

The DAS28–3(CRP) was included for comparative purposes only. Baseline DAS28–3(CRP) scores were somewhat higher than the mean DAS28–3(CRP) score of 3.96 observed for patients changing treatment (a surrogate for high disease activity) in the GRACE study [11]; however, DAS28–3(CRP) scores in this study were reduced below this level following 3 months of treatment. It should be noted, however, that this measure was developed and validated for rheumatoid arthritis and there are several reasons why it is inappropriate as a composite measure for assessing PsA, particularly as it measures only articular outcomes and excludes joints of the foot and ankle, potentially missing important inflammatory disease [27].

All reported effect size and standardized response mean values were greater than 0.80, the value generally taken to indicate a large treatment effect or response [3]. The largest effect size was observed at all time points and treatments for the composite endpoint PASDAS; this is consistent with findings reported for golimumab [3]. Effect size and standardized response mean generally showed increases with time on treatment, indicating that the composite endpoints demonstrated time-dependent improvement, as might be expected. Analysis of the percentage of PASDAS responders over time also demonstrated the ability of the PASDAS instrument to detect treatment-related changes in PsA disease activity.

The definition of MDA using the criteria applied in this analysis and in previous tofacitinib publications [9, 10] has utility for identifying treatment response and as such may be used as a target to guide treatment decisions [16]. When the standardized slope coefficients of the composite endpoints (STBs) from a multiple logistic regression model were compared, the change in PASDAS had the largest magnitude of association with MDA response among all the composite endpoints examined, suggesting that it had the strongest predictive ability compared with DAPSA and CPDAI; CPDAI had the lowest predictive ability of the endpoints.

The differing findings with respect to tofacitinib treatment for the three disease-specific composite endpoints considered in this analysis could have resulted from the different composition of the endpoints evaluated. The PASDAS and CPDAI both include assessment of the skin manifestations of PsA (the PASDAS by inclusion of the patient's global "arthritis and psoriasis" VAS) and the severity of enthesitis and dactylitis as well as TJC and SJC. DAPSA, however, is focused on TJC and SJC, with no consideration of skin disease, enthesitis, or dactylitis and an arthritis-focused global score. The PASDAS and CPDAI also both incorporate PROs; the PASDAS incorporates the PCS score of the SF-36v2 acute, and the CPDAI the DLQI and ASQoL. In this analysis, the PASDAS appeared to be the most sensitive to improvements in the signs and symptoms of PsA related to treatment with tofacitinib and adalimumab; the effect size observed with the PASDAS was higher than for any other endpoint at all time points in both studies. The ability of the PASDAS to detect change in these two studies might reflect the components of the measure; skin manifestations, enthesitis, dactylitis, and PROs all appeared to be sensitive to treatment-related changes in OPAL Broaden and OPAL Beyond, although the adoption of a hierarchical testing scheme for key secondary endpoints precluded demonstration of significance for all measures and time points [9, 10]. The CPDAI also incorporates skin, enthesitis, dactylitis, and PROs but appeared less sensitive to treatment differences than PASDAS though with generally higher effect size and standardized response mean than DAPSA. Inclusion of the axial disease domain in CPDAI (which does not feature in the other composite endpoints assessed) could offer an explanation as to why tofacitinib had the least impact on this composite; it may be that axial disease responds to a lesser extent than the other domains to treatment with tofacitinib and this may have impacted the final composite score. The CPDAI may also be less responsive because of the way it is constructed: the CPDAI is essentially a categorical measure re-expressed as a continuous scale and the hierarchical thresholds may blunt responsiveness. As previously discussed, the utility of DAS28–3(CRP) is limited because of the

small number of components included in the composite and the lack of inclusion of measures of skin disease, enthesitis, dactylitis, or PROs.

It is clear from these analyses that PASDAS has superior performance in this context and it has already been reported that the consensus view is that PASDAS should be the outcome measure of choice in PsA clinical trials [28]. The DAPSA is easier to evaluate but there are arguments against this measure; PsA is a complex multifaceted disease which requires appropriate evaluation across domains, and measures such as the DAPSA, though easy to perform in practice, do not fulfill this function. In terms of clinical practice, the PASDAS does provide a challenge in both acquiring the data and processing the result: the first challenge represents the general case of clinical assessment in PsA; the second challenge is easily overcome by the use of predefined spreadsheets and web-based resources.

This analysis had a number of limitations. The OPAL Broaden and OPAL Beyond studies were not designed for evaluation of the composite endpoints' longitudinal validity and sensitivity to change. In addition, for the calculation of effect size and standardized response mean, only patients with greater than or equal to 3% psoriasis BSA affected at baseline were included, with no missing values of the composite endpoints across multiple visits. Consequently, patient numbers were relatively low in some cases; CPDAI data were available for only 63% and 52% of patients receiving tofacitinib 10 mg BID in OPAL Broaden at month 12 and OPAL Beyond at month 6, respectively, and effect size and standardized response mean were calculated in only 47–64% of patients. Also, there was no adjustment for multiplicity; therefore, the P values reported for comparison with placebo should be considered nominal.

Conclusions

Overall, while the merits of specific composite measures for assessing PsA status are under discussion [29], this evaluation of three different composite scales for the assessment of tofacitinib efficacy in PsA supports the use of sensitive composite measures, particularly PASDAS, for the evaluation of efficacy of treatments that impact multiple PsA disease domains.

Abbreviations

ACR20: Greater than or equal to 20% improvement according to the criteria of the American College of Rheumatology; ASQoL: Ankylosing Spondylitis Quality of Life; BID: Twice daily; BSA: Body surface area; CPDAI: Composite Psoriatic Disease Activity Index; CRP: C-reactive protein; csDMARD: Conventional synthetic disease-modifying anti-rheumatic drug; DAPSA: Disease Activity Index for Psoriatic Arthritis; DAS28–3(CRP) : 3-component Disease Activity Score using 28 joints with C-reactive protein; DLQI: Dermatology Life Quality Index; FAS: Full analysis set; GRACE: GRAPPA Composite Exercise; GRAPPA: Group for Research and Assessment of Psoriasis and Psoriatic Arthritis; HAQ-DI: Health Assessment Questionnaire-Disability Index; IR: Inadequate responders; JAK: Janus kinase; LEI: Leeds Enthesitis Index; LS: Least squares; MDA: Minimal disease activity; OPAL: Oral Psoriatic Arthritis triaL; PASDAS: Psoriatic Arthritis Disease Activity Score; PASI: Psoriasis Area and Severity Index; PCS: Physical component summary; PRO: Patient-reported outcome; PsA: Psoriatic arthritis; Q2W: Once every 2 weeks; SC: Subcutaneous; SD: Standard deviation; SE: Standard error; SF-36v2: 36-item short-form survey version 2; SJC: Swollen joint count; TJC: Tender joint count; TNFi: Tumor necrosis factor inhibitor; VAS: Visual analog scale

Acknowledgments
The authors thank the patients who participated in the OPAL Broaden, OPAL Beyond, and OPAL Balance clinical studies. Medical writing support under the guidance of the authors was provided by Richard Knight, of CMC Connect, a division of Complete Medical Communications Ltd (Macclesfield, UK), and Carole Evans, on behalf of CMC Connect, and was funded by Pfizer Inc (New York, NY, USA) in accordance with Good Publication Practice (GPP3) guidelines (Ann Intern Med. 2015;163:461–4).

Funding
This study was funded by Pfizer Inc. Pfizer authors were involved in the design of the study; collection, analysis, and interpretation of data; and writing the manuscript.

Authors' contributions
All authors were involved in the analysis and interpretation of data and in critically revising the manuscript for important intellectual content. All authors agree to be accountable for all aspects of the work and read and approved the final manuscript to be published.

Consent for publication
Not applicable.

Competing interests
PH has received research grants from AbbVie, Janssen, and Pfizer Inc and has received personal fees from AbbVie, Amgen, Janssen, Pfizer Inc, and UCB. LCC has received research grants from AbbVie, Celgene, Janssen, Novartis, and Pfizer Inc and has received personal fees from AbbVie, Amgen, BMS, Celgene, Galapagos, Janssen, Lilly, MSD, Novartis, Pfizer Inc, Prothena, and UCB. OF has received grants from AbbVie, BMS, and Pfizer Inc and has received personal fees from BMS, Celgene, Janssen, Novartis, Pfizer Inc, and UCB. PN has received grants or fees for participating as a speaker or in advisory boards from AbbVie, BMS, Janssen, Lilly, MSD, Novartis, Pfizer Inc, Roche, Sanofi, and UCB. ERS has received grants or personal fees for participating as speaker or in advisory boards from AbbVie, BMS, GlaxoSmithKline, Janssen, Lilly, Novartis, Pfizer Inc, Roche, Sandoz, and UCB. MEH has received consultant or personal fees for participating in advisory boards from AbbVie, Genzyme/Sanofi, Janssen, Lilly, Novartis, and UCB. MAH, KSK, TH, JW, and EK are employees of Pfizer Inc and hold stock/stock options in Pfizer Inc.

Author details
[1]Leeds Institute of Rheumatic and Musculoskeletal Medicine, University of Leeds, 2nd Floor Chapel Allerton Hospital, Chapeltown Road, Leeds LS7 4SA, UK. [2]Nuffield Department of Orthopaedics Rheumatology and Musculoskeletal Sciences, University of Oxford, Windmill Road, Oxford OX3 7LD, UK. [3]Department of Rheumatology, St Vincent's University Hospital, 196 Merrion Road, Elm Park, Dublin D04 T6F4, Ireland. [4]Department of Medicine, University of Queensland, St Lucia, Brisbane QLD 4072, Australia. [5]El Hospital Italiano se encuentra ubicado en Tte. Gral. Juan Domingo Perón 4190, C.A.B.A. Buenos Aires, Argentina. [6]Cleveland Clinic Lerner Research Institute, N building, 9620 Carnegie Avenue, Cleveland, OH 44106, USA. [7]Pfizer Inc, 280 Shennecossett Rd, Groton, CT 06340, USA. [8]Pfizer Inc, 500 Arcola Rd, Collegeville, PA 19426, USA.

References
1. Coates LC, Kavanaugh A, Mease PJ, Soriano ER, Laura Acosta-Felquer M, Armstrong AW, et al. Group for Research and Assessment of Psoriasis and Psoriatic Arthritis 2015 treatment recommendations for psoriatic arthritis. Arthritis Rheumatol. 2016;68:1060–71.
2. FitzGerald O, Haroon M, Giles JT, Winchester R. Concepts of pathogenesis in psoriatic arthritis: genotype determines clinical phenotype. Arthritis Res Ther. 2015;17:115.
3. Helliwell PS, Kavanaugh A. Comparison of composite measures of disease activity in psoriatic arthritis using data from an interventional study with golimumab. Arthritis Care Res (Hoboken). 2014;66:749–56.
4. Acosta Felquer ML, Ferreyra Garrott L, Marin J, Catay E, Scolnik M, Scaglioni V, et al. Remission criteria and activity indices in psoriatic arthritis. Clin Rheumatol. 2014;33:1323–30.
5. Sankoh AJ, Li H, D'Agostino RB Sr. Use of composite endpoints in clinical trials. Stat Med. 2014;33:4709–14.
6. Schoels M. Psoriatic arthritis indices. Clin Exp Rheumatol. 2014;32:S109–S12.
7. Orbai AM, de Wit M, Mease P, Shea JA, Gossec L, Leung YY, et al. International patient and physician consensus on a psoriatic arthritis core outcome set for clinical trials. Ann Rheum Dis. 2017;76:673–80.
8. Meyer DM, Jesson MI, Li X, Elrick MM, Funckes-Shippy CL, Warner JD, et al. Anti-inflammatory activity and neutrophil reductions mediated by the JAK1/JAK3 inhibitor, CP-690,550, in rat adjuvant-induced arthritis. J Inflamm (Lond). 2010;7:41.
9. Mease P, Hall S, Fitzgerald O, van der Heijde D, Merola JF, Avila-Zapata F, et al. Tofacitinib or adalimumab versus placebo for psoriatic arthritis. N Engl J Med. 2017;377:1537–50.
10. Gladman D, Rigby W, Azevedo VF, Behrens F, Blanco R, Kaszuba A, et al. Tofacitinib for psoriatic arthritis in patients with an inadequate response to TNF inhibitors. N Engl J Med. 2017;377:1525–36.
11. Helliwell PS, FitzGerald O, Fransen J, Gladman DD, Kreuger GG, Callis-Duffin K, et al. The development of candidate composite disease activity and responder indices for psoriatic arthritis (GRACE project). Ann Rheum Dis. 2013;72:986–91.
12. Mumtaz A, Gallagher P, Kirby B, Waxman R, Coates LC, Veale JD, et al. Development of a preliminary composite disease activity index in psoriatic arthritis. Ann Rheum Dis. 2011;70:272–7.
13. Madsen OR. Is DAS28-CRP with three and four variables interchangeable in individual patients selected for biological treatment in daily clinical practice? Clin Rheumatol. 2011;30:1577–82.
14. Husted JA, Cook RJ, Farewell VT, Gladman DD. Methods for assessing responsiveness: a critical review and recommendations. J Clin Epidemiol. 2000;53:459–68.
15. Bhatti IP, Lohano HD, Pirzado ZA, Jafri IA. A logistic regression analysis of the ischemic heart disease risk. J Applied Sci. 2006;6:785–8.
16. Coates LC, Fransen J, Helliwell PS. Defining minimal disease activity in psoriatic arthritis: a proposed objective target for treatment. Ann Rheum Dis. 2010;69:48–53.
17. Helliwell PS, FitzGerald O, Fransen J. Composite disease activity and responder indices for psoriatic arthritis: a report from the GRAPPA 2013 meeting on development of cutoffs for both disease activity states and response. J Rheumatol. 2014;41:1212–7.
18. Kavanaugh A, McInnes IB, Mease PJ, Hall S, Chinoy H, Kivitz AJ, et al. Efficacy of subcutaneous secukinumab in patients with active psoriatic arthritis stratified by prior tumor necrosis factor inhibitor use: results from the randomized placebo-controlled FUTURE 2 study. J Rheumatol. 2016;43:1713–7.
19. Chatzidionysiou K, Kristensen LE, Eriksson J, Askling J, van Vollenhoven R. Effectiveness and survival-on-drug of certolizumab pegol in rheumatoid arthritis in clinical practice: results from the national Swedish register. Scand J Rheumatol. 2015;44:431–7.
20. Bykerk VP, Ostor AJ, Alvaro-Gracia J, Pavelka K, Ivorra JA, Graninger W, et al. Tocilizumab in patients with active rheumatoid arthritis and inadequate responses to DMARDs and/or TNF inhibitors: a large, open-label study close to clinical practice. Ann Rheum Dis. 2012;71:1950–4.
21. Coates LC, Mahmood F, Emery P, Conaghan PG, Helliwell PS. The dynamics of response as measured by multiple composite outcome tools in the TIght COntrol of inflammation in early Psoriatic Arthritis (TICOPA) trial. Ann Rheum Dis. 2017;76:1688–92.

22. Salaffi F, Ciapetti A, Carotti M, Gasparini S, Gutierrez M. Disease activity in psoriatic arthritis: comparison of the discriminative capacity and construct validity of six composite indices in a real world. Biomed Res Int. 2014;2014:528105.
23. Coates LC, Helliwell PS. Defining low disease activity states in psoriatic arthritis using novel composite disease instruments. J Rheumatol. 2016;43:371–5.
24. Chimenti MS, Triggianese P, Conigliaro P, Tonelli M, Gigliucci G, Novelli L, et al. A 2-year observational study on treatment targets in psoriatic arthritis patients treated with TNF inhibitors. Clin Rheumatol. 2017;36:2253–60.
25. Schoels MM, Aletaha D, Alasti F, Smolen JS. Disease activity in psoriatic arthritis (PsA): defining remission and treatment success using the DAPSA score. Ann Rheum Dis. 2016;75:811–8.
26. Acosta Felquer ML, Szentpetery A, Elmamoun M, Gallagher P, FitzGerald O, Soriano ER. Composite Psoriatic Disease Activity Index (CPDAI), defining remission and disease activity states using data from daily clinical practice [abstract]. Arthritis Rheumatol. 2016;68(suppl 10). https://acrabstracts.org/abstract/composite-psoriatic-disease-activity-index-cpdai-defining-remission-and-disease-activity-states-using-data-from-daily-clinical-practice/. Accessed 16 Oct 2018.
27. Coates LC, FitzGerald O, Gladman DD, McHugh N, Mease P, Strand V, et al. Reduced joint counts misclassify patients with oligoarticular psoriatic arthritis and miss significant numbers of patients with active disease. Arthritis Rheum. 2013;65:1504–9.
28. Coates LC, FitzGerald O, Merola JF, Smolen J, van Mens LJJ, Bertheussen H, et al. Group for Research and Assessment of Psoriasis and Psoriatic Arthritis/Outcome Measures in Rheumatology Consensus-Based Recommendations and Research Agenda for Use of Composite Measures and Treatment Targets in Psoriatic Arthritis. Arthritis Rheumatol. 2018;70:345–55.
29. Smolen JS, Schöls M, Braun J, Dougados M, FitzGerald O, Gladman DD, et al. Treating axial spondyloarthritis and peripheral spondyloarthritis, especially psoriatic arthritis, to target: 2017 update of recommendations by an international task force. Ann Rheum Dis. 2018;77:3–17.

13

Induction of chronic destructive arthritis in SCID mice by arthritogenic fibroblast-like synoviocytes derived from mice with antigen-induced arthritis

Oliver Frey[1,2,3*†], Marion Hückel[1†], Mieczyslaw Gajda[1], Peter K. Petrow[1] and Rolf Bräuer[1]

Abstract

Background: Fibroblast-like synoviocytes (FLSs) from patients with rheumatoid arthritis (RA) are autonomously activated to maintain inflammation and joint destruction in co-transplantation models. To elucidate inducing mechanisms involved in this altered behavior, the arthritogenic potential of FLSs from murine antigen-induced arthritis (AIA) were investigated in a transfer model.

Methods: FLSs were isolated, expanded in vitro, and transferred into knee joint cavities of severe combined immunodeficient (SCID) mice. Their arthritogenic capacity was assessed by monitoring joint swelling and evaluation of histological parameters 70 to 100 days after transfer.

Results: FLSs from AIA mice were able to transfer arthritis into recipient SCID mice. FLS transfer induced a chronic arthritis with recruitment of inflammatory cells and marked cartilage destruction. Long-lasting inflammation was not required for imprinting of arthritogenicity in FLSs since cells isolated from acute arthritic joints were fully competent to transfer arthritis. We also observed arthritogenic potential in FLSs isolated from contralateral non-arthritic joints in our monoarticular arthritis model.

Conclusions: We show that the transformation of FLSs into arthritogenic cells occurs early in arthritis development. This challenges current hypotheses on the role of these cells in arthritis pathogenesis and opens up the way for further mechanistic studies.

Keywords: Arthritis, Synovial fibroblast, Joint destruction

Background

Rheumatoid arthritis (RA) is a chronic inflammatory disease that primarily affects the joints. Key histological features of RA are infiltration by cells from the innate and the adaptive immune system, hyperplasia of the synovial membrane, and destruction of cartilage and adjacent bone [1, 2]. Fibroblast-like synoviocytes (FLSs) are the dominant cell type in the hyperplastic synovial membrane and are thought to play a key role in the pathogenesis of RA. Via their production of different inflammatory cytokines and chemokines, they can recruit inflammatory cells and sustain their persistence in inflamed joints. FLSs also produce matrix-degrading enzymes such as matrix metalloproteases (MMPs) and cathepsins and are thereby directly involved in joint destruction. A remarkable feature of FLSs is their ability to maintain their activated phenotype in tissue culture or upon engraftment in severe combined immunodeficient (SCID) mice [3–5]. Early models used transplantation of whole RA synovial tissue to study the inflammatory and destructive features of synovial cells in an in vivo environment [6–8]. Since synovial membranes of RA patients contain a mixture of different cell types, in later studies FLSs were isolated prior to transfer into SCID mice [9, 10]. In such chimeric models, FLSs attach to and invade the co-implanted cartilage, and they recruit

* Correspondence: o.frey@imd-berlin.de
†Oliver Frey and Marion Hückel contributed equally to this work.
[1]Institute of Pathology, University Hospital, Jena, Germany
[2]Institute of Clinical Chemistry and Laboratory Medicine, University Hospital, Am Klinikum 1, D-07743 Jena, Germany
Full list of author information is available at the end of the article

inflammatory cells. Furthermore, destructive fibroblasts migrate to and destroy unaffected cartilage co-transplanted in other anatomical locations upon transfer in immunodeficient mice [11]. Thus, although this model does not reflect all aspects of the complex pathogenesis of RA, it fosters the view that a permanent and autonomous activation of FLSs is central to disease progression.

Since the immunological process which finally triggers RA can precede the clinical disease onset by many years, the cascade of events eventually leading to FLS activation and disease cannot be reconstructed from patient material. Thus, animal models are clearly needed for a better understanding of the contribution of fibroblasts to chronic inflammation and joint destruction in arthritis. So far, there is only one published study using cloned immortalized FLSs confirming the observation of an arthritogenic behavior of FLSs in a tumor necrosis factor (TNF)-transgenic mouse model [5]. It is unknown whether this behavior can also be imprinted to non-immortalized FLSs isolated from arthritic wild-type mice.

Based on the above-mentioned studies using FLSs from patients with RA, it is widely assumed that the arthritis-promoting effect of these cells is the consequence of long-standing chronic inflammation. This has not yet been proven experimentally, and we therefore aimed to elucidate if chronic inflammation is mandatory for arthritogenic transformation of FLSs in our mouse model. If an acute (short-term) arthritis were sufficient to induce persistent changes in FLS behavior, it could be hypothesized that these cells are rather accomplices than villains in the induction and perpetuation of chronic arthritis. Thus, our study aimed at answering some fundamental questions of the biology of FLSs for the pathogenesis of arthritis.

We used antigen-induced arthritis (AIA), which is induced by intraarticular injection of an antigen into the knee joint cavity of animals preimmunized with the same antigen. This model was chosen because of its 100% incidence and the well-documented time course of pathogenic changes upon arthritis triggering [12, 13]. These features allows for a systematic study of FLS behavior isolated from arthritic as well as non-arthritic knee joints.

Methods
Animals and arthritis induction
Female C57BL/6 mice aged 6–12 weeks were immunized 21 and 14 days before arthritis induction by subcutaneous injection of 100 µg methylated bovine serum albumin (mBSA, Sigma, Deisenhofen, Germany) in 50 µl saline, emulsified in 50 µl complete Freund's adjuvant (CFA; Sigma), supplemented with 2.0 mg/ml heat-killed *Mycobacterium tuberculosis* (strain H37RA, Becton Dickinson, Heidelberg, Germany). At the same time, mice were injected with 5×10^8 heat-killed *Bordetella pertussis* bacteria (Chiron Behring, Marburg, Germany). On day 0,

arthritis was induced by a single injection of 100 µg mBSA in 25 µl saline into the right knee joint cavity. The left knee joint was left untreated. The animals were sacrificed, and the knees were dissected for the preparation of synovial cells in acute (before day 7) or chronic phase (after day 7) of AIA.

BALB/c SCID mice (Harlan Winkelmann, Borchen, Germany) aged 6–8 weeks were used as recipients. The SCID mice were housed in isolated cages at the Central Animal Facility, University Hospital Jena.

All experiments were approved by the appropriate governmental authority (Thüringer Landesamt für Verbraucherschutz) and conducted in accordance with institutional and state guidelines.

Preparation of FLSs
FLSs were obtained by explant cultures from synovial tissue dissected from the knee joints of normal, immunized, or arthritic mice (at different time points after arthritis induction) as previously described in [14]. The tissue was digested with 0.1% trypsin (Boehringer Mannheim, Germany) in phosphate-buffered saline (PBS) for 30 min and after washing, digested with 0.1% collagenase P (Boehringer) in PBS for an additional 2 h. The culture was maintained in Dulbecco's modified Eagle's medium (DMEM), completed with 10 mM 4-(2-hydroxyethyl)-1-piperazineethanesulfonic acid (HEPES), 1 mM sodium pyruvate (all from Gibco BRL, Gaithersburg, MD, USA), 100 U/ml penicillin (Jenapharm, Jena, Germany), 0.1 mg/ml streptomycin (Grünenthal, Stolberg, Germany), 2 mM glutamine (Gibco), and 20% fetal calf serum (FCS; Gibco) for 7 days at 5% CO_2 and 37 °C. Medium exchange took place each day. Synovial cells emerged from explanted synovium within 7 days. Confluent FLSs were detached by digestion with 0.25% trypsin/0.02% ethylenediaminetetraacetic acid (EDTA; Gibco) and subcultured in complete DMEM supplemented with 10% FCS. Synovial cells were repeatedly passaged to enrich FLSs and to deplete macrophages [10, 15]. For some experiments we depleted macrophages from the cell cultures after the first passage with magnetic cell sorting using anti-CD11b (clone 5C6; Serotec, Oxford, UK) followed by anti-rat Dynabeads® (10 beads/cell; Dynal, Hamburg, Germany). The separation was achieved using a Magnetic Particle Concentrator (Dynal MPC®). All FLS preparations used for transfer experiments contained > 95% fibroblasts by their typical spindle-shaped morphology.

Cell cultures were routinely screened for infection with mycoplasma (*Mycoplasma orale, M. arginini, M. hyorhinis,* and *M. laidlawii)* with an enzyme-linked immunosorbent assay (ELISA) detection kit (Roche Diagnostics, Mannheim, Germany), according to the manufacturer's instructions.

Cell transfer and monitoring of arthritis development

FLSs of the third to the fifth passage were harvested subsequently using 0.25% trypsin/0.02% EDTA in PBS and washed and suspended in PBS at a final concentration of 1.2×10^7 cell/ml; then 25 µl (3×10^5 cells) of this suspension were injected into the knee joint cavity of recipient SCID mice.

Development of clinical arthritis in SCID mice was monitored by measuring the mediolateral knee joint diameter with an Oditest vernier caliper (Kroeplin Längenmesstechnik, Schlüchtern, Germany). Knee joint swelling was expressed as the difference between the right (injected) and left (untreated) knees.

For histological assessment of arthritis severity [14], SCID mice were sacrificed 70–100 days after cell transfer (time indicated in results). Total knee joints were removed and fixed in 4.5% Tris-buffered formalin. After decalcification with 15% EDTA, embedding in paraffin, and sectioning, slides were stained with hematoxylin and eosin (H&E). A minimum of three sections (2 µm) from three different levels of the knee joints were evaluated blindly by at least two different observers (MG, PKP) for the degree of inflammation and joint destruction. The severity of inflammation was evaluated on a 0–3 point scale indicating lining layer hyperplasia and cellular infiltration (0: none, 1: mild, 2: moderate, 3: strong changes). The severity of degradation was assessed by scoring pannus formation and chondrocyte necrosis as well as cartilage and bone erosion. A final arthritis score was calculated for each animal by adding the scores for all four parameters (upper limit grade 12).

For the evaluation of proteoglycan loss, sections were stained with Safranin O. In this method, the degree of staining is inversely correlated with the loss of proteoglycans in the cartilage layers.

Statistics

All data shown are mean ± standard error of mean. Statistically significant differences were calculated using the non-parametric Mann-Whitney U test (two-tailed) with SPSS 22 (IBM). p values less than 0.05 were considered as statistically significant.

Results

Transfer of FLSs from C57BL/6 mice with AIA induce arthritis in SCID mice recipients

In order to investigate the arthritogenic potential of FLSs in vivo, these cells were injected into the knee joints of SCID mice. We followed arthritis development by measurement of the knee joint diameter and histological examination of the knee joints at the end point of the experiment. As shown in Fig. 1, FLSs from affected knee joints of mice with acute arthritis (isolated until day 7 post AIA induction) induced a slowly growing increase in joint swelling in the recipients. This surrogate parameter of joint inflammation was also found in recipients of FLSs from mice with chronic AIA (isolated after day 7), albeit to a lesser extent. We did not detect a similar knee joint swelling in SCID mice injected with PBS or FLSs isolated from naïve, non-arthritic mice, suggesting that the arthritogenic capacity is restricted to FLSs isolated from arthritic mice.

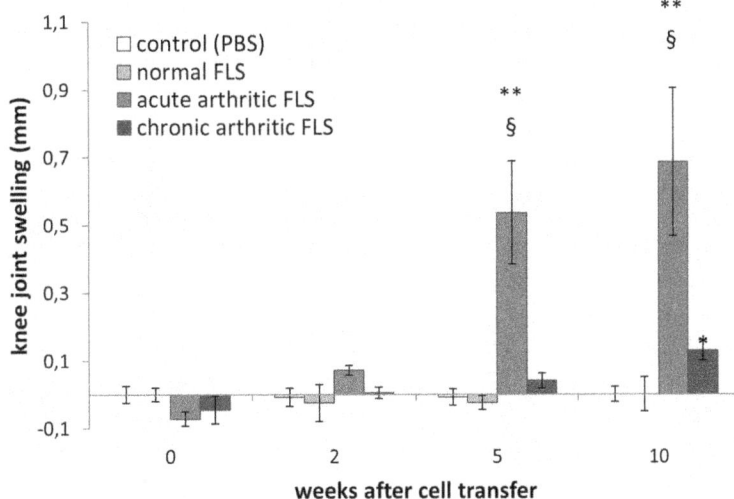

Fig. 1 Knee joint swelling in SCID mice after transfer of fibroblast-like synoviocytes (FLSs). FLSs from healthy C57BL/6 mice (normal FLSs, $n = 5$), from C57BL/6 mice with acute AIA (7 days, acute arthritic FLSs, $n = 7$), or from those with chronic AIA (21 days, chronic arthritic FLSs, $n = 11$) were transferred into the right knee joint cavity of SCID mice. Buffer was injected as a control (control, PBS, $n = 6$). Joint swelling was evaluated by differences between joint diameter of right knee (ispilateral) and left knee (contralateral) at day of measurement. All data shown are mean ± standard error of mean. (* $p < 0.05$ vs. PBS, ** $p < 0.01$ vs. PBS, § $p < 0.05$ vs. normal FLSs; Mann-Whitney U test.) Data shown are a representative example of at least two independent experiments per group

Histological evaluation of joint sections confirmed arthritis development observed by joint swelling. As shown in Fig. 2, injection of FLSs isolated from C57BL/6 mice with acute arthritis into SCID recipients resulted in cellular infiltration, hyperplasia of the synovial lining layer, pannus formation, and chondrocyte necrosis as well as cartilage and bone erosions. Safranin O staining revealed that the injection of arthritogenic cells also caused loss of proteoglycans. These typical histological signs of arthritis were not seen in recipients of FLSs isolated from naïve, non-arthritic mice. Semiquantitative scoring of histological arthritis severity showed a higher degree of inflammation and joint destruction, resulting in a higher total arthritis score, in the recipients from FLSs isolated from mice with acute compared to chronic arthritis (Fig. 3). Recipients of FLSs from naïve, non-arthritic mice showed only very limited signs of inflammation, while joint erosions were almost completely absent.

Thus, our data indicate that FLSs isolated from mice with AIA possess and maintain their arthritogenic potential without exogenous activation, a behavior which is similar to that of FLSs isolated from patients with RA. Remarkably, this arthritogenic potential of FLSs is induced early in the disease course and is not a consequence of long-lasting inflammation.

Depletion of macrophages prior to transfer had no influence on disease outcome

Our FLS cultures still contained approximately 20% CD11b⁺ macrophage-like cells after the third passage (data not shown). It is possible that these activated macrophages and not the FLSs contained in these preparations could trigger inflammation and joint destruction in the recipient SCID mice knee joints. We therefore depleted CD11b⁺ cells using immunobeads from FLS preparations from acutely arthritic AIA mice. Arthritogenicity of these pure FLS preparations (< 1% CD11b⁺, data not shown) were compared with unsorted FLS preparations in transfer experiments. The experiments were performed identically to those previously described. As shown in Fig. 4, we observed no differences in inflammatory changes or joint destruction upon histological examination of the recipient knee joints. These data show that the presence of macrophages has no effect on the arthritogenicity of FLS preparations from acutely arthritic joints from AIA mice. Furthermore, the small enrichment of fibroblasts in macrophage-depleted preparations did not lead to a significant increase of arthritis severity.

FLSs from contralateral (control) knee of AIA mice also show arthritogenic potential

Having demonstrated that the imprinting of arthritogenic behavior on FLSs occurs early during arthritis development, we next examined if interactions between fibroblasts and infiltrating cells are necessary for the induction of FLS aggressiveness. Since AIA is a monoarticular arthritis model, we are able to compare the arthritogenicity of FLS preparations from affected ipsilateral joints with the non-affected contralateral knee joints. Although the contralateral knee joint in AIA never shows histological abnormalities, FLS preparations from these joints were surprisingly potent inducers of arthritis. Semiquantitative scoring of end-point histology of the recipient knee joints showed significantly reduced inflammation but similar joint destruction in recipients of FLSs from ipsilateral and contralateral knee joints (Fig. 5).

Discussion

In this paper we show that FLSs isolated from knee joints of mice with AIA have the capacity to cause severe inflammation and destruction when injected intraarticularly into knee joints of SCID mice. Isolated FLSs express their arthritogenic potential even after several passages in vitro, indicating a long-lasting transformation to autonomous aggressor cells. This arthritogenicity was intrinsic to FLSs, since removal of contaminating macrophages did not affect arthritis severity in the recipients.

These features resemble the aggressive behavior of human FLSs from RA patients which upon co-transfer with engrafted cartilage into SCIID mice possess pro-inflammatory and pro-destructive activity [3, 9, 16]. In vitro studies have demonstrated a loss of contact inhibition as well as constitutive expression of cytokines and matrix-degrading enzymes as causative for the arthritogenicity of RA FLSs (for a review see [17]). However, the mechanisms leading to their transformation from cells with mainly homeostatic functions into cells with such an altered phenotype are still a matter of debate. Somatic mutations in genes regulating cellular functions like proliferation and apoptosis have been implicated in cell-autonomous aggressive behavior. Also, epigenetic alterations have been identified in RA FLSs, which may be imprinted by chronic exposure to inflammatory cytokines or cells [17]. Our findings presented here show that FLSs isolated from mice in the acute stage of AIA were already able to induce inflammation and joint destruction in the recipients. Compared to FLSs isolated from mice with chronic AIA they even induced a more severe arthritis in the recipients. This higher arthritogenicity of acute-stage FLSs might be related to their higher level of activation. Previous work from our group has demonstrated higher expression of matrix-degrading enzymes and concomitant maximal proteoglycan depletion in the acute stage of arthritis [18]. Taken together this indicates that the activation and transformation of FLSs is an early event in the disease course in AIA. An early upregulation of MMP-3 and MMP-9 activities has been described in TNF-overexpressing mice that develop arthritis [19], also

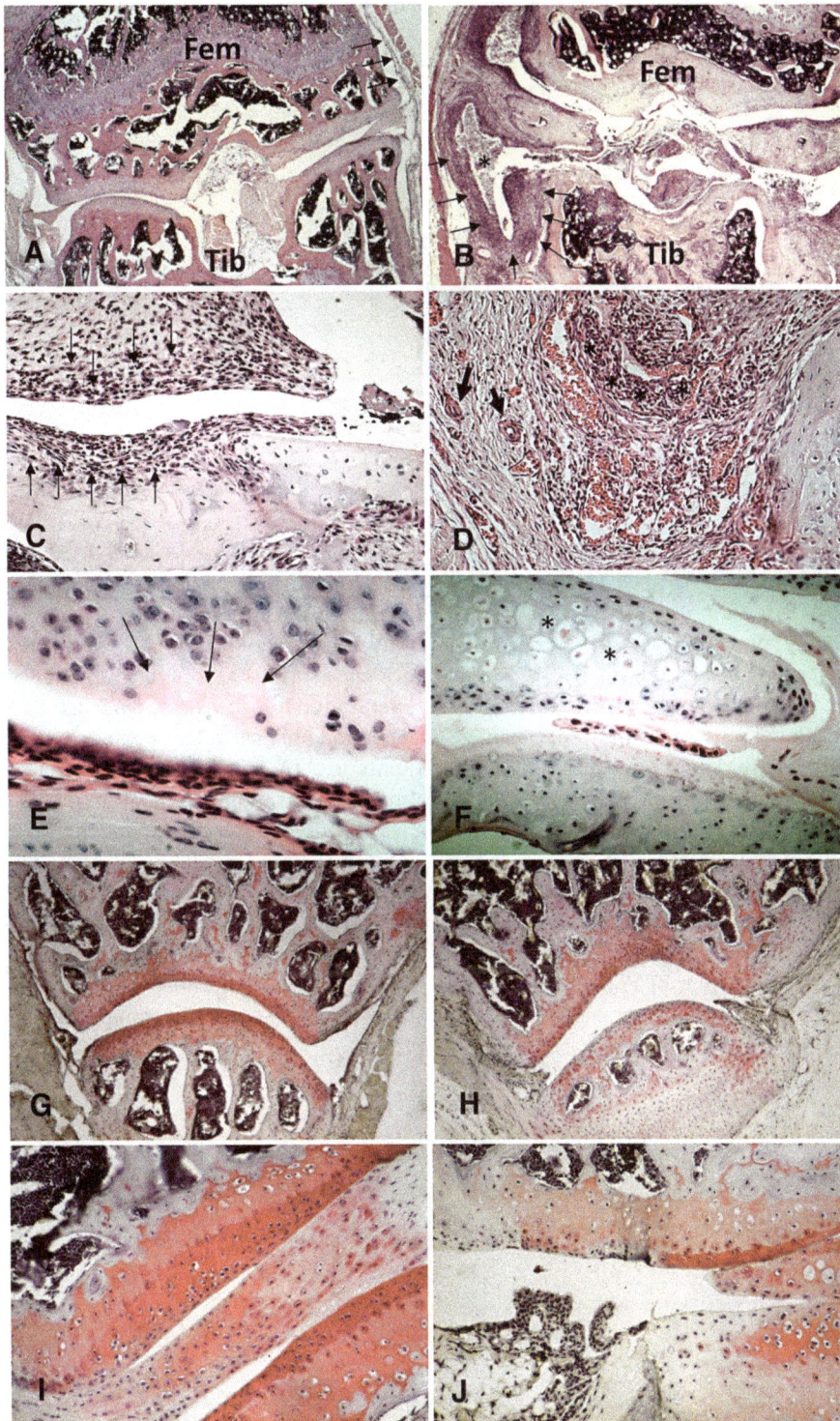

Fig. 2 Histological examination of knee sections from SCID mice. **a** Sections from healthy untreated knee joint (*Fem* femur, *Tib* Tibia). *Arrows* indicate a normal synovial membrane. **b** Knee joints 100 days after transfer of FLSs isolated from C57BL/6 mice with acute AIA. Shown is an overview of the inflamed and destructed joint (*Fem* femur, *Tib* tibia). *Arrows* indicate the hyperplastic and inflamed synovial membrane. *Asterisks* indicate the inflammatory exudate in the knee cavity. **c** and **d** Higher magnification to illustrate hyperplasia of the synovial lining layer and pannus formation (*arrows*) and inflammatory infiltration (*asterisks*) and neovascularization (*thick arrows*). **e** and **f** Cartilage erosions (*arrows*) and necrosis of chondrocytes (*asterisks*). Staining of proteoglycans with Safranin O in healthy knee joint sections (**g**, **i**) and arthritic knee joint of SCID mice (**h**, **j**) 100 days after cell transfer shows loss of proteoglycans in arthritic SCID joints. Sections **a–f** were stained with H&E, **g–j** with Safranin O. Magnifications: **a**, **b**, **g**, **h** 40×, **i**, **j** 100×, **c**, **d**, **f** 200×, **e** 400×

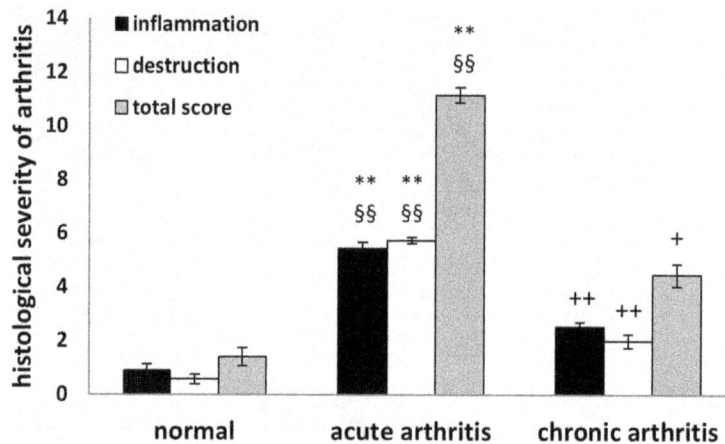

Fig. 3 Semiquantitative histologic scoring of inflammation, joint destruction, and total arthritis score in knee joint sections from SCID mice 70–100 days after transfer of FLSs. FLSs were isolated from non-immunized, non-arthritic mice (normal, $n = 9$), mice with acute arthritis (up to day 7 post AIA induction, $n = 13$), or mice with chronic AIA (isolated after day 7 post AIA induction, $n = 52$). Data are pooled from at least two experiments. Histological scoring was performed by two independent investigators on a 0–3 point scale for synovial lining layer hyperplasia, cellular infiltration, pannus formation, and cartilage invasion, giving a total score of 12. All data shown are mean ± standard error of mean (** $p < 0.001$ acute vs. normal, §§ $p < 0.001$ acute vs. chronic, + $p < 0.01$, ++ $p < 0.001$ chronic vs. normal, Mann-Whitney U test)

implying that FLS activation is an early event in arthritis pathogenesis and supporting our findings.

Although the activation and transformation of FLSs in RA might be multifactorial, our data imply that somatic mutations might not be an ultimate prerequisite for their arthritogenicity, but instead short-term activation through inflammatory mediators might be sufficient [3, 20–25].

Moreover, we have demonstrated that FLSs isolated from the contralateral, non-affected joints in AIA can induce inflammation and joint destruction in our transfer system. This intriguing and unexpected finding implies that activation and transformation of FLSs can occur in the absence of infiltrating inflammatory cells. Although

AIA is considered to be a monarthritis, several pieces of evidence suggest at least a partial affection of the contralateral joints. In previous work we have demonstrated a depletion of cartilage proteoglycans in non-affected joints in AIA in rats [26, 27]. We also detected macrophage activation by immunohistochemistry and near-infrared molecular imaging in the contralateral joint of arthritic mice [28], presumably as a consequence of the systemic macrophage activation in AIA [29]. Supernatants of synoviocyte cultures from contralateral joints of rats with AIA contained higher levels of interleukin (IL)-6 than those of healthy controls [30]. Although the exact reasons for activation of the

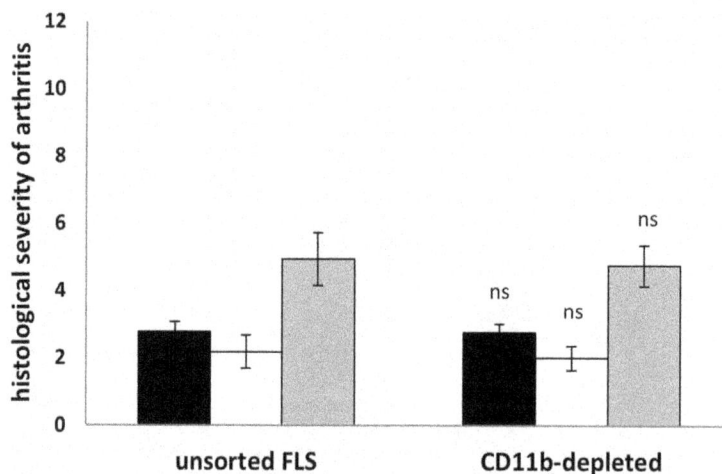

Fig. 4 Histological arthritis severity in recipient SCID mice that were intraarticularly injected with total unsorted FLSs or with CD11b-depleted FLSs (isolated 5 or 8 days post AIA induction). Cultures of depleted and non-depleted FLSs as well as cell transfer were done in parallel. Black bars: inflammation, white bars: joint destruction, grey bars: total arthritis score. All data shown are mean ± standard error of mean (total cells $n = 17$, depleted $n = 28$, ns no significant differences). Data are pooled from two independent experiments

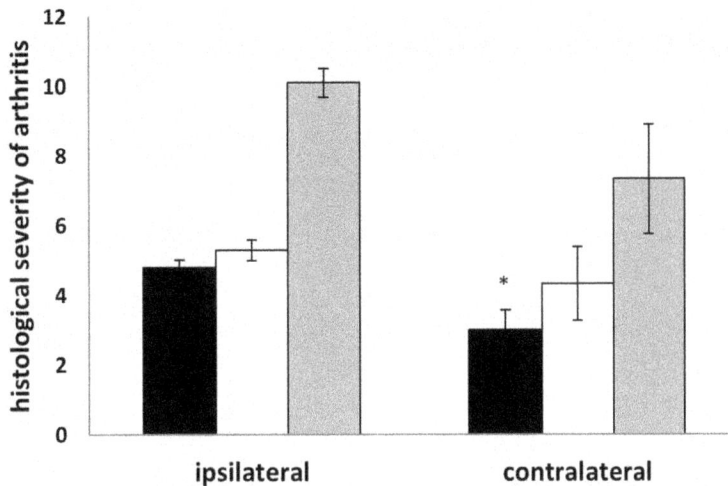

Fig. 5 Histological arthritis scoring after transfer of FLSs from the arthritic and contralateral knee joints of AIA mice. Cells were isolated and transferred in parallel, and the data shown are pooled from three independent experiments using FLSs from different time points (day 8 or 28) after AIA induction. Black bars: inflammation, white bars: joint destruction, grey bars: total arthritis score. All data shown are mean ± standard error of mean (ipsilateral $n = 10$, contralateral $n = 6$ (* $p < 0.05$ ipsilateral vs. contralateral)

contralateral FLSs in AIA remain elusive, this could be explained by elevated systemic levels of cytokines like TNF or IL-6 induced by immunization and intraarticular antigen challenge. Overexpression of TNF or enhanced IL-6 signaling due to a gain-of-function mutation of gp130 is sufficient to induce arthritis in mice [31, 32]. Strikingly, both cytokines can still induce joint inflammation when the expression of their receptor is restricted to mesenchymal cells such as FLSs [19, 32]. These data clearly demonstrate that activation of FLSs via cytokines is solely sufficient to induce arthritis.

Other activation stimuli could be delivered via neuronal mechanisms. Receptors for neurokinin 1 and bradykinin 2 are bilaterally upregulated in dorsal root ganglia of rats with AIA [27]. It has been shown that neurokinin 1 can transmit signals responsible for cartilage destruction at distal sites after induction of a unilateral local inflammation [33]. Unilateral arthritis also leads to bilateral hyperalgesia that in turn could trigger inflammation on the contralateral site via spinal reflexes [34]. Furthermore, the enhanced hippocampal neurogenesis found in AIA is mainly driven by immunization, not by localized inflammation [35]. Shenker et al. proposed that these contralateral effects in many models are mediated through neural mechanisms rather than reflecting a systemic or circulatory effect [36].

Regardless of whether the activation of FLSs is mediated via systemic or neuronal mechanisms, the fact that such a remote activation can occur is intriguing and could have implications for our understanding of RA pathogenesis. Assuming that such a remote activation of FLSs also occurs in humans, it is possible that FLS transformation is an early event in arthritis pathogenesis rather than a consequence of long-lasting local inflammation. In other words, FLS activation by such stimuli could be the missing link between systemic alterations of the immune system and joint-specific inflammation. Multiple animal models in which arthritis is induced by autoimmunity against ubiquitous antigens [37–40], by defective apoptosis [41], by a generally more autoreactive T cell repertoire [42], or by increased cytokine signaling [31, 43–45] provide evidence that the recognition of joint-specific antigens is not an absolute requirement for joint-specific inflammation (for a review see [46]). Taking into account that biomarkers of inflammation are upregulated years before clinical disease onset, such mechanisms could also be a pathogenic principle in human RA [47, 48].

While the FLSs from contralateral joints are nearly as equally potent inducers of inflammation and joint destruction as FLSs from arthritic AIA joints in our transfer system, there is little or no inflammation and only limited joint destruction in the joints from which the cells originate. This could be explained by an active counter-regulation in situ in the joints of the donor mice, which is intriguing, because the identification of such a regulatory mechanism could open up the way for new therapeutic approaches.

Conclusions

In summary, we have demonstrated in this report that FLSs from mice with experimental inflammatory AIA share important features with FLSs from patients with human RA. Therefore, this model is a valuable tool for experimental analyses of the molecular mechanisms of the pathogenic role of FLSs in the induction and joint destruction in chronic arthritis.

Abbreviations

AIA: Antigen-induced arthritis; FLS: Fibroblast-like synoviocyte; MMP: Matrix metalloprotease; RA: Rheumatoid arthritis; SCID: Severe combined immunodeficient; TNF: Tumor necrosis factor

Acknowledgements

We would like to thank Cornelia Hüttich and Renate Stöckigt for their excellent technical assistance.

Funding

RB was supported by the Deutsche Forschungsgemeinschaft (Br 1372/9), the Thuringian Ministry of Science, Research and Art (Grant B 378–01017), and the Interdisciplinary Center for Clinical Research (IZKF) Jena. OF received funding from the Deutsche Forschungsgemeinschaft (Priority Programme 1468 Immunobone) and from Novartis.

Authors' contributions

OF, MH, and RB conceived, designed, and interpreted the study. OF, MH, MG, and PKP performed data collection; OF and MH performed the statistical analysis. OF, MH, and RB drafted the manuscript. All authors read and approved the final manuscript.

Competing interests

The authors declare that they have no competing interests.

Author details

[1]Institute of Pathology, University Hospital, Jena, Germany. [2]Institute of Clinical Chemistry and Laboratory Medicine, University Hospital, Am Klinikum 1, D-07743 Jena, Germany. [3]Present address: Institute of Medical Diagnostics, Berlin, Germany.

References

1. Klareskog L, Catrina AI, Paget S. Rheumatoid arthritis. Lancet. 2009;373(9664): 659–72.
2. Firestein GS. Evolving concepts of rheumatoid arthritis. Nature. 2003; 423(6937):356–61.
3. Firestein GS. Invasive fibroblast-like synoviocytes in rheumatoid arthritis. Passive responders or transformed aggressors? Arthritis Rheum. 1996;39(11): 1781–90.
4. Noss EH, Brenner MB. The role and therapeutic implications of fibroblast-like synoviocytes in inflammation and cartilage erosion in rheumatoid arthritis. Immunol Rev. 2008;223:252–70.
5. Aidinis V, Plows D, Haralambous S, Armaka M, Papadopoulos P, Kanaki MZ, Koczan D, Thiesen HJ, Kollias G. Functional analysis of an arthritogenic synovial fibroblast. Arthritis Res. 2003;5(5):R140–57.
6. Geiler T, Kriegsmann J, Keyszer GM, Gay RE, Gay S. A new model for rheumatoid arthritis generated by engraftment of rheumatoid synovial tissue and normal human cartilage into SCID mice. Arthritis Rheum. 1994; 37(11):1664–71.
7. Sack U, Kuhn H, Kampfer I, Genest M, Arnold S, Pfeiffer G, Emmrich F. Orthotopic implantation of inflamed synovial tissue from RA patients induces a characteristic arthritis in immunodeficient (SCID) mice. J Autoimmun. 1996;9(1):51–8.
8. Sack U, Gunther A, Pfeiffer R, Genest M, Kinne J, Biskop M, Kampfer I, Krenn V, Emmrich F, Lehmann J. Systemic characteristics of chronic arthritis induced by transfer of human rheumatoid synovial membrane into SCID mice (human/murine SCID arthritis). J Autoimmun. 1999;13(3):335–46.
9. Müller-Ladner U, Kriegsmann J, Franklin BN, Matsumoto S, Geiler T, Gay RE, Gay S. Synovial fibroblasts of patients with rheumatoid arthritis attach to and invade normal human cartilage when engrafted into SCID mice. Am J Pathol. 1996;149(5):1607 15.
10. Lehmann J, Jungel A, Lehmann I, Busse F, Biskop M, Saalbach A, Emmrich F, Sack U. Grafting of fibroblasts isolated from the synovial membrane of rheumatoid arthritis (RA) patients induces chronic arthritis in SCID mice—A novel model for studying the arthritogenic role of RA fibroblasts in vivo. J Autoimmun. 2000;15(3):301–13.
11. Lefevre S, Knedla A, Tennie C, Kampmann A, Wunrau C, Dinser R, Korb A, Schnaker EM, Tarner IH, Robbins PD, et al. Synovial fibroblasts spread rheumatoid arthritis to unaffected joints. Nat Med. 2009;15(12):1414–20.
12. Frey O, Petrow PK, Gajda M, Siegmund K, Huehn J, Scheffold A, Hamann A, Radbruch A, Brauer R. The role of regulatory T cells in antigen-induced arthritis: aggravation of arthritis after depletion and amelioration after transfer of CD4+CD25+ T cells. Arthritis Res Ther. 2005;7(2):R291–301.
13. Huehn J, Siegmund K, Lehmann JC, Siewert C, Haubold U, Feuerer M, Debes GF, Lauber J, Frey O, Przybylski GK, et al. Developmental stage, phenotype, and migration distinguish naive- and effector/memory-like CD4+ regulatory T cells. J Exp Med. 2004;199(3):303–13.
14. Huckel M, Schurigt U, Wagner AH, Stockigt R, Petrow PK, Thoss K, Gajda M, Henzgen S, Hecker M, Brauer R. Attenuation of murine antigen-induced arthritis by treatment with a decoy oligodeoxynucleotide inhibiting signal transducer and activator of transcription-1 (STAT-1). Arthritis Res Ther. 2006;8(1):R17.
15. Armaka M, Gkretsi V, Kontoyiannis DL, Kollias G. A standardized protocol for the isolation and culture of normal and arthritogenic murine synovial fibroblasts. Protoc Exchange. 2009. https://doi.org/10.1038/nprot.2009.102.
16. Ritchlin C. Fibroblast biology; Effector signals released by synovial fibroblas in arthritis. Arthritis Res. 2000;2:356–60.
17. Bottini N, Firestein GS. Duality of fibroblast-like synoviocytes in RA: passive responders and imprinted aggressors. Nat Rev Rheumatol. 2013;9(1):24–33.
18. Schurigt U, Stopfel N, Huckel M, Pfirschke C, Wiederanders B, Brauer R. Local expression of matrix metalloproteinases, cathepsins, and their inhibitors during the development of murine antigen-induced arthritis. Arthritis Res Ther. 2005;7(1):R174–88.
19. Armaka M, Apostolaki M, Jacques P, Kontoyiannis DL, Elewaut D, Kollias G. Mesenchymal cell targeting by TNF as a common pathogenic principle in chronic inflammatory joint and intestinal diseases. J Exp Med. 2008;205(2):331–7.
20. Kontoyiannis D, Kollias G. Fibroblast biology. Synovial fibroblasts in rheumatoid arthritis: leading role or chorus line? Arthritis Res. 2000;2(5):342–3.
21. Karouzakis E, Gay RE, Gay S, Neidhart M. Epigenetic control in rheumatoid arthritis synovial fibroblasts. Nat Rev Rheumatol. 2009;5(5):266–72.
22. Kinne RW, Boehm S, Iftner T, Aigner T, Vornehm S, Weseloh G, Bravo R, Emmrich F, Kroczek RA. Synovial fibroblast-like cells strongly express jun-B and C-fos proto-oncogenes in rheumatoid- and osteoarthritis. Scand J Rheumatol Suppl. 1995;101:121–5.
23. Kinne RW, Liehr T, Beensen V, Kunisch E, Zimmermann T, Holland H, Pfeiffer R, Stahl HD, Lungershausen W, Hein G, et al. Mosaic chromosomal aberrations in synovial fibroblasts of patients with rheumatoid arthritis, osteoarthritis, and other inflammatory joint diseases. Arthritis Res. 2001;3(5):319–30.
24. Müller-Ladner U, Ospelt C, Gay S, Distler O, Pap T. Cells of the synovium in rheumatoid arthritis. Synovial fibroblasts. Arthritis Res Ther. 2007;9(6):223.
25. Pap T, Müller-Ladner U, Gay RE, Gay S. Fibroblast biology; Role of synovial fibroblasts in the pathogenesis of rheumatoid arthritis. Arthritis Res. 2000;2:361–7.
26. Meyer P, Burkhardt H, Palombo-Kinne E, Grunder W, Brauer R, Stiller KJ, Kalden JR, Becker W, Kinne RW. 123I-antileukoproteinase scintigraphy reveals microscopic cartilage alterations in the contralateral knee joint of rats with "monarticular" antigen-induced arthritis. Arthritis Rheum. 2000; 43(2):298–310.
27. Segond von Banchet GG, Petrow PK, Brauer R, Schaible HG. Monoarticular antigen-induced arthritis leads to pronounced bilateral upregulation of the expression of neurokinin 1 and bradykinin 2 receptors in dorsal root ganglion neurons of rats. Arthritis Res. 2000;2(5):424–7.
28. Hansch A, Frey O, Sauner D, Hilger I, Haas M, Malich A, Brauer R, Kaiser WA. In vivo imaging of experimental arthritis with near-infrared fluorescence. Arthritis Rheum. 2004;50(3):961–7.
29. Simon J, Surber R, Kleinstauber G, Petrow PK, Henzgen S, Kinne RW, Brauer R. Systemic macrophage activation in locally-induced experimental arthritis. J Autoimmun. 2001;17(2):127–36.
30. Mentzel K, Bräuer R. Matrix metalloproteinases, IL-6, and nitric oxide in rat antigen-induced arthritis. Clin Exp Rheumatol. 1998;16(3):269–76.
31. Keffer J, Probert L, Cazlaris H, Georgopoulos S, Kaslaris E, Kioussis D, Kollias G. Transgenic mice expressing human tumour necrosis factor: a predictive genetic model of arthritis. EMBO J. 1991;10(13):4025–31.

32. Murakami M, Okuyama Y, Ogura H, Asano S, Arima Y, Tsuruoka M, Harada M, Kanamoto M, Sawa Y, Iwakura Y, et al. Local microbleeding facilitates IL-6- and IL-17-dependent arthritis in the absence of tissue antigen recognition by activated T cells. J Exp Med. 2011;208(1):103–14.

33. Decaris E, Guingamp C, Chat M, Philippe L, Grillasca JP, Abid A, Minn A, Gillet P, Netter P, Terlain B. Evidence for neurogenic transmission inducing degenerative cartilage damage distant from local inflammation. Arthritis Rheum. 1999;42(9):1951–60.

34. Willis WD Jr. Dorsal root potentials and dorsal root reflexes: a double-edged sword. Exp Brain Res. 1999;124(4):395–421.

35. Leuchtweis J, Boettger MK, Niv F, Redecker C, Schaible HG. Enhanced neurogenesis in the hippocampal dentate gyrus during antigen-induced arthritis in adult rat—a crucial role of immunization. PLoS One. 2014;9(2):e89258.

36. Shenker N, Haigh R, Roberts E, Mapp P, Harris N, Blake D. A review of contralateral responses to a unilateral inflammatory lesion. Rheumatology (Oxford). 2003;42(11):1279–86.

37. Schubert D, Maier B, Morawietz L, Krenn V, Kamradt T. Immunization with glucose-6-phosphate isomerase induces T-cell dependent peripheral polyarthritis in genetically unaltered mice. J Immunol. 2004;172:4503–9.

38. Matsumoto I, Staub A, Benoist C, Mathis D. Arthritis provoked by linked T and B cell recognition of a glycolytic enzyme. Science. 1999;286(5445):1732–5.

39. Rankin AL, Reed AJ, Oh S, Cozzo Picca C, Guay HM, Larkin J 3rd, Panarey L, Aitken MK, Koeberlein B, Lipsky PE, et al. CD4+ T cells recognizing a single self-peptide expressed by APCs induce spontaneous autoimmune arthritis. J Immunol. 2008;180(2):833–41.

40. Ho PP, Lee LY, Zhao X, Tomooka BH, Paniagua RT, Sharpe O, BenBarak MJ, Chandra PE, Hueber W, Steinman L, et al. Autoimmunity against fibrinogen mediates inflammatory arthritis in mice. J Immunol. 2010;184(1):379–90.

41. Kawane K, Ohtani M, Miwa K, Kizawa T, Kanbara Y, Yoshioka Y, Yoshikawa H, Nagata S. Chronic polyarthritis caused by mammalian DNA that escapes from degradation in macrophages. Nature. 2006;443(7114):998–1002.

42. Sakaguchi N, Takahashi T, Hata H, Nomura T, Tagami T, Yamazaki S, Sakihama T, Matsutani T, Negishi I, Nakatsuru S, et al. Altered thymic T-cell selection due to a mutation of the ZAP-70 gene causes autoimmune arthritis in mice. Nature. 2003;426(6965):454–60.

43. Horai R, Saijo S, Tanioka H, Nakae S, Sudo K, Okahara A, Ikuse T, Asano M, Iwakura Y. Development of chronic inflammatory arthropathy resembling rheumatoid arthritis in interleukin 1 receptor antagonist-deficient mice. J Exp Med. 2000;191(2):313–20.

44. Atsumi T, Ishihara K, Kamimura D, Ikushima H, Ohtani T, Hirota S, Kobayashi H, Park SJ, Saeki Y, Kitamura Y, et al. A point mutation of Tyr-759 in interleukin 6 family cytokine receptor subunit gp130 causes autoimmune arthritis. J Exp Med. 2002;196(7):979–90.

45. Niki Y, Yamada H, Seki S, Kikuchi T, Takaishi H, Toyama Y, Fujikawa K, Tada N. Macrophage- and neutrophil-dominant arthritis in human IL-1 alpha transgenic mice. J Clin Invest. 2001;107(9):1127–35.

46. Sakaguchi S, Sakaguchi N. Animal models of arthritis caused by systemic alteration of the immune system. Curr Opin Immunol. 2005;17(6):589–94.

47. Rantapaa-Dahlqvist S, de Jong BA, Berglin E, Hallmans G, Wadell G, Stenlund H, Sundin U, van Venrooij WJ. Antibodies against cyclic citrullinated peptide and IgA rheumatoid factor predict the development of rheumatoid arthritis. Arthritis Rheum. 2003;48(10):2741–9.

48. Kokkonen H, Soderstrom I, Rocklov J, Hallmans G, Lejon K, Rantapaa Dahlqvist S. Up-regulation of cytokines and chemokines predates the onset of rheumatoid arthritis. Arthritis Rheum. 2010;62(2):383–91.

14

Immune complexes containing scleroderma-specific autoantibodies induce a profibrotic and proinflammatory phenotype in skin fibroblasts

Elena Raschi[1†], Cecilia Beatrice Chighizola[1,2,3*†] ⓘ, Laura Cesana[1], Daniela Privitera[1,2], Francesca Ingegnoli[2,4], Claudio Mastaglio[5], Pier Luigi Meroni[1,2,4] and Maria Orietta Borghi[1,2]

Abstract

Background: In systemic sclerosis (SSc), autoantibodies provide the most accurate tool to predict the disease subset and pattern of organ involvement. Scleroderma autoantibodies target nucleic acids or DNA/RNA-binding proteins, thus SSc immune complexes (ICs) can embed nucleic acids. Our working hypothesis envisaged that ICs containing scleroderma-specific autoantibodies might elicit proinflammatory and profibrotic effects in skin fibroblasts.

Methods: Fibroblasts were isolated from skin biopsies obtained from healthy subjects and patients with diffuse cutaneous SSc (dcSSc). ICs were purified by polyethylene-glycol precipitation from sera of SSc patients bearing different autoantibodies. ICs from patients with systemic lupus erythematosus (SLE) and primary anti-phospholipid syndrome (PAPS) and from normal healthy subjects (NHS) were used as controls. After incubation with ICs, fibroblasts were evaluated for ICAM-1 expression, interleukin (IL)-6, IL-8, monocyte chemoattractant protein (MCP)-1, matrix metalloproteinase (MMP)-2, tumor growth factor (TGF)-β1 and Pro-Collagenlα1 secretion, *collagen (col)lα1, mmp-1, toll-like receptor (tlr)2, tlr3, tlr4, tlr7, tlr8, tlr9, interferon (ifn)-α, ifn-β* and *endothelin-1* mRNA, and NFκB, p38MAPK and SAPK-JNK activation rate. Experiments were also performed after pretreatment with DNase I/RNase and NFκB/p38MAPK inhibitors.

Results: The antigenic reactivity for each SSc-IC mirrored the corresponding serum autoantibody specificity, while no positivity was observed in NHS-ICs or sera. SSc-ICs but not NHS-ICs increased ICAM-1 expression, stimulated IL-6, IL-8, MMP-2, MCP-1, TGF-β1 and Pro-Collagenlα1 secretion, upregulated *et-1, ifn-α, ifn-β, tlr2, tlr3* and *tlr4*, and activated NFκB, p38MAPK and SAPK-JNK. *tlr9* was significantly upregulated by ARA-ICs, *mmp-1* was significantly induced by ACA-ICs whereas *collα1* was not modulated by any SSc-ICs. SLE-ICs and PAPS-ICs significantly upregulated MMP-2 and activated NFκB, p38MAPK and SAPK-JNK. SLE-ICs and PAPS-ICs did not affect *collα1, mmp-1* and Pro-Collagenlα1. DNase I and RNase treatment significantly reduced the upregulation of study mediators induced by SSc-ICs. Pretreatment with NFκB/p38MAPK inhibitors suggested that response to anti-Th/To-ICs was preferentially mediated by p38MAPK whereas ATA-ICs, ACA-ICs and ARA-ICs engaged both mediators. In dcSSc fibroblasts, stimulation with SSc-ICs and NHS-ICs upregulated IL-6 and IL-8.

(Continued on next page)

---

* Correspondence: cecilia.chighizola@unimi.it
†Elena Raschi and Cecilia Beatrice Chighizola contributed equally to this work.
[1]Experimental Laboratory of Immunological and Rheumatologic Researches, IRCCS Istituto Auxologico Italiano, Via Zucchi 18, 20095 Cusano Milanino, Milan, Italy
[2]Department of Clinical Sciences and Community Health, University of Milan, Via Festa del Perdono 7, 20122 Milan, Italy
Full list of author information is available at the end of the article

(Continued from previous page)

Conclusions: These data provide the first demonstration of the proinflammatory and profibrotic effects of SSc-ICs on fibroblasts, suggesting the potential pathogenicity of SSc autoantibodies. These effects might be mediated by Toll-like receptors via the interaction with nucleic acid fragments embedded in SSc-ICs.

Keywords: Systemic sclerosis, Autoantibodies, Immune complexes, Toll-like receptors, Fibroblasts, Fibrosis, Inflammation

Background

Systemic sclerosis (SSc) is a chronic systemic auto-immune disease characterized by three cardinal processes: fibrotic derangement of the skin and visceral organs, endothelial damage and immune activation [1]. A hallmark feature of SSc is the production of autoantibodies: anti-nuclear antibodies (ANA) are detectable in more than 95% of patients at diagnosis [2]. SSc-specific autoantibodies typically precede disease onset, implicating they are not a mere reflection of the disease process [3]. Importantly, they provide the most accurate tool to predict disease subsets and the pattern of organ complications [4, 5]. Noteworthy, IgG transfer from SSc patients in skin-humanized SCID mice induced significant dermal fibrosis [6]. Despite these in-vivo data, the precise diagnostic accuracy and the strong prognostic role played by scleroderma-specific autoantibodies, scarce in-vitro evidence has been raised in support of their pathogenic potential. To date, available studies have mainly focused on anti-DNA topoisomerase I antibodies (ATA), that were demonstrated to bind to fibroblasts via surface-bound topoisomerase I inducing adhesion and activation of co-cultured monocytes [7, 8]. Antibodies against centromeric proteins (ACA) were reported to prevent the transactivation of the epidermal growth factor receptor and the subsequent secretion of interleukin (IL)-8 [9].

Immune complexes (ICs) are formed upon interaction between autoantibodies and soluble target antigens. ICs contribute to the pathogenesis of several autoimmune diseases, such as systemic lupus erythematosus (SLE), Sjögren's syndrome and rheumatoid arthritis [10–13]. Since the role of ICs in SSc has never been investigated, the aim of this study was to assess the proinflammatory and profibrotic effects of scleroderma ICs, using skin fibroblasts from healthy subjects as an in-vitro model. Since scleroderma autoantibodies engage nucleic acids or DNA/RNA-binding proteins as antigenic targets, SSc-ICs can embed nucleic acids [14]. The effects of SSc-ICs on target cells might thus be mediated by Toll-like receptors (TLRs) interacting with nucleic acid fragments. TLRs are expressed by many nonimmune cells, including fibroblasts, and are crucial in sensing pathogen-associated and damage-associated molecular patterns. In humans, 10 TLRs have been described:

TLR2 and TLR4 are involved in the recognition of microbial molecules; TLR3 recognizes double-stranded RNA; TLR7 and TLR8 bind single-stranded RNA; and TLR9 engages single-stranded DNA [15].

As a whole, the data presented in this study provide the first demonstration of the proinflammatory and profibrotic effects of SSc-ICs on healthy skin fibroblasts. The evidence raised in this work suggests that such effects might be ascribed to nucleic acid components of SSc-ICs via the interaction with TLRs on target cells. As a whole, these data shed new light on the pathogenic role of scleroderma-associated autoantibodies, potentially broadening our understanding of SSc etiopathogenesis.

Methods

Serum samples

Serum samples were obtained from 16 patients with SSc fulfilling the 2013 ACR/EULAR criteria [16]. All patients had ANA upon indirect immunofluorescence on HEp-2 cells, at a titer greater than 1:160, with staining patterns consistent with the antigenic specificity. Five patients carried ATA, five ACA, three anti-RNA polymerase III antibodies (ARA) and three anti-Th/To antibodies (anti-Th/To). The remaining autoantibody profile was negative. In all cases, antibody reactivities against scleroderma antigens were confirmed using two different techniques: line blot (EUROLINE-SSc profile kit; Euroimmun, Lubeck, Germany) and chemiluminescent immunoassays (QUANTA Flash; INOVA Diagnostics, San Diego, CA, USA). Seven patients were diagnosed with diffuse cutaneous SSc (dcSSc), and the remaining subjects had limited cutaneous involvement [17]. All patients were female, the median age was 48 years and the median disease duration from the first non-Raynaud's phenomenon symptom to blood withdrawal was 31 months. Two SLE patients were recruited: one patient carried anti-Sm, anti-U1 ribonucleoprotein (RNP) and anti-double stranded DNA antibodies; the other harbored anti-Sm [18]. Serum was also obtained from two subjects with primary anti-phospholipid syndrome (PAPS) and positive lupus anticoagulant test, anti-cardiolipin and anti-β2 glycoprotein I IgG antibodies [19]. Eight normal healthy subjects (NHS) with no autoimmune disease and negative autoantibody profile were enrolled. Serum samples were stored at − 20 °C.

Healthy skin fibroblast cell culture

Dermal fibroblasts were isolated from skin biopsies from eight NHS. Under local anesthesia with 1% xylocaine, 5-mm punch skin biopsies were performed in the distal forearm. Samples were minced into small pieces, and digested by collagenase type I (ThermoFisher Scientific Inc., Waltham, MA, USA) for 2 h at 37 °C with 5% CO_2. After centrifugation at $300 \times g$ for 10 min, pellets were resuspended in 1 ml D-MEM (Gibco-Life Technologies, Groningen, the Netherlands) supplemented with 20% fetal bovine serum (FBS; PAA-GE Healthcare, Buckinghamshire, UK), 2 mM glutamine (Sigma-Aldrich, Saint Louis, MO, USA), penicillin (100 U/ml)–streptomycin (100 μg/ml) (Sigma-Aldrich) and transferred into a T25 plate (Corning Incorporated, NY, USA). Cultures were maintained at 37 °C in 5% CO_2-humidified incubator until confluence. Nonadherent cells and dermal tissue were removed by washing, and established fibroblasts were passaged after trypsin/EDTA (ThermoFisher Scientific) release up to the eight passage. Cells were maintained in D-MEM with 10% FBS, 2 mM glutamine, penicillin (100 U/ml)–streptomycin (100 μg/ml) (ThermoFisher Scientific) or incubated overnight in D-MEM with 1% FBS before functional studies.

The purity of fibroblast culture was 98% as detected by flow cytometry using a mouse anti-human CD90 and a mouse anti-human CD45 antibodies–PE conjugated (BD Biosciences, San Jose, CA, USA).

Immune complexes

ICs were precipitated from sera of NHS and patients. Briefly, serum samples were mixed with ice-cold 5% polyethylene-glycol (PEG) 6000 (Sigma-Aldrich)–0.1 M EDTA (Bioscience, Inc., La Jolla, CA, USA) and incubated overnight at 4 °C. Samples were diluted three times with 2.5% PEG 6000 in RPMI (Euroclone S.p.A., Pero, Italy), layered on top of 2.5% PEG 6000 supplemented with 5% human serum albumin (Sigma-Aldrich) and centrifuged at $2100 \times g$ at 4 °C for 20 min. Pellets were dissolved in D-PBS to the initial serum volume and immediately used at 1:2 dilution [20].

The IC amount in PEG precipitates was quantified using Quanta Lite C1q CIC ELISA (INOVA Diagnostics), a sensitive and specific assay exploiting soluble IC binding to C1q [21, 22]. The presence of specific autoantibodies in PEG-precipitated ICs was tested using the commercial EUROLINE-SSc profile kit. The nucleic acid concentration (ng/μl) in IC preparations was evaluated by NanoPhotometer Pearl at 260 nm (Implen GmbH, München, Germany).

Every sample was used in triplicate, and each experiment was repeated twice using SSc-ICs isolated from all patients for each autoantibody specificity and control ICs.

The potential endotoxin contamination of IC preparations was ruled out by limulus amoebocyte lysate (LAL) gel-clot test (Pyrosate Kit, sensitivity 0.25 EU/ml; Associates of Cape Cod Incorporated, East Falmouth, MA, USA).

ICAM-1 expression

ICAM-1 surface levels were evaluated by home-made cell ELISA, as in previous studies on HUVECs [23]. Confluent fibroblast monolayers were rested in D-MEM with 1% FBS overnight in a 96-well plate.

After 24-h incubation with 100 μl/well of SSc-ICs, NHS-ICs, LPS (1 μg/ml; R&D Systems, Minneapolis, MN, USA), poly(I:C) (1 μg/ml; Sigma-Aldrich) or medium alone, cells were washed twice with HBSS (Sigma-Aldrich) and incubated for 60 min at room temperature with 100 μl/well of murine monoclonal IgG specific for human ICAM-1 (CD54; R&D Systems). The antibody was used at a final dilution of 1:500 in HBSS-FBS 2.5%. After two additional washes, cells were incubated for 90 min at room temperature with 100 μl of phosphatase-conjugated goat anti-mouse IgG (Cappel, Cochranville, PA, USA). The secondary antibody was used at a dilution of 1:1000 in HBSS–FBS 10%. After two washes with HBSS, 100 μl of the enzymatic substrate (p-nitrophenyl-phosphate in 0.05 M Mg-carbonate buffer pH 9.8; Sigma-Aldrich) was added. The optical density (OD) values were evaluated at 405 nm after 30 min of incubation by a semiautomatic reader (Titertek Multiskan MCC/340; Titertek Instruments Inc., Pforzheim, Germany).

IL-6, IL-8, matrix metalloproteinase-2, monocyte chemoattractant protein-1 and tumor growth factor protein secretion

IL-6, IL-8, matrix metalloproteinase (MMP)-2, monocyte chemoattractant protein (MCP)-1 and tumor growth factor (TGF)-β1 release was evaluated in culture supernatants after 48 h incubation with SSc-ICs, NHS-ICs or TLR synthetic agonists (LPS and poly(I:C)) by commercial ELISAs (R&D Systems).

Pro-CollagenIα1 secretion

Pro-CollagenIα1 secretion in culture supernatants was evaluated after 24 h incubation with SSc-ICs, NHS-ICs or recombinant human TGF-β1 (10 ng/ml; PreproTech, Rocky Hill, JN, USA) by the human Pro-CollagenIα1 DuoSet ELISA Kit (R&D Systems).

tlr2, tlr3, tlr4, tlr7, tlr8, tlr9, interferon-α, interferon-β, endothelin-1, collagenIα1 and mmp-1 mRNA expression levels

Total RNA from fibroblasts was purified using Trizol Reagent (ThermoFisher Scientific). Amplification Grade DNase I (ThermoFisher Scientific) was used to eliminate residual genomic DNA. A reverse transcription reaction was performed using the SuperScript™ First-Strand Synthesis

System for RT-PCR (ThermoFisher Scientific). Universal PCR Master Mix No AmpErase UNG (ThermoFisher Scientific) was used for quantitative RT-PCR by the ABIPR-ISM 7900 HT Sequence Detection System (ThermoFisher Scientific). Quantification of mRNA expression was performed with a TaqMan® Gene Expression Assay (Thermo-Fisher Scientific) for each target gene (Table 1). RT-PCR was performed after 24 h incubation with ICs. Expression levels of the target genes (*tlr2, tlr3, tlr4, tlr7, tlr8, tlr9, interferon (ifn)-α, ifn-β, endothelin (et)-1, collagenIα1 (coIα1)* and *mmp-1*) were determined by the comparative Ct method normalizing the target to the endogenous gene (*gapdh*). Relative values of the target to the reference were expressed as the fold change (RQ). The optimal time point to evaluate the mRNA levels of coIIα1 was set at 24 h based on a kinetics curve of the mRNA response to stimulation with TGF-β.

Nuclear factor kappa B, p38 mitogen activated kinase and SAPK-JNK activation rate

Fibroblast monolayers were incubated with SSc-ICs, NHS-ICs, poly(I:C) and LPS. Total proteins were isolated using RIPA Lysis Buffer added to Protease and Phosphatase inhibitor cocktail (Sigma-Aldrich). Protein concentration was evaluated using the BCA Protein Assay Kit (ThermoFisher Scientific). Proteins were fractionated by NuPAGE BIS–TRIS by 4–12% SDS-polyacrylamide precast gel electrophoresis and transferred to nitrocellulose using iBlot Transfer Stacks Nitrocellulose (ThermoFisher Scientific). Membranes were blocked for 2 h at room temperature in PBS/0.05% Tween 20 (PT) (Bio-Rad Laboratories, Hercules, CA, USA) containing 5% nonfat milk powder (Mellin, Milan, Italy), and incubated with anti-human nuclear factor kappa B (NFκB), anti-human phosphorylated NFκB (pNFκB), anti-human p38 mitogen activated kinase (p38MAPK), anti-human phosphorylated p38MAPK (pp38MAPK), anti-human SAPK-JNK or anti-human phosphorylated SAPK-JNK (anti-pSAPK-JNK) antibodies (Cell Signaling Technology, Danvers, MA,

USA). After washing, membranes were incubated in PT/5% nonfat milk powder plus HRP-conjugated secondary antibodies (MP Biomedicals, Santa Ana, CA, USA) and developed using the ECL Plus Detection System (ThermoFisher Scientific). Signals were detected using radiographic films (Kodak, Rochester, NY, USA). ImageJ software (LI-COR Biosciences, Lincoln, NE, USA) was used to analyze and quantify gels.

SLE and APS immune complexes

The protein secretion of MMP-2 and Pro-CollagenIα1, the mRNA levels of *coIα1* and *mmp-1*, and the activation rate of NFκB, p38MAPK, p54SAPK-JNK and p46SAPK-JNK were also evaluated in response to stimulation with ICs from SLE and PAPS sera.

DNase and RNase treatment

SSc-ICs were incubated for 1 h at 37 °C with recombinant DNase I or RNase (20 KU/ml and 8 μg/ml, respectively; Worthington Biochemical Corporation, Lakewood, NJ, USA) and then added to cells for 24 h. RT-PCR for *tlr2, tlr3, ifn-α* and *et-1* was then performed.

NFκB and p38MAPK inhibitors

Cells were preincubated for 1 h at 37 °C with inhibitors of NFκB (MG-132, 20 μmol; Sigma-Aldrich) and p38MAPK (SB202190, 20 μmol; Cell Signaling Technology). The expression levels of IL-6 and the activation rates of NFκB and p38MAPK were assessed by western blot analysis. IL-8, TGF-β1 and Pro-CollagenIα1 were measured by commercial ELISA kits in culture supernatants.

Scleroderma skin fibroblast cell culture

Dermal fibroblasts were isolated from two patients with dcSSc and cultured following the same procedures described for healthy fibroblasts. IL-6 and IL-8 secretion levels were assessed in culture supernatants after 48 h incubation with SSc-ICs, NHS-ICs or TLR synthetic agonists (LPS and poly(I:C)) by commercial ELISAs (R&D Systems).

Statistical analysis

Descriptive statistics were used to calculate the mean and standard deviation (SD). Since our data were derived from in-vitro experiments conducted under high controlled conditions and originated from a high number of cells, ANOVA was used to compare different experimental conditions, and post-hoc comparisons were assessed by Dunnett's test. With regards to nonhomogeneity of variance assumption, Welch's correction was applied when required. Paired or unpaired *t* tests were performed to compare mean values between two groups. All analyses were performed with GraphPad Prism 5.01. $p < 0.05$ was considered significant.

Table 1 TaqMan® Gene Expression Assays

Gene	TaqMan® Gene Expression ID
tlr2	Hs01872448_s1
tlr3	Hs01551078_m1
tlr4	Hs00152939_m1
tlr7	Hs01933259_s1
tlr8	Hs00152972_m1
tlr9	Hs00370913_s1
ifn-α	Hs00855471_g1
ifn-β	Hs01077958_s1
et-1	Hs00174961_m1
colla1	Hs00164004_m1
mmp-1	Hs00899658_m1
gapdh	Hs99999905_m1

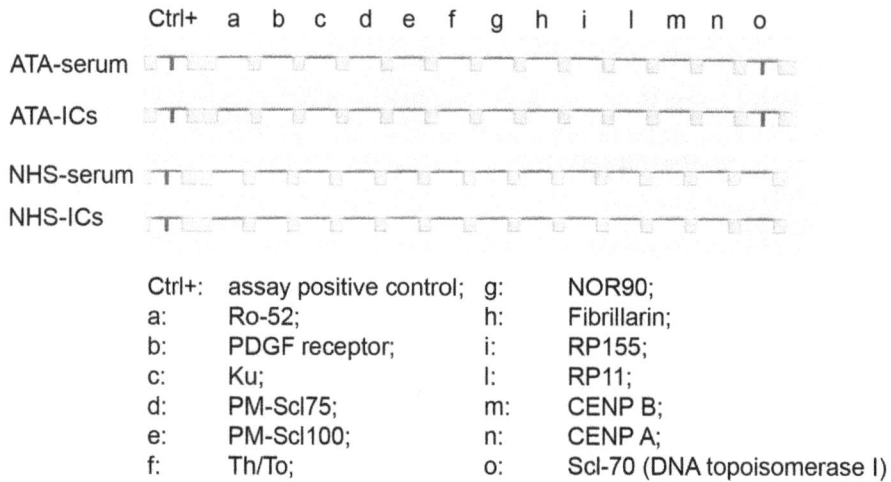

| | Ctrl+ | a | b | c | d | e | f | g | h | i | l | m | n | o |

ATA-serum
ATA-ICs
NHS-serum
NHS-ICs

Ctrl+:	assay positive control;	g:	NOR90;
a:	Ro-52;	h:	Fibrillarin;
b:	PDGF receptor;	i:	RP155;
c:	Ku;	l:	RP11;
d:	PM-Scl75;	m:	CENP B;
e:	PM-Scl100;	n:	CENP A;
f:	Th/To;	o:	Scl-70 (DNA topoisomerase I)

Fig. 1 TaqMan® Gene Expression assays against SSc-specific antigens of PEG-precipitated ICs and corresponding sera evaluated by EUROLINE-SSc profile kit. One ATA-IC and one NHS-IC presented as representative assay. CTR+, assay-positive control. a, Ro-52; b, PDGF receptor; c, Ku; d, PM-Scl75; e, PM-Scl100; f, Th/To; g, NOR90; h, Fibrillarin; i, RP155; I, RP11; m, CENP B; n, CENP A; o, Scl-70 (DNA topoisomerase I). ATA anti-DNA topoisomerase I antibodies, IC immune complex, NHS normal healthy subjects

The approval of the Institutional Review Board of Istituto G. Pini, Milan, Italy was obtained; all subjects provided written informed consent.

Results

Immune complex characterization

Quanta Lite C1q CIC ELISA confirmed that all PEG-precipitated preparations contained ICs. SSc preparations exhibited significantly higher IC amounts compared to NHS (50.77 ± 9.8 versus 5.95 ± 2.02, $p < 0.01$, $t = 4.477$; cutoff 10.8 Eq/ml).

Using the EUROLINE-SSc profile kit on PEG-precipitated preparations, reactivity against SSc-specific antigens for each SSc-IC mirrored the corresponding serum autoantibody specificity. No reactivity was observed in NHS-ICs (Fig. 1).

To identify the optimal IC dilution in functional studies, a dose–response curve (1:2–1:64) was performed by cell ELISA for ICAM-1 expression on the fibroblast surface. A 1:2 dilution was selected as this allowed the highest response without affecting cell viability (Fig. 2).

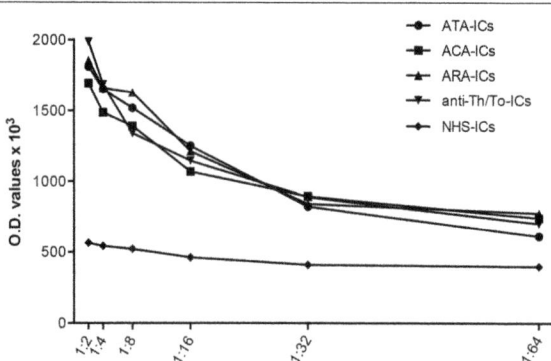

Fig. 2 Dose–response dilution curve for ICAM-1 expression on fibroblast cell surface. Fibroblasts exposed to serial two-fold dilutions (from 1:2 to 1:64) of SSc-ICs and NHS-ICs, and ICAM-1 evaluated by cell ELISA. anti-Th/To anti-Th/To antibodies, ATA anti-DNA topoisomerase I antibodies, IC immune complex, NHS normal healthy subjects, OD optical density

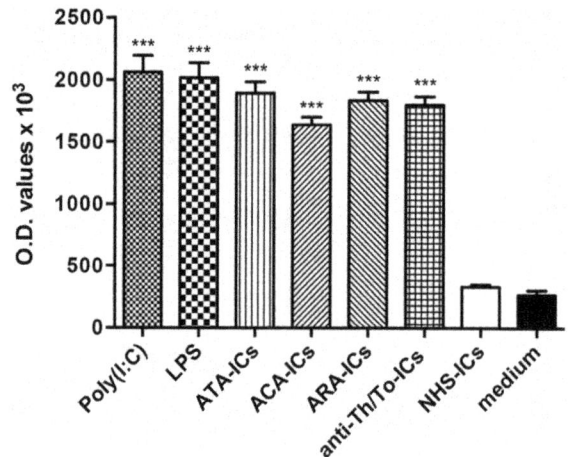

Fig. 3 ICAM-1 expression on fibroblasts stimulated with SSc-ICs or NHS-ICs. Fibroblasts exposed to SSc-ICs or NHS-ICs (1:2 dilution). Poly(I:C) and LPS, at concentration of 1 µg/ml, used as positive controls. ***$p < 0.0001$ versus medium. ACA anti-centromeric protein antibodies, anti-Th/To anti-Th/To antibodies, ARA anti-RNA polymerase III antibodies, ATA anti-DNA topoisomerase I antibodies, IC immune complex, LPS lipopolysaccharide, NHS normal healthy subjects, OD optical density, poly(I:C) polyinosinic-polycytidylic acid

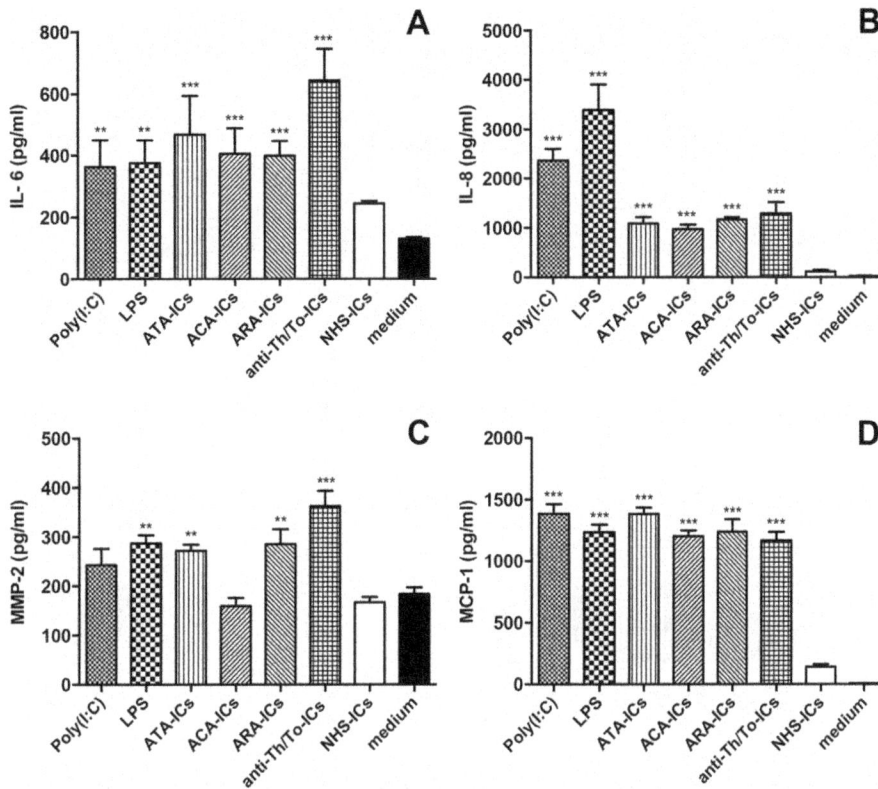

Fig. 4 IL-6, IL-8, MMP-2 and MCP-1 levels in culture supernatants from fibroblasts incubated with SSc-ICs or NHS-ICs. Fibroblasts exposed to SSc-ICs or NHS-ICs (1:2 dilution). Poly(I:C) and LPS, at concentration of 1 µg/ml, used as positive controls. **a** IL-6; **b** IL-8; **c** MMP-2; **d** MCP-1. **$*p < 0.001$, $***p < 0.0001$ versus medium. ACA anti-centromeric protein antibodies, anti-Th/To anti-Th/To antibodies, ARA anti-RNA polymerase III antibodies, ATA anti-DNA topoisomerase I antibodies, IC immune complex, IL interleukin, LPS lipopolysaccharide, MCP monocyte chemoattractant protein, MMP matrix metalloproteinase, NHS normal healthy subjects, poly(I:C) polyinosinic-polycytidylic acid

ICAM-1 expression

SSc-ICs significantly induced ICAM-1 expression on fibroblast monolayers compared to medium. No increase in ICAM-1 expression was observed with NHS-ICs. Poly(I:C) and LPS elicited a significant increase in ICAM-1 protein levels compared to medium (Fig. 3).

IL-6, IL-8, MMP-2 and MCP-1 secretion

All SSc-ICs, LPS and poly(I:C) upregulated IL-6 levels compared to medium. Conversely, NHS-ICs did not have any effect (Fig. 4a). All SSc-ICs, poly(I:C) and LPS elicited a significant rise in IL-8 levels compared to medium (Fig. 4b). Fibroblasts incubated with NHS-ICs exhibited IL-8 levels similar to cells treated with medium alone. ATA-ICs, ARA-ICs, anti-Th/To-ICs and LPS significantly upregulated MMP-2 levels compared to medium. ACA-ICs, poly(I:C) and NHS-ICs did not induce a significant increase in MMP-2 protein levels (Fig. 4c).

All SSc-ICs, poly(I:C) and LPS significantly upregulated MCP-1. NHS-ICs did not elicit a significant increase in MCP-1 protein levels (Fig. 4d).

et-1 and ifn mRNA expression

LPS, ATA-ICs, ACA-ICs and anti-Th/To-ICs, but not ARA-ICs, significantly upregulated et-1 levels compared to the medium, while NHS-ICs and poly(I:C) did not exert any effect (Fig. 5a).

ATA-ICs, ACA-ICs and anti-Th/To-ICs significantly upregulated mRNA levels of ifn-α. Poly(I:C), LPS, ARA-ICs and NHS-ICs did not significantly modulate ifn-α mRNA (Fig. 5b). Poly(I:C), ATA-ICs, ACA-ICs and anti-Th/To-ICs drove a significant increase of mRNA levels of ifn-β. Stimulation with LPS, ARA-ICs and NHS-ICs did not significantly affect mRNA of ifn-β compared to culture medium (Fig. 5c).

TGF-β1 and Pro-CollagenIα1 secretion, and colla1 and mmp-1 mRNA expression

All SSc-ICs significantly increased TGF-β1 levels compared to medium alone, while NHS-ICs did not exert any effect (Fig. 6a). All SSc-ICs and TGF-β1 significantly upregulated Pro-CollagenIα1 secretion in supernatants compared to medium alone. NHS-ICs did not affect protein levels (Fig. 6b). SSc-ICs and NHS-ICs did not

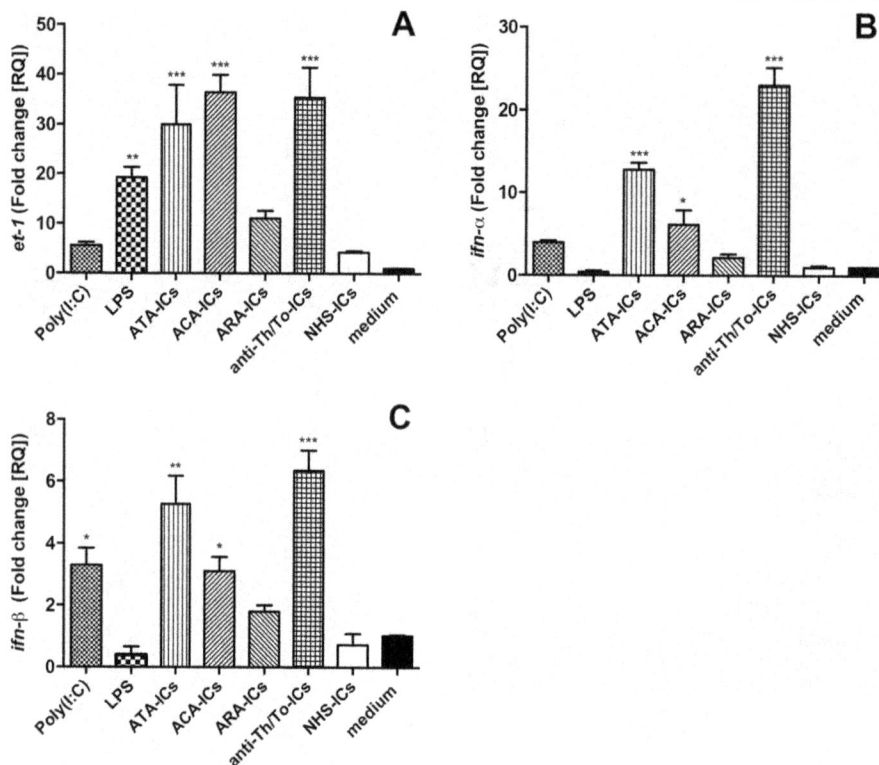

Fig. 5 *et-1*, *ifn-α* and *ifn-β* mRNA expression levels in fibroblasts stimulated with SSc-ICs or NHS-ICs. Fibroblasts exposed to SSc-ICs or NHS-ICs (1:2 dilution). Poly(I:C) and LPS, at concentration of 1 µg/ml, used as controls. **a** *et-1*; **b** *ifn-α*; **c** *ifn-β*. *$p < 0.01$, **$p < 0.001$, ***$p < 0.0001$ versus medium. ACA anti-centromeric protein antibodies, anti-Th/To anti-Th/To antibodies, ARA anti-RNA polymerase III antibodies, ATA anti-DNA topoisomerase I antibodies, et-1 endothelin-1, IFN interferon, IC immune complex, LPS lipopolysaccharide, NHS normal healthy subjects, poly(I:C) polyinosinic-polycytidylic acid

modulate *collα1* mRNA expression. Conversely, TGF-β1 significantly increased *collα1* mRNA levels (Fig. 6c). ACA-ICs drove a significant upregulation of *mmp-1* while all the other SSc-ICs as well as NHS-ICs and TGF-β1 did not significantly affect *mmp-1* mRNA levels (Fig. 6d).

tlr mRNA expression

All SSc-ICs, but not NHS-ICs, and both TLR agonists drove a significant increase in *tlr2* mRNA as compared to medium (Fig. 7a). Similarly, all SSc-ICs, but not NHS-ICs, induced a significant *tlr3* upregulation; an increase in *tlr3* mRNA was observed with poly(I:C) and LPS (Fig. 7b). LPS, ACA-ICs and ARA-ICs induced a significant upregulation in *tlr4* mRNA levels. Conversely, ATA-ICs, anti-Th/To-ICs, NHS-ICs and poly(I:C) did not affect *tlr4* mRNA levels (Fig. 7c). *tlr9* expression was significantly modulated by ARA-ICs and poly(I:C). Differently, ATA-ICs, ACA-ICs, anti-Th/To-ICs, NHS-ICs and LPS did not affect *tlr9* mRNA levels (Fig. 7d).

tlr7 and *tlr8* mRNA could not be detected in fibroblasts.

Intracellular signaling pathways

ATA-ICs, ARA-ICs, anti-Th/To-ICs and LPS significantly activated NFκB compared to the medium. Conversely, ACA-ICs and NHS-ICs did not elicit NFκB phosphorylation (Fig. 8a). All SSc-ICs, but not NHS-ICs, and LPS activated p38MAPK and p54SAPK-JNK (Fig. 8b, c). ATA-ICs, ARA-ICs, anti-Th/To-ICs and LPS induced a significant increased phosphorylation rate of p46SAPK-JNK. ACA-ICs and NHS-ICs did not exert any effect on the phosphorylation rate of p46SAPK-JNK (Fig. 8d).

Immune complexes from SLE and PAPS

SLE-ICs and PAPS-ICs phosphorylated NFκB (Fig. 9a), p38MAPK (Fig. 9b), p54SAPK-JNK (Fig. 9c) and p46SAPK-JNK (Fig. 9d). SLE-ICs and PAPS-ICs did not induce a significant upregulation of the mRNA levels of *collα1* (Fig. 10a) and *mmp-1* (Fig. 10b) or of the secretion of Pro-CollagenIα1 (Fig. 10c). SLE-ICs and PAPS-ICs, as well as LPS, significantly upregulated

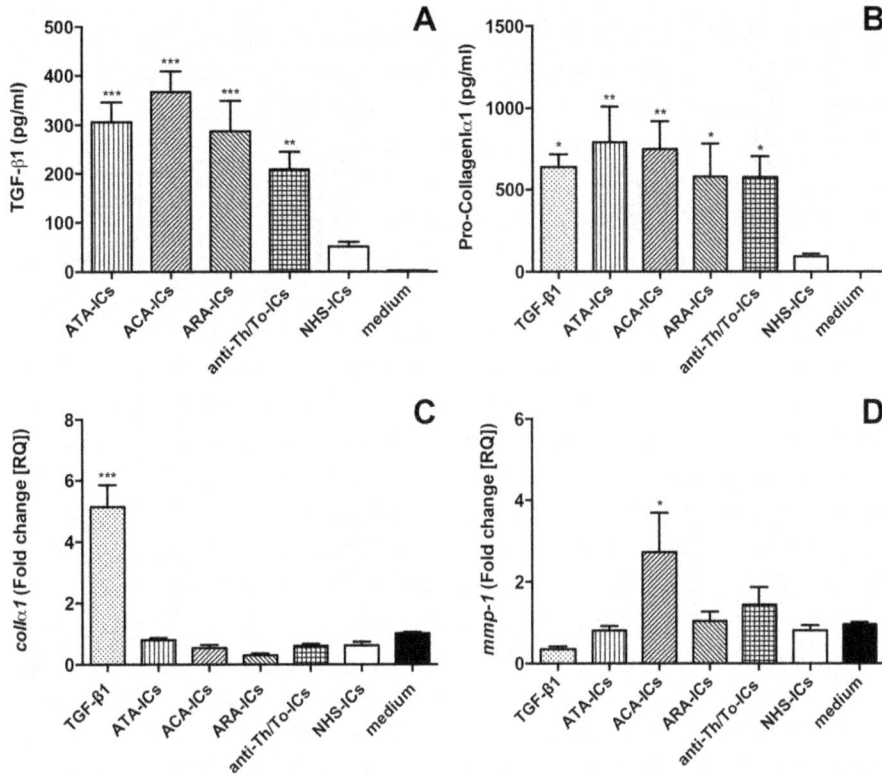

Fig. 6 TGF-β1 and Pro-Collagenlα1 secretion and *collα1* and *mmp-1* mRNA expression in fibroblasts stimulated with SSc-ICs or NHS-ICs. Fibroblasts exposed to SSc-ICs or NHS-ICs (1:2 dilution). TGF-β1 (10 ng/ml) used as positive control for collagen synthesis and secretion. **a** TGF-β1; **b** Pro-Collagenlα1; **c** *collα1*; **d** *mmp-1*. *p < 0.01, **p < 0.001, ***p < 0.0001 versus medium. ACA anti-centromeric protein antibodies, anti-Th/To anti-Th/To antibodies, ARA anti-RNA polymerase III antibodies, ATA anti-DNA topoisomerase I antibodies, collα1 collagenlα1, IC immune complex, MMP matrix metalloproteinase, NHS normal healthy subjects, TGF tumor growth factor

MMP-2 secretion compared to medium. NHS-ICs did not significantly affect MMP-2 levels (Fig. 10d).

Nucleic acid content

SSc-ICs contained a higher amount of nucleic acids compared to NHS-ICs (ssDNA 55.75 ± 16.41 ng/μl versus 43.11 ± 12.36 ng/μl ($p = 0.0470$, $t = 2.075$); dsDNA 81.06 ± 29.84 ng/μl versus 49.13 ± 13.51 ng/μl ($p = 0.0087$, $t = 2.867$); RNA 62.70 ± 22.67 ng/μl versus 37.14 ± 10.42 ng/μl ($p = 0.0086$, $t = 2.852$)).

DNase I and RNase pretreatment modulated the expression of study mediators induced by SSc-ICs. Both DNase I and RNase treatments prevented mRNA upregulation of *et-1* by ATA-ICs and ACA-ICs (Fig. 11a), *tlr2* by ACA-ICs and anti-Th/To-ICs (Fig. 11b), *ifn-α* by ATA-ICs and anti-Th/To-ICs (Fig. 11c), and *tlr3* by ATA-ICs, ACA-ICs, ARA-ICs and anti-Th/To-ICs (Fig. 11d). *et-1* upregulation by anti-Th/To-ICs was modulated by RNase only (Fig. 11a); *tlr2* mRNA expression enhancement observed with ATA-ICs and ARA-ICs was reduced by DNase I only (Fig. 11b). DNase I and

RNase treatments did not significantly affect study mediators when cells were incubated with NHS-ICs.

NFκB and p38MAPK inhibitors

The efficacy of NFκB and p38MAPK inhibitors was confirmed by western blot analysis (Fig. 12a, b). When cells were treated with NFκB inhibitor, the expression levels of IL-6 in response to stimulation with LPS as well as all SSc-ICs and NHS-ICs were not affected.

The inhibition of NFκB resulted in the significant modulation of TGF-β1 in response to LPS, ATA-ICs, ACA-ICs and ARA-ICs but not anti-Th/To-ICs and NHS-ICs (Fig. 13a). Pretreatment with NFκB inhibitor significantly downregulated the expression levels of Pro-Collagenlα1 induced by TGF-β1 and ARA-ICs but not ATA-ICs, ACA-ICs, anti-Th/To-ICs and NHS-ICs (Fig. 13b). Pretreatment with NFκB inhibitor led to the significant downregulation of the secretion levels of IL-8 induced by LPS, ATA-ICs and ACA-ICs but not ARA-ICs, anti-Th/To-ICs and NHS-ICs (Fig. 13c).

The inhibition of p38MAPK led to the significant modulation of TGF-β1 in response to LPS, ATA-ICs and anti-Th/

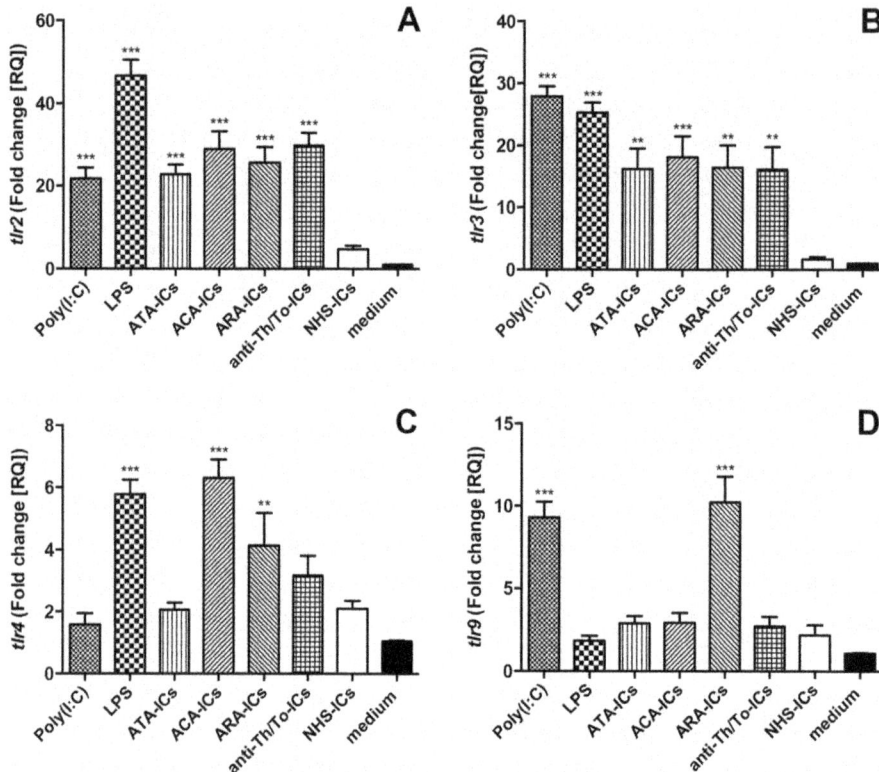

Fig. 7 *tlr* mRNA expression levels in fibroblasts stimulated with SSc-ICs or control NHS-ICs. Fibroblasts exposed to SSc-ICs or NHS-ICs (1:2 dilution). Poly(I:C) and LPS, at concentration of 1 μg/ml, used as controls. **a** *tlr2*; **b** *tlr3*; **c** *tlr4*; **d** *tlr9*. ****p* < 0.001, *****p* < 0.0001 versus medium. ACA anti-centromeric protein antibodies, anti-Th/To anti-Th/To antibodies, ARA anti-RNA polymerase III antibodies, ATA anti-DNA topoisomerase I antibodies, IC immune complex, LPS lipopolysaccharide, NHS normal healthy subjects, poly(I:C) polyinosinic-polycytidylic acid, TLR Toll-like receptor

To-ICs but not ACA-ICs, ARA-ICs and NHS-ICs (Fig. 14a). Pretreatment with p38MAPK inhibitor significantly down-regulated the expression levels of Pro-CollagenIα1 induced by TGF-β1 and anti-Th/To-ICs, but not ATA-ICs, ACA-ICs, ARA-ICs and NHS-ICs (Fig. 14b). Pretreatment with p38MAPK inhibitor resulted in the significant downregulation of IL-8 induced by LPS and ACA-ICs but not ATA-ICs, ARA-ICs, anti-Th/To-ICs and NHS-ICs (Fig. 14c). When cells were pretreated with p38MAPK inhibitor, the expression of IL-6 induced by LPS, ATA-ICs, ACA-ICs, ARA-ICs and anti-Th/To-ICs, but not NHS-ICs, was significantly affected (Fig. 14d).

IL-6 and IL-8 secretion in scleroderma fibroblasts

In fibroblasts from subjects with dcSSc, all ICs—those from SSc patients as well as NHS—upregulated both IL-6 and IL-8 as compared to medium. Even poly(I:C) and LPS elicited a significant raise in IL-6 and IL-8 levels compared to medium (Fig. 15a, b, respectively).

Discussion

To our knowledge, this is the first study investigating in vitro the pathogenic potential of ICs containing SSc-specific antibodies. The first relevant observation that emerged in this work consists of the confirmation of IC content in all PEG-precipitated preparations, with significantly higher IC amounts in the samples from SSc patients compared to NHS. Consistently, early works evaluating circulating ICs in serum samples from SSc patients evinced a positivity rate similar to SLE [24–27]. To note, the antigenic reactivity of each PEG-precipitated preparation mirrored the autoantibody specificity of the original serum, thus confirming that ICs contain scleroderma-specific autoantibodies. Most importantly, functional experiments showed that SSc-ICs can affect the functionality of skin fibroblasts, the main effectors of tissue fibrosis. In particular, the incubation with SSc-ICs modulated several molecules involved in the three cardinal scleroderma pathophysiologic processes: vascular dysfunction (ET-1 and IL-8), inflammation (ICAM-1, IL-6, IFNs and MCP-1) and fibrosis (TGF-β1 and Pro-CollagenIα1). Noteworthy, SSc-ICs affected the protein but not the mRNA levels of collagen, possibly due to the posttranscriptional regulatory mechanism of collagen metabolism [28]; this hypothesis should be confirmed in future experiments.

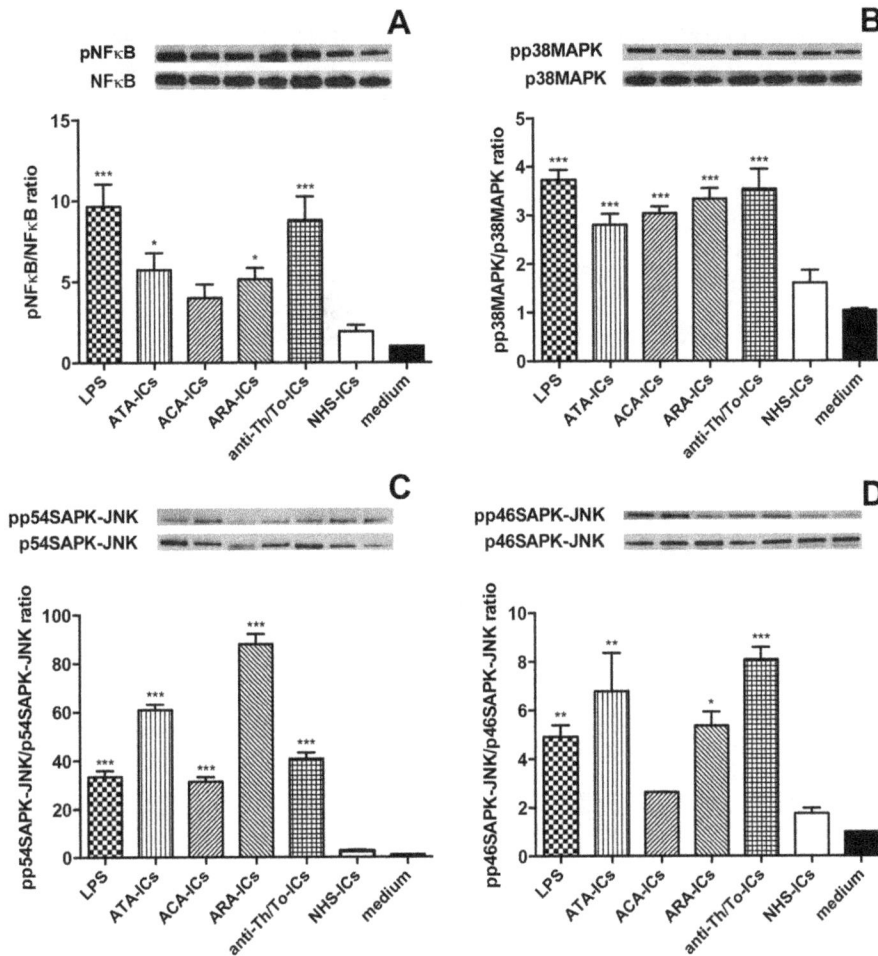

Fig. 8 Intracellular signaling pathways in fibroblasts stimulated with SSc-ICs or NHS-ICs. Fibroblasts exposed to SSc-ICs or NHS-ICs (1:2 dilution). LPS (1 μg/ml) used as control. **a** pNFκB/NFκB; **b** pp38MAPK/p38MAPK; **c** pp54SAPK-JNK/p54SAPK-JNK; **d** pp46SAPK-JNK/p46SAPK-JNK. Results expressed as ratio of phosphorylated to nonphosphorylated forms, evaluated using ImageJ software. Western blot images representative of single experiment. *$p < 0.01$, **$p < 0.001$, ***$p < 0.0001$ versus medium. ACA anti-centromeric protein antibodies, anti-Th/To anti-Th/To antibodies, ARA anti-RNA polymerase III antibodies, ATA anti-DNA topoisomerase I antibodies, IC immune complex, LPS lipopolysaccharide, MAPK mitogen activated kinase, NHS normal healthy subjects, NFκB nuclear factor kappa B, pNFκB phosphorylated NFκB, pp38MAPK phosphorylated p38MAPK, pp54SAPK-JNK phosphorylated p54SAPK-JNK, pp46SAPK-JNK phosphorylated p46SAPK-JNK

Another aspect that still needs elucidation is the role of type I IFNs. In our study, all SSc-ICs except ARA-ICs drove an interferogenic response, consistent with previous observations, such as the high IFN levels in scleroderma sera and skin samples and the IFN signature in peripheral blood cells and tissue macrophages from SSc patients [29, 30]. In particular, ATA-ICs significantly increased both IFN-α and IFN-β levels, in agreement with the already reported upregulation of IFNs elicited by ATA-positive sera in peripheral blood mononuclear cells [31, 32]. If the earlier cited authors proposed IFNs as early and prominent profibrotic mediators, it should be remembered that other investigators claimed an antifibrotic effect for IFNs, warranting further investigations [33, 34].

Our experiments suggest that SSc-ICs exert a specific pathogenic role in scleroderma, as compared to disease control ICs. Indeed, ICs from patients with autoimmune conditions other than SSc were tested: PAPS and SLE were identified as prototypical diseases. SLE is a systemic autoimmune disease characterized by a flourishing autoantibody production and a polymorphic clinical presentation [35]. APS is a systemic autoimmune condition characterized by vascular thrombosis and/or obstetric complications, in the persistent presence of circulating anti-phospholipid antibodies [36]. In both diseases, autoantibodies have been shown to exert a pathogenic role as well as a diagnostic one [37, 38]. Interestingly, in our study, SLE-ICs and PAPS-ICs did not modulate molecules

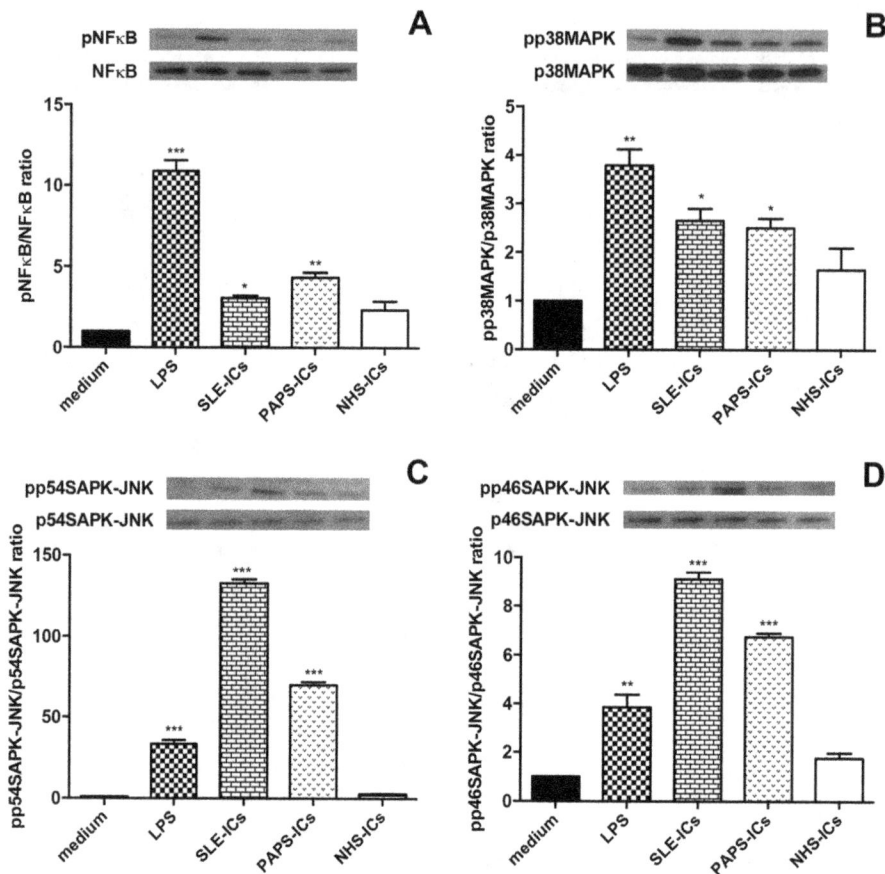

Fig. 9 Intracellular signaling pathways in fibroblasts stimulated with SLE-ICs, PAPS-ICs or NHS-ICs. Fibroblasts exposed to SLE-ICs, PAPS-ICs or NHS-ICs (1:2 dilution). LPS (1 μg/ml) used as control. **a** pNFκB/NFκB; **b** pp38MAPK/p38MAPK; **c** pp54SAPK-JNK/p54SAPK-JNK; **d** pp46SAPK-JNK/p46SAPK-JNK. Results expressed as ratio of phosphorylated to nonphosphorylated forms, evaluated using ImageJ software. Western blot images representative of single experiment. *$p < 0.01$, **$p < 0.001$, ***$p < 0.0001$ versus medium. IC immune complex, LPS lipopolysaccharide, MAPK mitogen activated kinase, NHS normal healthy subjects, NFκB nuclear factor kappa B, pNFκB phosphorylated NFκB, pp38MAPK phosphorylated p38MAPK, pp54SAPK-JNK phosphorylated p54SAPK-JNK, pp46SAPK-JNK phosphorylated p46SAPK-JNK, PAPS primary anti-phospholipid syndrome, SLE systemic lupus erythematosus

directly involved in fibrogenesis such as *mmp-1*, *collα1* and Pro-CollagenIα1. Both PAPS-ICs and SLE-ICs elicited a significant activation of intracellular mediators which are known to be involved in PAPS and SLE pathogenesis, such as NFκB, p38MAPK and SAPK-JNK [37, 38].

According to our data, the pathogenic effects of SSc-ICs on fibroblasts might be mediated by innate immunity sensors as TLRs. This hypothesis would allow overcoming one of the strongest objections against the pathogenicity of SSc autoantibodies, the intracellular localization of target antigens. Indeed, while dendritic and B cells could engage SSc autoantibodies via Fcγ receptor (FcγR), this is not the case of skin fibroblasts, which lack FcγR [39]. To note, genetic, in-vitro, in-vivo and ex-vivo findings are increasingly acknowledging TLRs as master players in SSc pathogenesis [40]. Consistently, SSc-ICs upregulated TLR expression, although

to a lower extent for *tlr9*. The recruitment of intracellular mediators downstream of TLRs was observed for SSc-ICs but not NHS-ICs, further suggesting the potential involvement of TLRs in driving the SSc-IC signal. We further investigated the contribution of intracellular mediators by pretreating fibroblast cells with NFκB and p38MAPK inhibitors. Data suggested that SSc-ICs might engage intracellular signaling pathways differently: response to anti-Th/To-ICs was preferentially mediated by p38MAPK. Conversely, stimulation with ATA-ICs, ACA-ICs and ARA-ICs appears to engage both intracellular mediators.

It could thus be proposed that TLRs on target cells might interact with SSc-ICs via the nucleic acid fragments. TLR2, which does not recognize nucleic acids, might recognize HMGB-1, which is incorporated in ICs and acts as an agonist for both TLR2 and TLR4 [41, 42].

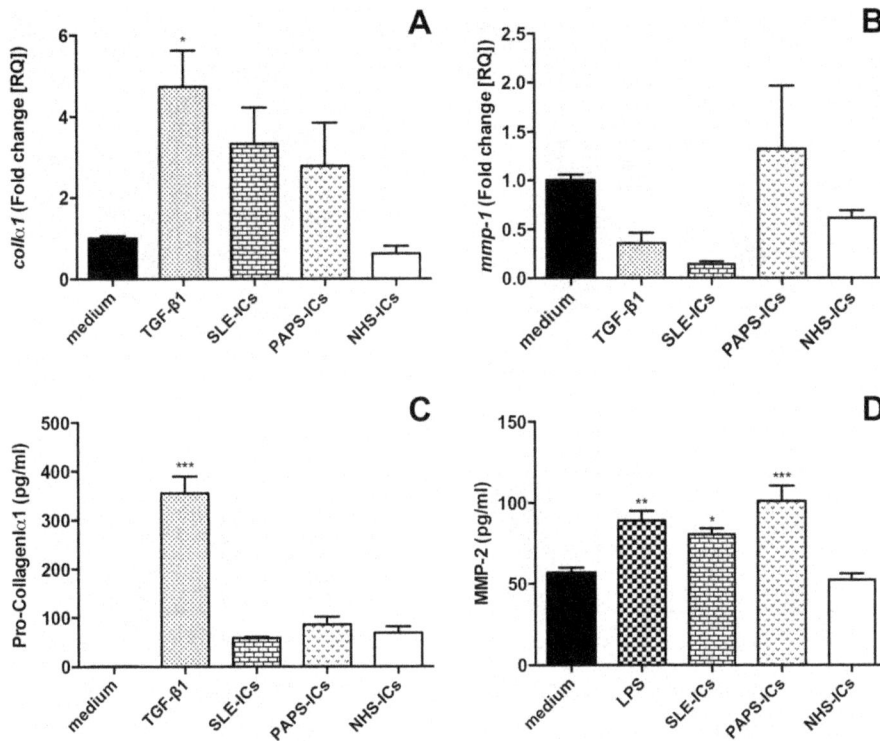

Fig. 10 *colla1* and *mmp-1* mRNA expression and Pro-Collagenlα1 and MMP-2 secretion in fibroblasts stimulated with SLE-ICs, PAPS-ICs or NHS-ICs. Fibroblasts exposed to PAPS-ICs, SLE-ICs or NHS-ICs (1:2 dilution). TGF-β1 (10 ng/ml) and LPS (1 µg/ml) used as positive control for collagen synthesis and secretion. **a** *colla1*; **b** *mmp-1*; **c** Pro-Collagenlα1; **d** MMP-2. *$p < 0.01$, **$p < 0.001$, ***$p < 0.0001$ versus medium. colla1 collagenlα1, IC immune complex, LPS lipopolysaccharide, MMP matrix metalloproteinase, NHS normal healthy subjects, PAPS primary anti-phospholipid syndrome, SLE systemic lupus erythematosus, TGF tumor growth factor

Our working hypothesis is suggested by the significant enrichment in nucleic acids of SSc-ICs compared to NHS-ICs. As further support, DNase I and RNase pretreatment prevented the upregulation of mediators induced by SSc-ICs, consistent with previous observations [31]. These data fit well with the recent evidence of elevated serum nucleosomes (histone proteins wrapped with DNA fragments) among SSc patients [43]. Nucleic acids embedded in ICs might be of endogenous nature: DNA and RNA residues are released from damaged and necrotic self-cells. Noteworthy, SSc patients exhibit increased DNA damage in peripheral blood cells [44]; the gene coding for *DNASE1L3*, an enzyme involved in DNA fragmentation during apoptosis, is one of the strongest susceptibility loci for SSc [45]. Nucleic acids from pathogens might also be included in ICs; interestingly, Epstein–Barr virus (EBV) was shown to infect most fibroblasts and endothelial cells in the skin of SSc patients [46].

Noteworthy, when fibroblasts from patients with dcSSc were used as an in-vitro model, we observed a significant difference in the modulation of IL-6 and IL-8 secretion levels in response to stimulation with all SSc-ICs as well as NHS-ICs. These findings are in agreement with the well-known hyperresponsiveness of scleroderma fibroblasts even to aspecific stimuli, prompting us to focus our research on healthy skin fibroblasts in order to reproduce the initiator phase of the disease.

As a whole, our findings allowed us to formulate a comprehensive hypothesis which postulates scleroderma-specific autoantibodies embedded in SSc-ICs as novel players in disease pathogenesis. The proposed pathogenic relevance of SSc-ICs fits well with the evidence that autoantibody positivity is the strongest predictor of progression into full-blown SSc [5]. Further support for the pathogenicity of autoantibodies comes from the striking temporal clustering and casual link between solid tumors and ARA-positive SSc [47, 48]. Indeed, the POLR3A locus, coding for the antigenic target of ARA, was altered in cancer tissue specimens from SSc patients carrying ARA, leading to the synthesis of an immunogenic enzyme resulting in T-cell-driven ARA production and SSc onset [49].

We reckon that several functional autoantibodies have already been described in SSc: anti-fibroblast antibodies (AFA), anti-endothelial cell antibodies, antibodies against platelet-derived growth factor receptor, etc. However, differently from SSc-specific antibodies,

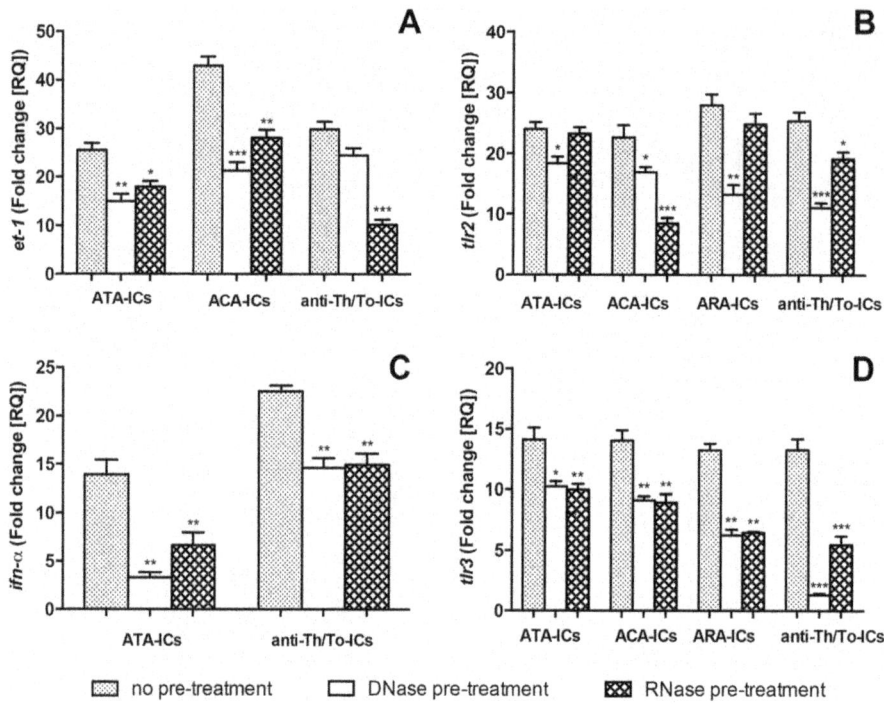

Fig. 11 *et-1*, *tlr2* and *tlr3* expression levels in fibroblasts stimulated with SSc-ICs or NHS-ICs pretreated with DNase/RNase. SSc-ICs treated with DNase I (20 KU/ml) or RNase (8 μg/ml) and then added to fibroblast cultures. **a** ATA-ICs, ACA-ICs and anti-Th/To-ICs on *et-1*; **b** ATA-ICs, ACA-ICs, ARA-ICs and anti-Th/To-ICs on *tlr2*; **c** ATA-ICs and anti-Th/To-ICs on *ifn-α*; **d** ATA-ICs, ACA-ICs, ARA-ICs and anti-Th/To-ICs on *tlr3*. *$p < 0.01$, **$p < 0.001$, ***$p < 0.0001$ versus medium. ACA anti-centromeric protein antibodies, anti-Th/To anti-Th/To antibodies, ARA anti-RNA polymerase III antibodies, ATA anti-DNA topoisomerase I antibodies, et-1 endothelin-1, IC immune complex, IFN interferon, TLR Toll-like receptor

most of these functional autoantibodies can be detected in a minority of patients' sera and present a poor specificity for scleroderma, being positive in many other autoimmune diseases and even in NHS [50]. In particular, AFA have been reported to upregulate ICAM-1,

IL-6, IL-1α, IL-1β, CCL2, CXCL8 and MMP-1, with partial exploitation of TLR4, whereas collagen and tissue inhibitor of MMP-1 were not affected [51, 52]. Interestingly, it has been suggested that anti-fibroblast activity might be mediated by ATA: AFA purified from

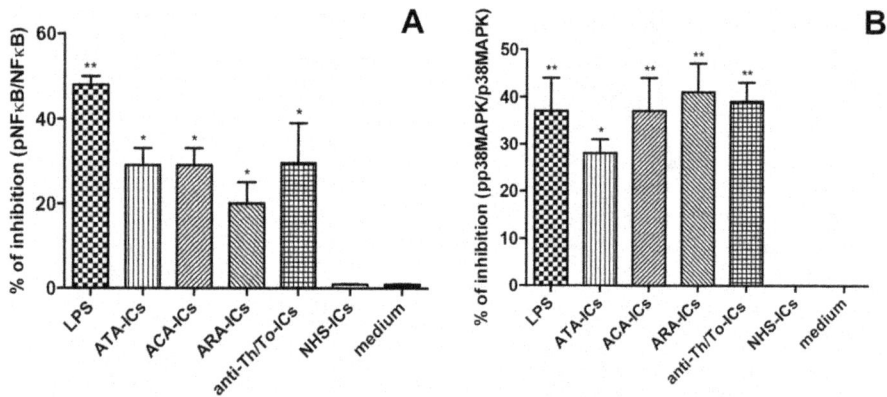

Fig. 12 Confirmation of efficacy of NFκB and p38MAPK inhibitors by western blot analysis. Cells preincubated for 1 h at 37 °C with inhibitors of NFκB and p38MAPK. Fibroblasts exposed to SSc-ICs or NHS-ICs (1:2 dilution). LPS (1 μg/ml) used as control. Results expressed as percentage of inhibition of activated (**a**) NFκB and (**b**) p38MAPK (expressed as ratio of phosphorylated to nonphosphorylated forms). *$p < 0.01$, **$p < 0.001$ versus medium. ACA anti-centromeric protein antibodies, anti-Th/To anti-Th/To antibodies, ARA anti-RNA polymerase III antibodies, ATA anti-DNA topoisomerase I antibodies, IC immune complex, LPS lipopolysaccharide, NFκB nuclear factor kappa B, NHS normal healthy subjects, MAPK mitogen activated kinase, pp38MAPK phosphorylated p38MAPK

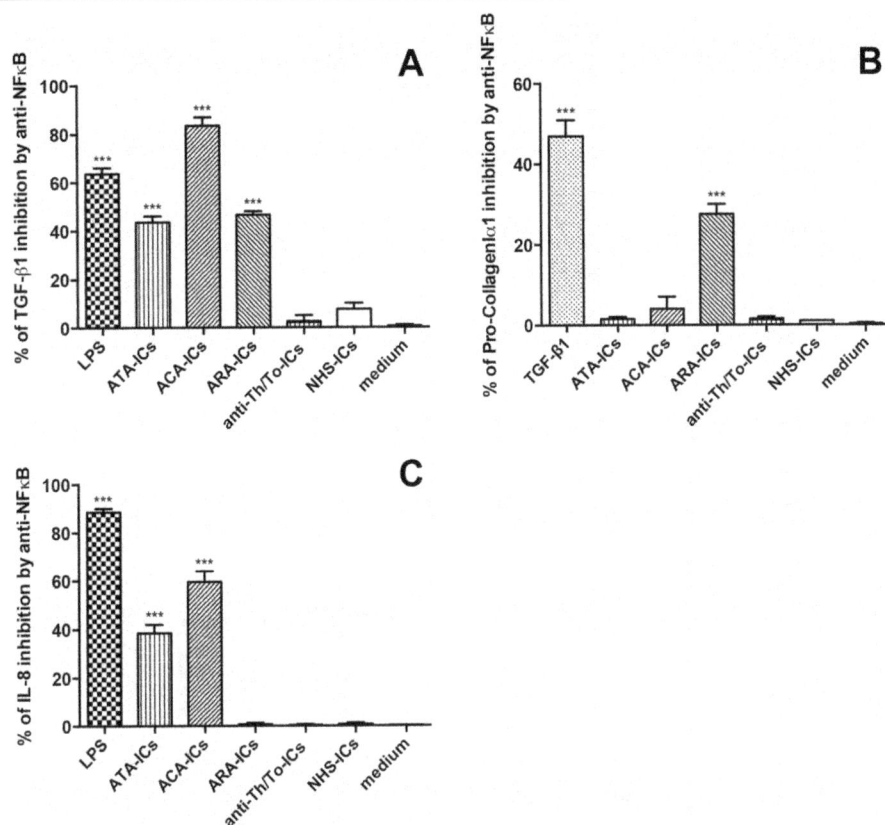

Fig. 13 TGF-β1, Pro-collagenIα1 and IL-8 in fibroblasts pretreated with NFκB inhibitor and incubated with SSc-ICs or NHS-ICs. Fibroblasts pretreated with MG-132 (20 μmol), an NFκB inhibitor, and then exposed to SSc-ICs or NHS-ICs (1:2 dilution). LPS (1 μg/ml) and TGF-β1 (10 ng/ml) used as positive controls. Results expressed as percentage of inhibition of **a** TGF-β1, **b** Pro-CollagenIα1 and **c** IL-8 in untreated versus MG-132-treated cells. ***$p < 0.0001$ versus medium. ACA anti-centromeric protein antibodies, anti-Th/To anti-Th/To antibodies, ARA anti-RNA polymerase III antibodies, ATA anti-DNA topoisomerase I antibodies, IC immune complex, IL interleukin, LPS lipopolysaccharide, NFκB nuclear factor kappa B, NHS normal healthy subjects, TGF tumor growth factor

SSc patients strongly reacted with topoisomerase I and AFA positivity at high titers correlated with pulmonary involvement and death [7].

We acknowledge that our work presents intrinsic limitations. Being an in-vitro study, it might be oversimplistic, not allowing adequate reproduction of the complexity of scleroderma pathogenesis. It would be intriguing to test the effects of scleroderma ICs on endothelial cells, macrophages and lymphocytes, some of the mosaic of cells contributing to the many processes that underpin fibrogenesis. In this regard, we have preliminarily observed that endothelial cells stimulated with SSc-ICs secrete a significantly higher amount of TGF-β1, which might in turn act on fibroblasts, hence promoting the acquisition of a profibrotic phenotype (unpublished data). Indeed, further in-vitro experiments using cell cocultures (e.g., endothelial cells and fibroblasts, fibroblasts and macrophages, etc.) should be performed in order to reproduce the multifaceted cellular orchestra implicated in scleroderma etiopathogenesis. We reckon that a major limitation of this study is the scarce number of

samples for each autoantibody specificity [53]. However, the limited patient cohort does not impinge the robustness of the conclusions of this study, whose aim was to provide the first proof-of-concept of IC involvement in the pathophysiology of SSc. In addition, some of the autoantibodies under investigation, such as ARA and anti-Th/To, are quite uncommon in the Italian SSc population [53], thus preventing the collection of a broader number of samples. Nevertheless, we believe this study offers important insights into scleroderma pathophysiology: the effects of SSc-ICs should be appropriately confirmed using samples from a wider cohort of SSc patients and the intracellular mediators engaged by SSc-ICs should be further characterized.

It would be tempting to postulate that the different modulation of some study mediators that emerged upon stimulation with the different scleroderma ICs might account for the characteristic clinical phenotype associated with each autoantibody profile; however, the differential response to SSc-ICs reacting with various antigens might be ascribed to the IC contents of the preparations.

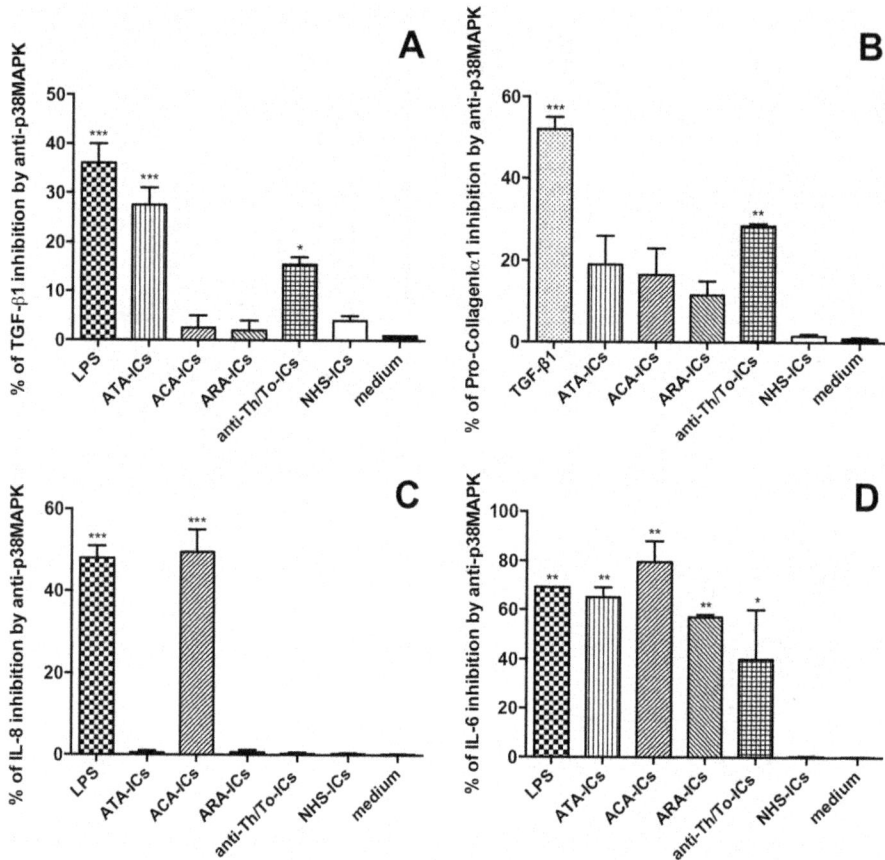

Fig. 14 TGF-β1, Pro-collagenIα1, IL-8 and IL-6 in fibroblasts pretreated with p38MAPK inhibitor and incubated with SSc-ICs or NHS-ICs. Fibroblasts pretreated with SB202190 (20 µmol), a p38MAPK inhibitor, and then exposed to SSc-ICs or NHS-ICs (1:2 dilution). LPS (1 µg/ml) and TGF-β1 (10 ng/ml) used as positive controls. Results expressed as percentage of inhibition of **a** TGF-β1, **b** Pro-CollagenIα1, **c** IL-8 and **d** IL-6 in untreated versus SB202190-treated cells. *$p < 0.01$, **$p < 0.001$, ***$p < 0.0001$ versus medium. ACA anti-centromeric protein antibodies, anti-Th/To anti-Th/To antibodies, ARA anti-RNA polymerase III antibodies, ATA anti-DNA topoisomerase I antibodies, IC immune complex, IL interleukin, LPS lipopolysaccharide, NHS normal healthy subjects, MAPK p38 mitogen activated kinase, TGF tumor growth factor

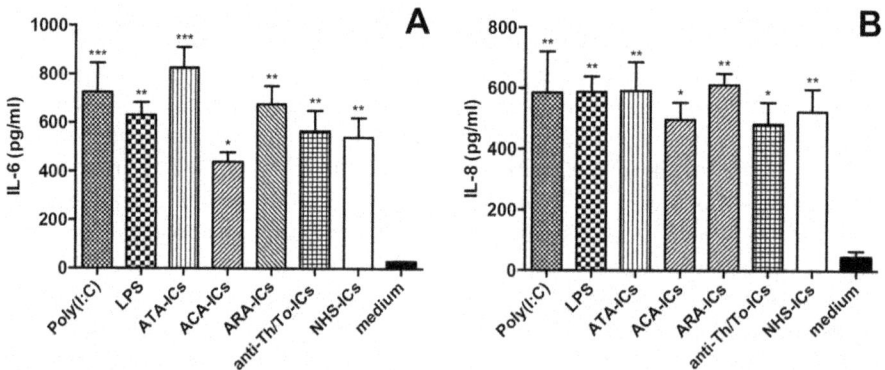

Fig. 15 IL-6 and IL-8 in culture supernatants from dcSSc fibroblasts incubated with SSc-ICs or NHS-ICs. dcSSc fibroblasts exposed to SSc-ICs or NHS-ICs (1:2 dilution). Poly(I:C) and LPS, at concentration of 1 µg/ml, used as positive controls. **a** IL-6; **b** IL-8. *$p < 0.01$, **$p < 0.001$, ***$p < 0.0001$ versus medium. ACA anti-centromeric protein antibodies, anti-Th/To anti-Th/To antibodies, ARA anti-RNA polymerase III antibodies, ATA anti-DNA topoisomerase I antibodies, IC immune complex, IL interleukin, LPS lipopolysaccharide, NHS normal healthy subjects, poly(I:C) polyinosinic-polycytidylic acid

Unfortunately, normalization of the IC content of our preparations could not be performed as PEG precipitates should be used fresh.

As a whole, the data presented in this work might impact our current understanding of SSc pathogenesis: SSc-ICs could provide an additional player in the complex interplay between autoimmunity, vascular damage and excessive fibroblast activation culminating in tissue fibrosis in the initiator phase of the disease. The relevance of SSc-ICs might account for the strong diagnostic and prognostic role scleroderma autoantibodies exert. Autoantibody production might be favored by environmental factors together with a predisposing genetic milieu, documented by the strong association with HLA assets and polymorphisms in TLRs and downstream mediators. Hopefully, further characterizing the pathogenic role of scleroderma autoantibodies could allow developing novel therapeutic strategies for a still barely treatable disease.

Conclusion

This study shows that sera from scleroderma patients contain ICs and proposes for the first time the potential pathogenicity of SSc-ICs. Indeed, using skin fibroblasts from NHS as an in-vitro model, we observed that SSc-ICs can trigger proinflammatory and profibrotic mediators. These effects might be mediated by TLRs via interaction with nucleic acid fragments embedded in SSc-ICs. Our data suggest that SSc-ICs might be a novel player in the pathogenesis of scleroderma, fitting well with the diagnostic and prognostic role of SSc-specific autoantibodies.

Abbreviations

ACA: Anti-centromeric protein antibodies; AFA: Anti-fibroblast antibodies; ANA: Anti-nuclear antibodies; anti-Th/To: Anti-Th/To antibodies; ARA: Anti-RNA polymerase III antibodies; ATA: Anti-DNA topoisomerase I antibodies; colIα1: CollagenIα1; DMEM: Dulbecco's modified Eagle's medium; EBV: Epstein–Barr virus; et-1: Endothelin-1; FBS: Fetal bovine serum; FcγR: Fcγ receptor; HBSS: Hank's balanced salt solution; IC: Immune complex; IFN: Interferon; IL: Interleukin; LAL: Lymulus amoebocyte lysate; LPS: Lipopolysaccharide ; MCP: Monocyte chemoattractant protein; MMP: Matrix metalloproteinase; NFκB: Nuclear factor kappa B; NHS: Normal healthy subjects; OD: Optical density; PT: PBS/0.05% Tween 20; p38MAPK: p38 mitogen activated kinase; PAPS: Primary anti-phospholipid syndrome; PEG: Polyethylene-glycol; pNFκB: Phosphorylated nuclear factor kappa B; Poly(I:C): Polyinosinic-polycytidylic acid; pp38MAPK: Phosphorylated p38MAPK ; RNP: Ribonucleoprotein ; RQ: Fold change ; RT-PCR: Real-time PCR ; SD: Standard deviation; SLE: Systemic lupus erythematosus; SSc: Systemic sclerosis; TGF: Tumor growth factor; TLR: Toll-like receptor

Acknowledgements

The authors are grateful to Dr Carlo Chizzolini, Dr Marvin J. Fritzler and Dr Minoru Satoh for critical revision of the manuscript. The authors acknowledge Dr Paola Lonati for support in the preparation of figures and Dr Roberta De Matteis for the useful contribution to the in-vitro experiments.

Funding

This work was supported by Ricerca Corrente 2013, IRCCS Istituto Auxologico Italiano to PLM and by Progetto Azione A Giovani Ricercatori, Department of Clinical Sciences and Community Health, University of Milan to CBC.

Authors' contributions

ER, CBC, PLM and MOB designed the experiments and wrote the manuscript. FI, CBC, CM and PLM were responsible for patient enrollment and follow-up. ER, LC and DP performed the in-vitro experiments. ER, CBC and DP ran the statistical analysis of the data. All authors reviewed and approved the final version of the manuscript.

Competing interests

The authors declare that they have no competing interests.

Author details

[1]Experimental Laboratory of Immunological and Rheumatologic Researches, IRCCS Istituto Auxologico Italiano, Via Zucchi 18, 20095 Cusano Milanino, Milan, Italy. [2]Department of Clinical Sciences and Community Health, University of Milan, Via Festa del Perdono 7, 20122 Milan, Italy. [3]Allergology, Clinical Immunology and Rheumatology Unit, IRCCS Istituto Auxologico Italiano, Piazzale Brescia 20, 20149 Milan, Italy. [4]Division of Rheumatology, ASST G. Pini, Piazza C Ferrari 1, 20122 Milan, Italy. [5]Rheumatology Unit, Ospedale Moriggia-Pelascini, Via Pelascini 3, 22015 Gravedona, Como, Italy.

References

1. Denton CP, Khanna D. Systemic sclerosis. Lancet. 2017;390:1685–99.
2. Mehra S, Walker J, Patterson K, Fritzler MJ. Autoantibodies in systemic sclerosis. Autoimmun Rev. 2013;12:350–4.
3. Kayser C, Fritzler MJ. Autoantibodies in systemic sclerosis: unanswered questions. Front Immunol. 2015;6:167.
4. Nihtyanova SI, Denton CP. Autoantibodies as predictive tools in systemic sclerosis. Nat Rev Rheumatol. 2010;6:112–6.
5. Valentini G, Marcoccia A, Cuomo G, Vettori S, Iudici M, Bondanini F, et al. Early systemic sclerosis: analysis of the disease course in patients with marker autoantibody and/or capillaroscopic positivity. Arthritis Care Res. 2014;66:1520–7.
6. Luchetti MM, Moroncini G, Jose Escamez M, Svegliati Baroni S, Spadoni T, Grieco A, et al. Induction of scleroderma fibrosis in skin-humanized mice by administration of anti-platelet-derived growth factor receptor agonistic autoantibodies. Arthritis Rheumatol. 2016;68:2263–73.
7. Hénault J, Tremblay ML, Clement I, Raymond Y, Senecal J-L. Direct binding of anti-DNA topoisomerase I autoantibodies to the cell surface of fibroblasts in patients with systemic sclerosis. Arthritis Rheum. 2004;50:3265–74.
8. Hénault J, Robitaille G, Senécal J-L, Raymond Y. DNA topoisomerase I binding to fibroblasts induces monocyte adhesion and activation in the presence of anti–topoisomerase I autoantibodies from systemic sclerosis patients. Arthritis Rheum. 2006;54:963–73.
9. Robitaille G, Christin M-S, Clément I, Senécal J-L, Raymond Y. Nuclear autoantigen CENP-B transactivation of the epidermal growth factor receptor via chemokine receptor 3 in vascular smooth muscle cells. Arthritis Rheum. 2009;60:2805–16.
10. Rönnelid J, Tejde A, Mathsson L, Nilsson-Ekdahl K, Nilsson B. Immune complexes from SLE sera induce IL10 production from normal peripheral blood mononuclear cells by an FcgammaRII dependent mechanism: implications for a possible vicious cycle maintaining B cell hyperactivity in SLE. Ann Rheum Dis. 2003;62:37–42.
11. Mathsson L, Ahlin E, Sjöwall C, Skogh T, Rönnelid J. Cytokine induction by circulating immune complexes and signs of in-vivo complement activation in systemic lupus erythematosus are associated with the occurrence of anti-Sjögren's syndrome A antibodies. Clin Exp Immunol. 2007;147:513–20.
12. Bendaoud B, Pennec YL, Lelong A, Le Noac'h JF, Magadur G, Jouquan J, et al. IgA-containing immune complexes in the circulation of patients with primary Sjögren's syndrome. J Autoimmun. 1991;4:177–84.
13. Manivel VA, Sohrabian A, Wick MC, Mullazehi M, Håkansson LD, Rönnelid J. Anti-type II collagen immune complex-induced granulocyte reactivity is associated with joint erosions in RA patients with anti-collagen antibodies. Arthritis Res Ther. 2015;17:8.

14. Czubaty A, Girstun A, Kowalska-Loth B, Trzcińska AM, Purta E, Winczura A, et al. Proteomic analysis of complexes formed by human topoisomerase I. Biochim Biophys Acta. 2005;1749:133–41.

15. Ewald SE, Barton GM. Nucleic acid sensing toll-like receptors in autoimmunity. Curr Opin Immunol. 2011;23:3–9.

16. van den Hoogen F, Khanna D, Fransen J, Johnson SR, Baron M, Tyndall A, et al. 2013 classification criteria for systemic sclerosis: an American College of Rheumatology/European League Against Rheumatism collaborative initiative. Ann Rheum Dis. 2013;72:1747–55.

17. LeRoy EC, Black C, Fleischmajer R, Jablonska S, Krieg T, Medsger TA Jr, et al. Scleroderma (systemic sclerosis): classification, subsets and pathogenesis. J Rheumatol. 1988;15:202–5.

18. Hochberg MC. Updating the American College of Rheumatology revised criteria for the classification of systemic lupus erythematosus. Arthritis Rheum. 1997;40:1725.

19. Miyakis S, Lockshin MD, Atsumi T, Branch DW, Brey RL, Cervera R, et al. International consensus statement on an update of the classification criteria for definite antiphospholipid syndrome (APS). J Thromb Haemost. 2006;4:295–306.

20. Pontes-de-Carvalho LC, Lannes-Vieira J, Giovanni-de-Simone S, Galvão-Castro B. A protein A-binding, polyethylene glycol precipitation-based immunoradiometric assay. Application to the detection of immune complexes and C3 in human sera and of private antigens in cross-reacting parasite extracts. J Immunol Methods. 1986;89:27–35.

21. Stanilova SA, Slavov ES. Comparative study of circulating immune complexes quantity detection by three assays-CIF-ELISA, C1q-ELISA and anti-C3 ELISA. J Immunol Methods. 2001;253:13–21.

22. Ahlin E, Mathsson L, Eloranta ML, Jonsdottir T, Gunnarsson I, Rönnblom L, et al. Autoantibodies associated with RNA are more enriched than anti-dsDNA antibodies in circulating immune complexes in SLE. Lupus. 2012;21:586–95.

23. Del Papa N, Guidali L, Sala A, Buccellati C, Khamashta MA, Ichikawa K, et al. Endothelial cells as target for antiphospholipid antibodies. Human polyclonal and monoclonal anti-beta 2-glycoprotein I antibodies react in vitro with endothelial cells through adherent beta 2-glycoprotein I and induce endothelial activation. Arthritis Rheum. 1997;40:551–61.

24. Seibold JR, Medsger TA, Winkelstein A, Kelly RH, Rodnan GP. Immune complexes in progressive systemic sclerosis (scleroderma). Arthritis Rheum. 1982;25:1167–73.

25. Hughes P, Cunningham J, Day M, Fitzgerald JC, French MA, Wright JK, et al. Immune complexes in systemic sclerosis; detection by C1q binding, K-cell inhibition and Raji cell radioimmunoassays. J Clin Lab Immunol. 1983;10:133–8.

26. Siminovitich K, Klein M, Pruzanski W, Wilkinson S, Lee P, Yoon SJ, et al. Circulating immune complexes in patients with progressive systemic sclerosis. Arthritis Rheum. 1982;25:1174–9.

27. French MA, Harrison G, Penning CA, Cunningham J, Hughes P, Rowell NR. Serum immune complexes in systemic sclerosis: relationship with precipitating nuclear antibodies. Ann Rheum Dis. 1985;44:89–92.

28. Schwarz RI. Collagen I and the fibroblast: high protein expression requires a new paradigm of post-transcriptional, feedback regulation. Biochem Biophys Rep. 2015;3:38–44.

29. Johnson ME, Mahoney JM, Taroni J, Sargent JL, Marmarelis E, Wu MR, et al. Experimentally-derived fibroblast gene signatures identify molecular pathways associated with distinct subsets of systemic sclerosis patients in three independent cohorts. PLoS One. 2015;10: e0114017.

30. Tan FK, Zhou X, Mayes MD, Gourh P, Guo X, Marcum C, et al. Signatures of differentially regulated interferon gene expression and vasculotrophism in the peripheral blood cells of systemic sclerosis patients. Rheumatology (Oxford). 2006;45:694–702.

31. Kim D, Peck A, Santer D, Patole P, Schwartz SM, Molitor JA, et al. Induction of interferon-alpha by scleroderma sera containing autoantibodies to topoisomerase I: association of higher interferon-alpha activity with lung fibrosis. Arthritis Rheum. 2008;58:2163–73.

32. Eloranta M-L, Franck-Larsson K, Lövgren T, Kalamajski S, Rönnblom A, Rubin K, et al. Type I interferon system activation and association with disease manifestations in systemic sclerosis. Ann Rheum Dis. 2010;69:1396–402.

33. Agarwal SK, Wu M, Livingston CK, Parks DH, Mayes MD, Arnett FC, et al. Toll-like receptor 3 upregulation by type I interferon in healthy and scleroderma dermal fibroblasts. Arthritis Res Ther. 2011;13:R3.

34. Fang F, Ooka K, Sun X, Shah R, Bhattacharyya S, Wei J, et al. A synthetic TLR3 ligand mitigates profibrotic fibroblast responses by inducing autocrine IFN signaling. J Immunol. 2013;191:2956–66.

35. Oku K, Atsumi T. Systemic lupus erythematosus: nothing stale her infinite variety. Mod Rheumatol. 2018;27:1–20. https://doi.org/10.1080/14397595.2018.1494239.

36. Schreiber K, Sciascia S, de Groot PG, Devreese K, Jacobsen S, Ruiz-Irastorza G, Salmon JE, Shoenfeld Y, Shovman O, Hunt BJ. Antiphospholipid syndrome. Nat Rev Dis Primers. 2018;4:17103.

37. Tsokos GC, Lo MS, Costa Reis P, Sullivan KE. New insights into the immunopathogenesis of systemic lupus erythematosus. Nat Rev Rheumatol. 2016;22(12):716–30.

38. Meroni PL, Borghi MO, Grossi C, Chighizola CB, Durigutto P, Tedesco F. Obstetric and vascular antiphospholipid syndrome: same antibodies but different diseases? Nat Rev Rheumatol. 2018;14(7):433–40. https://doi.org/10.1038/s41584-018-0032-6.

39. Gessner JE, Heiken H, Tamm A, Schmidt RE. The IgG Fc receptor family. Ann Hematol. 1998;76:231–48.

40. Bhattacharyya S, Varga J. Emerging roles of innate immune signaling and toll-like receptors in fibrosis and systemic sclerosis. Curr Rheumatol Rep. 2015;17:474–9.

41. Yu M, Wang H, Ding A, Golenbock DT, Latz E, Czura CJ, et al. HMGB1 signals through toll-like receptor (TLR) 4 and TLR2. Shock. 2006;26:174–9.

42. Sun W, Jiao Y, Cui B, Gao X, Xia Y, Zhao Y. Immune complexes activate human endothelium involving the cell-signaling HMGB1-RAGE axis in the pathogenesis of lupus vasculitis. Lab Investig. 2013;93:626–38.

43. Yoshizaki A, Taniguchi T, Saigusa R, Fukasawa T, Ebata S, Numajiri H, et al. Nucleosome in patients with systemic sclerosis: possible association with immunological abnormalities via abnormal activation of T and B cells. Ann Rheum Dis. 2016;75(10):1858–65. https://doi.org/10.1136/annrheumdis-2015-207405.

44. Palomino GM, Bassi CL, Wastowski IJ, Xavier DJ, Lucisano-Valim YM, Crispim JC, et al. Patients with systemic sclerosis present increased DNA damage differentially associated with DNA repair gene polymorphisms. J Rheumatol. 2014;41:458–65.

45. Mayes MD, Bossini-Castillo L, Gorlova O, Martin JE, Zhou X, Chen WV, et al. Immunochip analysis identifies multiple susceptibility loci for systemic sclerosis. Am J Hum Genet. 2014;94:47–61.

46. Farina A, Cirone M, York M, Lenna S, Padilla C, Mclaughlin S, et al. Epstein-Barr virus infection induces aberrant TLR activation pathway and fibroblast-myofibroblast conversion in scleroderma. J Invest Dermatol. 2014;134:954–64.

47. Shah AA, Rosen A, Hummers L, Wigley F, Casciola-Rosen L. Close temporal relationship between onset of cancer and scleroderma in patients with RNA polymerase I/III antibodies. Arthritis Rheum. 2010;62:2787–95.

48. Moinzadeh P, Fonseca C, Hellmich M, Shah AA, Chighizola C, Denton CP, et al. Association of anti-RNA polymerase III autoantibodies and cancer in scleroderma. Arthritis Res Ther. 2014;16:1–10.

49. Joseph CG, Darrah E, Shah AA, Skora AD, Casciola-Rosen LA, Wigley FM, et al. Association of the autoimmune disease scleroderma with an immunologic response to cancer. Science. 2014;343:152–7.

50. Kill A, Riemekasten G. Functional autoantibodies in systemic sclerosis pathogenesis. Curr Rheumatol Rep. 2015;17:34.

51. Fineschi S, Cozzi F, Burger D, Dayer JM, Meroni PL, Chizzolini C. Anti-fibroblast antibodies detected by cell-based ELISA in systemic sclerosis enhance the collagenolytic activity and matrix metalloproteinase-I production in dermal fibroblasts. Rheumatol. 2007;46:1779–85.

52. Fineschi S, Goffin L, Rezzonico R, Cozzi F, Dayer JM, Meroni PL, et al. Antifibroblast antibodies in systemic sclerosis induce fibroblasts to produce profibrotic chemokines, with partial exploitation of toll-like receptor 4. Arthritis Rheum. 2008;5:3913–23.

53. Ceribelli A, Cavazzana I, Franceschini F, Airò P, Tincani A, Cattaneo R, et al. Anti-Th/To are common antinucleolar autoantibodies in Italian patients with scleroderma. J Rheumatol. 2010;37:2071–5.

15

I do not want to suppress the natural process of inflammation: new insights on factors associated with non-adherence in rheumatoid arthritis

Valentin Ritschl[1,2,7], Angelika Lackner[3], Carina Boström[4,5], Erika Mosor[1], Michaela Lehner[2], Maisa Omara[1], Romualdo Ramos[1], Paul Studenic[2], Josef Sebastian Smolen[2,6] and Tanja Alexandra Stamm[1*] ⓘ

Abstract

Background: It is estimated that 50–70% of patients with rheumatoid arthritis (RA) are non-adherent to their recommended treatment. Non-adherent patients have a higher risk of not reaching an optimal clinical outcome. We explored factors associated with nonadherence from the patient's perspective.

Methods: Four hundred and fifty-nine RA patients (346 (75.4%) females; mean age 63.0 ± 14.8 years) who failed to attend follow-up visits in two rheumatology centres were eligible to participate in a qualitative interview study. We used this strategy to identify patients who were potentially non-adherent to medicines and/or non-pharmacological interventions. By means of meaning condensation analysis, we identified new and some already well known insights to factors associated with non-adherence. We used the capability, opportunity, and motivation model of behaviour (COM-B) model as a frame of reference to classify the factors.

Results: Forty-three of 131 patients (32.8%) who agreed to participate in the qualitative interviews were found to be non-adherent. New insights on factors associated with non-adherence included strong opinions of patients, such as pain being considered as an indicator of hard work and something to be proud of, or inflammation being a natural process that should not be suppressed; feeling not to be in expert's hands when being treated by a physician/ health professional; the experience of excessive self-control over the treatment; and rheumatologists addressing only drugs and omitting non-pharmacological aspects. The COM-B model comprehensively covered the range of our findings.

Conclusions: The new insights on factors associated with non-adherence allow a better understanding of this phenomenon and can substantially enhance patient care by helping to develop targeted interventions.

Keywords: Qualitative research, Deep understanding of patients' perspectives, Rehabilitation

Background

Rheumatoid arthritis (RA) is a chronic inflammatory disease characterized by destructive synovitis [1]. RA has an important impact on daily functioning including work capacity, social participation, and quality of life [2, 3]. The main target of treatment is to control disease activity [4], to reduce symptoms, to decrease the daily impact of the patients' condition, and to increase the feeling of a return to normality [5].

Disease-modifying anti-rheumatic drugs (DMARDs) reduce disease activity and radiological progression and improve long-term functional outcome in patients with RA [6]. However, it is estimated that 50–70% of patients with RA are non-adherent. These patients do not follow the recommended treatment/prescriptions [7–10]. Many of these will not achieve an optimal clinical outcome, since not taking medication as recommended is associated with more frequent disease flares and increased disability [11, 12]. Therefore, improving adherence enhances the efficacy of medical

* Correspondence: tanja.stamm@meduniwien.ac.at
[1]Section for Outcomes Research, Centre for Medical Statistics, Informatics, and Intelligent Systems, Medical University of Vienna, Spitalgasse 23, 1090 Vienna, Austria
Full list of author information is available at the end of the article

treatments and reduces hospitalisation and the subsequent healthcare costs associated with RA [8, 9, 13–16].

Non-adherence is a phenomenon which exists independent of age, gender, socio-economic status, health condition, setting, and/or prognosis [7, 17]. Furthermore, non-adherence can occur in the initial treatment phase (late or non-initiation of the prescribed treatment) and/or in the later treatment phases (sub-optimal implementation of the dosing regimen or early discontinuation of the treatment) [8, 18]. Non-pharmacological methods are associated with even lower adherence rates compared with medication because they often include life-style modifications and thus require changes in behaviour and habits of daily routine which are difficult to achieve [19].

The complexity of non-adherence is addressed by the psychological theory of planned behaviour [20], which posits that attitudes, subjective norms (i.e. expectations of others), and behavioural control are determinants of our intentions and subsequent actions. More specifically, scholars have recently suggested frameworks such as the capability, opportunity, and motivation model of behaviour (COM-B) [21] to describe patient (non-)adherence. The COM-B is a comprehensive model designed to understand human behaviour and includes capability (the physical and psychological capacity to be adherent, such as memory or comprehension of disease and treatment), opportunity (the physical and social factors to make adherent behaviour possible or prompt it such as access to healthcare facilities and regime complexity), and motivation (brain processes that energise and direct behaviour, such as perception of illness and beliefs about treatment) [22]. The model acknowledges that behaviour is part of an interacting, dynamic system involving these three components to determine a person's behaviour and, in this particular case, medical adherence. This is in accordance with the International Classification of Functioning, Disability and Health (ICF) put forth by the World Health Organization (WHO) [23]. While the contextual factors of the ICF are designed to explain functioning in a health-related context, the COM-B focuses on behaviours in any context that influences a person's engagement in activities and participation. The COM-B provides a more in-depth understanding than other widely used models such as the necessity-concerns framework [24, 25] and binary models of intentional and unintentional non-adherence by including not only patient's beliefs, but also physical, cognitive, and environmental determinants of behaviour [26]. A further advantage of the COM-B model when compared with other approaches is its applicability in interventions, such as evidence-based behavioural change techniques [27, 28]. The model has garnered support in recent literature [29, 30].

According to the WHO, the perspective of patients, including motivation, values, beliefs, and needs, are essential factors that influence non-adherence [9, 31]. However, there is still a lack of deep qualitative data regarding the range and variability of motivations of patients not to adhere. Furthermore, some studies did not differentiate between early and late phases of treatment [32], while others did not explore reasons why patients with RA did not show up for regular follow-up visits [30, 33, 34]. In the area of non-pharmacological methods, the knowledge on the perspectives of patients is even more limited; only case reports [35–46] exist, and no studies have systematically investigated the perspective of these patients in greater depth. None of the cited studies cover the multi-faceted nature of non-adherence as described in the model above [9]. The rigorous use of qualitative research methods is an ideal means to investigate the perspective of patients in a scientific, systematic way. Qualitative research methods investigate in depth the perspectives, motivations, values, beliefs, and needs of patients [47]. The findings of qualitative studies can inform subsequent quantitative models at a later stage.

In the present study, we therefore aimed to explore factors associated with non-adherence regarding medication and non-pharmacological methods from the perspective of patients with RA covering the earlier and later phases of treatment. Furthermore, we aimed to systematically report for the first time self-reported reasons for non-adherence to follow-up visits in a large sample.

Methods
Study design
Our study was performed in two parts. First, we identified potentially non-adherent patients and extracted their clinical data retrospectively using a database query at two rheumatology centres in Austria. Second, we invited these patients to participate in a qualitative interview. Based on the qualitative interviews, patients were assigned to having been non-adherent when they reported that they had stopped seeing a rheumatologist and/or were taking less than approximately 80% of the medication (steroids and DMARDs) prescribed [9]. From the perspectives of the non-adherent patients, we identified factors associated with non-adherence. We compared these factors with the literature to triangulate our findings, and we used the COM-B model [21] as a frame of reference to classify the factors we identified. The ethical committees of each institution approved the study (EK 1082/2015 (Vienna) and 27–324 ex 14/15 (Graz)). Reporting of the qualitative results was done according to the COREQ guidelines (Additional file 1: Supplement S1).

Identification of patients and extraction of clinical data

To identify potentially non-adherent patients, retrospective, observational data from patients with RA (EULAR/ACR criteria) [48] were selected from the databases of two rheumatology centres in Austria (Graz and Vienna); inclusion criteria were: 1) non-attenders to follow-up visits at the rheumatology centre over a time period of at least 9 months; 2) had a minimum of four visits; and 3) at least one prescribed DMARD. The identification of non-adherent patients was an essential aspect of our study. We therefore selected potentially non-adherent patients based on the fact that they did not attend regular follow-ups. This was considered a new and different identification strategy in contrast to asking patients consecutively in the outpatient clinic whether they were adherent or not because we expected a large number of socially desirable answers. To further reduce such reporting bias during the qualitative interviews, all interviews were performed by health professionals (VR, male, MMSc, health scientist with a background in occupational health and therapy, as well as assistive technologies; and AL, female, PhD, MSc, nursing scientist) who were not involved in the patient care or otherwise related to the patients. The following data were extracted from the last clinical visit of each patient: swollen joint counts (SJC32) and tender joint counts (TJC32) using 32 joint counts, erythrocyte sedimentation rate (ESR; mm/h), C-reactive protein (CRP; mg/l), anti-citrullinated protein antibodies (ACPA; U/ml), rheumatoid factor (RF; U/ml) [49], score of the Health Assessment Questionnaire (HAQ) [50, 51], patient global assessments (PGA) and evaluator global assessments (EGA), and pain using 10-cm visual analogue scale (VAS). Clinical and Simplified Disease Activity Indices (CDAI and SDAI) [52–54] were also calculated.

After comparing our data with the clinical case records and the death data registry to eliminate potential other reasons for non-adherence, such as significant other disease or death, we contacted all identified, remaining patients via telephone, informed them about the purpose and procedures of the study, documented self-reported reasons for non-adherence to the follow-up visits, and invited them to participate in a qualitative semi-structured interview (conducted from April 2015 to February 2016). If a patient gave oral and written consent to participate in this study an appointment for a one-time, one-on-one interview was made according to the preferences of the patient either in the course of a (second) scheduled telephone call or a face-to-face interview at the clinic. In case patients could not be reached, two researchers (VR and AL) tried to contact these patients three times at different time points in a day. If this procedure was not successful, they were considered not reachable.

Data collection

An interview guide was developed for the semi-structured individual interviews using the capability, opportunity, and motivation of the COM-B model [21] as a frame of reference. The interview guide was reviewed and adapted by the patient research partner (ML). Questions focused on the current status of rheumatology care of each patient, potential reasons for non-attendance to the follow-up visits and non-adherence to prescribed DMARDs and/or non-pharmacological methods. Examples of interview questions were as follows: "Please describe your experience from your last visit at the rheumatology centre?" (COM-B domain: motivation); "Which reasons prevented you from regular follow-up visits at the rheumatology centre?" (COM-B domain: motivation, opportunity); "Which medications were prescribed at your last visit in our centre and which of these do you still take?" (COM-B domain: opportunity); "Have you experienced any side effects due to your medication?" (COM-B domain: motivation, capability/body structures and functions); "What was your experience with non-pharmacological prescriptions/instructions?" (COM-B domain: motivation, capability/body structures and functions); and "Did you implement any of these recommendations in your daily life?" (COM-B domain: motivation, opportunity). The whole interview guideline is depicted in Additional file 1: Supplement S2.

Qualitative data analysis

Qualitative data were analysed using a meaning condensation analysis [47]. First, the audiotaped interviews were transcribed. If participants provided information during the first telephone contact, field notes were taken. The transcripts and potential field notes taken during the interviews were read through to gain an overview of the collected data. Second, the data was divided into meaning units (defined as specific units of text, a few words, or a few sentences with a common meaning). Meaning units represented the range of patient experiences. In a third final step, the concepts contained in the meaning units were identified. An example to illustrate the procedure of the qualitative analysis is shown in Additional file 1: Supplement S3. The concepts depict the factors associated with non-adherence identified in our study.

Subsequently, we assigned so-called "time-tags", when patients explicitly mentioned a specific time in their treatment course of the disease when an event of interest occurred, and "pharmacological versus non-pharmacological tags", when patients specifically related aspects to one type of intervention, e.g. adherence may be different in taking medication compared with performing and motivating oneself to perform exercises. Thereafter, we linked the factors extracted from the qualitative analysis to the domains of the COM-B model [21], namely capability, opportunity, and motivation.

Based on the qualitative interviews, patients were assigned to having been either adherent (having self-reported regular rheumatology visits in another centre or with a rheumatologist and were taking approximately 80% of the medication related to glucocorticoids and DMARDs as prescribed) or non-adherent (having stopped seeing a rheumatologist and/or taking less than approximately 80% of the medications related to steroids and DMARDs as prescribed) [9].

To ensure accuracy and rigour of the qualitative analysis, all interviews were performed according to a pre-determined interview guide; 25% of the results were reviewed by a second researcher (either TAS, EM, or MO) who have extensive experience in the field of qualitative research prior to the present project [47, 55, 56]. In addition, a patient research partner (ML) reviewed the results. In case of disagreement, the results were discussed (by VR, TAS, EM, MO, and ML) until consensus was achieved to obtain a common understanding about the meaning of the data and depth of the concepts.

Descriptive statistics

To summarize categorical variables, we used absolute frequencies and percentages. Discrete or continuous variables were described in terms of mean and standard deviation. The analysis was conducted using SPSS 24 (IBM) [57].

Results

Patient characteristics and reasons for non-adherence to regular follow-up visits

Of the 459 identified patients, 32 (7%) had died; 4 (0.9%) had a predominant other disease, including malignancies (1; 0.2%), dementia (2; 0.4%), or were in palliative care (1; 0.2%); 134 patients (29.2%) could not be reached; 27 patients (5.9%) rejected participation in the qualitative interview; and 131 (28.5%) did not fulfil the inclusion criteria due to documentation errors despite the fact that they had been identified in the database query (Fig. 1). A total of 131 (28.5%) patients agreed to participate in the qualitative study. Interview duration ranged from a few sentences up to a maximum of 32 min.

Based on the qualitative interviews, 43 (32.8%) of the 131 patients were classified as non-adherent and 88 (67.2%) were found to be adherent. Of the 88 adherent patients, 37 (42.0%) changed the centre or rheumatologist, 34 (38.6%) had extended (annual) intervals at the clinic, and 17 (19.3%) were incorrectly identified as non-adherent because of documentation errors. The characteristics of the adherent and non-adherent

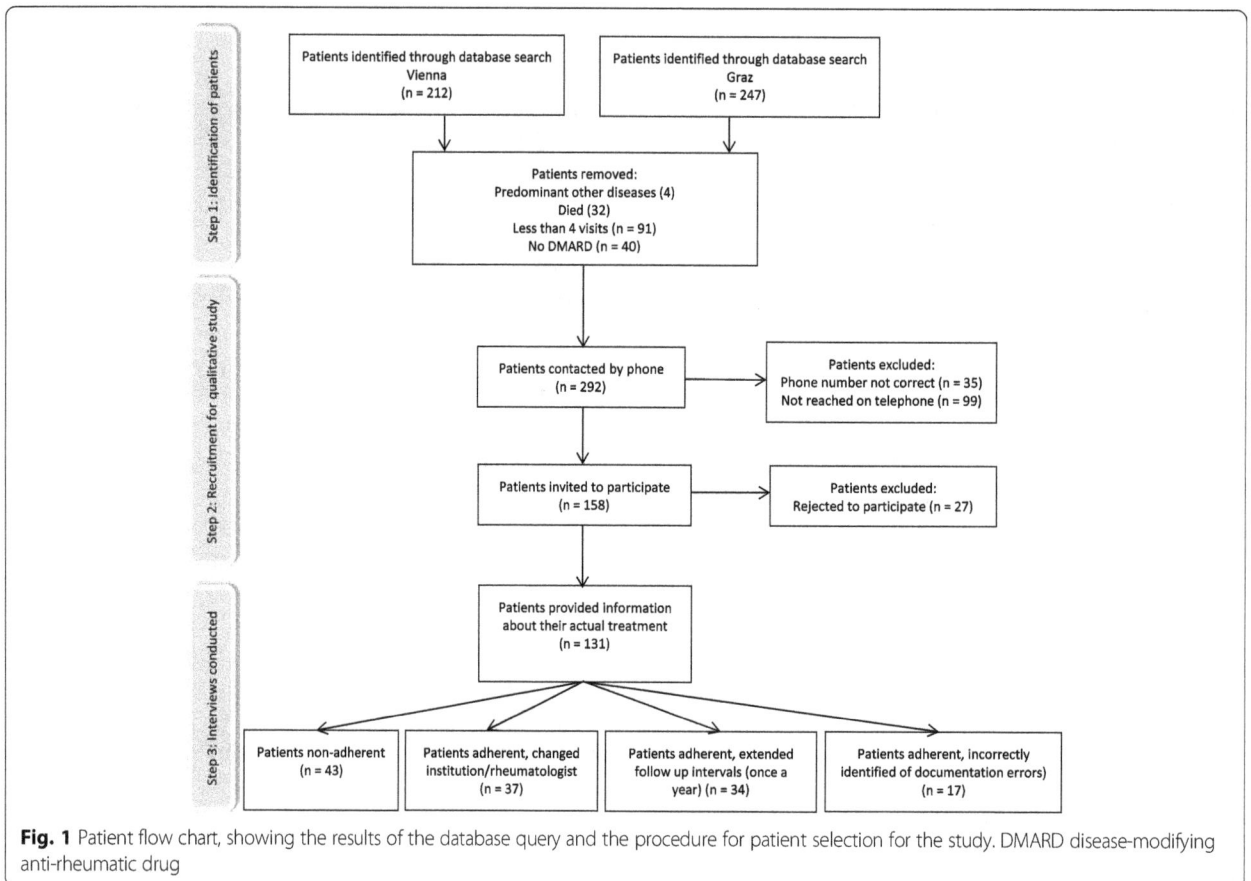

Fig. 1 Patient flow chart, showing the results of the database query and the procedure for patient selection for the study. DMARD disease-modifying anti-rheumatic drug

Table 1 Baseline characteristics of the adherent and non-adherent subgroups

	Non-adherent[a]	Adherent[b]	p value
Number of patients[c], n (%)	43 (32.8%)	88 (67.2%)	–
Female, n (%)	36 (83.7%)	73 (83.0%)	0.912
Age (years), mean (±SD)	58.3 (±13.1)	64.1 (±13.3)	**0.014**
Disease duration (years)[d], mean (±SD)	10.9 (±7.6)	12.4 (±9.3)	0.792
Treatment duration (years)[e], mean (±SD)	9.5 (±7.3)	8.8 (±7.2)	0.549
HAQ, mean (±SD)	0.9 (±0.8)	0.7 (±0.7)	0.233
SDAI, mean (±SD)	10.0 (±8.7)	6.9 (±6.4)	0.078
CDAI, mean (±SD)	9.2 (±8.2)	7.1 (±7.6)	0.121
PGA VAS[f], mean (±SD)	29.8 (±24.7)	27.8 (±26.7)	0.453
EGA VAS[g], mean (±SD)	14.7 (±16.2)	12.2 (±15.5)	0.325
Pain VAS[h], mean (±SD)	30.4 (±25.3)	28.8 (±28.2)	0.554
SJC32, mean (±SD)	2.8 (±4.3)	1.4 (±2.3)	0.128
TJC32, mean (±SD)	5.3 (±6.5)	2.6 (±5.0)	**0.008**
RF positive, n (%)	19 (44.2%)	46 (52.3%)	0.437

Data were extracted from the last clinical visit of each patient

Metric variables are shown in terms of mean and standard deviation. For nominal variables, absolute and relative frequencies were calculated

The p-value was calculated using Chi-Square test for nominal variables, and the Mann-Whitney U Test for ordinal and metric variables; significant results are highlighted in bold

CDAI Clinical Disease Activity Index, EGA evaluator global assessment, HAQ Health Assessment Questionnaire, PGA patient global assessment, RF rheumatoid factor, SDAI Simplified Disease Activity Index, SJC32 swollen joint count using a 32-joint count, TJC32 tender joint count using a 32-joint count, VAS visual analogue scale

[a]Patients were classified as non-adherent when they reported a change in intake of medication or other prescription without consulting a professional, or when they reported taking less than approximately 80% of the medication (steroids and disease-modifying anti-rheumatic drugs (DMARDs)) as prescribed, or missing appointments occasionally (out of 131 patients; patients who died or had other predominant diseases (n = 36) were not assigned to the subgroups adherent or non-adherent)

[b]Patients were classified as adherent when they reported following the treatment plan and visiting the outpatient clinic (or any other institute/health professional) as recommended (out of 131 patients; patients who died or had other predominant diseases (n = 36) were not assigned to the subgroups adherent or non-adherent)

[c]Total n = 131 patients; patients who died or had other predominant diseases (n = 36) were not assigned to the subgroups adherent or non-adherent

[d]Disease duration refers to the time duration between the first symptoms reported by the patient and the last visit at the centres

[e]Treatment duration refers to the time duration between the first and the last visit when the patients presented themselves at the centres

[f]Patient self-report measure using a 100-mm VAS [53]

[g]In addition to the PGA, EGA integrates subjective and objective measures obtained by the evaluator [53]

[h]Measured using a 100-mm VAS

patients who participated in the qualitative interviews are presented in Table 1. Baseline characteristics of patients who agreed to participate in the qualitative interviews and the non-participating individuals are depicted in Additional file 1: Supplement S4.

Factors associated with non-adherence known from the literature

The following concepts confirmed earlier findings from the literature [8, 30, 32–35, 37–40, 43–46, 58], with patients being non-adherent: 1) if they did not understand the purpose of the treatment, did not experience a benefit and/or experienced adverse events and/or toxicity; 2) if the proposed treatment plan was experienced as being too time consuming, including necessary waiting times, and requiring too much effort to be implemented in daily life; 3) if a lack of support of the environment occurred; and 4) if patients were not actively involved in a shared decision-making process. A non-adherent patient described that a shared decision about her medication treatment had not taken place:

"If the doctor does not listen to me or does not take my opinion into account when deciding about the medication that I should take, then I change the amount of the medication myself and I potentially lie to him"; participant no. 182 (female, age 34, Vienna)

Factors associated with non-adherence known from the literature together with quotes from the interviews are shown in Table 2.

New insights on factors associated with non-adherence

Four new concepts emerged in our study that have not been reported so far in the literature (Table 3). The first new aspect referred to a patient's strong opinion, meaning that values or beliefs that people accepted without any doubts inhibited adherence; pain, for example, was considered to be a necessary part of life in older age which should not be reduced because it was experienced as a reference for hard (manual) work during different phases of the patient's life. Similarly, another participant

Table 2 Factors associated with non-adherence which are known from the literature and were confirmed in our study

No.	Factors	Description	Quotation	Domains of the COM-B model
1	Lack of understanding the purpose; no benefit and/or adverse events	Patients were less likely to follow treatment instructions if they did not understand the purpose of the treatment, did not experience a benefit, and/or experienced adverse events and/or toxicity.	If I experience that it [the medication/intervention] doesn't help or if I do not understand the purpose, he [the rheumatologist] must accept that the instructions are not being followed (participant no. 182, female, age 34, Vienna). I stopped taking the medication by myself because of severe diarrhoea. I did not wait for an appointment to consult a doctor (participant no. 29, female, age 57, Vienna). I am getting older and older—the age is increasingly affecting my health. Sometimes I am afraid to do the exercises because everything is more or less deteriorating—the muscles and the bones (participant no. 110, female, age 70, Vienna).	Capability; body structures and functions
2	Implementation requirements	Patients were less likely to follow treatment instructions if the proposed treatment plan was experienced as being too time consuming, including necessary waiting times, and requiring too much effort to be implemented in daily life.	I was personally involved in building a medical centre and therefore I had no time for regular appointments. I was very glad that I did not have to spend a whole morning at the clinic, but instead was able to solve things easier and faster by consulting friends (physicians, but not rheumatologists). I thought that it was not important to see a rheumatologist any more (participant no. 126, female, age 38, Vienna). I still do my exercises—or correctly spoken again. I have exercises I should do every day. I don't do the exercises at the moment. I'm very lazy. And now I thought I could start again (participant no. 110, female, age 72, Vienna).	Motivation
3	Lack of supportive environmental factors	Patients were less likely to follow treatment instructions if lack of support of the environment occurred.	My mother cannot speak German. She missed the last appointment. She was not able to make a new appointment and I didn't have time to make an appointment for her. Then I totally forgot, and that's why she didn't come to the outpatients-clinic (daughter of participant no. 74, female, age 55, Vienna, who translated during the interview). You actually have an appointment but, nevertheless, you have to wait a long time. I was afraid if I said too often that I could not come [to work], I might lose my job (participant no. 143, male, age 47, Vienna). Meeting different doctors every time is aggravating (participant no. 29, female, age 57, Vienna).	Opportunity
4	Lack of shared decision-making	Patients were less likely to follow treatment instructions if they were not actively involved in a shared decision-making process.	The young doctors at the outpatient clinic were very annoying. They have no empathy. Rheumatism also has a lot to do with the soul of a patient. If young doctors consider themselves more important and think to you know everything better than the patient—that won't work at all (participant no. 45, female, age 57, Vienna). At my last visit to the outpatient clinic, I felt I was not being taken seriously and I had the feeling that the outpatient clinic is not patient-centred, but instead pharmaceutical company-centred (participant no. 37, female, age 70, Graz).	Opportunity

The capability, opportunity, and motivation model of behaviour (COM-B) model [21] was used as a frame of reference

Table 3 New insights on factors associated with non-adherence

No.	Factors	Description	Quotation	Domains of the COM-B model
1	Patient's strong opinion, similar to a dogma	"Patient's dogma", meaning that strong opinions, values, or beliefs that people accept without any doubts facilitated non-adherence.	*I am 77 years old now, always worked hard and long hours. I raised 6 children and I was never unemployed. It is no wonder that I am in pain. It indicates that I have been working hard all my life* (participant no. 150, female, age 76, Vienna). *I don't like drugs. Drugs made me sick. I never really recovered from that sickness drugs made me. I stopped taking medication. I have now bought a magnetic field mat, changed my diet and now I have no pain anymore* (participant no. 48, female, age 56, Graz).	Motivation
2	Feeling not to be in expert's hands when being treated by a physician/health professional	Patients searched for the best and most trustworthy physician/health professional. They had less trust in physicians/health professionals when: physicians appeared to be young regarding their age; when physicians disagreed with the opinions of other physicians; or when a physician consulted another physician for advice.	*At the outpatient clinic, two doctors said different things—then I was confused what I should do. Then, I decided not to come to the next appointment anymore* (participant no. 28, female, age 43, Graz). *The young, unexperienced doctors always want to prescribe drugs [DMARDs], but if that does not work then they are immediately at a loss, do not know what to do and then I simply do not feel well* (participant no. 165, male, age 70, Vienna).	Motivation
3	Excessive self-control	Patients who perceived excessive self-control over the treatment were less adherent.	*When the symptoms are more severe I go to see the doctor, but if they are only mild then I treat them by myself, because I know what will help anyway* (participant no. 182, female, age 34, Vienna). *It has been a long time since I was at the outpatient clinic. The drug made me uncomfortable. I vomited a lot. I never stopped taking it, because I need it. But I reduced it by myself to half the amount that the doctor had prescribed. The reduction did not affect the pain and I stopped feeling uncomfortable* (participant no. 170, female, age 45, Vienna).	Opportunity, with a negative connotation (not using the opportunity)
4	Missing a holistic approach	Some patients did not feel properly taken care of if physicians only prescribed medicines without addressing non-pharmacological aspects of treatment, including life-style advice, physical activity and diet, as well as alternative therapies.	*All I got at the outpatients clinic was medication. Nothing else. I did water gymnastics with my daughter—that was very beneficial for me, as well as mud treatments* (participant no. 99, female, age 56, Vienna). *There are also recommendations, for example regarding diet. That is never mentioned. Also regarding sports. The patients have to find out these things for themselves. They are only instructed us regarding medication here* (participant no. 182, female, age 34, Vienna).	Motivation

The capability, opportunity, and motivation model of behaviour (COM-B) model [21] was used as a frame of reference
DMARD disease-modifying anti-rheumatic drug

(no. 2, female, age 40, Graz) considered inflammation to be a natural process that should not be suppressed:

"I did not want to do this [take the prescribed medication] *anymore. I decided that I do not always want to suppress the inflammation. I want to leave the inflammation as it is, because it is a natural process. I do not want an infusion every month that, moreover, costs so much money, which in fact only supports the*

pharmaceutical companies. Doctors are brainwashed by the pharmaceutical companies, otherwise they would not prescribe these drugs."

Second, patients felt they were not the hands of experts when being treated by a physician/health professional. This was reported when the treating physicians appeared to be inexperienced which was associated with physicians being perceived either as young regarding their age (participant no. 165, male, age 70, Vienna) or if a rheumatologist asked senior consultants or colleagues for advice during the consultation with the patient. Third, patients who perceived excessive self-control over their treatment were likely to be non-adherent. Participant no. 21 (female, age 57, Vienna) said:

"I just started to reduce the medication on my own. And no difference was noticeable. I reduced it myself for a very long time and nothing worse happened. And that's the reason why I haven't been to the outpatient clinic for so long, because I have it under control anyway."

Fourth, some patients did not feel properly taken care of if the rheumatologist prescribed medicines only without giving advice on daily life issues and non-pharmacological aspects of treatment. New insights on factors associated with non-adherence together with quotes from the interviews are shown in Table 3.

Differences between medicine and non-pharmacological non-adherence

Most concepts were related to both non-adherence to medicines and non-adherence to non-pharmacological methods. However, their degree of influence was different. For example, the impact of the concept "non-adherence due to too much effort and time required" was described by patients who reported long waiting times at the rheumatology clinic. However, even greater efforts were described to implement non-pharmacological methods in daily life. Wearing splints, performing exercises, modifying life-style and/or changing daily habits were experienced to be more time consuming, were perceived as needing substantial changes of habits, and were reported to be more difficult to be included in daily patterns than taking medications. As an example, participant no. 168 (female, age 69, Vienna) explained:

"I was told to do full-body exercises [in German: Ganzkörperübungen]. I do these according to my own decision. (...) There are so many things going on in my life. When I have little time, I consider them [the exercises] not so important. And then I just don't do them."

Strong opinions of patients were primarily found with regards to medications. Patients stopped following treatment instructions because it was not in line with their preferences, values, and beliefs, e.g. pain or inflammation were seen as natural processes, and physicians were considered to be influenced by industry. Environmental factors outside the control of the patients were mentioned regardless of medicines or non-pharmacological

interventions. As an example, participant no. 99 (female, age 55, Vienna) argued:

"I do not drive and I have to wait until he [my husband] is well again to bring me to the clinic. (...) Initially, I wanted to take the ambulance, but it costs a lot of money and I cannot afford that."

Time perspective in relation to treatment phase

Some factors associated with non-adherence were more frequently perceived by the patients in the earlier phases of the disease (all included patients had at least four visits and one DMARD prescription), while others were found more relevant in later phases of the disease. For example, not understanding the purpose or not experiencing a potential benefit were associated with non-adherence especially in the early stages of RA, as patients perceived a potential worsening of the disease, adverse events of medications, and/or no benefits of the treatment. The concept regarding excessive self-control was found in the later phases of treatment only.

Time perspective in relation to age

A time perspective emerged in relation to age. Some patients considered themselves too old to do exercises (participant no. 110, female, age 70, Vienna; Table 2), while other patients argued that they were too young to take medication. An example is participant no. 115 (female, age 50, Vienna):

"It was the hopelessness, a bit, that drove me away. When you are in your mid-thirties and they [the rheumatologists] tell you that you have to take strong medication all your life. There must be another way; I do not want to poison my body for such a long time."

Discussion

We identified new and unexpected insights on factors associated with non-adherence regarding pharmacological and non-pharmacological methods in patients with RA by means of qualitative research. Moreover, we systematically described reasons for non-adherence to clinical follow-up visits, and linked them to the COM-B model. Qualitative research is a means to elicit meanings of concepts to individual patients and thus to explore reasons and motivation for behaviour [47]. We therefore decided to first start with a qualitative analysis rather than setting out to explore the influence of clinical variables on non-adherence in a statistical model. Furthermore, each individual perspective adds to the range of experiences collected. While qualitative research does not produce representative results for all patients, it allows us to better understand potential reasons for the behaviour of non-adherent patients and gives us tools to explore these in other patients. The COM-B model comprehensively covered the range of our findings. Other theories and models, such as the necessity-concerns framework [24, 25], include only parts of the concepts that emerged from our study, e.g. patients' lack of understanding regarding the purpose of a medication or non-pharmacological method. In contrast, environmental factors, e.g. lack of supportive environmental factors, were not covered. The concept of lack of supportive environmental factors was linked to opportunity of the COM-B model. While the needs and concerns of patients have an important influence on increasing or decreasing adherence rates, other factors, such as the environment, also impact on adherence. The WHO stated that the common belief that patients themselves are solely responsible for adherence is misleading and excludes other potentially influencing factors [9]. In this sense, our study provides additional evidence to support this WHO statement.

Some findings that emerged in our qualitative analysis have already been mentioned in the literature. We already know that patient beliefs [25, 30, 33, 34, 59], patient trust [33, 34], and self-control [60], for example, influence adherence. However, we could describe these findings in greater depth regarding the perspective of patients and their motivations not to adhere to follow-up visits and recommended treatment. While beliefs, expectations, and perceptions about medication and illness have been reported in some studies [30, 33, 34, 59], quality and theoretical depth of these concepts, such as the role of pain, inflammation, or of the pharmaceutical industry from the perspective of patients, were added in our study. Therefore, the factors found in our study can contribute substantially to the ongoing debate on how and what to assess regarding (non-)adherence from the perspective of patients.

Personalized medicine claims that we need stratified interventions relevant to subgroups of patients based on biomarkers. In addition to biomarkers, psycho-social markers, including personal attitudes, strong opinions, cultural values and norms, environmental factors, and so forth, derived from qualitative data such as from our study, could be used to further stratify patients. The idea of stratifying patients for tailored patient information and education is an obvious consequence from our findings. However, a large body of research on interventions to increase adherence found that most of these interventions were not successful, although some of them have already used tailored information and targeted interventions [61]. According to the findings of our study, interventions could address different components. Interventions could target the way physicians and/or health professionals interact with patients, and care processes could be standardised to avoid disagreement and to guide younger, less experienced personnel. Furthermore, the range of patient experiences might be used as examples that could be explicitly addressed in the interactions

with patients. Moreover, a complex phenomenon, such as adherence, might require multi-component interventions to successfully change human behaviour [9]. Multi-component interventions were found to be more effective in clinical trials than interventions that focused on single components only [54].

The time perspective detected in our analysis relates to two different aspects. First, patients reported differences between concepts that are important in early versus late phases of treatment. Second, a relationship with age occurred. From this we could conclude that non-adherence might not be stable throughout a patient's lifetime, but might change in relation to experiences, values, beliefs, and the needs of patients over time. Interventions specifically targeted to the values, beliefs, and needs of a patient in certain phases of their disease course may thus be essential to sustainably influence adherence over a lifetime.

A limitation of our study is that the results are based on the perspectives of patients who were non-adherent to follow-up visits. We are aware that this is a specific subpopulation of non-adherent patients. It is very likely that some people regularly come to the outpatient clinic and are still non-adherent to their medication. These people might have other drivers for their non-adherence compared with the patients who do not show up at the outpatient clinic regularly. However, we needed this approach to identify a substantial number of patients potentially non-adherent to medicines and non-pharmacological treatment as simply asking patients would lead to socially desirable answers. In addition, future studies could explore the perspectives and motivations of those patients who have been adherent for several years. Our findings could then be compared with the perspectives of these adherent patients.

Conclusions

In conclusion, new insights on factors associated with non-adherence allow a better understanding of this phenomenon and can substantially enhance patient care by helping to develop targeted interventions. Clinicians could explicitly address the issues during a consultation or in a patient education session. Furthermore, these new insights on factors can contribute substantially to the ongoing debate on how and what to assess regarding non-adherence from the perspective of patients.

Funding
This work was partly supported by a peer-reviewed research grant from AbbVie (grant number 10587/FA 716D0408). AbbVie reviewed and approved the study protocol, but was not involved in data gathering, nor in the analyses or the preparation of the manuscript.

Authors' contributions

VR and TAS were involved in the planning of the study conception and design. VR, AL, ML, PS, JSS, and TAS were involved in the recruitment of patients. VR, AL, CB, EM, ML, MO, RFR, JSS, and TAS contributed substantially to analysis and interpretation of data. All authors were involved in drafting the article and revising it critically for important content, and all authors read and approved the final manuscript.

Consent for publication

The present manuscript does not contain any individual person's data, such as individual details, images, or videos.

Competing interests

PS has received speaker fees from AbbVie, Lilly, and SOBI, and has provided remunerated expert advice to Lilly and Roche. JSS has received grants for his institution from Abbvie, Lilly, MSD, Pfizer, and Roche and has provided remunerated expert advice to and/or had speaking engagements for Abbvie, Amgen, Astra-Zeneca, Astro, BMS, Boehringer-Ingelheim, Celgene, Celltrion, Chugai, Gilead, Glaxo, ILTOO, Janssen, Lilly, Medimmune, MSD, Novartis-Sandoz, Pfizer, Roche, Samsung, Sanofi, and UCB. TAS has received speaker fees from AbbVie, Janssen, MSD, Novartis, and Roche, and grant support from AbbVie. The remaining authors declare that they have no competing interests.

Author details

[1]Section for Outcomes Research, Centre for Medical Statistics, Informatics, and Intelligent Systems, Medical University of Vienna, Spitalgasse 23, 1090 Vienna, Austria. [2]Division of Rheumatology, Department of Medicine 3, Medical University of Vienna, Vienna, Austria. [3]Department of Rheumatology, Medical University of Graz, Styria, Austria. [4]Division of Physiotherapy, Department of Neurobiology, Karolinska Institute, Care Sciences and Society (NVS), Huddinge, Sweden. [5]Karolinska University Hospital, Stockholm, Sweden. [6]Department of Internal Medicine, Centre for Rheumatic Diseases, Hietzing Hospital, Vienna, Austria. [7]Division of Occupational Therapy, University of Applied Sciences FH Campus Wien, Vienna, Austria.

References

1. Helmick CG, et al. Estimates of the prevalence of arthritis and other rheumatic conditions in the United States. Part I. Arthritis Rheum. 2008;58(1):15–25.
2. Franke L, et al. Cost-of-illness of rheumatoid arthritis and ankylosing spondylitis. Clin Experiment Rheumatol. 2009;27(4, Suppl. 55):118–23.
3. Loza E, et al. Multimorbidity: prevalence, effect on quality of life and daily functioning, and variationof this effect when one condition is a rheumatic disease. Semin Arthritis Rheum. 2009;38(4):312–9.
4. Smolen JS, et al. Treating rheumatoid arthritis to target: recommendations of an international task force. Ann Rheum Dis. 2010;69(4):631–7.
5. van Tuyl LH, et al. The patient perspective on remission in rheumatoid arthritis: 'You've got limits, but you're back to being you again'. Ann Rheum Dis. 2015;74(6):1004–10.
6. Jones G, et al. The effect of treatment on radiological progression in rheumatoid arthritis: a systematic review of randomized placebo-controlled trials. Rheumatology. 2003;42(1):6–13.
7. Haynes RB, et al. Interventions for enhancing medication adherence. Cochrane Database Syst Rev. 2005;4:CD000011.
8. Van Den Bemt BJ, Zwikker HE, Van Den Ende CH. Medication adherence in patients with rheumatoid arthritis: a critical appraisal of the existing literature. Expert Rev Clin Immunol. 2012;8(4):337–51.
9. World Health Organisation. Adherence to long-term therapies: evidence for action. Switzerland: World Health Organisation; 2003.
10. DiMatteo MR. Variations in patients' adherence to medical recommendations: a quantitative review of 50 years of research. Med Care. 2004;42(3):200–9.
11. Contreras-Yáñez I, et al. Inadequate therapy behavior is associated to disease flares in patients with rheumatoid arthritis who have achieved remission with disease-modifying antirheumatic drugs. Am J Med Sci. 2010;340(4):282–90.
12. Viller F, et al. Compliance to drug treatment of patients with rheumatoid arthritis: a 3 year longitudinal study. J Rheumatol. 1999;26(10):2114–22.
13. López-González R, et al. Adherence to biologic therapies and associated factors in rheumatoid arthritis, spondyloarthritis and psoriatic arthritis: a systematic literature review. Clin Exp Rheumatol. 2015;33:559–69.
14. Borah BJ, et al. Trends in RA patients' adherence to subcutaneous anti-TNF therapies and costs. Curr Med Res Opin. 2009;25(6):1365–77.
15. Curkendall S, et al. Compliance with biologic therapies for rheumatoid arthritis: do patient out-of-pocket payments matter? Arthritis Care Res. 2008;59(10):1519–26.
16. Lathia U, Ewara EM, Nantel F. Impact of adherence to biological agents on health care resource utilization for patients over the age of 65 years with rheumatoid arthritis. Patient Preference Adherence. 2017;11:1133.
17. Vermeire E, et al. Patient adherence to treatment: three decades of research. A comprehensive review. J Clin Pharm Ther. 2001;26(5):331–42.
18. Vrijens B, et al. A new taxonomy for describing and defining adherence to medications. Br J Clin Pharmacol. 2012;73(5):691–705.
19. Veehof MM, et al. Determinants of the use of wrist working splints in rheumatoid arthritis. Arthritis Rheum. 2008;59(4):531–6.
20. Ajzen I. From intentions to actions: a theory of planned behavior, in action control - From Cognition to Behavior, J. Kuhl and J. Beckmann, Editors. Berlin Heidelberg: Springer; 1985. p. 11–39.
21. Jackson C, et al. Applying COM-B to medication adherence: a suggested framework for research and interventions. Eur Health Psychol. 2014;16(1):7–17.
22. Michie S, Van Stralen MM, West R. The behaviour change wheel: a new method for characterising and designing behaviour change interventions. Implement Sci. 2011;6(1):42.
23. World Health Organization, International classification of functioning, disability, and health: ICF. 2001: Version 1.0. Geneva: World Health Organization.
24. Horne R. Treatment perceptions and self regulation. In: Cameron L, Leventhal H, editors. The self-regulation of health and illness behaviour. London: Routledge; 2003. p. 138–53.
25. Horne R, Weinman J, Hankins M. The beliefs about medicines questionnaire: the development and evaluation of a new method for assessing the cognitive representation of medication. Psychol Health. 1999;14(1):1–24.
26. Patton DE, et al. Theory-based interventions to improve medication adherence in older adults prescribed polypharmacy: a systematic review. Drugs Aging. 2017;34(2):97–113.
27. Easthall C, Barnett N. Using theory to explore the determinants of medication adherence; moving away from a one-size-fits-all approach. Pharmacy. 2017;5(3):50.
28. Michie S, et al. The behavior change technique taxonomy (v1) of 93 hierarchically clustered techniques: building an international consensus for the reporting of behavior change interventions. Ann Behav Med. 2013;46(1):81–95.
29. Brown T, et al. Final report for the IMAB-Q study: validation and feasibility testing of a novel questionnaire to identify barriers to medication adherence. Norwich: The University of East Anglia; 2017. p. 54. 2018
30. Voshaar M, et al. Barriers and facilitators to disease-modifying antirheumatic drug use in patients with inflammatory rheumatic diseases: a qualitative theory-based study. BMC Musculoskelet Disord. 2016;17(1):442.
31. Treharne G, Lyons A, Kitas G. Medication adherence in rheumatoid arthritis: effects of psychosocial factors. Psychol Health Med. 2004;9(3):337–49.
32. Popa-Lisseanu MGG, et al. Determinants of treatment adherence in ethnically diverse, economically disadvantaged patients with rheumatic disease. J Rheumatol. 2005;32(5):913–9.
33. Brandstetter S, et al. 'The lesser of two evils...'—views of persons with rheumatoid arthritis on medication adherence: a qualitative study. Psychol Health. 2016;31(6):675–92.
34. Pasma A, et al. Facilitators and barriers to adherence in the initiation phase of disease-modifying antirheumatic drug (DMARD) use in patients with arthritis who recently started their first DMARD treatment. J Rheumatol. 2015;42(3):379–85.
35. Hammond A, Young A, Kidao R. A randomised controlled trial of occupational therapy for people with early rheumatoid arthritis. Ann Rheum Dis. 2004;63(1):23–30.
36. Barry M, et al. Effect of energy conservation and joint protection education in rheumatoid arthritis. Rheumatology. 1994;33(12):1171–4.
37. Waggoner CD, LeLieuvre RB. A method to increase compliance to exercise regimens in rheumatoid arthritis patients. J Behav Med. 1981;4(2):191–201.
38. Vervloesem N, et al. Are personal characteristics associated with exercise participation in patients with rheumatoid arthritis? A cross-sectional explorative survey. Musculoskelet Care. 2012;10(2):90–100.
39. de Jong Z, et al. Long-term follow-up of a high-intensity exercise program in patients with rheumatoid arthritis. Clin Rheumatol. 2009;28(6):663–71.

40. Van den Ende C, et al. Comparison of high and low intensity training in well controlled rheumatoid arthritis. Results of a randomised clinical trial. Ann Rheum Dis. 1996;55(11):798–805.

41. Taal E, et al. Health status, adherence with health recommendations, self-efficacy and social support in patients with rheumatoid arthritis. Patient Educ Couns. 1993;20(2–3):63–76.

42. Niedermann K, et al. Six and 12 months' effects of individual joint protection education in people with rheumatoid arthritis: a randomized controlled trial. Scand J Occup Ther. 2012;19(4):360–9.

43. Mayoux-Benhamou A, et al. Influence of patient education on exercise compliance in rheumatoid arthritis: a prospective 12-month randomized controlled trial. J Rheumatol. 2008;35(2):216–23.

44. Häkkinen A, Sokka T, Hannonen P. A home-based two-year strength training period in early rheumatoid arthritis led to good long-term compliance: a five-year follow-up. Arthritis Care Res. 2004;51(1):56–62.

45. Feinberg J. Effect of the arthritis health professional on compliance with use of resting hand splints by patients with rheumatoid arthritis. Arthritis Rheumatol. 1992;5(1):17–23.

46. Nordgren B, et al. An outsourced health-enhancing physical activity programme for people with rheumatoid arthritis: exploration of adherence and response. Rheumatology. 2014;54(6):1065–73.

47. Stamm TA, et al. Concepts of functioning and health important to people with systemic sclerosis: a qualitative study in four European countries. Ann Rheum Dis. 2011;70(6):1074–9.

48. Aletaha D, et al. 2010 rheumatoid arthritis classification criteria: an American College of Rheumatology/European League Against Rheumatism collaborative initiative. Arthritis Rheumatol. 2010;62(9):2569–81.

49. Nell-Duxneuner V, et al. Autoantibody profiling in patients with very early rheumatoid arthritis: a follow-up study. Ann Rheum Dis. 2010;69(01):169–74.

50. Fries JF, et al. Measurement of patient outcome in arthritis. Arthritis Rheum. 1980;23(2):137–45.

51. Bruhlmann P, Stucki G, Michel BA. Evaluation of a German version of the physical dimensions of the Health Assessment Questionnaire in patients with rheumatoid arthritis. J Rheumatol. 1994;21(7):1245–9.

52. Aletaha D, et al. Acute phase reactants add little to composite disease activity indices for rheumatoid arthritis: validation of a clinical activity score. Arthritis Res Ther. 2005;7(4):R796–806.

53. Aletaha D, Smolen J. The Simplified Disease Activity Index (SDAI) and the Clinical Disease Activity Index (CDAI): a review of their usefulness and validity in rheumatoid arthritis. Clin Exp Rheumatol. 2005;23(5):100–8.

54. Aletaha D, et al. Remission and active disease in rheumatoid arthritis: defining criteria for disease activity states. Arthritis Rheum. 2005;52(9):2625–36.

55. Stack RJ, et al. Perceptions of risk and predictive testing held by the first-degree relatives of patients with rheumatoid arthritis in England, Austria and Germany: a qualitative study. BMJ Open. 2016;6(6):e010555.

56. van Beers-Tas MH, et al. Initial validation and results of the Symptoms in Persons At Risk of Rheumatoid Arthritis (SPARRA) questionnaire: a EULAR project. RMD Open. 2018;4(1):e000641.

57. IBM Corp., IBM SPSS Statistics for Windows (Version 24). Released 2016, IBM Corp.: NY.

58. Van Den Bemt BJ, Van Lankveld WG. How can we improve adherence to therapy by patients with rheumatoid arthritis? Nat Rev Rheumatol. 2007; 3(12):681.

59. Morgan C, et al. The influence of behavioural and psychological factors on medication adherence over time in rheumatoid arthritis patients: a study in the biologics era. Rheumatology. 2015;54(10):1780–91.

60. Brus H, et al. Determinants of compliance with medication in patients with rheumatoid arthritis: the importance of self-efficacy expectations. Patient Educ Couns. 1999;36(1):57–64.

61. Zwikker HE, et al. Effectiveness of a group-based intervention to change medication beliefs and improve medication adherence in patients with rheumatoid arthritis: a randomized controlled trial. Patient Educ Couns. 2014;94(3):356–61.

62. Tong A, Sainsbury P, Craig J. Consolidated criteria for reporting qualitative research (COREQ): a 32-item checklist for interviews and focus groups. Int J Qual Health Care. 2007;19(6):349–57.

16

T-cell costimulation blockade is effective in experimental digestive and lung tissue fibrosis

Gonçalo Boleto[1,2], Christophe Guignabert[3,4], Sonia Pezet[1], Anne Cauvet[1], Jérémy Sadoine[5], Ly Tu[3,4], Carole Nicco[1], Camille Gobeaux[6], Frédéric Batteux[1], Yannick Allanore[1,2] and Jérôme Avouac[1,2*] 🆔

Abstract

Background: We aimed to investigate the efficacy of abatacept in preclinical mouse models of digestive involvement, pulmonary fibrosis, and related pulmonary hypertension (PH), mimicking internal organ involvement in systemic sclerosis (SSc).

Methods: Abatacept has been evaluated in the chronic graft-versus-host disease (cGvHD) mouse model (abatacept 1 mg/mL for 6 weeks), characterized by liver and intestinal fibrosis and in the Fra-2 mouse model (1 mg/mL or 10 mg/mL for 4 weeks), characterized by interstitial lung disease (ILD) and pulmonary vascular remodeling leading to PH.

Results: In the cGvHD model, abatacept significantly decreased liver transaminase levels and markedly improved colon inflammation. In the Fra-2 model, abatacept alleviated ILD, with a significant reduction in lung density on chest microcomputed tomography (CT), fibrosis histological score, and lung biochemical markers. Moreover, abatacept reversed PH in Fra-2 mice by improving vessel remodeling and related cardiac hemodynamic impairment. Abatacept significantly reduced fibrogenic marker levels, T-cell proliferation, and M1/M2 macrophage infiltration in lesional lungs of Fra-2 mice.

Conclusion: Abatacept improves digestive involvement, prevents lung fibrosis, and attenuates PH. These findings suggest that abatacept might be an appealing therapeutic approach beyond skin fibrosis for organ involvement in SSc.

Keywords: Pulmonary fibrosis, Pulmonary hypertension, Gastrointestinal tract involvement, Systemic sclerosis, Abatacept

Background

Systemic sclerosis (SSc) is a rare life-threatening condition of autoimmune origin [1] defined by pathological fibrosis of the skin and internal organs [2]. T cells represent a major component of the infiltrate in the early inflammatory stage of the disease, exhibiting an activated phenotype with CD4+ T cells predominating over CD8+ T cells [3].

Cytotoxic T lymphocyte-associated molecule (CTLA)-4 is an immunoregulatory membrane receptor resulting in the downregulation of T-cell responses by inhibiting the costimulatory interactions of CD28-B7 [4]. We have recently shown that abatacept both prevents and induces regression of inflammation-driven dermal fibrosis in two complementary mouse models of SSc [5]. Preliminary clinical data have suggested benefits of abatacept on inflammatory joint involvement [6] and skin fibrosis [7] in SSc patients, and a randomized controlled trial is ongoing (NCT02161406). However, SSc prognosis depends on major organ involvement. Pulmonary complications including interstitial lung disease (ILD) and pulmonary hypertension (PH) remain the largest causes of mortality in SSc [1]. Digestive involvement is very frequent in SSc patients and can also lead to severe malabsorption.

We hypothesized that, beyond skin effects, abatacept may be efficient for the treatment of organ damage, in particular digestive, lung, and vessel fibrosis. Our aim was to assess the effects of abatacept in mouse models mimicking severe organ damage characterizing SSc.

---

* Correspondence: javouac@me.com; jerome.avouac@aphp.fr
[1]Université Paris Descartes, Sorbonne Paris Cité, INSERM U1016, Institut Cochin, CNRS UMR8104, Paris, France
[2]Université Paris Descartes, Sorbonne Paris Cité, Service de Rhumatologie A, Hôpital Cochin, 27 rue du Faubourg Saint Jacques, 75014 Paris, France
Full list of author information is available at the end of the article

Methods

Animals

Thirteen-week-old male and female C57BL6/J mice and 6-week-old female BALB/c mice were purchased from Janvier Laboratory (Le Genest Saint Isle, France). Thirteen-week-old male and female Fra-2 transgenic mice (SA5446 D-H3/FRA-2 (Tg4)) were obtained from a collaboration established with Sanofi Genzyme [8, 9]. B10.D2-enhanced green fluorescent protein (eGFP) mice were provided by Colette Kanellopoulos-Langevin, CDTA–CNRS–Orléans, France. All mice were housed in ventilated cages with sterile food and water ad libitum. All animals were treated in accordance with the Guide for the Care and Use of Laboratory Animals as adopted by INSERM, and approval was granted by the Ethics Committee of our University.

Pharmacological treatment

Abatacept (CTLA-4-Ig) was provided by Bristol-Myers Squibb, and purified human IgG1 (MP Biomedicals, Illkirch, France) was used as a negative control. Abatacept at two different concentrations (1 mg/mL and 10 mg/mL) and control IgG1 were dissolved in 0.9% NaCl and injected every other day intraperitoneally at a dose of 100 µg/mouse, as used previously [10]. A dose of 1 mg/mL was used in the chronic graft-versus-host disease (cGvHD) model since it has been shown to be effective in this setting in a previous report [5]. To assess a potential dose effect of abatacept, two different dose regimens were used in the Fra-2 transgenic mouse model. The dosage of the drug was not adjusted to body weight. Both doses of abatacept, 1 mg/mL (3 mg/kg) and 10 mg/mL (30 mg/kg) were physiological since abatacept has been administered in preclinical studies up to 50 mg/kg in rodents without any sign of toxicity.

In the cGvHD model, treatment with abatacept or IgG1 started 5 days after transplantation and the outcome was analyzed after 6 weeks.

In Fra-2 mice, treatment started at the age of 13 weeks and the outcome was analyzed after 4 weeks.

Murine sclerodermatous cGvHD

cGvHD was induced in BALB/c mice (H-2 d) by grafting allogeneic transplantation of 1×10^6 bone marrow cells and 2×10^6 splenocytes from 7-week-old to 8-week-old male B10.D2-eGFP mice (H-2 d), as previously described [5, 11, 12]. Recipient mice develop an inflammation-driven fibrosis resembling the early inflammatory stages of SSc which is responsible for liver and gastrointestinal tract damage. Intraperitoneal injections of abatacept 1 mg/mL ($n = 12$ mice) or control IgG1 ($n = 12$ mice) were performed every other day, starting 5 days after transplantation, which corresponds to a preventative setting. The outcome was analyzed after 6 week. Mice undergoing

syngeneic transplantation of bone marrow cells and splenocytes served as controls ($n = 8$).

Serum alanine aminotransferase and aspartate aminotransferase activities in the cGvHD model

Serum activity of alanine aminotransferase (ALT) and aspartate aminotransferase (AST) were used as markers of hepatocyte cytolysis. AST and ALT activities were quantified using a standard clinical automatic analyzer (Modular PP, Roche Diagnostics, Meylan, France).

Histopathologic assessment of colon involvement in the cGvHD model

Fixed colon biopsies were embedded in paraffin. A 5-mm thick tissue section was stained with hematoxylin and eosin [13]. Slides were examined by standard bright-field microscopy (Nikon Eclipse 80i, Tokyo, Japan). The severity of colon involvement was semiquantitatively assessed on a scale of 0–4 according to the method described by Blazar et al. [14] by two examiners (GB and SP) blinded to the genotype and the treatment. The grading criteria were as follows: grade 0, normal; grade 0.5, occasional necrotic crypt cell, minimal infiltration in lamina propria and submucosa; grade 1, necrotic cells in up to 15% of crypts, minor infiltration of up to 20% of lamina propria (1- to 2-cell thickness in intermucosal areas and submucosa); grade 1.5, necrotic cells in up to 15% of crypts, minor infiltration of less than or equal to one-third of the lamina propria (1- to 2-cell thickness in intermucosal areas and submucosa); grade 2, necrotic cells in ≤ 25% of crypts, infiltration of less than or equal to one-third of the lamina propria (3-cell thickness in intermucosal areas and submucosa); grade 2.5, necrotic cells in 25% to 50% of crypts, infiltration of less than or equal to one-third of lamina propria (3- to 4-cell thickness in intermucosal areas and submucosa); grade 3, necrotic cells in greater than 50% of crypts, infiltration of lamina propria (5- to 6-cell thickness in intermucosal areas and submucosa) with loss of ≤ 25% of goblet cells; grade 3.5, necrotic cells in greater than 50% of crypts, infiltration of lamina propria resulting in displacement of ≤ 50% of mucosa with loss of 50% of goblet cells; and grade 4, necrotic cells in greater than 50% of crypts, infiltration of lamina propria resulting in displacement of greater than 50% of mucosa with loss of 75% to 100% of goblet cells.

Effects of abatacept in the Fra-2 model

Transgenic mice expressing the fra-2 gene under control of the ubiquitous major histocompatibility complex class I antigen H2Kb promoter display systemic fibrosis, microangiopathy, and PH. These manifestations follow a similar temporal sequence as seen in human SSc. The presence of typical capillary changes, pulmonary fibrosis, and PH is unique among murine models for SSc. A significant decrease in capillary density occurs from weeks 12–13 [15]. In the lungs, obliteration of pulmonary arteries, accompanied by perivascular inflammatory infiltrates, becoming apparent at an age of 12–13 weeks precedes the onset of fibrosis by 2–3 weeks [16]. Regarding the occurrence of PH, Fra-2 transgenic mice develop severe vascular remodeling of pulmonary arteries resembling human SSc-PH. Histological features typical for SSc-PH, such as intimal thickening with concentric laminar lesions, medial hypertrophy, perivascular inflammatory infiltrates, and adventitial fibrosis, are frequently detected [9, 17].

Three groups of Fra-2 transgenic mice and one group of C57BL/6 mice were treated by intraperitoneal injections of abatacept 1 mg/mL ($n = 8$ Fra-2 mice), abatacept 10 mg/mL ($n = 8$ Fra-2 mice), or control IgG1 ($n = 6$ Fra-2 mice and 5 C57BL/6 mice) every other day, starting at the age of 13 weeks. Injections were performed for 4 weeks. Mice were killed by cervical dislocation at the age of 17 weeks.

It is important to note that, at week 13, lung fibrosis is not present in this model [18], which means that our therapeutic approach for this outcome was preventative. On the other hand, obliteration of pulmonary arteries is usually detected at week 12 in Fra-2 mice [15, 16], which supports a curative approach of PH.

Assessment of fibrosing alveolitis by chest microcomputed tomography in the Fra-2 model

Fibrosing alveolitis of mice was evaluated using microcomputed tomography (microCT) 2 days before sacrifice, as previously reported [19]. CT images were obtained with a Perkin Elmer's Quantum FX system (Caliper Life Sciences). The animals were placed in the supine position on the CT table. Mice were sedated with 3–4% isoflurane anesthesia at 0.5–1.5 L/min for induction by a nose cone. Anesthesia was maintained with 2.5–3% isoflurane at 400–800 mL/min during the acquisition. During image acquisition, thoracic breathing movements were recorded, detecting the up- and downward movement of the thorax. Images were acquired throughout the spontaneous respiratory cycle. Only images acquired during expiration were analyzed. Images were acquired with the following parameters: 90 kV x-ray source voltage, 160 µA current. Total scanning time was approximately 4.5 min per mouse choosing from the list mode made by the constructor with the gating parameter. Tomograms were reconstructed using Rigaku software. The analysis starts with the isolation of lung tissue by manually drawing a volume of interest. Analysis of lung density and drawing was performed with Ctan Brucker software. Lung density was measured in Hounsfield Units (HU) after calibration. A phantom

calibration was made on the acquisition Rigaku software: a water-filled 1.5-mL tube inside a 2-mL tube was scanned. Based on full-stack histograms of a manually delimited volume of interest containing only water or air, the mean grayscale index of water was set at 0 HU, and the grayscale index of air was set at –1000 HU. This value was reported in the Ctan Brucker software. Means of lung density of both groups were achieved by evaluation of all CT scans acquired from the apices to the bases of the lungs. Furthermore, the volume of functional lung parenchyma corresponding to functional residual capacity (FRC) was manually drawn by excluding the fibrosis area and vessels. Percentages of FRC on total lung volumes were calculated. The CT expert (JS) was blinded to the background of the mice, to the treatment, and to the results of the histological assessment.

Histopathologic assessment of fibrosing alveolitis in the Fra-2 model

Paraffin-embedded lung sections (5 µm) were stained with hematoxylin and eosin. The severity of fibrosing alveolitis was semiquantitatively assessed according to the method described by Ashcroft et al. by two examiners blinded to the genotype and the treatment (SP and AC) [19, 20]. Lung fibrosis was graded on a scale of 0 to 8 by examining randomly chosen fields of the left upper lobe. The grading criteria were as follows: grade 0, normal lung; grade 1, minimal fibrous thickening of alveolar walls; grade 3, moderate thickening of walls without obvious damage; grade 5, increased fibrosis with definite damage and formation of fibrous bands; grade 7, severe distortion of structure and large fibrous areas; and grade 8, total fibrous obliteration. Grades 2, 4, and 6 were used as intermediate stages between these criteria. This analysis was performed two examiners (SP and AC) in blinded manner. All images were taken with a Lamina multilabel slide scanner.

Collagen measurements in Fra-2 transgenic mice

The collagen content in lesional lung samples, taken from the same lobe for each mouse, was explored by hydroxyproline assay, as previously described [5, 9]. Briefly, each sample was hydrolyzed and titrated to a pH of 7. This solution was combined with chloramine T and p-dimethylaminobenzaldehyde in perchloric acid and read at 557 nm with a spectrophotometer (Molecular Devices, Sunnyvale, CA). This experiment was performed for two samples per mouse analyzed.

Nonlinear microscopy and second harmonic generation processing in Fra-2 transgenic mice

A multiphoton inverted stand Leica SP5 microscope (Leica Microsystems Gmbh, Wetzlar, Germany) was used for tissue imaging. A Ti:Sapphire Chameleon Ultra

(Coherent, Saclay, France) with a center wavelength at 810 nm was used as the laser source for second harmonic generation (SHG) and two-photon excited fluorescence (TPEF) signals. The laser beam was circularly polarized to ensure isotropic excitation of the sample regardless of the orientation of fibrillar collagen. A Leica Microsystems HCX IRAPO 25×/0.95 W objective was used to excite and collect SHG and TPEF. Signals were detected in epi-collection through a 405/15-nm and a 525/50 bandpass filter, respectively, by NDD PMT detectors (Leica Microsystems) with a constant voltage supply, at constant laser excitation power, allowing direct comparison of SHG intensity values. Two fixed thresholds were chosen to distinguish biological material from the background signal (TPEF images) and specific collagen fibers (SHG images). SHG score was established by comparing the area occupied by the collagen relative to the sample surface. Image processing and analysis (thresholding and SHG scoring) were performed using ImageJ homemade routines (https://imagej.nih.gov/ij/) as previously described [8]. Results were normalized to control C57/BL6 mice.

Lung biomarker measurement in Fra-2 transgenic mice

Selected fibrogenic markers were quantified by enzyme-linked immunosorbent assay (ELISA) in lesional lungs of Fra-2 transgenic mice. Proteins were extracted from lesional lungs, taken from the same specific lobe for each mouse, with Tissue Protein Extraction Reagent (T-PER®; Thermo Fischer Scientific, Villebon Sur Yvette, France) with Halt Protease Inhibitor Single-Use Cocktail, EDTA-free (Thermo Fischer Scientific). Total proteins were dosed by the BCA technique. All proteins were quantified in lesional lungs with mouse ELISA kits according to the instructions of the manufacturers. The detection limit was > 10 pg/mL. The following markers were assayed based on their relevance in the pathogenesis of SSc and animal models of SSc [2, 21–23] and on previous experience with these markers in the Fra-2 mouse model [19]: transforming growth factor (TGF)-β1, osteopontin (OPN), monocyte chemoattractant protein (MCP)-1, and TIMP metallopeptidase inhibitor-1 (TIMP-1) (all from R&D systems, Lille, France). Results are expressed as amount of biomarker per mg total tissue protein.

Immunostaining of lesional lung sections

Immunofluorescence and immunohistochemistry were performed after antigen retrieval and blocking with 2% bovine serum albumin (BSA) for 1 h at room temperature.

Type 1 (M1) and type 2 (M2) macrophages were detected by immunofluorescence in lesional lung sections. To detect M1 macrophages, sections were incubated with goat inducible nitric oxide synthase (iNOS)

antibodies (Invitrogen, Paris, France; dilution 1:200), monoclonal CD11c antibodies (Abcam, Cambridge, UK; dilution 1:20), and monoclonal F4/80 antibodies (Abcam; dilution 1:100) overnight at 4 °C. To detect M2 macrophages, lesional lung sections were incubated with polyclonal cMAF antibodies (Santa Cruz, San Diego, CA; dilution 1:50), polyclonal arginase antibodies (Santa Cruz; dilution 1:200), and F4/80 [24]. Additional stainings by immunofluorescence included Ki-67 (polyclonal antibodies, dilution 1:550; Abcam) and CD3 (monoclonal antibodies, dilution 1:50; Abcam) to identify proliferative T cells. The following secondary antibodies were used for 1 h at room temperature [25]: Alexa-Fluor-labeled donkey anti-rabbit 488 (1:200), donkey anti-goat 594 (1:100), chicken anti-rat 647 (1:200), and goat anti-hamster 594 (1:100) (all from Life Technologies, Darmstadt, Germany). All sections were counterstained with DAPI.

We also performed immunohistochemistry in lesional colon sections for CD45 (polyclonal antibodies, dilution 1:200; Novus, Lille, France) to quantify inflammatory cells and Annexin-V (polyclonal antibodies, 1:100; Abcam) to detect apoptotic/necrotic cells. Polyclonal horseradish peroxidase-labeled goat anti-rabbit immunoglobulins were used as secondary antibodies (1:200; Agilent Technologies, Les Ulis, France). Staining was visualized with DAB peroxidase substrate solution (Sigma-Aldrich, Darmstadt, Germany).

All images were captured with a Lamina multilabel slide scanner (PerkinElmer, Villebon Sur Yvette, France). Cell quantification was performed by two independent investigators (GB and SP) according an automated counting method using the ImageJ software.

Hemodynamic measurements and assessment of vessel remodeling in Fra-2 transgenic mice

Right ventricular systolic pressure (RVSP) and heart rate were determined in unventilated mice under isoflurane anesthesia (1.5–2.5%, 2 L O_2/min) using a closed chest technique, by introducing a catheter (1.4-F catheter; Millar Instruments Inc., Houston, TX) into the jugular vein and directing it to the right ventricle [26–28]. After all the hemodynamic assessments were completed, blood was collected by direct cardiac puncture and sacrificed by exsanguination. The heart and lungs were then removed en bloc and right ventricular hypertrophy (RVH) was determined by the Fulton index measurement (right ventricle/left ventricle plus septum (RV/LV + S)) [26–28]. The pulmonary circulation was flushed with 5 mL buffered saline at 37 °C, and then the left lung was prepared for morphometric analyses and the right lung was quickly harvested, immediately snap-frozen in liquid nitrogen and kept at −80 °C.

Morphometric analyses were performed on paraffin-embedded lung sections stained using hematoxylin and eosin and alpha smooth muscle actin (α-SMA). α-SMA was detected by incubation with monoclonal anti-α-SMA antibody (clone 1A4; Dako Glostrup, Denmark) at a dilution of 1:100 overnight at 4 °C. A Vectastain ABC kit was the used according to the manufacturer's instructions (Vector Laboratories, Burlingame, CA) and slides were then counterstained with hematoxylin (Sigma-Aldrich). The percentage of wall thickness ((2 × medial wall thickness/external diameter) × 100) and of muscularized vessels were determined as previously described [29]. All morphometric analyses were performed by one observer (CG) blinded to genotype and treatment conditions.

Statistics

All data are expressed as median values ± interquartile range (IQR). Multiple group comparisons were analyzed using a post-hoc Dunnett's test. The Mann-Whitney U test was used for a two-group comparison. $P < 0.05$ (all two-sided) was considered significant.

Results

Abatacept alleviates liver cytolysis and gut involvement in experimental cGvHD

Treatment of allogeneic mice with abatacept led to a significant reduction in ALT (24%, $P = 0.014$) and AST

levels (61%, $P < 0.001$) compared with IgG1-treated allogeneic mice (Additional file 1A, B). Pathological analysis of the colon revealed reduced inflammatory cell infiltration in the lamina propria, necrotic crypt cells, and loss of goblet cells in allogeneic abatacept-treated mice compared with IgG1-treated mice (Fig. 1a). A significant 47% reduction in the histological score, evaluating inflammatory change, was observed in allogeneic mice treated with abatacept ($P = 0.019$) (Fig. 1b). Consistent with this observation, submucosal CD45$^+$ inflammatory cell infiltration and the number of annexin V-positive dead cells were markedly reduced in allogeneic abatacept-treated mice (Additional file 2A, B).

Abatacept alleviates lung fibrosis in the Fra-2 mouse model

Mice treated with abatacept 10 mg/mL showed decreased lung density to levels similar to control C57BL/6 mice when assessed by chest microCT (Fig. 2a, b). The FRC significantly improved in both groups of abatacept-treated mice, with similar values to control C57BL/6 mice (Fig. 2c).

Lung specimens from IgG1-treated mice exhibited features of fibrosing alveolitis (Fig. 3a). On treatment with abatacept, a significant 79% reduction of the lung fibrosis score was observed at a dose of 10 mg/mL compared

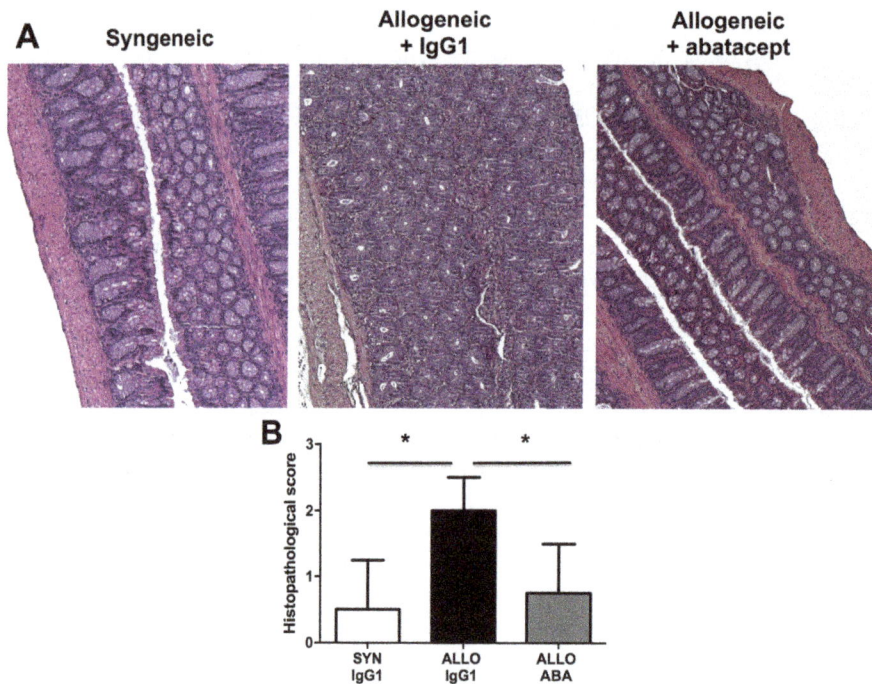

Fig. 1 Abatacept prevents cGvHD-associated colon involvement. **a** Representative 5-mm thick colon sections stained by hematoxylin and eosin showing syngeneic BALB/c mice and cGvHD mice treated by control IgG1 or abatacept 1 mg/mL. Submucosal infiltration by mononuclear cells and destruction of crypts in abatacept-treated cGvHD mice are decreased when compared with IgG1-treated cGvHD mice. **b** Histological score of colon involvement decreased significantly upon treatment with abatacept 1 mg/mL in cGvHD mice compared with IgG1-treated cGvHD mice. A total of 32 mice were used (12 allogeneic (ALLO) control IgG1-treated mice, 12 abatacept (ABA) 1 mg/mL-treated mice, and 8 control syngeneic (SYN) BALB/c mice). Values are the median ± IQR. Statistics are from post-hoc Dunnett's multiple comparison test. *$P < 0.05$

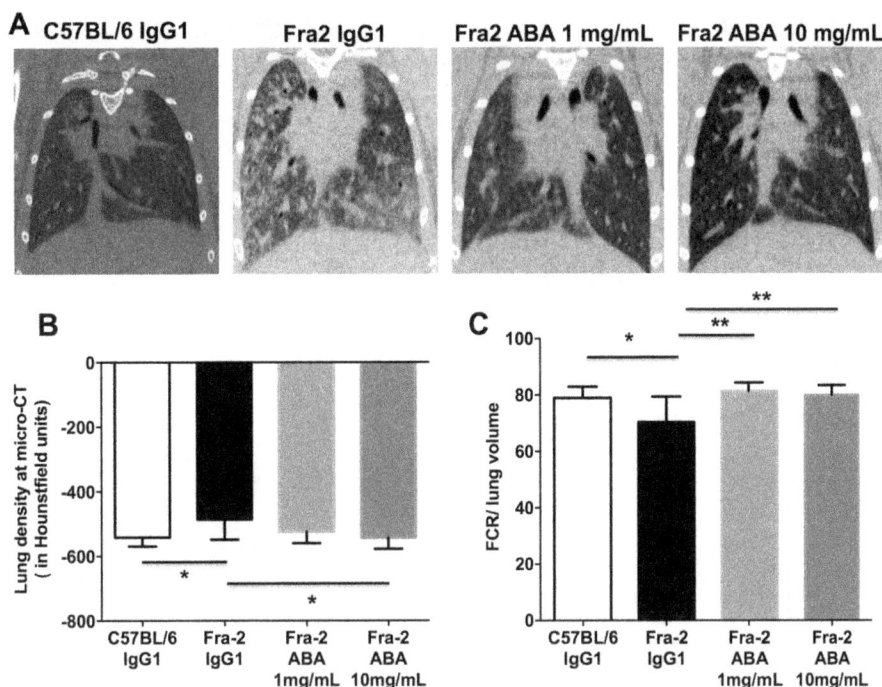

Fig. 2 Abatacept protects against fibrosing alveolitis in the Fra-2 mouse model. Evaluation by CT-scan. **a** Treatment with abatacept (ABA) prevents lung fibrosis in Fra-2 transgenic mice; representative pictures of microcomputed tomography. **b** Decreased lung density at microcomputed tomography (micro-CT) in Fra-2 transgenic mice treated with abatacept 10 mg/mL compared with control IgG1-treated mice. **c** Reduced residual lung volume, expressed as the percentage of functional residual capacity (FRC) on total lung volume in Fra-2 transgenic mice treated with abatacept 1 mg/mL and 10 mg/mL compared with control IgG1-treated mice. A total of 27 mice were used (5 C57BL/6 mice, 6 Fra-2 control IgG1, 8 Fra-2 abatacept 1 mg/mL, and 8 Fra-2 abatacept 10 mg/mL). Values are the median ± IQR. Statistics are from post-hoc Dunnett's multiple comparison test. *$P < 0.05$, **$P < 0.01$

with mice treated with IgG1 ($P = 0.009$) (Fig. 3a, b). Consistent with CT and histological analysis, hydroxyproline content was also reduced by 31% in lung specimens from mice treated with abatacept 10 mg/mL ($P = 0.044$) (Fig. 3c).

SHG showed a preferential perivascular distribution of fibrosis in IgG1-treated mice, which was consistent with fibrosing alveolitis (Additional file 3A). Scoring of fibrillar collagen deposits confirmed a significant decrease in collagen scoring in Fra-2 mice receiving abatacept 10 mg/mL compared with Fra-2 mice treated with IgG1 (Additional file 3B).

Treatment with abatacept 10 mg/mL markedly reduced lung protein levels of MCP1 by 79% ($P = 0.043$), OPN by 87% ($P = 0.039$), and TGF-β by 69% ($P = 0.013$). Levels of TGF-β were also reduced by 61% on treatment with abatacept 1 mg/mL ($P = 0.037$) (Additional file 4A–D).

Abatacept reverses PH in the Fra-2 mouse model

On treatment with abatacept 10 mg/mL, a substantial reduction of RVSP (28.1 ± 1.5 mmHg vs. 36.0 ± 5.1 mmHg, $P = 0.037$) was observed compared with IgG1-treated mice (Fig. 4a). RVH was also significantly decreased with abatacept 1 mg/mL (0.29 ± 0.01% vs. 0.33 ± 0.01%, $P = 0.037$)

and 10 mg/mL (0.29 ± 0.01% vs. 0.33 ± 0.01%, $P = 0.037$) (Fig. 4b). Likewise, abatacept 1 mg/mL and abatacept 10 mg/mL were associated with a significant decrease in percentage medial wall thickness (Fig. 4c, d) and number of muscularized distal pulmonary arteries (Fig. 4c, e).

Abatacept reduces T-cell proliferation and M1/M2 macrophage infiltration in lesional lungs

To evaluate the effects of abatacept on T-cell proliferation, we detected the expression of the proliferation marker Ki-67 in lesional lungs (Fig. 5a). The ratio of T cells expressing Ki-67 to total CD3-positive T cells was found significantly decreased by 21% ($P = 0.009$) and 29% ($P = 0.001$) in mice treated with abatacept 1 mg/mL and 10 mg/mL, respectively, compared with mice receiving control IgG1 (Fig. 5a, b).

To evaluate whether abatacept influences the outcome of Fra-2 mice by regulating infiltration of M1/M2 macrophages, we quantified the number of proinflammatory M1 macrophages and profibrotic M2 macrophages in lesional lungs (Fig. 6a, b). The ratio of M1 and M2 macrophages to total macrophages dramatically decreased in mice treated with abatacept 1 mg/mL (by 72%, $P < 0.001$, and 93%, $P < 0.001$, respectively) and 10 mg/mL (by 58%,

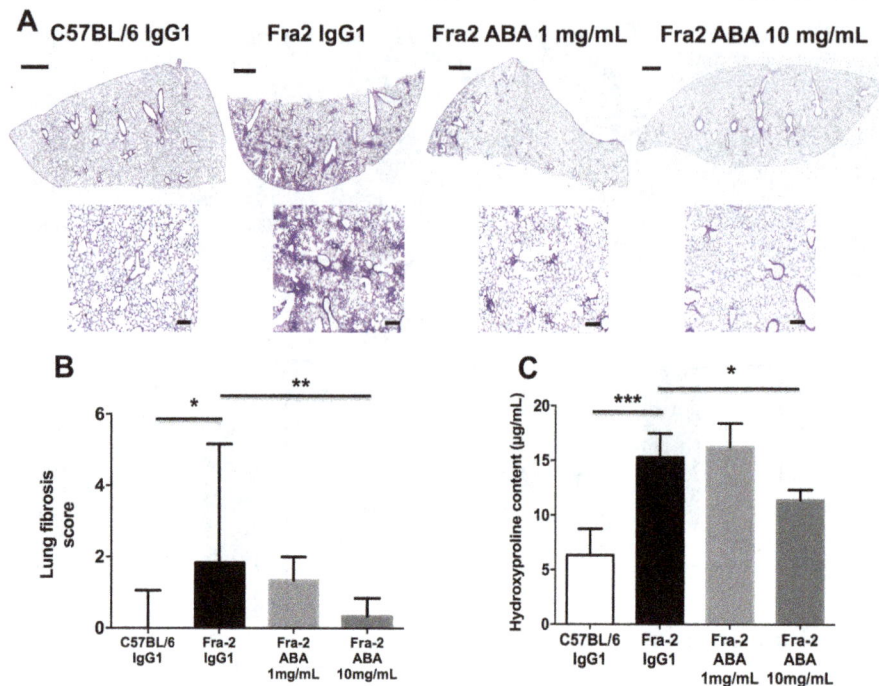

Fig. 3 Abatacept 10 mg/mL prevents lung fibrosis in Fra-2 transgenic mice. Evaluation by histology. **a** Treatment with abatacept (ABA) 10 mg/mL prevents lung fibrosis in Fra-2 transgenic mice; representative lung sections stained by hematoxylin and eosin. Scale bars = 100 μm. **b** Histological lung fibrosis score decreased significantly on treatment with abatacept 10 mg/mL compared with mice receiving abatacept 1 mg/mL and control IgG1-treated mice. **c** Hydroxyproline content in lesional lungs of Fra-2 mice markedly decreased on treatment with abatacept 10 mg/mL compared with mice receiving abatacept 1 mg/mL and control IgG1-treated mice. A total of 27 mice were used (5 C57BL/6 mice, 6 Fra-2 control IgG1, 8 Fra-2 abatacept 1 mg/mL, and 8 Fra-2 abatacept 10 mg/mL). Values are the median ± IQR. Statistics are from post-hoc Dunnett's multiple comparison test. *$P < 0.05$, **$P < 0.01$, ***$P < 0.001$

$P = 0.003$, and 70%, $P < 0.001$, respectively) compared with those injected with control IgG (Fig. 6c, d).

Discussion

In this study, we demonstrate how the inhibition of T-cell costimulation reduces the severity of SSc organ damage in two complementary experimental models. Abatacept was well tolerated in both mouse models with no weight loss during the whole treatment period (control IgG1 +1.50 ± 1.12 g, abatacept 1 mg/mL +1.13 ± 1.35 g, and abatacept 10 mg/mL +0.97 ± 1.07 g).

Abatacept prevents liver and colon damage in the cGvHD model. As in the early stages of human SSc, this model is characterized by dense inflammatory infiltrates in affected organs (skin, liver, gastrointestinal tract), composed of mononuclear cells, T cells, and monocyte-macrophages, which contribute to the initial activation of resident fibroblasts by the release of profibrotic mediators. However, the degree of persistent cellular infiltrate is rather more than is typical of human SSc [30, 31].

Fra-2 transgenic mice are characterized by features of human vasculopathy, including PH, paralleled by fibrosing alveolitis similar to that seen in patients with SSc. Abatacept substantially improves parameters evaluating

both interstitial lung inflammation and fibrosis in this mouse model, supporting the concept that the beneficial effects of abatacept are not only restricted to inflammatory changes. Abatacept also markedly alleviates vascular remodeling and signs of PH.

These results extend previous findings observed in experimental models of inflammation-driven fibrosis [5, 32, 33] and hypersensitivity pneumonitis [34]. Targeting T cell-mediated responses made it possible to interfere with tissue remodeling leading to lung fibrosis and PH in the Fra-2 model [18], in line with the attenuation, upon T-cell costimulation blockade, of cardiac hypertrophy and fibrosis that were observed in experimental models of systemic hypertension and pathological cardiac hypertrophy [35, 36].

It is noteworthy that, despite the efficacy of abatacept 1 mg/mL in the cGvHD model and the positive signal observed on several parameters with this dose in Fra-2 mice, significant improvements in the Fra-2 model were mostly reached with the dose of 10 mg/mL. The contribution of T cells for disease phenotype may partly explain this result. In the cGvHD, the role of T cells is preponderant [37]. In Fra-2 transgenic mice, although inflammatory infiltrates seem to contribute to disease

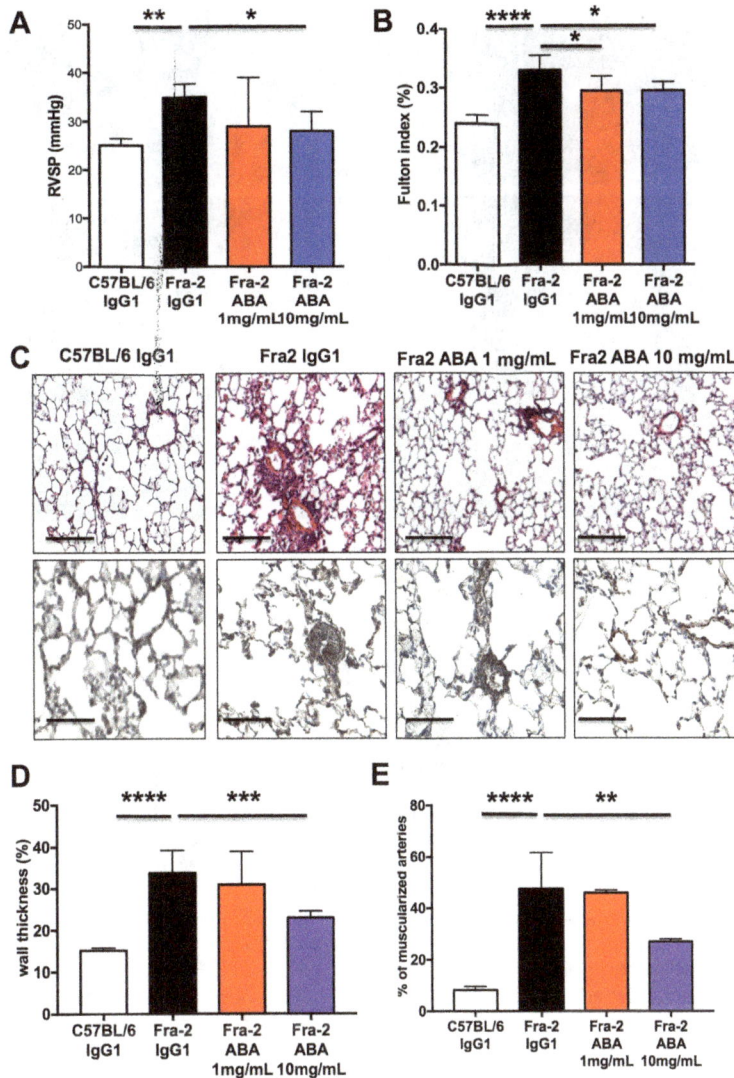

Fig. 4 Abatacept alleviates pulmonary hypertension in Fra-2 transgenic mice. **a** Right ventricular systolic pressure (RVSP) and **b** right ventricular hypertrophy assessed by the Fulton index. **c** Representative images of hematoxylin and eosin staining (upper row) and representative images of α-smooth muscle actin (α-SMA) immunohistostaining (lower row) showing a substantial reduction in the percentage of medial wall thickness (**d**) and a significant reduction in the percentage of distal artery muscularization (**e**) in Fra-2 mice treated with abatacept (ABA) 1 mg/mL and 10 mg/mL compared with control IgG1-treated mice. Scale bars = 100 μm. A total of 27 mice were used (5 C57BL/6 mice, 6 Fra-2 control IgG1, 8 Fra-2 abatacept 1 mg/mL, and 8 Fra-2 abatacept 10 mg/mL). Values are the median ± IQR. Statistics are from post-hoc Dunnett's multiple comparison test. *$P < 0.05$, **$P < 0.01$, ***$P < 0.001$, ****$P < 0.0001$

pathogenesis, their implication seems less fundamental, since reciprocal bone marrow reconstitution experiments and the assessment of Fra-2 mice lacking functional B and T lymphocytes showed that T and B cells are not essential for the pathogenesis of pulmonary fibrosis [18].

It is difficult to speculate on organ-specific differences in treatment response with abatacept, which depends on the dose received and the mouse model. The dose of 1 mg/mL seems relevant to treat inflammation-driven skin fibrosis given the positive results observed with this dose in bleomycin-induced dermal fibrosis and cGvHD [5].

Higher doses appear necessary to treat more severe organ complications such as ILD and PH.

The benefit conferred by abatacept treatment may be that it targets T-cell costimulation and thus their optimal activation. Furthermore, targeting costimulation requires the targeting of CD80/CD86-bearing macrophages and B cells, which contributes to the therapeutic effect, affecting T cell-associated B cell and macrophage responses [38]. Fibrosis formation requires the combined action of Th2 cells and innate immune cells. In the Fra-2 mouse model, we identified an intense M1-polarized innate response, which we speculate subsequently switches to an

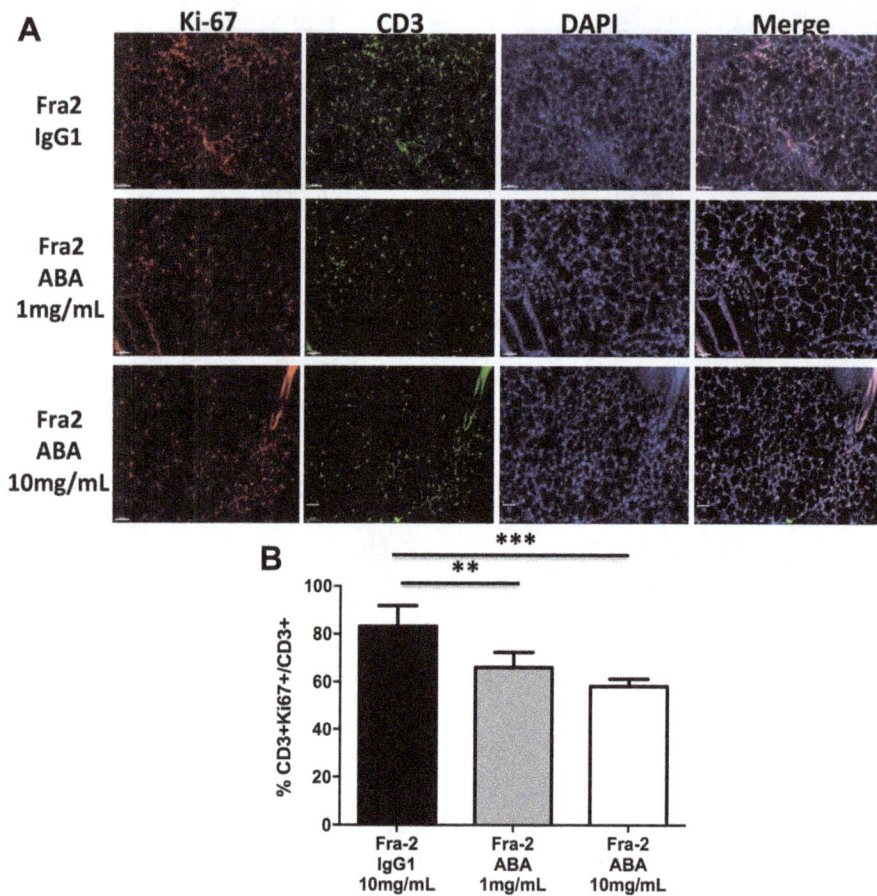

Fig. 5 Abatacept reduces T-cell proliferation in lesional lungs of Fra-2 transgenic mice. **a** Representative lung sections stained by the proliferation marker Ki-67 and CD3 to quantify the number of proliferative T cells. **b** Abatacept (ABA) significantly reduced the number of proliferative CD3$^+$Ki-67$^+$ cells reported on the total number of CD3$^+$ cells. A total of 22 mice were used (6 Fra-2 control IgG1, 8 Fra-2 abatacept 1 mg/mL, and 8 Fra-2 abatacept 10 mg/mL). Values the median ± IQR. Statistics are from post-hoc Dunnett's multiple comparison test. **$P < 0.01$, ***$P < 0.001$

M2/Th2 polarization which plays a central role in the pathogenesis of fibrosis. We observed that abatacept led to a marked reduction of both inflammatory M1 and profibrotic M2 macrophage infiltrates. In addition, abatacept has been recently shown in inflammation-driven dermal fibrosis to regulate T-cell activation and infiltration, as well as the production of proinflammatory and profibrotic cytokines, leading to decreased resident fibroblast activation and reduced excessive collagen production [5]. Inhibition of activation and infiltration of T cells and macrophages may reduce cell proliferation and death [39], which is in line with decreased T-cell proliferation observed in lesional lungs of Fra-2 mice with abatacept treatment.

Our study has several limitations that deserve consideration. Liver involvement is a classical feature of preclinical and human cGvHD but is not usually affected in SSc. We used ALT/AST serum levels only to assess liver involvement, without complementary histologic evaluation. The merit of a cell-counting method on lesional tissue may appear less consistent than cell quantification performed by flow cytometry. However, we have developed a robust proficiency with this automated counting method, which was performed by two experienced independent investigators [5, 8, 19]. Lung compliance was not directly measured, but was indirectly reflected by the evaluation of FRC. It is also noteworthy that the impact of abatacept on survival in both mouse models has not been assessed.

Conclusions

Taken together, our findings demonstrate how the inhibition of proinflammatory T-cell function, along with effects on macrophages (Additional file 5), yields significant therapeutic benefits in models of SSc organ damage. T-cell costimulation blockade might be therapeutically exploited to treat SSc patients with visceral organ involvement. The benefit of this strategy should

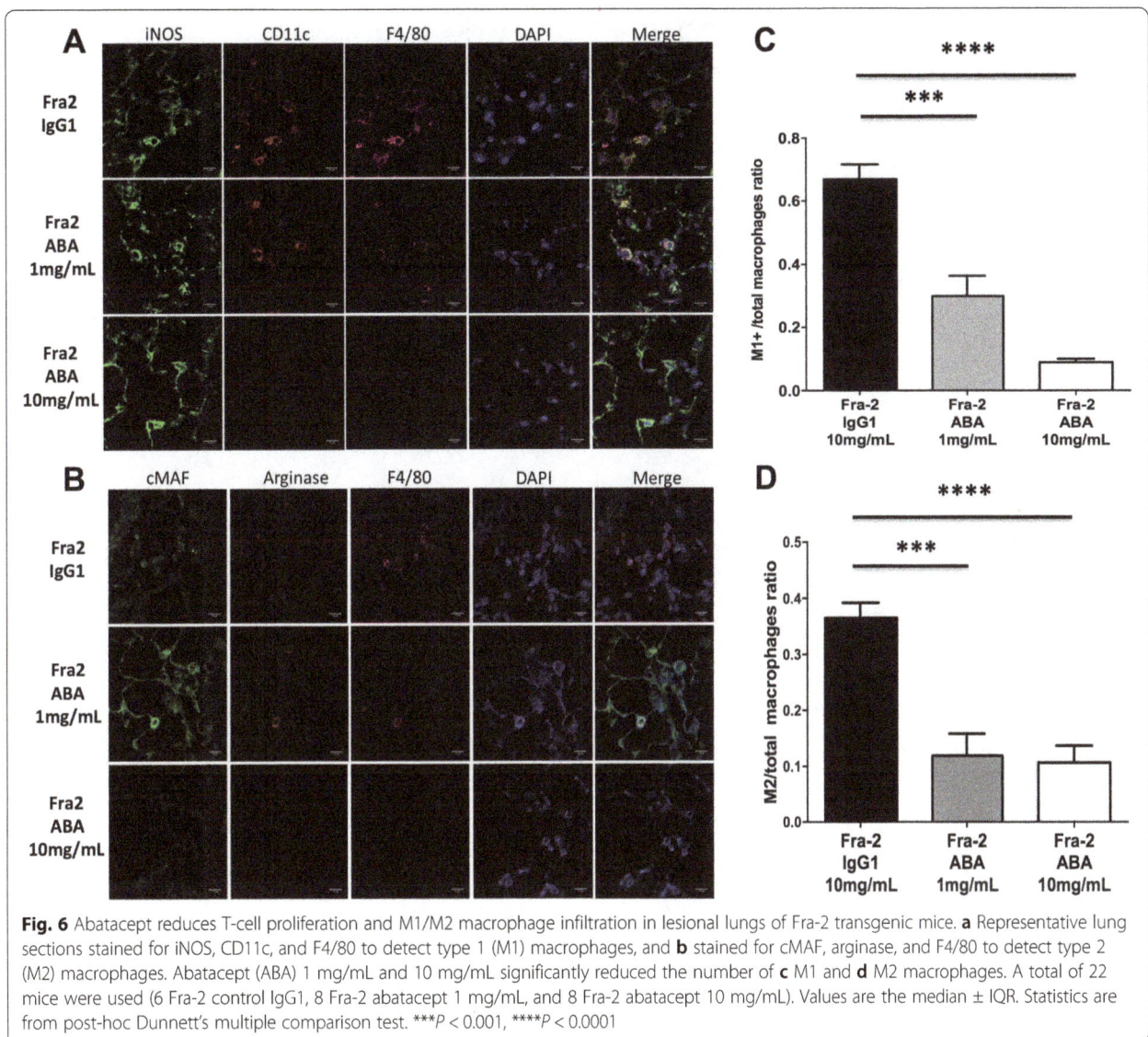

Fig. 6 Abatacept reduces T-cell proliferation and M1/M2 macrophage infiltration in lesional lungs of Fra-2 transgenic mice. **a** Representative lung sections stained for iNOS, CD11c, and F4/80 to detect type 1 (M1) macrophages, and **b** stained for cMAF, arginase, and F4/80 to detect type 2 (M2) macrophages. Abatacept (ABA) 1 mg/mL and 10 mg/mL significantly reduced the number of **c** M1 and **d** M2 macrophages. A total of 22 mice were used (6 Fra-2 control IgG1, 8 Fra-2 abatacept 1 mg/mL, and 8 Fra-2 abatacept 10 mg/mL). Values are the median ± IQR. Statistics are from post-hoc Dunnett's multiple comparison test. ***$P < 0.001$, ****$P < 0.0001$

be further compared with classical immunosuppressive approaches and emerging direct antifibrotic therapies. There is a strong rationale to evaluate T cell-targeting strategies in SSc given the importance of T cells in the early and inflammatory stages of the disease and accumulating preclinical evidence of a beneficial effects of targeted immunotherapy targeting T-cell costimulatory pathways, including OX40L, DNAM-1, or CTLA-4 [5, 8, 40]. In addition, a therapeutic approach for T cell-mediated diseases would target antigen-specific T cells involved in the disease, without leading to generalized immunosuppression. As a drug already in clinical use, and given its favorable safety profile in this study and in rheumatic patients, abatacept may be more translationally relevant than other means for targeting T cells currently being explored for the treatment of SSc.

Additional files

Additional file 1: Abatacept prevents cGvHD-associated liver involvement. Serum alanine aminotransferase (ALT) (A) and serum aspartate aminotransferase (AST) (B) levels were substantially reduced in the serum of abatacept-treated cGvHD mice compared with control IgG1-treated cGvHD mice. A total of 32 mice were used (12 allogeneic control IgG1-treated mice, 12 abatacept 1 mg/mL-treated mice, and 8 control syngeneic BALB/c mice). Values are the median ± IQR. Statistics are from post-hoc Dunnett's multiple comparison test. *$P < 0.05$, **$P < 0.01$. ALLO allogeneic, cGvHD chronic graft-versus-host disease, SYN syngeneic.

Additional file 2: Abatacept alleviates gut involvement in experimental cGvHD. Representative images of inflammatory cell infiltration in lesional colon sections assessed by immunohistochemistry for CD45 (A). Increased submucosal CD45+ cell infiltration was detected in IgG1-treated cGvHD mice (A and B). CD45+ cell infiltration was markedly reduced in allogeneic cGvHD mice receiving abatacept (A and B). Representative images of cell death evaluation in lesional colon sections assessed by immunohistochemistry for Annexin-V (C). Cell death was prominent in

IgG1-treated allogeneic cGvHD mice and was markedly reduced upon treatment with abatacept (C and D). A total of 32 mice were used (12 allogeneic control IgG1-treated mice, 12 abatacept 1 mg/mL-treated mice, and 8 control syngeneic BALB/c mice). Values are the median ± IQR. Statistics are from post-hoc Dunnett's multiple comparison test. *$P < 0.05$, **$P < 0.01$, ****$P < 0.0001$. ALLO allogeneic, cGvHD chronic graft-versus-host disease, SYN syngeneic.

Additional file 3: Abatacept alleviates lung fibrosis in the Fra-2 mouse model. Representative images of second harmonic generation (SHG) performed to evaluate the accumulation of fibrillar collagen (A). SHG showed fibrillar collagen in Fra-2 mice treated with IgG1 (in pink), but not in mice receiving abatacept 10 mg/mL (A and B). Scale bar = 50 µm. Second harmonic scores were higher in Fra-2 mice receiving IgG1 or abatacept 1 mg/mL compared with Fra-2 mice treated by abatacept 10 mg/mL. A total of 27 mice were used (5 C57BL/6 mice, 6 Fra-2 control IgG1, 8 Fra-2 abatacept 1 mg/mL, and 8 Fra-2 abatacept 10 mg/mL). Values are the median ± IQR. Statistics are from post-hoc Dunnett's multiple comparison test. *$P < 0.05$.

Additional file 4: Abatacept decreases levels of fibrogenic markers in lesional lungs of Fra-2 transgenic mice. Protein levels of MCP1 (A) and osteopontin (OPN) (B) were markedly reduced on treatment with abatacept 10 mg/mL. Protein levels of TGF-β (C) were significantly reduced on treatment with 1 mg/mL and 10 mg/mL abatacept compared with control IgG1-treated mice in lesional lungs of Fra-2 transgenic mice. A trend was observed for decreased concentrations of TIMP1 (D) in abatacept-treated mice. A total of 27 mice were used (5 C57BL/6 mice, 6 Fra-2 control IgG1, 8 Fra-2 abatacept 1 mg/mL, and 8 Fra-2 abatacept 10 mg/mL). Values are the median ± IQR. Statistics are from post-hoc Dunnett's multiple comparison test. *$P < 0.05$.

Additional file 5: Abatacept alleviates inflammation-driven fibrosis by suppressing the immune response. Schematic cartoon of the mechanism of action of abatacept in systemic sclerosis (SSc) based on results presented in this study and previously published results in skin fibrosis [5]. In the early stages of SSc, T cells are activated through their TCR and receive costimulation via CD28 from CD80/CD86-expressing antigen-presenting cells. The full activation of T cells enhances the activation of dermal/lung fibroblasts through the action of proinflammatory and/or profibrotic cytokines (IL-6, IL-10). This also involves the proinflammatory action of macrophages. During abatacept treatment, the drug blocks CD80/CD86-mediated costimulation by macrophages and B cells, leading to inhibition of T-cell activation, proliferation, and/or infiltration. The effects on macrophages lead to lower maturation and infiltration. B-cell infiltration is also reduced. As a consequence of the effect on T cells, B cells, and macrophages, the progression of dermal, lung, and vessel fibrosis is blocked.

Abbreviations
ALT: Alanine aminotransferase; AST: Aspartate aminotransferase; cGvHD: Chronic graft-versus-host disease; CT: Computed tomography; CTLA: Cytotoxic T lymphocyte-associated molecule; FRC: Functional residual capacity; ILD: Interstitial lung disease; MCP: Monocyte chemoattractant protein; OPN: Osteopontin; PH: Pulmonary hypertension; RVH: Right ventricular hypertrophy; RVSP: Right ventricular systolic pressure; SHG: Second harmonic generation; SSc: Systemic sclerosis; TGF: Transforming growth factor; TPEF: Two-photon excited fluorescence

Acknowledgements
We thank M. Andrieu (cytometry and immunobiology facility), M. Favier (morphology and histology facility), and P. Bourdoncle (cellular imaging: confocal microscopy facility) of the Institut Cochin, Paris, France, and Prof. Catherine Chaussain, EA2496, Université Paris Descartes, Faculté de Chirurgie Dentaire, Montrouge, France.

Funding
The study drug was supplied by Bristol-Myers Squibb, Co. Bristol-Myers Squibb was not involved in the study design, data acquisition, data analysis, or writing of the manuscript.

Authors' contributions
JA and YA designed the study. GB, JA, CG, LT, SP, JS, AC, and CN conducted all experiments. GB, JA, CG, SP, JS, AC, and YA analyzed the data generated. GB, JA, CG, SP, JS, AC, FB, and YA wrote/drafted and revisited the manuscript. GB, YA, CG, LT, JS, CN, SP, AC, FB, and JA gave the final approval for the manuscript. All authors read and approved the final manuscript.

Consent for publication
Not applicable.

Competing interests
JA has had a consultancy relationship and/or has received research funding for the treatment of systemic sclerosis from Actelion, Roche, Pfizer, and Bristol-Myers Squibb. YA has had a consultancy relationship and/or has received research funding for the treatment of systemic sclerosis from Actelion, Bayer, Biogen Idec, Bristol-Myers Squibb, Genentech/Roche, Inventiva, Medac, Pfizer, Sanofi Genzyme, Servier, and UCB. The remaining authors declare that they have no competing interests.

Author details
Université Paris Descartes, Sorbonne Paris Cité, INSERM U1016, Institut Cochin, CNRS UMR8104, Paris, France. [2]Université Paris Descartes, Sorbonne Paris Cité, Service de Rhumatologie A, Hôpital Cochin, 27 rue du Faubourg Saint Jacques, 75014 Paris, France. [3]INSERM UMR_S 999, Le Plessis-Robinson, France. [4]Université Paris-Sud, Université Paris-Saclay, Le Kremlin-Bicêtre, France. [5]EA 2496 Pathologie, Imagerie et Biothérapies Orofaciales, UFR Odontologie, Université Paris Descartes and PIDV, PRES Sorbonne Paris Cité, Montrouge, France. [6]Clinical Chemistry Laboratory, Cochin and Hôtel-Dieu Hospitals, Paris, France.

References
1. Elhai M, Meune C, Boubaya M, Avouac J, Hachulla E, Balbir-Gurman A, et al. Mapping and predicting mortality from systemic sclerosis. Ann Rheum Dis. 2017;76(11):1897–905.
2. Varga J, Pasche B. Transforming growth factor beta as a therapeutic target in systemic sclerosis. Nat Rev Rheumatol. 2009;5(4):200–6.
3. Gu YS, Kong J, Cheema GS, Keen CL, Wick G, Gershwin ME. The immunobiology of systemic sclerosis. Semin Arthritis Rheum. 2008;38(2):132–60.
4. Carreno BM, Bennett F, Chau TA, Ling V, Luxenberg D, Jussif J, et al. CTLA-4 (CD152) can inhibit T cell activation by two different mechanisms depending on its level of cell surface expression. J Immunol. 2000;165(3):1352–6.
5. Ponsoye M, Frantz C, Ruzehaji N, Nicco C, Elhai M, Ruiz B, et al. Treatment with abatacept prevents experimental dermal fibrosis and induces regression of established inflammation-driven fibrosis. Ann Rheum Dis. 2016;75:2142–9.
6. Elhai M, Meunier M, Matucci-Cerinic M, Maurer B, Riemekasten G, Leturcq T, et al. Outcomes of patients with systemic sclerosis-associated polyarthritis and myopathy treated with tocilizumab or abatacept: a EUSTAR observational study. Ann Rheum Dis. 2013;72(7):1217–20.
7. Chakravarty EF, Martyanov V, Fiorentino D, Wood TA, Haddon DJ, Jarrell JA, et al. Gene expression changes reflect clinical response in a placebo-controlled randomized trial of abatacept in patients with diffuse cutaneous systemic sclerosis. Arthritis Res Ther. 2015;17:159.
8. Elhai M, Avouac J, Hoffmann-Vold AM, Ruzehaji N, Amiar O, Ruiz B, et al. OX40L blockade protects against inflammation-driven fibrosis. Proc Natl Acad Sci U S A. 2016;113(27):E3901–10.
9. Avouac J, Guignabert C, Hoffmann-Vold AM, Ruiz B, Dorfmuller P, Pezet S, et al. Role of Stromelysin 2 (matrix metalloproteinase 10) as a novel mediator of vascular remodeling underlying pulmonary hypertension associated with systemic sclerosis. Arthritis Rheum. 2017;69(11):2209–21.
10. Yue D, Brintnell W, Mannik LA, Christie DA, Haeryfar SM, Madrenas J, et al. CTLA-4Ig blocks the development and progression of citrullinated fibrinogen-induced arthritis in DR4-transgenic mice. Arthritis Rheum. 2010;62(10):2941–52.

11. Kavian N, Marut W, Servettaz A, Laude H, Nicco C, Chereau C, et al. Arsenic trioxide prevents murine sclerodermatous graft-versus-host disease. J Immunol. 2012;188(10):5142–9.

12. Morin F, Kavian N, Marut W, Chereau C, Cerles O, Grange P, et al. Inhibition of EGFR tyrosine kinase by erlotinib prevents sclerodermatous graft-versus-host disease in a mouse model. J Invest Dermatol. 2015;135(10):2385–93.

13. Blazar BR, Taylor PA, Linsley PS, Vallera DA. In vivo blockade of CD28/CTLA4: B7/BB1 interaction with CTLA4-Ig reduces lethal murine graft-versus-host disease across the major histocompatibility complex barrier in mice. Blood. 1994;83(12):3815–25.

14. Blazar BR, Taylor PA, Panoskaltsis-Mortari A, Yagita H, Bromberg JS, Vallera DA. A critical role for CD48 antigen in regulating alloengraftment and lymphohematopoietic recovery after bone marrow transplantation. Blood. 1998;92(11):4453–63.

15. Maurer B, Busch N, Jungel A, Pileckyte M, Gay RE, Michel BA, et al. Transcription factor fos-related antigen-2 induces progressive peripheral vasculopathy in mice closely resembling human systemic sclerosis. Circulation. 2009;120(23):2367–76.

16. Eferl R, Hasselblatt P, Rath M, Popper H, Zenz R, Komnenovic V, et al. Development of pulmonary fibrosis through a pathway involving the transcription factor Fra-2/AP-1. Proc Natl Acad Sci U S A. 2008;105(30): 10525–30.

17. Maurer B, Reich N, Juengel A, Kriegsmann J, Gay RE, Schett G, et al. Fra-2 transgenic mice as a novel model of pulmonary hypertension associated with systemic sclerosis. Ann Rheum Dis. 2012;71(8):1382–7.

18. Maurer B, Distler JH, Distler O. The Fra-2 transgenic mouse model of systemic sclerosis. Vasc Pharmacol. 2013;58(3):194–201.

19. Avouac J, Konstantinova I, Guignabert C, Pezet S, Sadoine J, Guilbert T, et al. Pan-PPAR agonist IVA337 is effective in experimental lung fibrosis and pulmonary hypertension. Ann Rheum Dis. 2017;76(11):1931–40.

20. Ashcroft T, Simpson JM, Timbrell V. Simple method of estimating severity of pulmonary fibrosis on a numerical scale. J Clin Pathol. 1988;41(4):467–70.

21. Distler JH, Akhmetshina A, Schett G, Distler O. Monocyte chemoattractant proteins in the pathogenesis of systemic sclerosis. Rheumatology (Oxford). 2009;48(2):98–103.

22. Frost J, Ramsay M, Mia R, Moosa L, Musenge E, Tikly M. Differential gene expression of MMP-1, TIMP-1 and HGF in clinically involved and uninvolved skin in South Africans with SSc. Rheumatology (Oxford). 2012;51(6):1049–52.

23. Wu M, Schneider DJ, Mayes MD, Assassi S, Arnett FC, Tan FK, et al. Osteopontin in systemic sclerosis and its role in dermal fibrosis. J Invest Dermatol. 2012;132(6):1605–14.

24. Barros MH, Hauck F, Dreyer JH, Kempkes B, Niedobitek G. Macrophage polarisation: an immunohistochemical approach for identifying M1 and M2 macrophages. PLoS One. 2013;8(11):e80908.

25. Avouac J, Palumbo K, Tomcik M, Zerr P, Dees C, Horn A, et al. Inhibition of activator protein 1 signaling abrogates transforming growth factor beta-mediated activation of fibroblasts and prevents experimental fibrosis. Arthritis Rheum. 2012;64(5):1642–52.

26. Guignabert C, Alvira CM, Alastalo TP, Sawada H, Hansmann G, Zhao M, et al. Tie2-mediated loss of peroxisome proliferator-activated receptor-gamma in mice causes PDGF receptor-beta-dependent pulmonary arterial muscularization. Am J Physiol Lung Cell Mol Physiol. 2009;297(6):L1082–90.

27. Ricard N, Tu L, Le Hiress M, Huertas A, Phan C, Thuillet R, et al. Increased pericyte coverage mediated by endothelial-derived fibroblast growth factor-2 and interleukin-6 is a source of smooth muscle-like cells in pulmonary hypertension. Circulation. 2014;129(15):1586–97.

28. Huertas A, Tu L, Thuillet R, Le Hiress M, Phan C, Ricard N, et al. Leptin signalling system as a target for pulmonary arterial hypertension therapy. Eur Respir J. 2015;45(4):1066–80.

29. Le Hiress M, Tu L, Ricard N, Phan C, Thuillet R, Fadel E, et al. Proinflammatory signature of the dysfunctional endothelium in pulmonary hypertension. Role of the macrophage migration inhibitory factor/CD74 complex. Am J Respir Crit Care Med. 2015;192(8):983–97.

30. Soare A, Ramming A, Avouac J, Distler J. Updates on animal models of systemic sclerosis. J Scleroderma Relat Disord. 2016;1(3):266–76.

31. Beyer C, Schett G, Distler O, Distler JH. Animal models of systemic sclerosis: prospects and limitations. Arthritis Rheum. 2010;62(10):2831–44.

32. Claman HN, Jaffee BD, Huff JC, Clark RA. Chronic graft-versus-host disease as a model for scleroderma. II. Mast cell depletion with deposition of immunoglobulins in the skin and fibrosis. Cell Immunol. 1985;94(1):73–84.

33. Via CS, Rus V, Nguyen P, Linsley P, Gause WC. Differential effect of CTLA4Ig on murine graft-versus-host disease (GVHD) development: CTLA4Ig prevents both acute and chronic GVHD development but reverses only chronic GVHD. J Immunol. 1996;157(9):4258–67.

34. Israel-Assayag E, Fournier M, Cormier Y. Blockade of T cell costimulation by CTLA4-Ig inhibits lung inflammation in murine hypersensitivity pneumonitis. J Immunol. 1999;163(12):6794–9.

35. Wang H, Kwak D, Fassett J, Hou L, Xu X, Burbach BJ, et al. CD28/B7 deficiency attenuates systolic overload-induced congestive heart failure, myocardial and pulmonary inflammation, and activated T cell accumulation in the heart and lungs. Hypertension. 2016;68(3):688–96.

36. Kallikourdis M, Martini E, Carullo P, Sardi C, Roselli G, Greco CM, et al. T cell costimulation blockade blunts pressure overload-induced heart failure. Nat Commun. 2017;8:14680.

37. Eisenberg RA, Via CS. T cells, murine chronic graft-versus-host disease and autoimmunity. J Autoimmun. 2012;39(3):240–7.

38. Wenink MH, Santegoets KC, Platt AM, van den Berg WB, van Riel PL, Garside P, et al. Abatacept modulates proinflammatory macrophage responses upon cytokine-activated T cell and toll-like receptor ligand stimulation. Ann Rheum Dis. 2012;71(1):80–3.

39. Davis PM, Nadler SG, Stetsko DK, Suchard SJ. Abatacept modulates human dendritic cell-stimulated T-cell proliferation and effector function independent of IDO induction. Clin Immunol. 2008;126(1):38–47.

40. Avouac J, Elhai M, Tomcik M, Ruiz B, Friese M, Piedavent M, et al. Critical role of the adhesion receptor DNAX accessory molecule-1 (DNAM-1) in the development of inflammation-driven dermal fibrosis in a mouse model of systemic sclerosis. Ann Rheum Dis. 2013;72(6):1089–98.

17

Downregulation of miRNA17–92 cluster marks Vγ9Vδ2 T cells from patients with rheumatoid arthritis

Giuliana Guggino[1], Valentina Orlando[2], Laura Saieva[3], Piero Ruscitti[4], Paola Cipriani[4], Marco Pio La Manna[2], Roberto Giacomelli[4], Riccardo Alessandro[3], Giovanni Triolo[1], Francesco Ciccia[1], Francesco Dieli[2,3] and Nadia Caccamo[2,3]* (iD)

Abstract

Background: We aimed to evaluate the phenotype, function, and microRNA (miRNA)17–92 cluster expression in Vγ9Vδ2 T-cell subsets and the correlation with immune response in rheumatoid arthritis (RA) patients.

Methods: Peripheral blood from 10 early RA untreated patients and 10 healthy donors (HD) was obtained. Polyclonal Vγ9Vδ2 T-cell lines were generated and analysed by flow cytometry. Analysis of miRNA17–92 cluster expression was performed by real-time polymerase chain reaction (RT-PCR), and expression of mRNA target genes was also studied.

Results: A remarkable change in the distribution of Vγ9Vδ2 T-cell functional subsets was observed in the peripheral blood of RA patients compared with HD, with an expansion of effector subsets and reduction of naive cells which was accompanied by modifications in proinflammatory cytokine expression. Vγ9Vδ2 T cells with a T_{EM} (effector memory) phenotype and producing proinflammatory cytokines were correlated with disease activity score (DAS28). The comparison of miRNA expression among Vγ9Vδ2 T-cell subsets from RA patients and HD showed a lower level of miR-106a-5p and miR-20a-5p, and a higher level of miR-21a-5p, among Vγ9Vδ2 T_{EM} cells, and a lower level of miR-19b-3p among Vγ9Vδ2 T_{CM} (central memory) cells was also found. These differentially expressed miRNAs correlated with higher levels of expression of interleukin (IL)-8, IL-6, and PDCD4 genes.

Conclusions: Our results provide evidence for a role of miR-106a, miR-19-3p, miR-20a, and miR-21a in the regulation of Vγ9Vδ2 T-cell function in RA patients and suggest the possibility that the miRNA17–92 family and Vγ9Vδ2 T cells contribute to the pathogenesis of RA.

Keywords: γδ T cells, Rheumatoid arthritis, Inflammatory cytokines, miRNA17–92

Background

MicroRNAs (miRNAs) are non-coding RNAs (ncRNAs) of around 22 nucleotides in length which play significant roles in regulating gene expression [1, 2]. The miRNA17–92 family is a well-known miRNA cluster involved in health and disease [3] which has long been considered only for its oncogenic role, being in fact known as the first 'oncomir' [4]. Several studies have demonstrated a role for this cluster in normal development, immune disease, cardiovascular disease, and many age-related conditions [4]. The cluster is able to maintain a homeostatic setting under physiological conditions essential for the control of inflammatory reactions. Therefore, abnormal expression of this miRNA has been related to several immune disease such as rheumatoid arthritis (RA), and altered miRNA production/expression has been involved in RA pathogenesis [5].

* Correspondence: nadia.caccamo@unipa.it
Giuliana Guggino and Valentina Orlando contributed equally to this work.
Francesco Dieli and Nadia Caccamo are joint senior authors on this work.
[2]Central Laboratory of Advanced Diagnosis and Biomedical Research (CLADIBIOR), Azienda Ospedaliera Universitaria Policlinico P. Giaccone, Palermo, Italy
[3]Dipartimento di Biopatologia e Biotecnologie Mediche, Università di Palermo, Palermo, Italy
Full list of author information is available at the end of the article

The miRNA17–92 cluster appears as a key factor in the inflammatory pathways activated during RA in synovial cells. It has been widely recognized that an abnormal activation of CD4$^+$ lymphocytes producing proinflammatory cytokines (i.e. interleukin (IL)-8, IL-6, IL-17, and tumour necrosis factor (TNF)-α) has a role in RA [6–8], but current studies have also shown that γδ T lymphocytes promote the onset and progression of RA [9]. RA patients show an imbalance between effector subsets (T helper (Th)1, Th17, and γδ T cells) and regulatory T (Treg) cells which likely determines an alteration of homeostasis and favouring a proinflammatory environment [10].

miRNA-mediated RNA interference is emerging as a crucial mechanism in the control of differentiation and function of several lymphocyte subsets, such as γδ T cells, but their specific roles remain to be addressed.

Although the differentiation into various effector subsets and functions of T lymphocytes have been extensively studied, the molecular mechanisms of the differentiation of T-cell subsets and the acquisition of effector function are not completely understood.

We were aimed to evaluate phenotype, effector functions, and miRNA17–92 expression in Vγ9Vδ2 T cells of RA patients compared with healthy donors (HD).

Methods

Patients

Heparinized peripheral blood from 10 RA patients (age 40 (range 28–50) years, two female, eight male) and 10 HD (age 43 (27–51) years, three female, seven male) was obtained for this study. Patients fulfilled the 1987 criteria of the American College of Rheumatology (ACR) for RA. All the patients, classified as having an early RA (ERA; disease duration 1.7 years (range 5 months to 2 years), were disease-modifying anti-rheumatic drug (DMARD; methotrexate, leflunomide)-naive and had not received prednisone or equivalent for at least 2 weeks before blood collection. Eight out of the 10 patients were anti-citrullinated protein antibody (ACPA)-positive. Increased levels of erythrocyte sedimentation rate (30.4 ± 15.7 mm/h) and C-reactive protein (0.69 ± 1.2 mg/dl) were also found in all patients. The study was approved by the Ethical Committee of the University Hospital in Palermo where the patients were recruited. Informed consent was signed by all participants.

γδ T cell identification

Peripheral blood mononuclear cells (PBMC) were obtained by density gradient centrifugation using Ficoll-Hypaque (Pharmacia Biotech, Uppsala, Sweden).

Fc receptor blocking was performed with human immunoglobulin (Sigma; 3 μg/ml final concentration) followed by surface staining with different fluorochrome-conjugated antibodies to study the phenotype and the cytokine production by Vγ9Vδ2 T cells.

The following fluorescein isothiocyanate (FITC)-, phycoerythrin (PE)-, PE-Cy5-, PE-Cy7-, allophycocyanin (APC)-, and APC-Cy7-conjugated anti-human monoclonal antibodies (mAbs) were used to characterise the Vγ9Vδ2 T-cell population: live/dead-FITC, anti-CD45-APCH7 (clone2D1), anti-CD3-PECy7 (clone SK7), anti-TCRVδ2-PE (clone B6), anti-CD27-APC (clone MT271), and anti-CD45RA peridinin chlorophyll protein (PerCP)-Cy5.5 (clone HI100). Expression of surface markers was determined by flow cytometry on a FACS-Canto II Flow Cytometer with the use of FlowJo software (BD Biosciences).

For the intracellular cytokine assay, PBMC (10^6/ml) were stimulated with ionomycin (Sigma, St. Louis, MO, USA; 1 μg/ml final concentration) and phorbolmyristate acetate (PMA; Sigma; 150 ng/ml final concentration). Cells were cultured in a humidified incubator at 37 °C with 5% CO_2 for 6 h in the presence of 5 μg/ml Brefeldin A (Sigma, St. Louis, MO, USA). Following incubation, PBMC were harvested, washed in phosphate-buffered saline (PBS) containing 1% fetal calf serum (FCS) and 0.1% sodium azide, and then stained as follows: live/dead-FITC, anti-CD45-APCH7 (clone 2D1), anti-CD3-PECy7 (clone SK7), anti-TCRVδ2-PE (clone B6), in incubation buffer (PBS, 1% FCS, 0.1% sodium azide) for 30 min at 4 °C.

Subsequently, PBMC were washed, fixed, and permeabilized (Cytofix/Cytoperm Kit, BD Pharmingen) according to the manufacturer's instructions and stained for intracellular cytokines with conjugated anti-IFN-γ-APC (clone 25723.11), anti-IL-8-APC (cloneE8N1), and anti-IL-6-APC (clone MQ2-13A5) mAbs. Isotype-matched control mAbs were used. All mAbs were obtained from BD (San Josè, CA, USA) except IL-8 (from Biolegend, San Diego, CA, USA). Cells were washed, fixed in 1% paraformaldehyde, and at least 1×10^6 lymphocytes were acquired using a FACSCanto II Flow Cytometer (BD Biosciences) after gating by forward (FSC) and side scatter (SSC) plots. FACS plots were analysed using FlowJo software (version 6.1.1; Tree Star, Ashland, OR, USA). Negative controls were obtained by staining PBMC in the absence of any stimulation. Cut-off values for a positive response were pre-determined to be in excess of 0.01% responsive cells. Results below this value were considered negative and set to zero [11]. Values found using isotype control mAbs were subtracted in all the samples analysed. The gating strategy used for the phenotype distribution of Vγ9Vδ2 T cells and for the evaluation of the intracellular cytokine content was made starting with the initial lymphocyte gate (SSC vs FSC), followed by gating on single cells, live/dead cells vs CD45, CD3 vs Vγ9Vδ2 T cells, followed by further surface or intracellular molecules.

Generation of γδ T-cell lines

Polyclonal Vγ9Vδ2 T-cell lines were generated by first enriching PBMC using a γδ T-cell isolation kit (Miltenyi Biotec, Bergisch Gladbach, Germany), followed by sorting single Vγ9Vδ2 T cells through a FACSAria I Cell Sorter (BD Biosciences) with specific mAbs. Sorted cells at the concentration of 2×10^4 were then cultured into each well of round-bottomed plates, containing 2×10^4 irradiated (40 Gy from a caesium source) allogeneic PBMC, plus zoledronic acid (2 μM) and 200 U/ml recombinant IL-2 (Proleukin, Novartis Pharma) [12]. Growing T-cell lines were expanded in 200 U/ml IL-2 and re-stimulated every 3 days. Cells were collected after 2 weeks and sorted according to their phenotype into four different subsets: naive (T_{naive}; CD45RA$^+$CD27$^+$), central memory (T_{CM}; CD45RA$^-$CD27$^+$), effector memory (T_{EM}; CD45RA$^-$CD27$^-$), and terminally differentiated effector memory (T_{EMRA}; CD45RA$^+$CD27$^-$).

RNA purification and miRNA expression analysis

For analysis of miRNA17–92 among total Vγ9Vδ2 T cells and the different cell subsets, total RNA containing miRNA was purified using an miRNeasy mini-kit (Qiagen). miRNA labelling, hybridization, scanning, and expression profiling was performed using miRCURY LNA microarray service (Exiqon).

Real-time polymerase chain reaction (RT-PCR) analysis of the whole population of Vγ9Vδ2 T cells

Total RNA was extracted from γδ T-cell lines derived from RA patients and HD with the miRNeasy Mini Kit (Qiagen) isolation kit according to the manufacturer's instructions. The quality of RNA was accessed with a Nano-Drop 1000 Spectrophotometer V3.7 (Thermo Scientific). The obtained RNA was subsequently used as a template for cDNA generation. For this purpose, a reverse transcription reaction was performed with miScript II RT Kit (Qiagen; 300 ng of RNA per reaction) following the manufacturer's protocol. The resulting cDNA was used to conduct an RT-PCR reaction with miScript SYBR Green PCR Kit (Qiagen) applying primers specific for hsa-miR-21a-5p, hsa-miRNA-hsa-miR-19a-3p, hsa-miR-19b-3p, hsa-miR-20a-5p, and hsa-miR-106a-5p (commercially available from QIAGEN) in a Rotor-Gene Q system. The expression level of RNU6 was used as an endogenous control.

RT-PCR was also performed to evaluate IL-8, IL-6, and programmed cell death 4 (PDCD4) mRNA using the commercially available Illustra RNAspin Mini Isolation Kit (GE Healthcare, Little Chalfont, Buckinghamshire, UK) according to the manufacturer's instructions. For quantitative TaqMan RT-PCR, master mix and TaqMan gene expression assays for *GAPDH* (glyceraldehyde 3-phosphate dehydrogenase, Hs99999905_m1) control and target genes were obtained from Applied Biosystems. Samples were run in duplicate using the Step-One Real-Time PCR system (Applied Biosystems, Foster City, CA, USA). Relative changes in gene expression between paired patients before and after treatment were determined using the $\Delta\Delta C_t$ method. Levels of the target transcript were normalized to a GAPDH endogenous control constantly expressed in both groups (ΔC_t). For $\Delta\Delta C_t$ values, additional subtractions were performed between untreated and treated samples ΔC_t values. Final values were expressed as fold of induction (FOI).

Statistical analysis

miRNA microarray data were analysed by miRCURY LNA microarray service (Exiqon). Data were normalized using the non-parametric regression method, LOESS. Unsupervised two-way clustering of miRNAs and samples was performed on $\log_2$ (Hy3/Hy5) ratios (with each sample versus the common reference pool) to produce a heat map. Heat map expression data were displayed using Gene-E software developed by Joshua Gould (http://www.broadinstitute.org/cancer/software/GENE-E). Hierarchical clustering using one minus Pearson's correlation was applied to samples and genes/miRNAs. Global or relative map colours were applied using the minimum and maximum values in the data. Network analysis to identify miRNA targets using gene and miRNA expression data was performed using MIR@NT@N [13].

Obtained C_t values were used to calculate expression levels of tested miRNAs with the $2^{\Delta\Delta Ct}$ method in two groups, each composed of HD and RA patients. To assess the statistical significance of observed differences, independent student t tests and Mann Whitney tests were performed on all groups and p values *$p \leq 0.05$, **$p \leq 0.01$, and ***$p \leq 0.001$ were considered as significant, very significant, and extremely significant, respectively.

The normal distribution of the data was assessed by a Shapiro-Wilk normality test. Analysis of variance (ANOVA) was performed as part of the data analysis, and these data are reported as a heat map.

Results

Skewed distribution of circulating Vγ9Vδ2 T cells in RA patients

Although the mean frequency of peripheral blood Vγ9Vδ2 T cells was similar in RA patients and HD (Fig. 1a), a remarkable change in their phenotype distribution was observed. T_{EMRA} and T_{CM} cells were the major Vγ9Vδ2 T-cell subset in the peripheral blood of RA patients, while T_{naive} and T_{CM} cells were the dominant

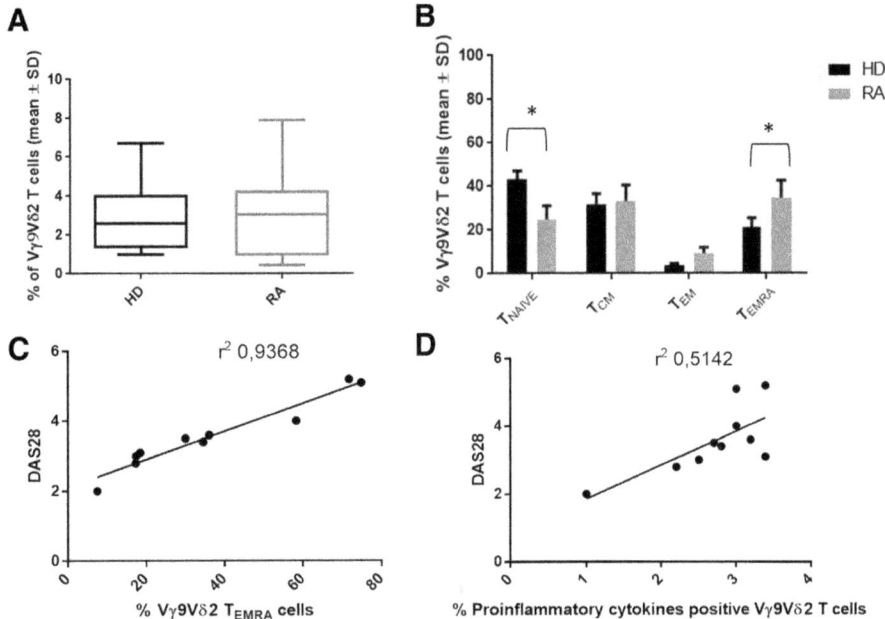

Fig. 1 Percentage and phenotype distribution of Vγ9Vδ2 T cells in rheumatoid arthritis (RA) patients and healthy donors (HD) and correlation of T terminally differentiated effector memory (T_{EMRA}) cells and cytokines production with activity disease score (DAS) in RA patients. **a** Percentage of Vγ9Vδ2 T cells evaluated in peripheral blood of HD (black box) and RA patients (grey box). **b** Phenotype distribution of Vγ9Vδ2 T cells in HD (black column) and RA patients (grey column). *$p < 0.05$. **c** Correlation between DAS28 activity scores and the percentage of Vγ9Vδ2 T_{EMRA} cells. **d** Correlation between DAS28 activity scores and the percentage of Vγ9Vδ2 T cells expressing proinflammatory cytokines. T_{CM} T central memory, T_{EM} T effector memory, T_{naive} T naive

populations in HD; other Vγ9Vδ2 T-cell subsets were poorly represented in both patients and controls (Fig. 1b). Moreover, we found a statistically significant decrease in T_{naive} and an increase in T_{EMRA} cells when RA patients were compared with HD (Fig. 1b). Most notably, in RA patients the DAS28 activity scores was directly correlated with the percentage of Vγ9Vδ2 T cells with a T_{EMRA} phenotype (Fig. 1c) and expressing the proinflammatory cytokines interferon (IFN)-γ, IL-6, and IL-8 (Fig. 1d).

We then analysed the ability of Vγ9Vδ2 T cells to produce proinflammatory cytokines, such as IFN-γ, IL-6, and IL-8, by intracellular FACS analysis ex vivo and after short-term in-vitro stimulation with ionomycin and PMA. The left hand panels in Fig. 2 show the gating strategy used to select Vγ9Vδ2 T cells and the sequential gating on lymphocytes, single live cells, live/dead cells/ CD45[+] and CD3[+] cells vs Vγ9Vδ2 T cells. Figure 2a and b show representative intracellular FACS analysis of Vγ9Vδ2 T cells producing IFN-γ, IL-6, and IL-8 in one representative RA patient ex vivo and after ionomycin and PMA stimulation, while Fig. 2c and d show a representative HD ex vivo and after ionomycin and PMA stimulation.

Figure 2e shows that the percentage of Vγ9Vδ2 T-cell response for the production of total proinflammatory

cytokines (IFN-γ, IL-6, and IL-8) in RA patients was significantly elevated compared with HD. Figure 2f and g show the cumulative mean percentage of each cytokine-producing Vγ9Vδ2 T cells in 10 RA patients and 10 HD ex vivo and after stimulation with ionomycin and PMA, respectively.

Expression of miRNA17–92 in Vγ9Vδ2 T-cell subsets

Vγ9Vδ2 T-cell lines were obtained from RA patients and HD after two weeks of in-vitro culture and were used either as a total population or were further sorted into different naive, memory, and effector subsets for miRNA17–92 expression analysis. Figure 3 shows the heat map of the miRNA expression profile for five RA patients and five HD. When comparing the groups within 'group' using a one-way ANOVA, five miRNAs were found to be differentially expressed using a cut-off p value < 0.05.

miRNA levels were evaluated as the fold increase or decrease comparing RA patients with HD in the four subsets of Vγ9Vδ2 T cells, where they displayed different expression levels: T_{EM} cells showed lower levels of miR-106a-5p and miR-20a-5p and higher level of miR-21a-5p, while significantly lower levels of miR-19 were found in T_{CM} and T_{EMRA} cells (Fig. 4a). Figure 4a

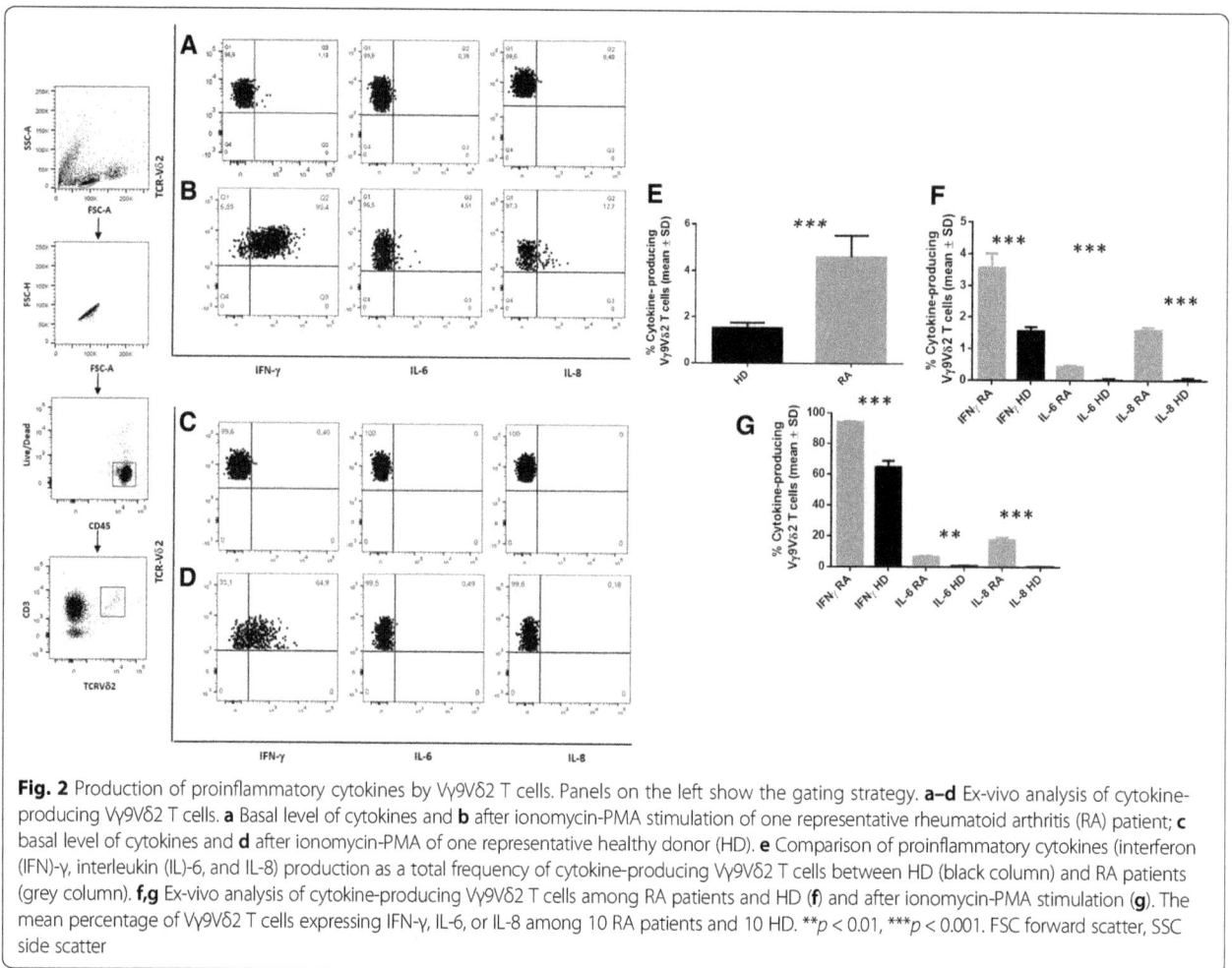

Fig. 2 Production of proinflammatory cytokines by Vγ9Vδ2 T cells. Panels on the left show the gating strategy. **a–d** Ex-vivo analysis of cytokine-producing Vγ9Vδ2 T cells. **a** Basal level of cytokines and **b** after ionomycin-PMA stimulation of one representative rheumatoid arthritis (RA) patient; **c** basal level of cytokines and **d** after ionomycin-PMA of one representative healthy donor (HD). **e** Comparison of proinflammatory cytokines (interferon (IFN)-γ, interleukin (IL)-6, and IL-8) production as a total frequency of cytokine-producing Vγ9Vδ2 T cells between HD (black column) and RA patients (grey column). **f,g** Ex-vivo analysis of cytokine-producing Vγ9Vδ2 T cells among RA patients and HD (**f**) and after ionomycin-PMA stimulation (**g**). The mean percentage of Vγ9Vδ2 T cells expressing IFN-γ, IL-6, or IL-8 among 10 RA patients and 10 HD. *******p* < 0.01, ********p* < 0.001. FSC forward scatter, SSC side scatter

and b show cumulative data from 10 RA patients and 10 HD in the different subsets (Fig. 4a) and in the total Vγ9Vδ2 T-cell population (Fig. 4b), respectively. We did not find any significant differences in miRNA expression in the T$_{naive}$ subset from RA patients and HD. All the other tested miRNAs did not show any significant modulation in all the samples studied (data not shown). The same trend of miRNA expression in selected subsets was also detected when analysing the total Vγ9Vδ2 T-cell population, indicating that the expression of these miRNAs could represent a specific signature of the whole Vγ9Vδ2 T lymphocyte compartment (Fig. 4b).

To further assess the accuracy of the miRNA signature of Vγ9Vδ2 T-cell lines as a determinant to discriminate between RA patients and HD, receiver operating characteristic (ROC) curves and cross-over plots were produced. As shown in Fig. 5a, the different miRNAs distinguish RA patients from HD, with the best accuracy for miR-106a (area under the curve (AUC) 0.95, *p* < 0.030, with 91.04% and 93.55% sensitivity and specificity, respectively).

Correlation of miRNA expression with cytokine and cell survival gene expression

Several miRNAs play a role in the regulation of cytokine gene expression and on the regulation of genes that are involved in cell survival. Therefore, we analysed if the different miRNA profiles found in patients with RA could be correlated with the expression of genes involved in the modulation of the immune response.

The comparison of the mRNA levels of the inflammatory cytokines IL-6, IL-8, and PDCD4 gene between RA patients and HD showed statistical significance in terms of fold increase in RA patients (Fig. 6a). Since IL-17 plays a (controversial) role in the pathogenesis of RA [14], we also evaluated IL-17 mRNA levels among γδ T cells, but we found that IL-17 mRNA levels were undetectable in γδ T cells from RA patients and HD (data not shown). Therefore, and considering the important role of miR-106a, miR-19a-3p, and miR-20a-5pin targeting IL-8 and IL-6 genes and the well-known over-expression of IL-6 and IL-8 in RA synovial tissue, we correlated the expression of IL-6, IL-8, and PDCD4

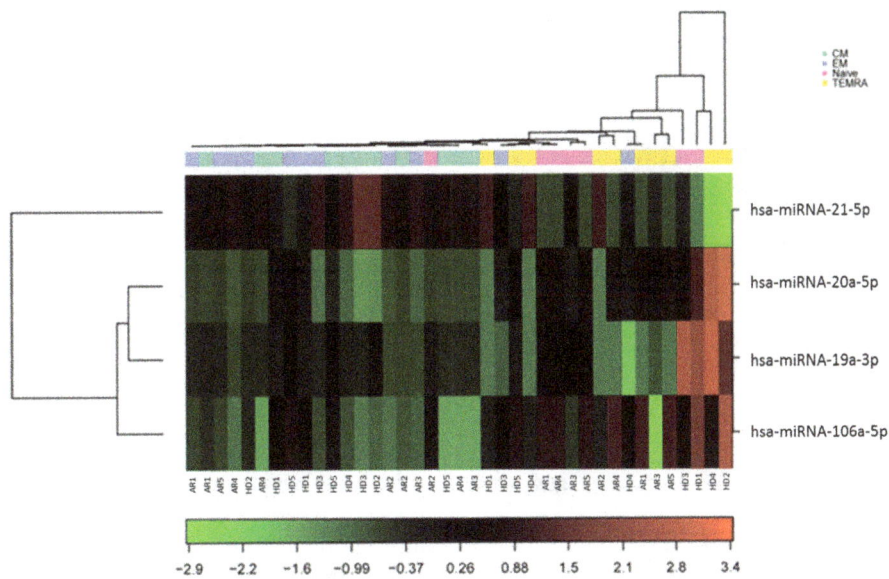

Fig. 3 Heat map of the different miRNA expression profiles for each RA patient and HD. The heat map diagram shows the result of the two-way hierarchical clustering of miRNAs in samples from five RA patients and five HD. Each row represents one miRNA, and each column represents one sample. The miRNA clustering tree is shown on the left. The colour scale shown at the bottom illustrates the relative expression level of an miRNA across all samples: red represents an expression level above mean, and green represents an expression lower than the mean. The clustering is performed on all samples, and miRNAs displayed are the large-magnitude changes that are also statistically significant on the five out of 19 miRNAs with the highest standard deviation. Normalized (dCq) values have been used for the analysis. CM central memory, EM effector memory, TEMRA T terminally differentiated effector memory

mRNA with these miRNAs and also with miR-19b-3p and miR-21a-5p that were found to be statistically significant in RA patients. Lower levels of miR-106a expression correlated with high levels of IL-8 mRNA in RA patients compared with controls (Fig. 6b), and lower levels of miR-19a-3p correlated with high levels of expression of IL-6 mRNA. An inverse correlation between the expression of miR-21a and the anti-apoptotic gene PDCD4 was also found in RA patients compared with HD (Fig. 6b). We did not find any significant correlation of the above cytokines and PDCD4 gene expression when comparing miR-19b-3p and miR-20a-5p (data not shown). Overall, these data highlight the role of miRNA in patients with RA in the production of inflammatory cytokines, and on the ability of Vγ9Vδ2 T cells to survive and display a potentially pathological role.

Discussion

The role of miRNA17–92 has been evaluated in different human immune cells such as B, T, and natural killer (NK) lymphocytes, macrophages, and dendritic cells, but its role in γδ T cells is not well understood. The aim of the present study was to investigate the different expression of members of the miRNA17–92 family among Vγ9Vδ2 T-cell subsets from healthy donors and patients with RA [15]. We found lower levels of miR-106a,

miR-19a, miR-19b, and miR-20a expression, and a higher level of miR-21a expression in RA patients compared with HD, either in the different subsets or in the total γδ T-cell population.

Vγ9Vδ2 T-cell subsets are characterized by distinct migratory routes and display different functional properties depending on the microenvironment due to their high plasticity [16–18].

The role of Vγ9Vδ2 T cells has been investigated under physiological and pathological conditions such as infections, autoimmunity, or cancer. Therefore, we aimed to evaluate the role of the miRNA17–92 cluster on Vγ9Vδ2 T-cell functions in RA patients to uncover a biosignature of disease. The analysis of the phenotypic distribution and functional properties of γδ T cells showed remarkable changes in RA patients. In fact, T_{EMRA} and T_{CM} cells were the predominant Vγ9Vδ2 T-cell subsets in the peripheral blood of RA patients and these cells represented a relevant source of proinflammatory cytokines.

The comparison between the levels of proinflammatory cytokines and Vγ9Vδ2 T cells with the T_{EMRA} phenotype correlated with the severity of the disease.

Different miRNA17–92 levels were expressed both in the total population and in the different subsets of the Vγ9Vδ2 T-cell population.

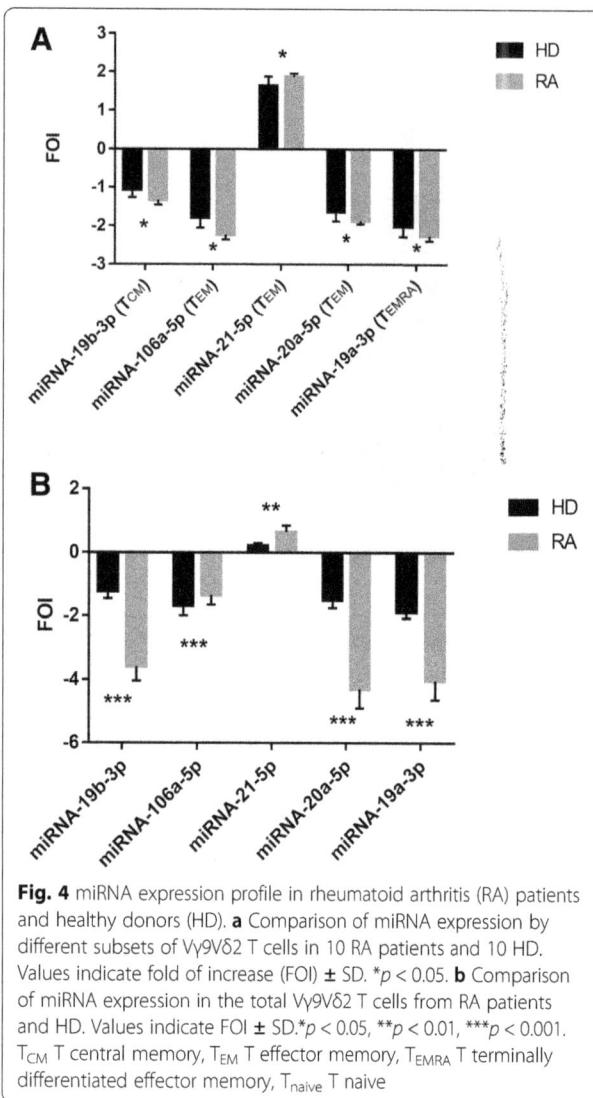

Fig. 4 miRNA expression profile in rheumatoid arthritis (RA) patients and healthy donors (HD). **a** Comparison of miRNA expression by different subsets of Vγ9Vδ2 T cells in 10 RA patients and 10 HD. Values indicate fold of increase (FOI) ± SD. *$p < 0.05$. **b** Comparison of miRNA expression in the total Vγ9Vδ2 T cells from RA patients and HD. Values indicate FOI ± SD.*$p < 0.05$, **$p < 0.01$, ***$p < 0.001$. T_{CM} T central memory, T_{EM} T effector memory, T_{EMRA} T terminally differentiated effector memory, T_{naive} T naive

Five out of 19 miRNAs displayed a large magnitude of change in RA patients. Therefore, to evaluate if the expression levels of these miRNAs could be considered as biomarkers of disease, we studied the accuracy by ROC curve analysis. The results demonstrated that the best performance was found for miR-106a, followed by miR-20a, miR-19a, miR-19b, and miR-21a.

Therefore, we correlated the IL-8 mRNA expression with miR-106, and IL6 mRNA levels with miR-19a levels to find direct evidence of the modulation of these two proinflammatory cytokines and their role in the contribution to inflammation and joint damage. Accordingly, lower levels of miR-19 in our RA patients correlated with the increase in IL-6, and this was in agreement with a previous study showing that treatment with IL-6 but not with TNF-α led to down-regulation of miRNA19 expression [19]. In-vitro studies have demonstrated that

IL-8 is a direct target of miR-106a, and an miR-106a inhibitor increases its production [20]. In the absence of miR-106a, fibroblast-like synoviocytes (FLS) from RA patients produce more IL-6 and IL-8, which contribute to inflammation and joint damage.

We have found that the lower levels of miR-106a, miR-20a, and miR-19 were accompanied by higher levels of miR-21a in RA patients.

We have found an inverse correlation of miR-21a levels with PDCD4 mRNA levels. The elevated levels of miR-21 could induce T-cell proliferation by negatively regulating PDCD4 gene expression [21], as observed in our RA patients, by causing the sustained production of proinflammatory cytokines by cells that upregulate the PDCD4 gene, which is correlated with a high survival rate. Since aberrant expression of miR-21 is related to increased susceptibility to immune-inflammatory disorders, an adequate expression of miR-21 might be critical for regulating normal immune responses. Evidence is now accumulating to support the therapeutic potential of miR-21 in autoimmune disorders.

Finally, the upregulation of miR-21 could be sustained by the contextual downregulation of miR-20a that could contribute to the lack of an anti-inflammatory property [22].

It has been demonstrated that higher levels of miR-21a occurs in all types of solid tumours, and additional studies showed elevated miR-21 expression also in leukaemias [23]. Interestingly, high levels of miR-21 may not only characterise cancer cells but also represent a common feature of cell stress as demonstrated by Xu et al. on the correlation between inflammation and cancer [24].

We do not know if the reduced expression of miR-20a could contribute to the lack of anti-inflammatory responses. miR-20a represses ASK1, a member of the kinase family that is activated in response to several stress signals, including lipopolysaccharide (LPS) or TNF-α. Activated ASK1, in turn, generates the production of reactive oxygen species (ROS) by a NADPH oxidase 4 (Nox4)-dependent mechanism, and consequently by decreasing the capacity of FLS to secrete IL-6 or matrix metalloproteinase (MMP)-3 [25].

Therefore, the decrease or increase in the tested miRNAs could impact at different stages of RA, with the production of proinflammatory cytokines and the maintenance of cells due to their high survival rate because of the negative regulation of PDCD4 altogether contributing to inflammation in RA patients.

It has been demonstrated that overexpression of miR-20a in human naive CD4+ T-helper cells inhibits TCR-mediated signalling and CD69 expression, and

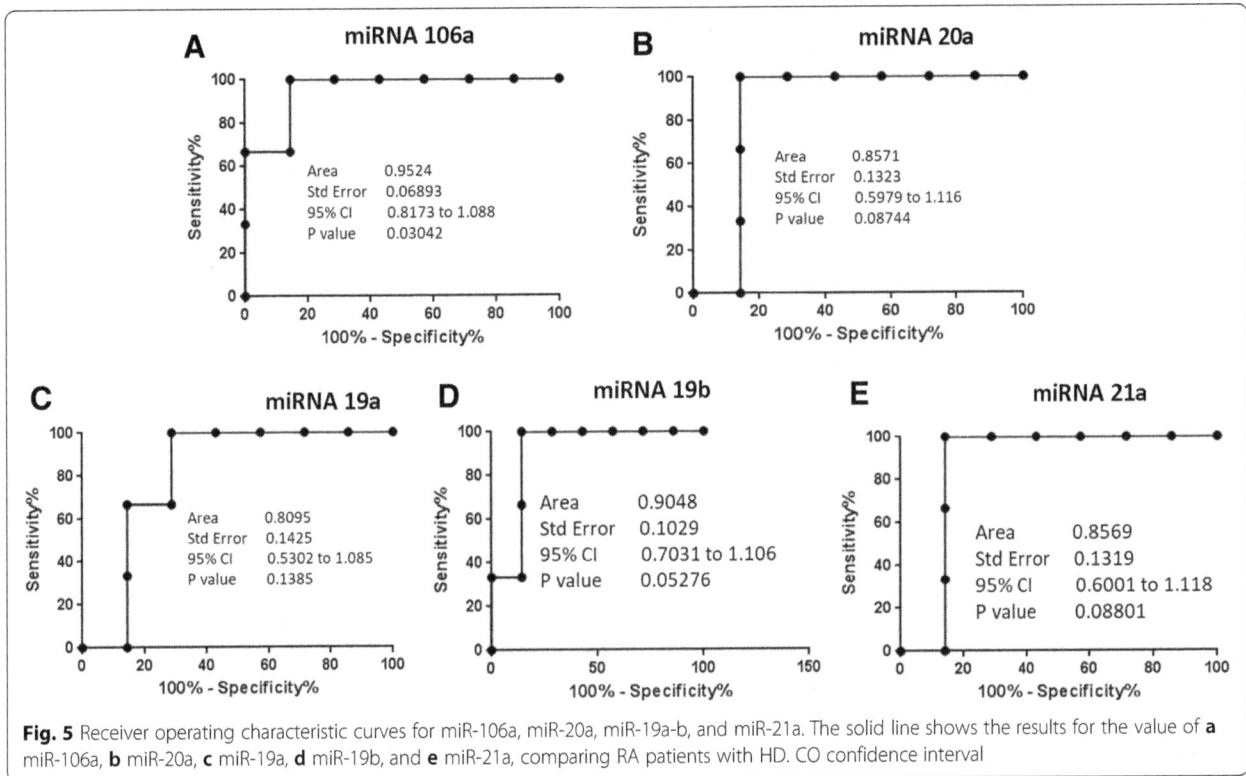

Fig. 5 Receiver operating characteristic curves for miR-106a, miR-20a, miR-19a-b, and miR-21a. The solid line shows the results for the value of **a** miR-106a, **b** miR-20a, **c** miR-19a, **d** miR-19b, and **e** miR-21a, comparing RA patients with HD. CO confidence interval

determines the decrease in production of cytokines such as IL-6 and IL-8 [22]. Therefore, we speculate that miR-20a could also be implicated in the control of proinflammatory cytokine production by γδ T cells.

Conclusions

Our results provide evidence for a role of miR-106a, miR-19a-b, miR-20a, and miR-21a in the regulation of Vγ9Vδ2 T-cell functions in RA patients and suggest the possibility that the miRNA17–92 family and γδ T cells

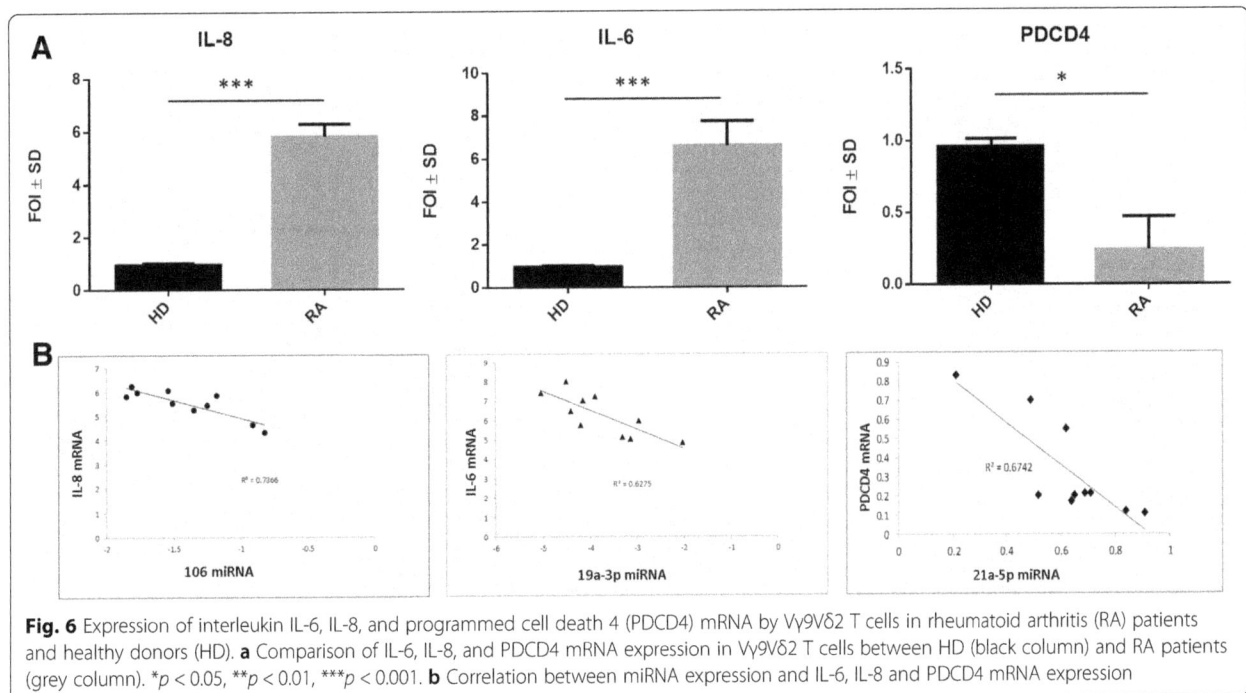

Fig. 6 Expression of interleukin IL-6, IL-8, and programmed cell death 4 (PDCD4) mRNA by Vγ9Vδ2 T cells in rheumatoid arthritis (RA) patients and healthy donors (HD). **a** Comparison of IL-6, IL-8, and PDCD4 mRNA expression in Vγ9Vδ2 T cells between HD (black column) and RA patients (grey column). *$p < 0.05$, **$p < 0.01$, ***$p < 0.001$. **b** Correlation between miRNA expression and IL-6, IL-8 and PDCD4 mRNA expression

could be involved and contribute to the pathogenesis of RA. This study has the limitation of a low number of patients studied, and hence the role of γδ T cells should be investigated in a larger cohort of patients, including analysis of γδ T cells at the site of disease. Moreover, additional miRNA silencing experimental approaches are needed to prove the role of these miRNAs in the regulation of Vγ9Vδ2 T cells [26].

Abbreviations

ACPA: Anti-citrullinated protein antibody; APC: Allophycocyanin; DMARD: Disease-modifying anti-rheumatic drug; FITC: Fluorescein isothiocyanate; HD: Healthy donors; mAbs: Monoclonal antibodies; miRNA: MicroRNA; ncRNA: Non-coding RNA; PBMC: Peripheral blood mononuclear cells; PDCD4: Programmed cell death 4; PE: Phycoerythrin; PerCP: Peridinin chlorophyll protein; PMA: Phorbolmyristate acetate; RA: Rheumatoid arthritis; RT-PCR: Real-time polymerase chain reaction; T_{CM}: T central memory; T_{EM}: T effector memory; T_{EMRA}: T terminally differentiated effector memory; Th : T helper; T_{naive}: T naive; Treg: Regulatory T

Acknowledgments

Part of this study has been presented as a poster at the EULAR 2017 meeting (Madrid), and the XI National Congress of the Italian Society of Immunology, Clinical Immunology, and Allergology 2017 meeting (Bari).

Funding

This work was supported by grants from the University of Palermo (ATE 0381 to NC).

Authors' contributions

GG study conception and design, data interpretation, literature search, figure creation, writing, paper revision, and acceptance; VO data interpretation, data collection, paper revision, and acceptance; LS data collection, data interpretation, literature search, paper revision, and acceptance; PR data interpretation, literature search, paper revision, and acceptance; PC data collection, literature search, paper revision, and acceptance; MPLM data collection, data interpretation, paper revision, and acceptance; RG literature search, paper revision, and acceptance; RA literature search, paper revision, and acceptance; GT data interpretation, literature search, paper revision, and acceptance; FC data collection, data interpretation, literature search, paper revision, and acceptance; FD data collection, literature search, paper revision, and acceptance, financial support for the experiments; NC study conception and design, data collection, data interpretation, literature search, paper revision, and acceptance. All authors gave final approval for submitting the manuscript for review and agree to be accountable for all aspects of the work.

Consent for publication

Informed consent was obtained from each patient and control.

Competing interests

The authors declare that they have no competing interests.

Author details

[1]Dipartimento Biomedico di Medicina Interna e Specialistica, Sezione di Reumatologia, Università di Palermo, Palermo, Italy. [2]Central Laboratory of Advanced Diagnosis and Biomedical Research (CLADIBIOR), Azienda Ospedaliera Universitaria Policlinico P. Giaccone, Palermo, Italy. [3]Dipartimento di Biopatologia e Biotecnologie Mediche, Università di Palermo, Palermo, Italy. [4]Division of Rheumatology, Department of Biotechnological and Applied Clinical Science, School of Medicine, University of L'Aquila, L'Aquila, Italy.

References

1. Bartel DP. MicroRNAs: genomics, biogenesis, mechanism, and function. Cell. 2004;116(2):281–97.
2. Bartel DP. MicroRNAs: target recognition and regulatory functions. Cell. 2009;136(2):215–33.
3. Mogilyansky E, Rigoutsos I. The miR-17/92 cluster: a comprehensive update on its genomics, genetics, functions and increasingly important and numerous roles in health and disease. Cell Death Differ. 2013; 20(12):1603–14.
4. He L, Thomson JM, Hemann MT, Hernando-Monge E, Mu D, Goodson S, Powers S, Cordon-Cardo C, Lowe SW, Hannon GJ, et al. A microRNA polycistron as a potential human oncogene. Nature. 2005;435(7043):828–33.
5. Philippe L, Alsaleh G, Bahram S, Pfeffer S, Georgel P. The miR-17 approximately 92 cluster: a key player in the control of inflammation during rheumatoid arthritis. Front Immunol. 2013;4:70.
6. Georganas C, Liu H, Perlman H, Hoffmann A, Thimmapaya B, Pope RM. Regulation of IL-6 and IL-8 expression in rheumatoid arthritis synovial fibroblasts: the dominant role for NF-kappa B but not C/EBP beta or c-Jun. J Immunol. 2000;165(12):7199–206.
7. Hwang SY, Kim JY, Kim KW, Park MK, Moon Y, Kim WU, Kim HY. IL-17 induces production of IL-6 and IL-8 in rheumatoid arthritis synovial fibroblasts via NF-kappaB- and PI3-kinase/Akt-dependent pathways. Arthritis Res Ther. 2004;6(2):R120–8.
8. Matsuno H, Yudoh K, Katayama R, Nakazawa F, Uzuki M, Sawai T, Yonezawa T, Saeki Y, Panayi GS, Pitzalis C, et al. The role of TNF-alpha in the pathogenesis of inflammation and joint destruction in rheumatoid arthritis (RA): a study using a human RA/SCID mouse chimera. Rheumatology. 2002; 41(3):329–37.
9. Mitogawa T, Nishiya K, Ota Z. Frequency of gamma delta T cells in peripheral blood, synovial fluid, synovial membrane and lungs from patients with rheumatoid arthritis. Acta Med Okayama. 1992;46(5):371–9.
10. Dejaco C, Duftner C, Grubeck-Loebenstein B, Schirmer M. Imbalance of regulatory T cells in human autoimmune diseases. Immunology. 2006; 117(3):289–300.
11. Caccamo N, Guggino G, Joosten SA, Gelsomino G, Di Carlo P, Titone L, Galati D, Bocchino M, Matarese A, Salerno A, et al. Multifunctional CD4(+) T cells correlate with active Mycobacterium tuberculosis infection. Eur J Immunol. 2010;40(8):2211–20.
12. Cordova A, Toia F, La Mendola C, Orlando V, Meraviglia S, Rinaldi G, Todaro M, Cicero G, Zichichi L, Donni PL, et al. Characterization of human gammadelta T lymphocytes infiltrating primary malignant melanomas. PLoS One. 2012;7(11):e49878.
13. Le Bechec A, Portales-Casamar E, Vetter G, Moes M, Zindy PJ, Saumet A, Arenillas D, Theillet C, Wasserman WW, Lecellier CH, et al. MIR@NT@N: a framework integrating transcription factors, microRNAs and their targets to identify sub-network motifs in a meta-regulation network model. BMC Bioinformatics. 2011;12:67.
14. van Baarsen LGM, Lebre MC, van der Coelen D, Aarrass S, Tang MW, Ramwadhdoebe TH, Gerlag DM, Tak PP. Heterogeneous expression pattern of interleukin 17A (IL-17A), IL-17F and their receptors in synovium of rheumatoid arthritis, psoriatic arthritis and osteoarthritis: possible explanation for nonresponse to anti-IL-17 therapy? Arthritis Res Ther. 2014; 16(4):426.
15. Kuo G, Wu CY, Yang HY. MiR-17-92 cluster and immunity. J Formos Med Assoc. 2018.
16. Paul S, Singh AK, Shilpi LG. Phenotypic and functional plasticity of gamma-delta (gammadelta) T cells in inflammation and tolerance. Int Rev Immunol. 2014;33(6):537–58.
17. Vantourout P, Hayday A. Six-of-the-best: unique contributions of gammadelta T cells to immunology. Nat Rev Immunol. 2013;13(2):88–100.
18. Caccamo N, Todaro M, Sireci G, Meraviglia S, Stassi G, Dieli F. Mechanisms underlying lineage commitment and plasticity of human gammadelta T cells. Cell Mol Immunol. 2013;10(1):30–4.
19. Dou L, Meng X, Sui X, Wang S, Shen T, Huang X, Guo J, Fang W, Man Y, Xi J, et al. MiR-19a regulates PTEN expression to mediate glycogen synthesis in hepatocytes. Sci Rep. 2015;5:11602.
20. Hong Z, Hong H, Liu J, Zheng X, Huang M, Li C, Xia J. miR-106a is downregulated in peripheral blood mononuclear cells of chronic hepatitis B and associated with enhanced levels of interleukin-8. Mediat Inflamm. 2015; 2015:629862.
21. Liu S, Fang Y, Shen H, Xu W, Li H. Berberine sensitizes ovarian cancer cells to cisplatin through miR-21/PDCD4 axis. Acta Biochim Biophys Sin. 2013; 45(9):756–62.

22. Reddycherla AV, Meinert I, Reinhold A, Reinhold D, Schraven B, Simeoni L. miR-20a inhibits TCR-mediated signaling and cytokine production in human naive CD4+ T cells. PLoS One. 2015;10(4):e0125311.

23. Krichevsky AM, Gabriely G. miR-21: a small multi-faceted RNA. J Cell Mol Med. 2009;13(1):39–53.

24. Xu WD, Pan HF, Li JH, Ye DQ. MicroRNA-21 with therapeutic potential in autoimmune diseases. Expert Opin Ther Targets. 2013;17(6):659–65.

25. Philippe L, Alsaleh G, Pichot A, Ostermann E, Zuber G, Frisch B, Sibilia J, Pfeffer S, Bahram S, Wachsmann D, et al. MiR-20a regulates ASK1 expression and TLR4-dependent cytokine release in rheumatoid fibroblast-like synoviocytes. Ann Rheum Dis. 2013;72(6):1071–9.

26. Alivernini S, Kurowska-Stolarska M, Tolusso B, Benvenuto R, Elmesmari A, Canestri S, Petricca L, Mangoni A, Fedele AL, Di Mario C, et al. MicroRNA-155 influences B-cell function through PU.1 in rheumatoid arthritis. Nat Commun. 2016;7:12970.

18

Aberrant expression of interleukin-23-regulated miRNAs in T cells from patients with ankylosing spondylitis

Ning-Sheng Lai[1,2†], Hui-Chun Yu[1†], Chien-Hsueh Tung[1,2], Kuang-Yung Huang[1,2], Hsien-Bin Huang[3] and Ming-Chi Lu[1,2*] (iD)

Abstract

Background: Interleukin (IL)-23 can facilitate the differentiation of IL-17-producing helper T cells (Th17). The IL-23/IL-17 axis is known to play a key role in the immunopathogenesis of ankylosing spondylitis (AS). We hypothesized that the expression of microRNAs (miRNAs, miRs) would be regulated by IL-23 and that these miRNAs could participate in the immunopathogenesis of AS.

Methods: Expression profiles of human miRNAs in K562 cells, cultured in the presence or absence of IL-23 for 3 days, were analyzed by microarray. Potentially aberrantly expressed miRNAs were validated using T-cell samples from 24 patients with AS and 16 control subjects. Next-generation sequencing (NGS) was conducted to search for gene expression and biological functions regulated by specific miRNAs in the IL-23-mediated signaling pathway.

Results: Initial analysis revealed that the expression levels of 12 miRNAs were significantly higher, whereas those of 4 miRNAs were significantly lower, in K562 cells after coculture with IL-23 for 3 days. Among these IL-23-regulated miRNAs, the expression levels of miR-29b-1-5p, miR-4449, miR-211-3p, miR-1914-3p, and miR-7114-5p were found to be higher in AS T cells. The transfection of miR-29b-1-5p mimic suppressed IL-23-mediated signal transducer and activator of transcription 3 (STAT3) phosphorylation in K562 cells. After NGS analysis and validation, we found that miR-29b-1-5p upregulated the expression of angiogenin, which was also upregulated in K562 cells after coculture with IL-23. Increased expression of miR-29b-1-5p or miR-211-3p could enhance interferon-γ expression.

Conclusions: Among the miRNAs regulated by IL-23, expression levels of five miRNAs were increased in T cells from patients with AS. The transfection of miR-29b-1-5p mimic could inhibit the IL-23-mediated STAT3 phosphorylation and might play a role in negative feedback control in the immunopathogenesis of AS.

Keywords: Ankylosing spondylitis, IL-23, T cells, MicroRNAs, STAT3, Angiogenin

Background

Ankylosing spondylitis (AS) is a chronic inflammatory disease characterized by axial skeletal involvement leading to spine deformities, increased disability, and mortality [1, 2]. The pathogenesis of AS is complex, and earlier research focused on the misfolding of human leukocyte antigen B27 [3], a major genetic risk factor in AS [4].

Recent studies revealed that the genetic variant of interleukin (IL)-23 receptor (IL-23R) was associated with the risk of AS [5]. Serum level of IL-23 is elevated in patients with AS compared with control subjects [6]. Other studies have also demonstrated that IL-23/IL-17-related signaling pathways could play a critical role in the pathogenesis of AS [7]. Most importantly, targeting IL-17 is a novel therapy for AS [8].

MicroRNAs (miRNAs, miRs) are short noncoding RNA molecules of 21–24 base pairs that control the expression of multiple gene targets at the post-transcriptional level. They play a crucial role in regulating both the innate and adaptive immune responses. One of our previous studies

---
* Correspondence: e360187@yahoo.com.tw
†Ning-Sheng Lai and Hui-Chun Yu contributed equally to this work.
[1]Division of Allergy, Immunology and Rheumatology, Dalin Tzu Chi Hospital, Buddhist Tzu Chi Medical Foundation, No. 2, Minsheng RoadDalin, Chiayi 62247, Taiwan
[2]School of Medicine, Tzu Chi University, Hualien City, Taiwan
Full list of author information is available at the end of the article

showed that dysregulated miRNAs in T cells from patients with AS could participate in the inflammatory response [9]. Many studies have also reported that the expression of miRNAs in whole blood, peripheral blood mononuclear cells (PBMCs), or serum from patients with AS could participate in bone erosion, cytokine expression, and autophagy in the pathogenesis of AS [10].

Few studies have addressed the IL-23/IL-17 axis-related miRNAs and their possible roles in the immunopathogenesis of AS [11]. We believe that many additional miRNAs regulated by IL-23 could be found to be aberrantly expressed in T cells from patients with AS, and these miRNAs could participate in the IL-23-related signaling pathway. In this study, we hypothesized that IL-23-regulated miRNAs in T cells from patients with AS could alter the expression of downstream target molecules and thereby contribute to the immunopathogenesis of AS.

Methods

Cell culture

Among the human myeloid and lymphoid cell lines, the mRNA expression of IL-23R is more abundant in K562 cells than in Jurkat cells [12]. We chose K562 cells for this study. K562 cells, a human erythroleukemia line, purchased from the American Type Culture Collection (Manassas, VA, USA) were cultured in medium with or without the presence of IL-23 (20 ng/ml; Sigma-Aldrich, St. Louis, MO, USA) for 3 days according to previous studies [13, 14] with some modifications. These cells were used for subsequent analysis.

Isolation of T cells from patients and control subjects

A total of 24 patients fulfilling the Assessment of SpondyloArthritis international Society (ASAS) classification criteria [15] were recruited for this study. In addition, 16 healthy individuals were also recruited to serve as control subjects. Blood samples were collected just before taking oral medications and the administration of the next dose of biologic agent to minimize any effects of medications. All participants provided informed consent under a study protocol approved by the institutional review board of Dalin Tzu Chi Hospital, Buddhist Tzu Chi Medical Foundation (no. B10502002).

T cells were further purified by antihuman CD3-coated magnetic beads (IMag Cell Separation System; BD Biosciences, Franklin Lakes, NJ, USA), and the purities of T cells were all greater than 98% according to methods previously described [16].

Measurement of ankylosing spondylitis disease activity

The Ankylosing Spondylitis Disease Activity Score (ASDAS) based on C-reactive protein (CRP) was used to evaluate disease activity in this study [17]. ASDAS-CRP was calculated using the following formula: $0.121 \times$ back pain $+ 0.058 \times$ duration of morning stiffness $+ 0.110 \times$ patient global assessment $+ 0.073 \times$ peripheral pain or swelling $+ 0.579 \times \ln (CRP + 1)$.

RNA isolation for microarray and next-generation sequencing

Total RNA was extracted by using TRIzol® Reagent (Life Technologies, Carlsbad, CA, USA) according to the manufacturer's instructions. The purified RNA was quantified at optical density 260 nm using an ND-1000 spectrophotometer (NanoDrop Technologies/Thermo Scientific, Wilmington, DE, USA), and quality was evaluated using a Bioanalyzer 2100 (Agilent Technologies, Santa Clara, CA, USA) with the RNA 6000 Nano Kit (Agilent Technologies).

Microarray analysis of miRNAs

Total RNA (0.1 μg) was dephosphorylated and labeled with pCp-Cy3 by using the Agilent miRNA Complete Labeling and Hyb Kit (Agilent Technologies). Hybridization buffer (Agilent Technologies) was added to the labeled mixture to a final volume of 45 μl. The mixture was heated at 100 °C for 5 min and immediately cooled to 0 °C. Each 45-μl sample was hybridized onto an Agilent human miRNA Microarray R21 (Agilent Technologies) at 55 °C for 20 h. After hybridization, slides were washed in Gene Expression Wash Buffer at room temperature for 5 min and then in Gene Expression Wash Buffer 2 at 37 °C for 5 min (Agilent Technologies). Microarrays were scanned with an Agilent microarray scanner (model G2505C; Agilent Technologies) at 535 nm for Cy3. Feature Extraction software version 10.7.3.1 (Agilent Technologies) was used for image analysis. Microarray data were uploaded in the Gene Expression Omnibus (GEO) database of the National Center for Biotechnology Information [GEO:GSE118806].

Measurement of expression of miRNAs

A real-time PCR-based method was used to quantify the expression levels of miRNAs following a protocol described previously [18]. Expression of the U6 small nuclear RNA was used as an endogenous control for data normalization.

Measurement of expression of mRNAs

Expression levels of mRNA were quantified by real-time PCR using a one-step RT-PCR kit (TaKaRa, Shiga, Japan) on the ABI Prism 7500 Fast Real-Time PCR System (Applied Biosystems, Foster City, CA, USA). Conditions for the qPCR were 42 °C for 5 min and 95 °C for 10 s for RT, followed by 40 cycles of 95 °C for 5 s and 34 °C for 34 s. Expression of 18S ribosomal RNA was used as an endogenous control for data normalization.

Western blot analysis

Cells were lysed with 1% NP-40 (Sigma-Aldrich) in the presence of a proteinase inhibitor and phosphatase inhibitor cocktail (Sigma-Aldrich). Seventy micrograms of the cell lysates were electrophoresed and transferred to a polyvinylidene difluoride sheet (Sigma-Aldrich). The membranes were blocked with 1% skim milk solution and then incubated with the primary antibodies for signal transducer and activator of transcription 3 (STAT3), phosphorylated STAT3 (Cell Signaling Technology, Danvers, MA, USA) and angiogenin (ANG) (Santa Cruz Biotechnology, Dallas, TX, USA), followed by horseradish peroxidase-conjugated secondary antibodies (Cell Signaling Technology). The cognate molecules were visualized using an enhanced chemiluminescence reaction (GE Healthcare Life Sciences, Marlborough, MA, USA).

Transfection of miRNA

K562 cells (1×10^6/ml) were electroporated with 1 µg of scrambled oligonucleotides or miRNA mimics (Ambion/Thermo Fisher Scientific, Austin, TX, USA) using the Gene Pulser MXcell electroporation system (Bio-Rad Laboratories, Hercules, CA, USA) using the condition described previously [18] and then cultured at 37 °C with a humidified atmosphere containing 5% CO_2 for 24 h or 48 h for further analysis of miRNA expression or for Western blot analysis, respectively.

Next-generation sequencing

We transfected K562 cells with miR-29b-1-5p mimic or scrambled oligonucleotides and then cultured them at 37 °C under a humidified atmosphere containing 5% CO_2 for 48 h. The RNA was extracted according to the method described above. For the next-generation sequencing (NGS) analysis, all procedures were carried out according to the manufacturer's protocol (Illumina, San Diego, CA, USA). In brief, library construction of all samples was performed by using the Agilent Technologies SureSelect Strand Specific RNA Library Preparation Kit for 75 single-end sequencing on the Solexa platform (Illumina). The sequence was directly determined using sequencing-by-synthesis technology via the TruSeq SBS Kit (Illumina). Raw sequences were obtained from the Illumina Pipeline software bcl2fastq v2.0 and expected to generate 30 million reads (or Gb) per sample. The sequencing procedure was performed by Welgene Biotech (Taipei, Taiwan). For the results analysis, the generated sequences went through a filtering process to obtain qualified reads initially. Trimmomatics (Illumina) was implemented to trim or remove the reads according to the quality score. Qualified reads after filtering low-quality data were analyzed using TopHat/Cufflinks [19] for gene expression estimation. The gene expression level was calculated as fragments per kilobase of transcript per million mapped reads. For differential expression analysis, CummeRbund was employed to perform statistical analyses of gene expression profiles. The reference genome and gene annotations were retrieved from the Ensembl database.

Statistical analysis

Data are represented as the median and IQR or number (%) as appropriate. Simple and multiple linear regression analyses were used to calculate the correlation coefficients among different clinical parameters and expression levels of IL-23-regulated miRNAs in T cells of patients with AS. Statistical significance between patients with AS and control subjects was assessed using the Mann-Whitney U test. A P value < 0.05 was considered statistically significant. All analyses were performed with Stata software (StataCorp, College Station, TX, USA).

Results

Increased STAT3 phosphorylation in K562 cells after incubation with IL-23

First, we demonstrated that the phosphorylation ratio of STAT3, a key downstream signaling molecule of the IL-23

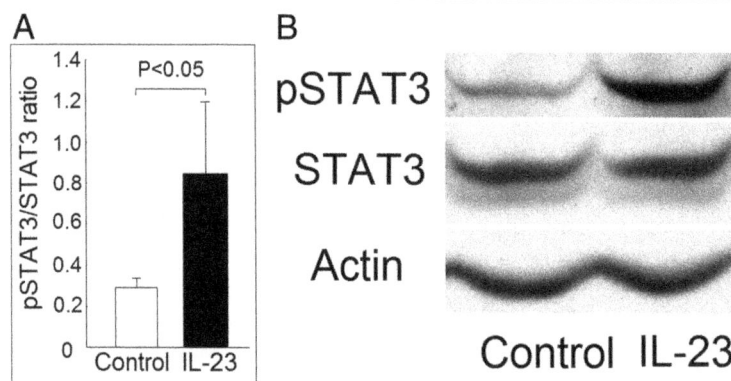

Fig. 1 Effect of interleukin (IL)-23 on signal transducer and activator of transcription 3 (STAT3) protein phosphorylation in K562 cells. **a** The phosphorylation ratio of STAT3 increased in K562 cells after coculture with IL-23 (20 ng/ml) for 3 days compared with those cocultured with medium (control) only. **b** A representative case

signaling pathway, was increased after coculture with IL-23 in K562 cells (Fig. 1a and b).

Identification of the IL-23-regulated miRNA expression in K562 cells

Expression profiles of miRNAs in K562 cells cocultured with or without IL-23 (20 ng/ml) for 3 days are displayed in Fig. 2a, with each scatter spot representing the mean of three adjusted miRNA levels from each group. The expression levels of 12 miRNAs (miR-1287-5p, miR-29b-1-5p, miR-6872-3p, miR-486-3p, miR-21-3p, miR-151a-3p, miR-4449, miR-211-3p, miR-6826-5p, miR-3132, miR-1914-3p,

and miR-7114-5p) were significantly higher, whereas the expression levels of 4 miRNAs (miR-7110-5p, miR-6869-5p, miR-642a-3p, and miR-1229-5p) were significantly lower, in K562 cells after coculture with IL-23 for 3 days ($P < 0.05$) (Fig. 2b).

Expression profiles of IL-23-regulated miRNAs in T cells from patients with AS and control subjects

Expression levels of the IL-23-regulated miRNAs were investigated in T cells from patients with AS and control subjects. The demographic and clinical data of the 24 patients with AS and 16 control subjects are presented

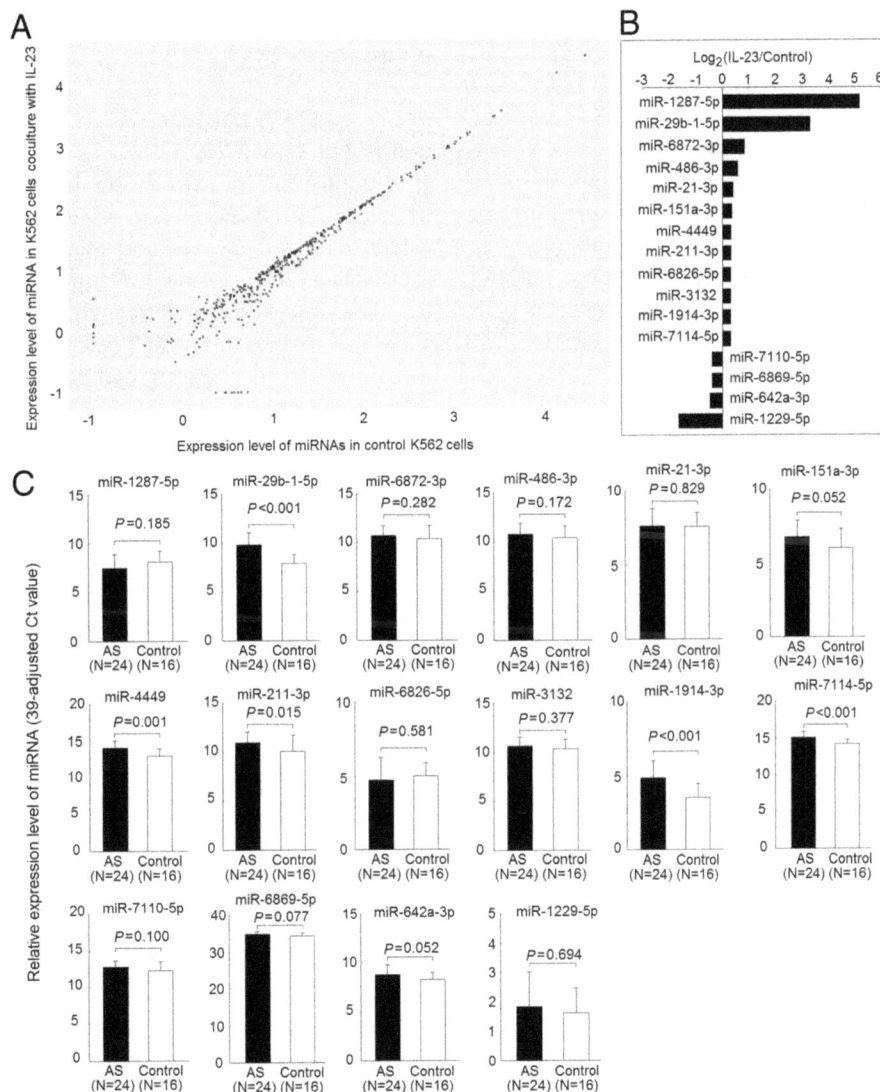

Fig. 2 Altered expression of interleukin (IL)-23-regulated microRNAs (miRNAs) in T cells from patients with ankylosing spondylitis (AS) and from healthy control subjects. **a** Expression profiles of miRNAs in K562 cells cocultured with or without IL-23 (20 ng/ml) for 3 days, evaluated using microarray analysis. Each scatter spot represents the mean raw signals of miRNA in three repeats of each treatment. **b** The expression levels of 12 miRNAs were significantly higher, whereas the expression levels of 4 miRNAs were significantly lower, in K562 cells after coculture with IL-23 for 3 days ($P < 0.05$). **c** Increased expression of miR-29b-1-5p, miR-4449, miR-211-3p, miR-1914-3p, and miR-7114-5p in AS T-cell miRNA, compared with normal T cells after validation

Table 1 Demographics and clinical data of patients with ankylosing spondylitis and healthy control subjects

	Patients with AS ($n = 24$)	Healthy control subjects ($n = 16$)	P value
Age (years)	39.5 (33.0–57.8)	39.0 (33.5–43.5)	0.313
Sex (M:F)	12:4	12:4	> 0.999
HLA-B27[+]	24 (100%)	–	
C-reactive protein (mg/dl)	0.24 (0.08–1.24)	–	
Medication			
NSAID	23 (95.8%)	–	
Salazopyrine	24 (100%)	–	
Anti-TNF therapy	14 (58.3%)	–	

Abbreviations: AS Ankylosing spondylitis, HLA Human leukocyte antigen, – Not determined, NSAID Nonsteroidal anti-inflammatory drugs, TNF Tumor necrosis factor

in Table 1. There were no differences in the distribution of age and sex between the two groups.

The expression of miR-29b-1-5p, miR-4449, miR-211-3p, miR-1914-3p, and miR-7114-5p ($P < 0.05$) was found to be higher in AS T cells than in controls (Fig. 2c). The fold changes of expression levels for these miRNAs compared with controls were as follows: miR-29b-1-5p, 3.71-fold, miR-4449, 2.13-fold, miR-211-3p, 1.85-fold; miR-1914-3p, 2.57-fold; and miR-7114-5p, 1.82-fold. After adjusting for age and sex, the expression levels of miR-29b-1-5p, miR-4449, miR-1914-3p, and miR-7114-5p miRNAs remained significantly higher in T cells from patients with AS than in those from control subjects.

Correlations of miRNA expression levels and clinical parameters in patients with AS

The relationships between various clinical parameters and the expression levels of miRNAs in AS T cells were investigated using regression analyses (Table 2). With simple linear regression analysis, expression levels of miR-7114-5p showed a trend of correlation with the use of anti-tumor necrosis factor (anti-TNF) therapy ($P = 0.099$). After adjusting for age and sex using multiple linear regression analysis, patients with AS receiving anti-TNF therapy showed a significant 1.56-fold increment ($P = 0.048$; 95% CI, 1.00–2.43) in miR-7114-5p expression compared with those who did not receive anti-TNF therapy. Because we found that the fold

changes of in miR-29b-1-5p expression level were the greatest among these IL-23-regulated miRNAs in T cells from patients with AS, we selected miR-29b-1-5p for subsequent analysis.

Decreased STAT3 phosphorylation in K562 cells after transfection of miR-29b-1-5p

We found that the expression levels of miR-29b-1-5p were significantly elevated in K562 cells 24 h after transfection with miR-29b-1-5p mimic compared with those transfected with scrambled oligonucleotides (as the control) (Fig. 3a). We found that the phosphorylation ratio of STAT3 decreased in K562 cells 48 h after transfection with miR-29b-1-5p mimic compared with the controls (Fig. 3b and c).

Search of genes regulated by miR-29b-1-5p using next-generation sequencing

To search for the expression of genes regulated by miR-29b-1-5p, we performed gene expression analysis using NGS after transfecting K562 cells with miR-29b-1-5p mimic or scrambled oligonucleotides. We found that mRNA expression levels of 10 genes were decreased, whereas the expression levels of 16 genes were increased, in K562 cells after transfection with miR-29b-1-5p mimic compared with those transfected with scrambled oligonucleotides ($P < 0.05$) (Fig 4a and b).

Table 2 Simple and multiple linear regression analyses for assessing the correlations among different clinical parameters and expression levels of IL-23-regulated miRNAs in T cells of patients with ankylosing spondylitis

	miR-7114-5p	miR-1914-3p	miR-211-3p	miR-4449	miR-29b-1-5p
Sex (M/F)	−0.112 (0.784)	0.317 (0.564)	0.473 (0.366)	0.294 (0.520)	−0.207 (0.731)
Age (per 10 years)	−0.085 (0.505)	0.021 (0.919)	0.030 (0.875)	−0.159 (0.337)	−0.031 (0.889)
CRP (per 1 mg/dl)	−0.005 (0.920)	0.008 (0.915)	0.073 (0.299)	0.054 (0.380)	0.020 (0.804)
Anti-TNF therapy (yes/no)	0.490 (0.099[a])	0.351 (0.466)	0.330 (0.474)	0.286 (0.475)	0.029 (0.965)
ASDAS-CRP	−0.194 (0.250)	−0.941 (0.727)	−0.121 (0.639)	0.230 (0.304)	0.278 (0.358)

Abbreviations: ASDAS Ankylosing Spondylitis Disease Activity Score, CRP C-reactive protein, TNF Tumor necrosis factor
Values are correlation coefficients and (P values) from simple linear regression analyses
[a]After adjusting for age and sex in the multiple linear regression analysis, patients with AS using anti-TNF therapy had a significant 1.56-fold increase ($P = 0.048$; 95% CI, 1.00–2.43) in miR-7114-5p expression compared with those who did not receive anti-TNF therapy

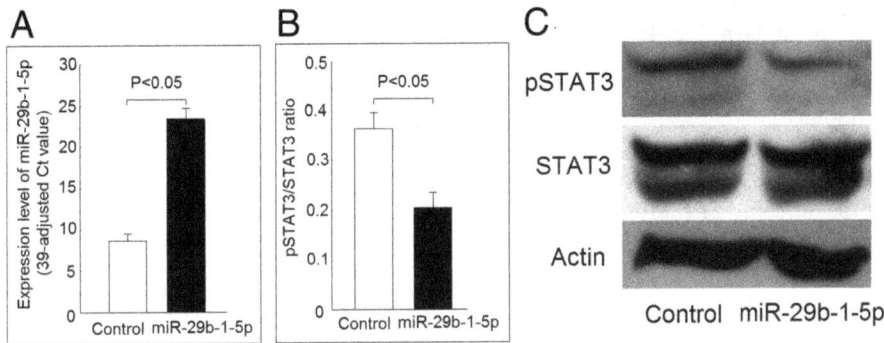

Fig. 3 Effect of miR-29b-1-5p on signal transducer and activator of transcription 3 (STAT3) protein phosphorylation in K562 cells. **a** Increased miR-29b-1-5p expression in K562 cells after transfection with miR-29b-1-5p mimic versus scramble oligonucleotides. **b** The phosphorylation ratio of STAT3 decreased in K562 cells after transfection with miR-29b-1-5p mimic compared with those transfected with scramble oligonucleotides after culturing with medium for 48 h. **c** A representative case

Involvement of miR-29b-1-5p-regulated genes in IL-23 signaling pathway

From among the previous identified miR-29b-1-5p regulated genes, we selected one downregulated gene, Fas apoptotic inhibitory molecule 2 (*FAIM2*), and three upregulated genes—phosphodiesterase 2A (*PDE2A*), cyclin-dependent kinase 15 (*CDK15*), and angiogenin (*ANG*)—that are potentially involved in the inflammatory responses for further analysis. The mRNA expression levels of *ANG*, but not *FAIM2*, *PDE2A*, or *CDK15*,

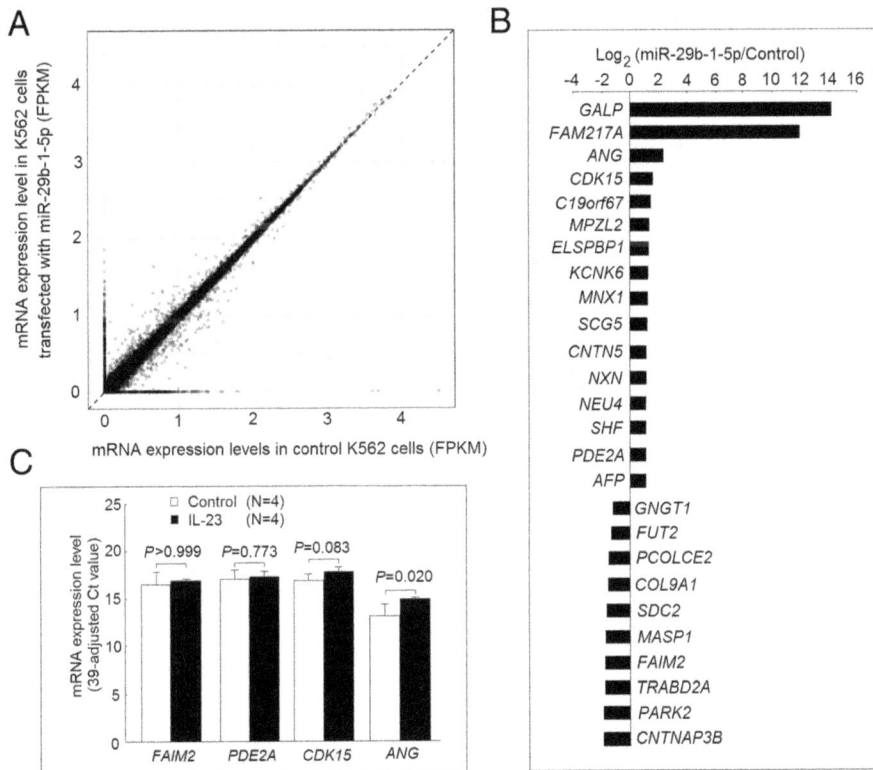

Fig. 4 Identification of miR-29b-1-5p-regulated genes. **a** Expression profiles of messenger RNAs (mRNAs) in K562 cells transfected with miR-29b-1-5p mimic or scramble oligonucleotides then cultured with medium for 48 h were evaluated using RNA-Seq transcriptome analysis. Each scatter spot represents the mean raw signals of microRNA (miRNA) in three repeats of each treatment. **b** The RNA expression levels of 16 genes were significantly higher, whereas the RNA expression levels of 10 genes were significantly lower, in K562 cells after being transfected with miR-29b-1-5p mimic for 48 h. **c** Four genes potentially involved in the inflammatory responses were selected for further analysis. The mRNA expression levels of *ANG* were significantly elevated in K562 cells after coculture with interleukin (IL)-23 (20 ng/ml) for 3 days (Fig. 3c)

were significantly elevated in K562 cells after coculture with IL-23 (20 ng/ml) for 3 days (Fig. 4c).

Protein expression of angiogenin

We confirmed that the protein expression of *ANG* was elevated in K562 cells after transfection with miR-29b-1-5p (Fig. 5a and b). The protein expression of *ANG* was also increased in K562 cells after coculture with IL-23 (Fig. 5c and d).

Effect of miRNAs on expression levels of proinflammatory cytokines

We further surveyed the effect of increased expression of miR-29b-1-5p or miR-211-3p on the expression of proinflammatory cytokines. We found that increased miR-29b-1-5p expression could increase interferon-γ (*IFN-γ*) expression, but not *IL-17A* or *TNF-α* expression, in K562 cells cultured with medium alone (Fig. 6a). The addition of IL-23 could increase the expression of IFN-γ in K562 cells, but the transfection of miR-29b-1-5p did not affect the *IFN-γ*, *IL-17A*, or *TNF-α* expression in K562 cells cultured with IL-23 (Fig. 6b and c). We also confirmed that the expression levels of miR-211-3p were dramatically increased in K562 cells after transfection with miR-211-3p mimic (Fig. 7a). Increased expression of miR-211-3p did not affect the *IFN-γ*, *IL-17A*, or *TNF-α* expression in K562 cells cultured with medium alone (Fig. 7b). The transfection of miR-211-3p enhanced the mRNA expression of *IFN-γ*, but not of *IL-17A* or *TNF-α*, in K562 cells cocultured with IL-23 (Fig. 7c).

Discussion

IL-23, a member of the IL-12 family, is a heterodimeric cytokine secreted by several types of immune cells, such as natural killer cells and dendritic cells [20]. Patients with AS have elevated serum IL-23 levels compared with control subjects [6]. In addition to AS, IL-23 is also involved in the pathogenesis of several other autoimmune diseases, such as inflammatory bowel disease and psoriasis, which all belong to the category of spondyloarthritis [21]. However, few studies have addressed the possible effect of IL-23 on the regulation of miRNA expression [22–24]. In this study, K562 cells instead of Jurkat cells were used as a platform for screening the IL-23-regulated miRNA expression because Jurkat cells had low expression levels of IL-23 receptor compared with K562 cells [12]. The differential expression levels of IL-23-regulated miRNAs were validated in T-cell samples from patients with AS and control subjects.

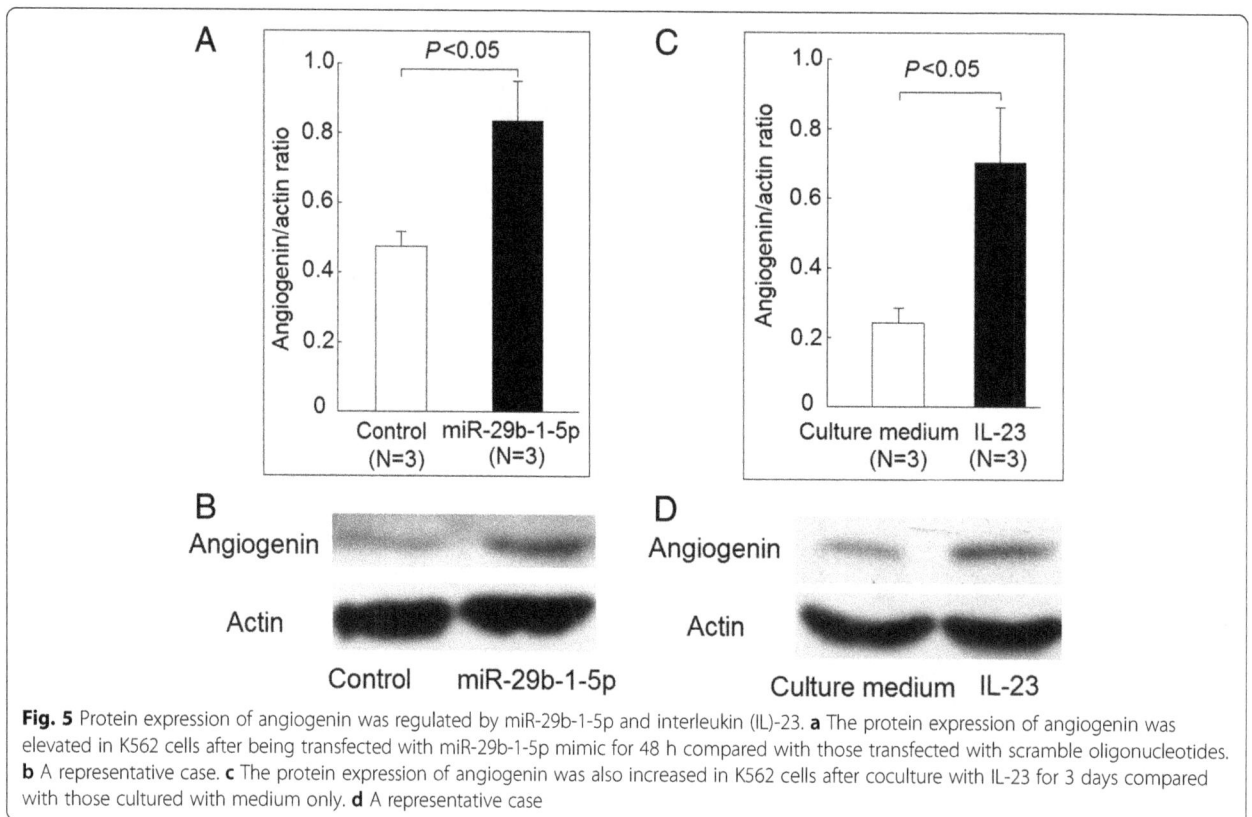

Fig. 5 Protein expression of angiogenin was regulated by miR-29b-1-5p and interleukin (IL)-23. **a** The protein expression of angiogenin was elevated in K562 cells after being transfected with miR-29b-1-5p mimic for 48 h compared with those transfected with scramble oligonucleotides. **b** A representative case. **c** The protein expression of angiogenin was also increased in K562 cells after coculture with IL-23 for 3 days compared with those cultured with medium only. **d** A representative case

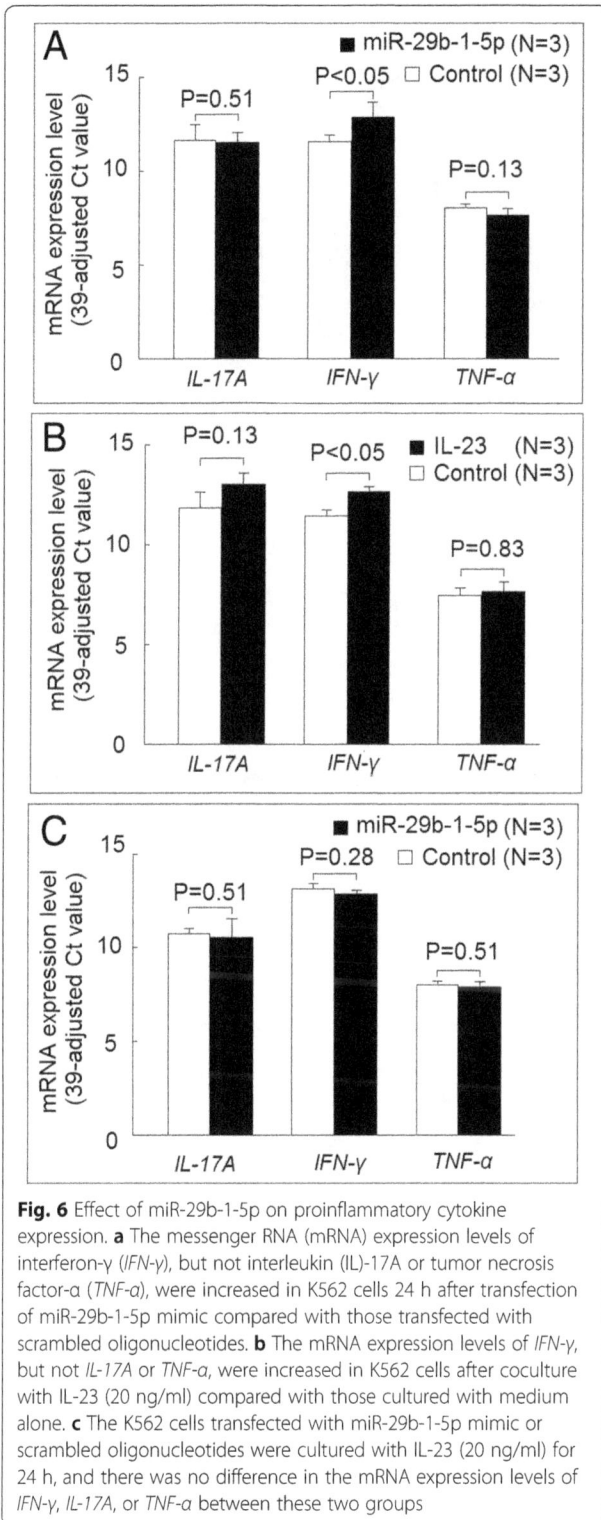

Fig. 6 Effect of miR-29b-1-5p on proinflammatory cytokine expression. **a** The messenger RNA (mRNA) expression levels of interferon-γ (*IFN-γ*), but not interleukin (IL)-17A or tumor necrosis factor-α (*TNF-α*), were increased in K562 cells 24 h after transfection of miR-29b-1-5p mimic compared with those transfected with scrambled oligonucleotides. **b** The mRNA expression levels of *IFN-γ*, but not *IL-17A* or *TNF-α*, were increased in K562 cells after coculture with IL-23 (20 ng/ml) compared with those cultured with medium alone. **c** The K562 cells transfected with miR-29b-1-5p mimic or scrambled oligonucleotides were cultured with IL-23 (20 ng/ml) for 24 h, and there was no difference in the mRNA expression levels of *IFN-γ*, *IL-17A*, or *TNF-α* between these two groups

Although several studies have attempted to identify the potential roles of miRNAs in the pathogenesis of AS using PBMCs, serum, plasma, or whole blood [10], few studies have addressed the role of miRNAs in T-cell

dysfunction of AS [6, 9–11, 25]. In this study, we found that the expression levels of five miRNAs (miR-29b-1-5p, miR-4449, miR-211-3p, miR-1914-3p, and miR-7114-5p) were higher in T cells from patients with AS. One of our earlier studies showed that three miRNAs were overexpressed in AS T cells [9]. In that study, only the expression levels of 270 miRNAs were explored. However, in the present study, we used a microarray that contained 2549 miRNA expression profiles. Therefore, a large number of miRNAs were expected to be found differentially expressed in AS T cells. In addition, miR-4449 is overexpressed in multiple myeloma [26], and it is interesting that the abnormal expression of IL-23 plays a role in the pathogenesis of multiple myeloma [27]. The role of other miRNAs deserves further study.

For the functional aspect of IL-23-regulated miRNAs, we found that the expression of miR-7114-5p was elevated in T cells from patients with AS. Anti-TNF therapy was associated with increased expression levels of miR-7114-5p. Milanez et al. found that the use of anti-TNF therapy in patients with AS did not affect the plasma level of IL-23 [28]. The use of anti-TNF therapy might indicate that these patients with AS had more severe or more active disease. We found that miR-29b-1-5p could suppress the phosphorylation of STAT3, a critical downstream transcription factor of the IL-23 signaling pathway that is required for Th17 cell differentiation [29]. Therefore, the increased expression of miR-29b-1-5p after exposure to IL-23 could be a negative feedback signal for the IL-23 signaling pathway. We found that increased *ANG* expression in K562 cells after transfection with miR-29b-1-5p mimic. We also confirmed that the addition of IL-23 or increased expression of miR-29b-1-5p could upregulate the protein expression of *ANG*. *ANG*, also known as ribonuclease 5, was initially known to induce new blood vessel formation. More recently, many biological functions, such as regulating cell proliferation, survival, migration, invasion, and/or differential are shown to be regulated by *ANG* [30, 31]. In inflammatory responses, ANG could inhibit the TANK-binding protein kinase 1-mediated nuclear factor-κB translocation, and this could suppress inflammatory responses [32]. Because IL-17 could enhance *ANG* expression in fibrocytes, it might play a role in the IL-23/IL-17-related signaling pathway [33]. Eleftheriadis et al. showed that ANG could inhibit T-cell apoptosis [34], and the biological function of *ANG* in T cells needs to be further explored.

Conclusions

The expression levels of miR-29b-1-5p, miR-4449, miR-211-3p, miR-1914-3p, and miR-7114-5p were shown

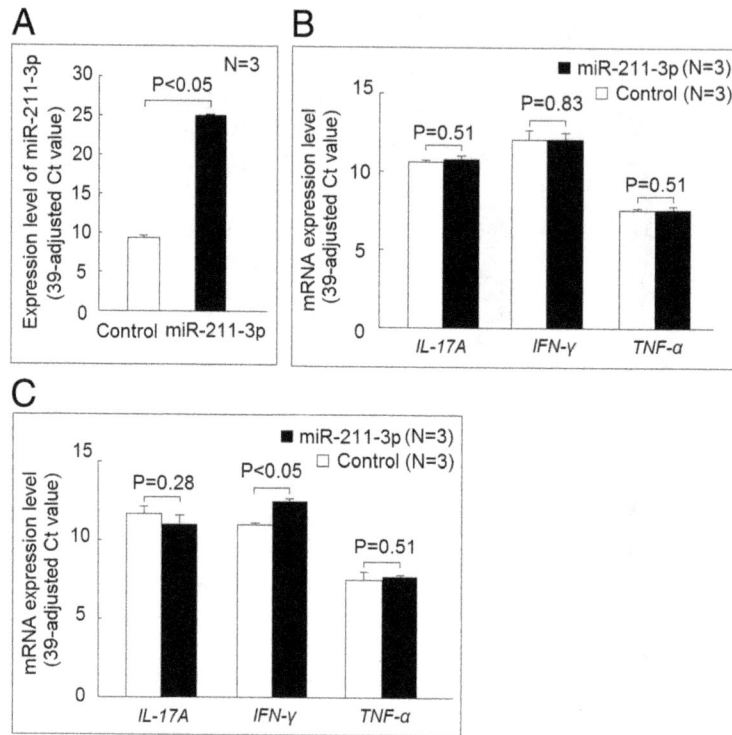

Fig. 7 Effect of miR-211-3p in proinflammatory cytokine expression. **a** The expression levels of miR-211-3p dramatically increased after transfection with miR-211-3p mimic compared with those transfected with scrambled oligonucleotides (control). **b** There were no differences in the mRNA expression levels of interferon-γ (*IFN-γ*), interleukin (IL)-17A, or tumor necrosis factor-α (*TNF-α*) in K562 cells 24 h after transfection of miR-211-3p mimic compared with those transfected with scrambled oligonucleotides. **c** The K562 cells transfected with miR-211-3p mimic or scrambled oligonucleotides were cultured with IL-23 (20 ng/ml) for 24 h. The mRNA expression levels of *IFN-γ*, but not *IL-17A* or *TNF-α*, were increased in those transfected with miR-211-3p mimic compared with the control

to be higher in AS T cells among the IL-23-regulated miR-NAs. Increased expression of miR-29b-1-5p could suppress IL-23-mediated STAT3 phosphorylation and increase *ANG* expression in the IL-23 signaling pathway.

Abbreviations
ANG: Angiogenin; AS: Ankylosing spondylitis; ASAS: Assessment of SpondyloArthritis international Society; ASDAS: Ankylosing Spondylitis Disease Activity Score; CDK15: Cyclin-dependent kinase 15; CRP: C-reactive protein; FAIM2: Fas apoptotic inhibitory molecule 2; HLA: Human leukocyte antigen; IFN-γ: Interferon-γ; IL: Interleukin; miRNAs: MicroRNAs; NSAID: Nonsteroidal anti-inflammatory drug; PBMC: Peripheral blood mononuclear cell; PDE2A: Phosphodiesterase 2A; STAT: Signal transducer and activator of transcription; TNF-α: Tumor necrosis factor-α

Acknowledgements
We thank Dr. Malcolm Koo for his writing assistance and statistical advice.

Funding
This work was supported by grants from the Ministry of Science and Technology (MOST 105-2314-B-303-020-MY2 and MOST 106-2314-B-303 -003) and Tzu Chi Medical Mission Project 105-01-02, Buddhist Tzu Chi Medical Foundation, Taiwan.

Authors' contributions
NSL, KYH, and MCL conceived of and designed the study. HCY and HBH performed the experiment. NSL, CHT, and MCL analyzed and interpreted the data. MCL wrote the paper. All authors revised the manuscript critically for important intellectual content, and all authors read and approved the final version to be published.

Consent for publication
Not applicable.

Competing interests
The authors declare that they have no competing interests.

Author details
[1]Division of Allergy, Immunology and Rheumatology, Dalin Tzu Chi Hospital, Buddhist Tzu Chi Medical Foundation, No. 2, Minsheng RoadDalin, Chiayi 62247, Taiwan. [2]School of Medicine, Tzu Chi University, Hualien City, Taiwan. [3]Department of Life Science and Institute of Molecular Biology, National Chung Cheng University, Minxiong, Chiayi, Taiwan.

References

1. Bakland G, Gran JT, Nossent JC. Increased mortality in ankylosing spondylitis is related to disease activity. Ann Rheum Dis. 2011;70:1921–5.

2. Sieper J, Poddubnyy D. Axial spondyloarthritis. Lancet. 2017;390:73–84.

3. Ranganathan V, Gracey E, Brown MA, Inman RD, Haroon N. Pathogenesis of ankylosing spondylitis - recent advances and future directions. Nat Rev Rheumatol. 2017;13:359–67.

4. Brewerton DA, Hart FD, Nicholls A, Caffrey M, James DC, Sturrock RD. Ankylosing spondylitis and HL-A 27. Lancet. 1973;1:904–7.

5. Wellcome Trust Case Control Consortium, Australo-Anglo-American Spondylitis Consortium (TASC), Burton PR, Clayton DG, Cardon LR, Craddock N, et al. Association scan of 14,500 nonsynonymous SNPs in four diseases identifies autoimmunity variants. Nat Genet. 2007;39:1329–37.

6. Wang Y, Luo J, Wang X, Yang B, Cui L. MicroRNA-199a-5p induced autophagy and inhibits the pathogenesis of ankylosing spondylitis by modulating the mTOR signaling via directly targeting Ras homolog enriched in brain (Rheb). Cell Physiol Biochem. 2017;42:2481–91.

7. Smith JA, Colbert RA. The interleukin-23/interleukin-17 axis in spondyloarthritis pathogenesis: Th17 and beyond. Arthritis Rheumatol. 2014;66:231–41.

8. Baeten D, Sieper J, Braun J, Baraliakos X, Dougados M, Emery P, et al. Secukinumab, an interleukin-17A inhibitor, in ankylosing spondylitis. N Engl J Med. 2015;373:2534–48.

9. Lai NS, Yu HC, Chen HC, Yu CL, Huang HB, Lu MC. Aberrant expression of microRNAs in T cells from patients with ankylosing spondylitis contributes to the immunopathogenesis. Clin Exp Immunol. 2013;173:47–57.

10. Mohammadi H, Hemmatzadeh M, Babaie F, Gowhari Shabgah A, Azizi G, Hosseini F, et al. MicroRNA implications in the etiopathogenesis of ankylosing spondylitis. J Cell Physiol. 2018;233:5564–73.

11. Chen L, Al-Mossawi MH, Ridley A, Sekine T, Hammitzsch A, de Wit J, et al. miR-10b-5p is a novel Th17 regulator present in Th17 cells from ankylosing spondylitis. Ann Rheum Dis. 2017;76:620–5.

12. Li Z, Wu F, Brant SR, Kwon JH. IL-23 receptor regulation by Let-7f in human CD4+ memory T cells. J Immunol. 2011;186:6182–90.

13. Oppmann B, Lesley R, Blom B, Timans JC, Xu Y, Hunte B, et al. Novel p19 protein engages IL-12p40 to form a cytokine, IL-23, with biological activities similar as well as distinct from IL-12. Immunity. 2000;13:715–25.

14. Sieve AN, Meeks KD, Lee S, Berg RE. A novel immunoregulatory function for IL-23: inhibition of IL-12-dependent IFN-γ production. Eur J Immunol. 2010;40:2236–47.

15. Rudwaleit M, Landewé R, van der Heijde D, Listing J, Brandt J, Braun J, et al. The development of Assessment of SpondyloArthritis international Society classification criteria for axial spondyloarthritis (part I): classification of paper patients by expert opinion including uncertainty appraisal. Ann Rheum Dis. 2009;68:770–6.

16. Lai NS, Yu HC, Tung CH, Huang KY, Huang HB, Lu MC. The role of aberrant expression of T cell miRNAs affected by TNF-α in the immunopathogenesis of rheumatoid arthritis. Arthritis Res Ther. 2017;19:261.

17. van der Heijde D, Lie E, Kvien TK, Sieper J, Van den Bosch F, Listing J, et al. ASDAS, a highly discriminatory ASAS-endorsed disease activity score in patients with ankylosing spondylitis. Ann Rheum Dis. 2009;68:1811–8.

18. Lu MC, Lai NS, Chen HC, Yu HC, Huang KY, Tung CH, et al. Decreased microRNA (miR)-145 and increased miR-224 expression in T cells from patients with systemic lupus erythematosus involved in lupus immunopathogenesis. Clin Exp Immunol. 2013;171:91–9.

19. Trapnell C, Roberts A, Goff L, Pertea G, Kim D, Kelley DR, et al. Differential gene and transcript expression analysis of RNA-seq experiments with TopHat and Cufflinks. Nat Protoc. 2012;7:562–78.

20. Li Y, Wang H, Lu H, Hua S. Regulation of memory T cells by interleukin-23. Int Arch Allergy Immunol. 2016;169:157–62.

21. Croxford AL, Mair F, Becher B. IL-23: one cytokine in control of autoimmunity. Eur J Immunol. 2012;42:2263–73.

22. Nakayama W, Jinnin M, Tomizawa Y, Nakamura K, Kudo H, Inoue K, et al. Dysregulated interleukin-23 signalling contributes to the increased collagen production in scleroderma fibroblasts via balancing microRNA expression. Rheumatology (Oxford). 2017;56:145–55.

23. Cocco C, Canale S, Frasson C, Di Carlo E, Ognio E, Ribatti D, et al. Interleukin-23 acts as antitumor agent on childhood B-acute lymphoblastic leukemia cells. Blood. 2010;116:3887–98.

24. Wang H, Chao K, Ng SC, Bai AH, Yu Q, Yu J, et al. Pro-inflammatory miR-223 mediates the cross-talk between the IL23 pathway and the intestinal barrier in inflammatory bowel disease. Genome Biol. 2016;17:58.

25. Hou C, Zhu M, Sun M, Lin Y. MicroRNA let-7i induced autophagy to protect T cell from apoptosis by targeting IGF1R. Biochem Biophys Res Commun. 2014;453:728–34.

26. Shen X, Ye Y, Qi J, Wu X, Ni H, Cong H, et al. Identification of a novel microRNA, miR-4449, as a potential blood based marker in multiple myeloma. Clin Chem Lab Med. 2017;55:748–54.

27. Giuliani N, Airoldi I. Novel insights into the role of interleukin-27 and interleukin-23 in human malignant and normal plasma cells. Clin Cancer Res. 2011;17:6963–70.

28. Milanez FM, Saad CG, Viana VT, Moraes JC, Périco GV, Sampaio-Barros PD, et al. IL-23/Th17 axis is not influenced by TNF-blocking agents in ankylosing spondylitis patients. Arthritis Res Ther. 2016;18:52.

29. Paradowska-Gorycka A, Grzybowska-Kowalczyk A, Wojtecka-Lukasik E, Maslinski S. IL-23 in the pathogenesis of rheumatoid arthritis. Scand J Immunol. 2010;71:134–45.

30. Lyons SM, Fay MM, Akiyama Y, Anderson PJ, Ivanov P. RNA biology of angiogenin: current state and perspectives. RNA Biol. 2017;14:171–8.

31. Sheng J, Xu Z. Three decades of research on angiogenin: a review and perspective. Acta Biochim Biophys Sin Shanghai. 2016;48:399–410.

32. Lee SH, Kim KW, Min KM, Kim KW, Chang SI, Kim JC. Angiogenin reduces immune inflammation via inhibition of TANK-binding kinase 1 expression in human corneal fibroblast cells. Mediators Inflamm. 2014;2014:861435.

33. Hayashi H, Kawakita A, Okazaki S, Yasutomi M, Murai H, Ohshima Y. IL-17A/F modulates fibrocyte functions in cooperation with CD40-mediated signaling. Inflammation. 2013;36:830–8.

34. Eleftheriadis T, Pissas G, Sounidaki M, Antoniadis N, Antoniadi G, Liakopoulos V, et al. Angiogenin is upregulated during the alloreactive immune response and has no effect on the T-cell expansion phase, whereas it affects the contraction phase by inhibiting CD4+ T-cell apoptosis. Exp Ther Med. 2016;12:3471–5.

19

The inflammatory response in the regression of lumbar disc herniation

Carla Cunha[1,2*] , Ana J. Silva[1,2], Paulo Pereira[3,4,5], Rui Vaz[1,3,4,5], Raquel M. Gonçalves[1,2,6] and Mário A. Barbosa[1,2,6]

Abstract

Lumbar disc herniation (LDH) is highly associated with inflammation in the context of low back pain. Currently, inflammation is associated with adverse symptoms related to the stimulation of nerve fibers that may lead to pain. However, inflammation has also been indicated as the main factor responsible for LDH regression. This apparent controversy places inflammation as a good prognostic indicator of spontaneous regression of LDH. This review addresses the molecular and cellular mechanisms involved in LDH regression, including matrix remodeling and neovascularization, in the scope of the clinical decision on conservative versus surgical intervention. Based on the evidence, a special focus on the inflammatory response in the LDH context is given, particularly in the monocyte/macrophage role. The phenomenon of spontaneous regression of LDH, extensively reported in the literature, is therefore analyzed here under the perspective of the modulatory role of inflammation.

Keywords: Low back pain, Spine, Intervertebral disc, Immunomodulation, Macrophages

Low back pain and lumbar disc herniation

Lumbar disc herniation (LDH) is a major contributor to low back pain and affects around 9% of all people worldwide, with a high associated economic burden and a tendency to increase as the population ages [1]. LDH has been associated with disruption of the annulus fibrosus (AF), extrusion of the nucleus pulposus (NP), and stimulation of nerve fibers, leading to pain. However, more recently, Rajasekaran et al. [2] suggested that disc herniation is more commonly the result of endplate junction failure than AF rupture. Herniated discs are found in 30–40% of asymptomatic people by imaging diagnostic tools [3].

The current treatments for LDH, as well as for degenerative disc disease in general, can be divided into conservative versus surgical approaches and the decision on which approach to use is variable and patient–clinician dependent. Symptoms originated by LDH may disappear without any surgical treatment and in some of these patients this is accompanied by a reduction of the size of disc herniation in imaging studies. This phenomenon is known as spontaneous hernia regression, which may be partial or complete. Clearly, this evidence is indicative of the paramount need to identify the mechanisms behind LDH regression and to develop predictive methods for detection of this phenomenon in clinical practice.

Clinical evidence of spontaneous LDH regression

Since the first report of spontaneous LDH regression [4] and of computed tomography (CT)-confirmed spontaneous LDH regression [5], documentation of this phenomenon has become broadly available in the literature. Imaging diagnostic tools such as magnetic resonance imaging (MRI) have a central role in confirming LDH regression and, although controversial for a significant number of years, it is now widely recognized that large-sized and sequestrated LDH tend to regress more than other LDH subtypes (Fig. 1). This regression may be partial or complete. The level most commonly affected by this phenomenon is L4–L5, which is also where LDH occurs more frequently [6]. The main hypothesis behind the initiation of spontaneous LDH regression has been described as the exposure of herniated disc material to the epidural vascular supply through the ruptured posterior longitudinal ligament (PLL) (Fig. 1).

* Correspondence: carla.cunha@ineb.up.pt
Carla Cunha and Ana J. Silva contributed equally to this work.
Raquel M. Gonçalves and Mário A. Barbosa contributed equally to this work.
[1]i3S—Instituto de Investigação e Inovação em Saúde, Universidade do Porto, Rua Alfredo Allen 208, 4200-135 Porto, Portugal
[2]INEB—Instituto de Engenharia Biomédica, Universidade do Porto, Rua do Campo Alegre 823, 4150-180 Porto, Portugal
Full list of author information is available at the end of the article

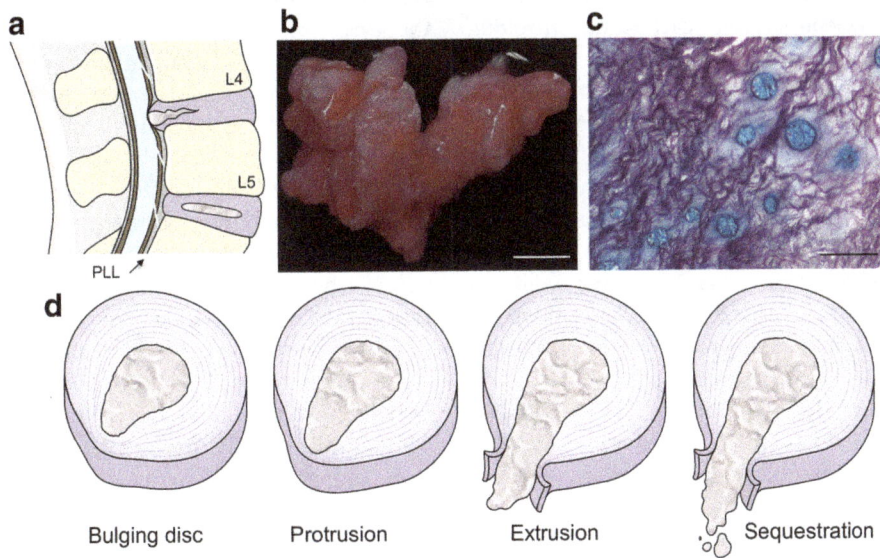

Fig. 1 a Schematic representation of typical L4–L5 hernia, with compression and possible rupture of posterior longitudinal ligament (PLL). **b** Human LDH fragment, obtained from patient who underwent microdiscectomy after informed consent and ethics committee approval from Centro Hospitalar São João. **c** Histological staining of tissue collected in (b), showing cell clusters producing proteoglycans (Alcian blue) embedded in a collagen matrix (Picrosirius red). **d** LDH is currently divided into four subtypes, according to MRI, as bulging disc (mildest form), protrusion, extrusion, and sequestration, the severest form of LDH. Proteoglycan-rich nucleus pulposus in center is surrounded by collagen-rich concentric rings of annulus fibrosus. Scale bars: (**b**) 3 cm, (**c**) 100 μm. Image credits: (**a**, **d**) used elements from Servier Medical Art; (**b**, **c**) unpublished

MRI analyses that allow precise quantifications of the decrease in herniation volume have shown that spontaneous LDH regression is more related to the presence of transligamentous extension and not so much to the initial size of herniation. Ahn et al. analyzed longitudinally in time 36 symptomatic herniated lumbar discs and showed that 25 of them decreased in size and that the most frequent herniation types that reduced in size were sequestered herniations (average decreases of 17%, 48%, and 82% for the subligamentous, transligamentous, and sequestered herniation groups, respectively). These results suggest that the PLL rupture is more important than the initial size of the hernia [7]. In Takada et al.'s study [8], all cases of sequestrated discs were completely resolved after 9 months, whereas extruded discs were only completely resolved after 12 months. On the other hand, disc protrusions showed little to no signs of regression after 12 months, most probably because of the patients' younger age and the abundance of collagen fibers and chondrocyte-like cells from the NP in these discs. The faster rate of radiographic resolution seen with sequestrated discs has been traditionally associated with dehydration and shrinkage, as the free fragment is no longer supplied with nutrients from the parent disc [9, 10]. Other authors postulate that sequestrated discs, unlike other LDH subtypes, trigger an inflammatory response characterized by neovascularization and immune cell-mediated degradation [11–13]. The subsequent increase in blood flow around free fragments explains why the periphery of disc sequestrations is enhanced with gadolinium (Gd) contrast, which is measured by MRI rim enhancement. In fact, Autio et al. [11] proposed that sequestrated discs with higher levels of Gd diethylenetriamine pentaacetic acid (Gd-DTPA) enhancement on MRI images served as predictors for their higher resorption rate. In this study, MRI of herniated patients was repeated throughout 12 months showing that a significant NP resorption occurred until 2 months after diagnosis and was more pronounced over the 1-year follow-up period. Higher resorption rates were associated with higher baseline scores of rim enhancement thickness, higher degree of herniated NP displacement in the Komori classification, and an age range of 41–50 years. The thickness of rim enhancement was a stronger determinant of spontaneous resorption than its extent. The extent of rim enhancement significantly correlated with the degree of disc displacement, being most pronounced in the case of sequesters.

Clinical decision on conservative versus surgical intervention for LDH

In order to understand spontaneous LDH regression, its prognostic factors, and its predictive outcomes, large cohorts have been conducted, namely the Maine Lumbar Spine Study [14], the Spine Patient Outcomes Research

Trial (SPORT) [15], and the Hague Spine Intervention Prognostic Study Group [16], each one enrolling hundreds of patients suffering from LDH. Interestingly, all of these studies indicate that early surgery achieves more rapid relief of LDH symptoms than conservative care but, in the long run, outcomes gradually become identical to conservative treatment. Many other systematic studies have consistently obtained similar results [17–20]. Buttermann [21] compared the LDH symptoms of patients after 6 weeks of conservative treatment (38 patients) with those who received epidural injections (20 patients) and found that both groups had similar outcomes, including the size of herniated NP.

Despite the evidence for spontaneous LDH regression, there is still much debate among clinicians concerning the efficacy of conservative vs nonconservative treatments. Initial management for patients with the sequestrated subtype of LDH may be conservative due to the higher likelihood and faster rate of resolution in comparison to the other LDH subtypes (reviewed in [6, 22]). Patients with intractable pain, neurological deficit, or bowel or bladder dysfunction, among other associated factors, remain candidates for earlier surgical intervention. However, it is still hard to predict which patients are more likely to benefit from conservative treatment and have higher probability of spontaneous regression of the disc herniation. It is therefore remarkably challenging to decide which patients to submit to surgery. Future large, prospective, randomized trials are required to better determine a set of specific clinical criteria, such as those defined by Chiu et al. [22], that may predict the surgery outcome. On a more mechanistic approach, finding molecular markers, possibly noninvasive ones, such as systemic markers, to predict the outcome of LDH would have a major impact on the clinical decision. These approaches are only starting to emerge, such as the study by Elkan et al. [23] in which high plasminogen activator inhibitor 1, a marker of fibrinolysis, analyzed in blood samples of patients with LDH, was fairly consistently associated with poor LDH surgery outcome.

Mechanisms behind LDH spontaneous regression

As already described, the spontaneous regression of IVD herniated tissue is well documented clinically, but the underlying mechanisms remain unclear. To the best of our knowledge, three theories have been proposed to explain the resorption of herniated material. The first theory proposes that the herniated disc fragment reduces in size due to gradual dehydration and shrinkage, which may explain the decrease of signal intensity of the disc in the follow-up MRI studies [9, 10]. The second hypothesis suggests that tension applied by the PLL leads to retraction of the herniated disc fragment back into the IVD space. This mechanism may explain the

cases where the herniated disc has an intact AF, but not the cases with completely extruded or migrated disc fragments [5]. Onel et al. [24] showed that under a static traction load of 45 kg, the herniated tissue retracted in 21 out of 30 LDH patients, while in two of them the herniated tissue has actually increased. The third theory, the most extensively studied with preclinical and clinical evidence to support it, is the gradual hernia resorption through enzymatic degradation and phagocytosis induced by an inflammatory reaction and neovascularization [11–13]. This inflammatory reaction is supposed to be triggered when the disc content extrudes into the epidural space and is then recognized as foreign. Depending on each individual clinical condition, it is possible that one specific mechanism or different combinations of the three may operate in spontaneous regression of the herniated disc tissue.

The privileged immunity of IVD

The IVD is the largest avascular organ in the human body and considered an immune-privileged site [25]. The NP appears to be particularly isolated from the immune system of the host, given its position between two cartilaginous endplates and inside the dense collagen fibrous structure of the AF. Additionally to this physiological barrier, the IVD cells also actively resist invasion by immune cells, due to the Fas ligand (FasL) expression, which is characteristic of immune-privileged sites [26]. FasL belongs to the tumor necrosis factor (TNF) family and is known to induce apoptosis by binding to its receptor, Fas. While Fas is expressed in a wide variety of cells, FasL expression is restricted to the surface of cytotoxic T cells, natural killer (NK) cells, tumor cells, and stromal cells of some immune-privileged sites. In immune-privileged sites, FasL of stromal cells binds to Fas receptor expressed on immune cells and infiltrating cells. This ligand–receptor binding induces apoptosis of the infiltrating immune cells, maintaining the immune-privileged condition of the tissue [27]. The immune-privileged environment of the NP is the pillar of the theory of the inflammatory reaction behind LDH resorption. This theory proposes that the extrusion of the NP tissue into the epidural space evokes an autoimmune reaction that leads to the infiltration of immune cells which will interact with IVD cells and secrete a variety of molecules initiating the hernia resorption process [11, 12, 28].

Macrophages as key players in LDH regression

Macrophages are indicated as the most important immune players in the resorption process of herniated discs. Numerous studies have found by immunohistochemistry the presence of macrophages in herniated IVD tissue specimens [29–32]. These cells have the capability to actively phagocyte the herniated tissue and process it in their lysosomes filled with collagen-degrading enzymes.

Macrophages also secrete lysosomal enzymes by exocytosis, which break down intercellular substances such as the disc matrix components proteoglycans and collagens [12, 33]. Furthermore, phagocytic activity of macrophages was observed in surgically removed samples of herniated NP through electron microscopy [12] and these immune cells are known to express scavenger receptors, such as CD36, which have been characterized as the main responsible molecules for the phagocytosis of apoptotic cells, highlighting the potential role of macrophages in hernia resorption [34]. Interestingly, in LDH histological samples, macrophage phagocytosis was observed more often in sequestration subtype LDH than subligamentous ones [35], in accordance with the clinical evidence showing that sequestered hernias are more likely to regress. Ikeda et al. [29] also observed more frequently the infiltration of macrophages and neovascularization along the margins of the transligamentous extruded disc material than in other subtypes of LDH.

Monocyte recruitment to IVD tissue
The exact mechanism by which monocytes are recruited to the IVD remains unclear, as reviewed previously [36]. However, it is known that the IVD endogenously includes inflammatory-like cells (i.e., cells with phagocytic capacity) and IVD cells are able to produce inflammatory mediators [36], which may themselves contribute to recruit other immune cells to the hernia site. In particular, monocyte chemoattractant protein (MCP)-1, a CC chemokine that contributes to the activation and recruitment of monocytes, has been extensively demonstrated to be produced by IVD cells [13, 37–40]. In particular, Yoshida et al. [13] developed a hernia model in which IVD cells produced proinflammatory cytokines as an initial response to disc herniation. These cytokines stimulate the production of MCP-1 by IVD cells, resulting in macrophage infiltration in herniated discs. The infiltrating monocyte-derived macrophages also produce MCP-1, increasing the monocyte recruitment to the IVD

[13]. Apart from macrophages, plasmacytoid dendritic cells have also been shown to be involved in LDH resorption [41]. Surgical material from transligamentous and subligamentous sequestrations was analyzed by flow cytometry and plasmacytoid dendritic cells were found to predominate over macrophages on transligamentous sequestrations, indicating that these cells may be involved in the initiation of the immune response [41].

Inflammatory cascades in LDH-implicating macrophages
Numerous studies analyzed immune mediators in LDH and especially implicating macrophages in LDH regression (Table 1). Shamji et al. [32] showed high expression levels of macrophage products like IL-4, IL-6, IL-12, and interferon gamma (IFN-γ) in herniated disc tissue. Other studies demonstrated that IVD tissue is also capable of spontaneously producing other molecules, such as the chemokines IL-8 and MCP-1, the main functions of which are chemotaxis of macrophages and angiogenesis [37]. Furthermore, Kang et al. [42] demonstrated that herniated discs release high levels of matrix metalloproteinases (MMPs), nitric oxide (NO), IL-6, and prostaglandin E2 (PGE2) and this production increases when the discs are stimulated with IL-1β, evidencing that IVD cells are biologically responsive to exogenous stimuli. Regarding IL-6, it has already been demonstrated in vitro that its production is induced when IVDs and macrophages are cocultured [43]. More recently, Takada et al. [44] showed that coculturing IVDs and macrophages upregulated IL-8, PGE2, and cyclooxygenase 2 (COX-2). In both studies, the mentioned biochemical mediators are mainly produced by macrophages. The latter study also showed that rat IVD autografts induced extensive macrophage infiltration in vivo, increasing the mRNA levels of TNF-α, IL-6, IL-8, and COX-2. TNF-α is required for IL-6 and PGE2 production, but not for IL-8 production, during IVD–macrophage interaction. Neutralization of TNF-α and IL-8 may be a valuable therapy for pain related with LDH [44]. Other studies

Table 1 Immune mediators implicating macrophages in LDH regression

Immune mediator	Sample	Species	Study
IL-6, NO, PGE2, MMP-3, MMP-2/MMP-9	Herniated IVD tissue	Human	Kang et al., 1997 [42]
IL-8, MCP-1	Herniated IVD tissue	Human	Burke et al., 2002 [37]
IL-4, IL-6, IL-12, IFN-γ	Herniated IVD tissue	Human	Shamji et al., 2010 [32]
MMP-3, MMP-7	Coculture of IVD and macrophages	Mouse	Haro et al., 2000 [45]
MMP-7, TNF-α	Coculture of IVD and macrophages	Mouse	Haro et al., 2000 [46]
MMP-3, MMP-7, TNF-α, VEGF	Coculture of IVD and macrophages	Mouse	Kato et al., 2004 [47]
IL-6	Coculture of IVD and macrophages	Rat	Takada et al., 2004 [43]
IL-8, PGE2, COX-2	Coculture of IVD and macrophages	Rat	Takada et al., 2012 [44]

COX-2 cyclooxygenase 2, IFN-γ interferon gamma, IL interleukin, IVD intervertebral disc, LDH lumbar disc herniation, MCP-1 monocyte chemoattractant protein-1, MMP matrix metalloproteinase, NO nitric oxide, PGE2 prostaglandin E2, TNF-α tumor necrosis factor alpha, VEGF vascular endothelial growth factor

have also analyzed the interaction between macrophages and IVD tissue using cocultures between macrophages and chondrocytes or whole IVD. Haro et al. demonstrated that the production of both MMP-3 and MMP-7 was strongly upregulated in IVD cell/macrophage coculture, MMP-3 being produced by both chondrocytes and macrophages while MMP-7 is produced predominantly by macrophages. Moreover, the authors also revealed that disc-derived MMP-3 is required for the physical degradation of disc tissues and for macrophage infiltration, which ultimately leads to hernia resorption [45]. In other studies, the same group demonstrated that MMP-7 released by macrophages contributes to the process of herniated disc resorption through the release of soluble TNF-α [46, 47]. TNF-α is a potent inducer of many MMPs, such as MMP-3, and also of vascular endothelial growth factor (VEGF) that is implicated in the neovascularization of herniated discs [47, 48]. The crucial role of MMP-7 in the initiation of herniated disc resorption resulted in the development of a recombinant human MMP-7 intradiscal therapy, which is in phase I/II clinical trials in the United States. This therapy avoids the side effects associated with surgery, such as nerve tissue damage [49].

Neovascularization in LDH resorption

Altogether, these studies provide evidence for a mechanism of LDH resorption associated with a cascade of inflammation, matrix remodeling, and angiogenesis. However, only few studies have specifically addressed neovascularization.

Usually, few blood vessels exist in the mature IVD. However, proliferation of new vessels has already been demonstrated at the margin of the herniated tissue and this is thought to be a major determinant of spontaneous regression of LDH [11, 50]. Several molecular mediators have been suggested to be involved in the neovascularization of LDH, including TNF-α, VEGF, and basic fibroblast growth factor (bFGF). As mentioned earlier, TNF-α can promote the expression of VEGF, which plays an essential role in the formation of new blood vessels, and some studies confirmed the presence of VEGF and VEGF receptors in human LDH tissue [48, 51]. Also, the interaction between macrophages and disc tissue leads to generation of inflammatory cytokines, which are known to be involved in the induction of angiogenesis. Haro et al. observed an increase in the mRNA and protein levels of VEGF when macrophages were in contact with disc tissue comparatively to the expression levels when they were cultured alone. This enhancement of the VEGF levels was apparently mediated by a TNF-α-dependent pathway since this effect was abrogated by the use of a TNF-α neutralizing antibody [48]. Using MRI in

humans, the presence of capillaries invading the hernia and monocyte-derived macrophages migrating out of these capillaries has been demonstrated [12]. Additionally, in an experimental model in rabbits, bFGF, a factor known to stimulate mitogenesis and chemotaxis of fibroblasts and capillary endothelial cells, as well as to stimulate angiogenesis, promoted the resorption of disc material. In this study, treatment with bFGF led to an increase in the number of newly formed vessels with a consequent higher infiltration of inflammatory cells (macrophages, lymphocytes, and fibroblasts), which contributed to the resorption process [52].

These studies reinforce the importance of the crosstalk between angiogenesis and inflammation, which ultimately leads to LDH regression.

Contribution of other immune response mediators

An autoimmune reaction is far more complex than the mere macrophage recruitment and neovascularization so far described. Indeed, apart from macrophages, other immune cells are present in LDH (Fig. 2). The complete understanding of the immune response associated with LDH regression has benefited to a great extent from in-vivo animal models. More than in-vivo evidence for LDH resorption, already thoroughly clinically demonstrated, animal models have been employed to unravel the underlying mechanisms of IVD regression. We have shown spontaneous regression of LDH in a rat IVD lesion model [53]. In this work, IVD lesion was induced by either 21-G or 25-G needle puncture and we have found that the size of the hernia formed was proportional to the needle gauge used. In both cases, hernias significantly diminish in volume from 2 to 6 weeks post injury. Also, we found that the number of CD68+ macrophages within the hernia as well as cell apoptosis within the tissue were both proportional to the hernia volume. Using the same model, we further confirmed that the number of CD68+ macrophages in the hernia was proportional to its size and hypothesized that only a certain number of macrophages will be recruited and activated per area of hernia, keeping the tissue homeostasis. Moreover, we have found that the systemic transplantation of rat bone marrow MSC resulted in a significant reduction in the size of the hernias formed 2 weeks post lesion and that the number of B lymphocytes surrounding the hernia increased [54]. In another study, a rabbit herniation model was developed, consisting of the introduction of a needle up to penetrating the PLL and then physically compressing to extrude the NP to the epidural space [13]. The herniated discs spontaneously reduced in size gradually up to 12 weeks post surgery. Infiltrating cells, mainly composed of macrophages, were observed from day 3. Immunohistochemically, IVD cells in the

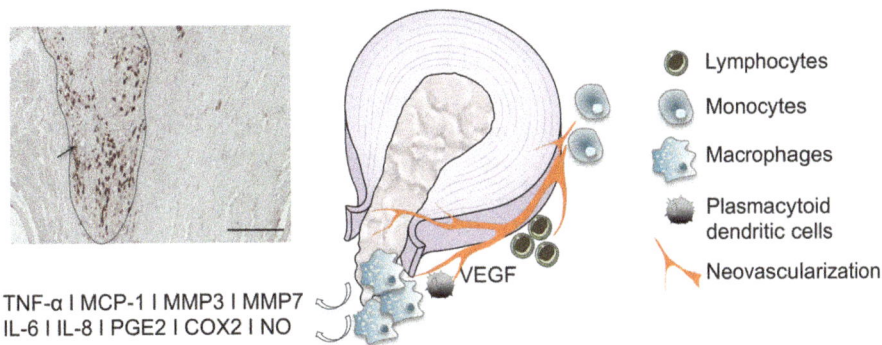

Fig. 2 Representative proposed mechanism of LDH resorption. Both herniated IVD tissue and macrophages produce tumor necrosis factor alpha (TNF-α), monocyte chemoattractant protein (MCP)-1, matrix metalloproteinases (MMPs), interleukin (IL)-6, IL-8, prostaglandin E2 (PGE2), cyclooxygenase 2 (COX2), and nitric oxide (NO), which contribute to the inflammatory reaction and resorption of the herniated tissue. Vascular endothelial growth factor (VEGF) induces blood vessel ingrowth and neovascularization, which support immune cell mobilization to hernia site. Insert: in rat model of IVD herniation, CD68+ macrophages localized within hernia (delimited by dashed line), which include a blood vessel (arrow). Scale bar: 100 μm. Image used elements from Servier Medical Art; insert: unpublished

herniated discs produced TNF-α and IL-1β on day 1, followed by MCP-1 on day 3.

Nevertheless, most of the current in-vivo LDH models are autotransplantation models in which IVDs are transplanted into subcutaneous or dorsal epidural spaces of the animals after laminectomy, with the scope of specifically analyzing the associated immune response. This is because it is still controversial whether the inflammatory response of the host is initiated simply by exposure to structural elements and compounds that are present in the disc cell membrane and matrix, by direct contact of the NP material with the immune system via an autoimmune response, or whether it is secondary to an auto-immune response. It has been shown previously that subcutaneously transplanted NP cell survival was reduced in association with an immunological reaction, by transplanting NP tissue into Lewis rats and into NOD mice, and that NK cells and macrophages were present around the outgrown NP tissues but no T cells were found [55]. Another study implanted autologous NP subcutaneously in pigs and activated T cells (CD4+ and CD8+) were found in the exudates in considerable number, as well as activated B cells expressing immunoglobulin kappa (Igκ). The results showed that NP attracts activated T and B cells [56].

What most of these studies show is that the immune system is able to respond to the intact healthy NP tissue. To analyze whether inflammation occurs in response to compounds secreted from viable cells in the NP or whether inflammation simply requires exposure to structural cell or matrix components, Rand et al. [57] used a mouse model in which the animal was exposed to disc tissue containing viable NP and AF cells, to disc tissue containing viable AF cells, or to disc tissue with no

viable cells. The three tissue preparations were inserted into the right lower peritoneal cavity. The devitalized tissue was intended to assess a possible effect of chemical irritants that may be present in the disc and that may induce inflammation. Macrophage recruitment occurred over the course of 1, 2, and 7 days post injury and only after exposure to viable disc tissue but not after exposure to devitalized disc components [57], indicating that macrophage recruitment occurred only in response to cell cues.

Most of the evidence for the inflammatory reaction around spontaneous hernia regression has been collected from animal studies. Despite this, some studies mostly involving immunohistochemistry analysis of clinical samples have confirmed the results obtained in animal experimentation. The presence of T and B lymphocytes on isolated human herniated discs was further confirmed by the same group [58]. Also, histological analyses of human herniated discs revealed the presence of infiltrated T cells [59]. Furthermore, in human herniated tissue, lymphocytes were found to be three times more abundant in sequestrated hernias than in extrusions, while no other inflammatory cells were seen in protrusions apart from macrophages [60]. In another study, the inflammatory infiltrate has been characterized by immunostaining in portions of herniated discs which underwent surgery for LDH. None of the 38 samples expressed the immunophenotypic markers of the lymphocyte (CD20, CD45RO, CD4, CD8, TCR), mature monocyte (CD33), or dendritic cell (CD1a, CD80, CD86, S100). However, an abundant infiltration of CD68+ cells that lacked CD33 with variable amounts of CD11b, CD11c, and CD40 was observed, likely representing a process of differentiation from monocytes to macrophages [61].

Conclusions

LDH spontaneous resorption is well documented clinically and in preclinical studies. Spine surgeons are becoming increasingly aware of this phenomenon and many recognize the usefulness of conservative treatment for LDH and advise patients accordingly. Different forms of nonsurgical treatments should be exhausted before considering surgery in acute stages of LDH, unless conservative treatment is contraindicated for reasons such as neurological deficit and intolerable pain despite administration of adequate pain medications.

It is clear that the inflammatory response that occurs associated with LDH is crucial to its spontaneous resorption. Therefore, inflammation in this specific clinical context is a good prognostic indicator and should not be halted. Still, it is exactly an inflammatory response that causes a harmful effect on the adjacent nerve roots, causing pain. The control of the inflammatory reaction in this setting is an important challenge when treating patients with LDH. The combination of knowledge from the biological mechanisms behind LDH resorption and the detailed personalized diagnosis will be the determinant to tailor treatment to each individual patient and may ultimately lead to reduction in costs to the health system.

Abbreviations

AF: Annulus fibrosus; IVD: Intervertebral disc; LDH: Lumbar disc herniation; MSC: Mesenchymal stem cells; NP: Nucleus pulposus

Acknowledgements

The figures used elements from Servier Medical Art, provided by Servier, licensed under a Creative Commons Attribution 3.0 unported license (http://smart.servier.com). The authors declare no potential conflict of interests.

Funding

This work was financed by project "Bioengineered Therapies for infectious diseases and tissue regeneration" (NORTE-01-0145-FEDER-000012), supported by Norte Portugal Regional Operational Programme (NORTE 2020), under the PORTUGAL 2020 Partnership Agreement, through the European Regional Development Fund (ERDF), by FEDER/COMPETE 2020 (POCI), Portugal 2020, and by Portuguese funds through FCT/MCTES in the framework of the project "Institute for Research and Innovation in Health Sciences" (POCI-01-0145-FEDER-007274). Cunha C and Gonçalves RM acknowledge FCT by their postdoc fellowship (SFRH/BDP/87071/2012) and FCT Investigator Grant (IF/00638/2014), respectively. Silva AJ acknowledges her fellowship under the framework of the project Norte-01-0145-FEDER-000012.

Authors' contributions

CC, AJS, RMG, and MAB conceived the study. CC, AJS, PP, RV, RMG, and MAB wrote the manuscript. All authors read and approved the final manuscript.

Consent for publication

Not applicable.

Competing interests

The authors declare that they have no competing interests.

Author details

[1]i3S—Instituto de Investigação e Inovação em Saúde, Universidade do Porto, Rua Alfredo Allen 208, 4200-135 Porto, Portugal. [2]INEB—Instituto de Engenharia Biomédica, Universidade do Porto, Rua do Campo Alegre 823, 4150-180 Porto, Portugal. [3]Department of Neurosurgery, Centro Hospitalar São João, Porto, Portugal. [4]Department of Clinical Neurosciences and Mental Health, Faculty of Medicine, University of Porto, Porto, Portugal. [5]Neurosciences Center, CUF Porto Hospital, Porto, Portugal. [6]ICBAS—Instituto de Ciências Biomédicas Abel Salazar, Universidade do Porto, Rua Jorge Viterbo Ferreira 228, 4050-313 Porto, Portugal.

References

1. Hoy D, March L, Brooks P, Blyth F, Woolf A, Bain C, et al. The global burden of low back pain: estimates from the Global Burden of Disease 2010 study. Ann Rheum Dis. 2014;73(6):968–74 PubMed PMID: 24665116.
2. Rajasekaran S, Bajaj N, Tubaki V, Kanna R, Shetty A. ISSLS Prize winner: The anatomy of failure in lumbar disc herniation: an in vivo, multimodal, prospective study of 181 subjects. Spine. 2013;38(17):1491–500.
3. Brinjikji W, Luetmer PH, Comstock B, Bresnahan BW, Chen LE, Deyo RA, et al. Systematic literature review of imaging features of spinal degeneration in asymptomatic populations. AJNR Am J Neuroradiol. 2015;36(4):811–6 PubMed PMID: 25430861. Pubmed Central PMCID: 4464797.
4. Key J. Intervertebral disk lesions are the most common cause of low back pain with or without sciatica. Ann Surg. 1945;121(4):534–9.
5. Teplick JG, Haskin ME. Spontaneous regression of herniated nucleus pulposus. AJR Am J Roentgenol. 1985;145(2):371–5 PubMed PMID: 3875236.
6. Macki M, Hernandez-Hermann M, Bydon M, Gokaslan A, McGovern K, Bydon A. Spontaneous regression of sequestrated lumbar disc herniations: literature review. Clin Neurol Neurosurg. 2014;120:136–41.
7. Ahn S, Ahn M, Byun W. Effect of the transligamentous extension of lumbar disc herniations on their regression and the clinical outcome of sciatica. Spine. 2000;25:475–80.
8. Takada E, Takahashi M, Shimada K. Natural history of lumbar disc hernia with radicular leg pain: spontaneous MRI changes of the herniated mass and correlation with clinical outcome. J Orthop Surg. 2001;9(1):1–7 PubMed PMID: 12468836.
9. Henmi T, Sairyo K, Nakano S, Kanematsu Y, Kajikawa T, Katoh S, et al. Natural history of extruded lumbar intervertebral disc herniation. J Med Investig. 2002;49(1–2):40–3 PubMed PMID: 11901758.
10. Slavin KV, Raja A, Thornton J, Wagner FC Jr. Spontaneous regression of a large lumbar disc herniation: report of an illustrative case. Surg Neurol. 2001; 56(5):333–6 discussion 7. PubMed PMID: 11750011.
11. Autio RA, Karppinen J, Niinimaki J, Ojala R, Kurunlahti M, Haapea M, et al. Determinants of spontaneous resorption of intervertebral disc herniations. Spine. 2006;31(11):1247–52 PubMed PMID: 16688039.
12. Kobayashi S, Meir A, Kokubo Y, Uchida K, Takeno K, Miyazaki T, et al. Ultrastructural analysis on lumbar disc herniation using surgical specimens: role of neovascularization and macrophages in hernias. Spine. 2009;34(7): 655–62 PubMed PMID: 19333096.
13. Yoshida M, Nakamura T, Sei A, Kikuchi T, Takagi K, Matsukawa A. Intervertebral disc cells produce tumor necrosis factor alpha, interleukin-1beta, and monocyte chemoattractant protein-1 immediately after herniation: an experimental study using a new hernia model. Spine. 2005; 30(1):55–61 PubMed PMID: 15626982.
14. Atlas SJ, Keller RB, Wu YA, Deyo RA, Singer DE. Long-term outcomes of surgical and nonsurgical management of lumbar spinal stenosis: 8 to 10 year results from the Maine Lumbar Spine Study. Spine. 2005;30(8):936–43 PubMed PMID: 15834339.
15. Lurie JD, Tosteson TD, Tosteson AN, Zhao W, Morgan TS, Abdu WA, et al. Surgical versus nonoperative treatment for lumbar disc herniation: eight-year results for the Spine Patient Outcomes Research Trial. Spine. 2014;39(1): 3–16 PubMed PMID: 24153171. Pubmed Central PMCID: 3921966.

16. Peul WC, van den Hout WB, Brand R, Thomeer RT, Koes BW, Leiden—The Hague Spine Intervention Prognostic Study Group. Prolonged conservative care versus early surgery in patients with sciatica caused by lumbar disc herniation: two year results of a randomised controlled trial. BMJ. 2008; 336(7657):1355–8 PubMed PMID: 18502911. Pubmed Central PMCID: 2427077.

17. Hahne AJ, Ford JJ, McMeeken JM. Conservative management of lumbar disc herniation with associated radiculopathy: a systematic review. Spine. 2010; 35(11):E488–504 PubMed PMID: 20421859.

18. Jacobs W, Tulder M, Arts M, Rubinstein S, Middelkoop M, Ostelo R, et al. Surgery versus conservative management of sciatica due to a lumbar herniated disc: a systemic review. Eur Spine J. 2011;20:513–22.

19. Martinez-Quinones JV, Aso-Escario J, Consolini F, Arregui-Calvo R. Spontaneous regression from intervertebral disc herniation. Propos of a series of 37 cases. Neurocirugia. 2010;21(2):108–17 PubMed PMID: 20442973. Regresion espontanea de hernias discales intervertebrales. A proposito de una serie de 37 casos.

20. Weber H. Lumbar disc herniation. A controlled, prospective study with ten years of observation. Spine. 1983;8(2):131–40 PubMed PMID: 6857385.

21. Buttermann G. Lumbar disc herniation regression after successful epidural steroid injection. J Spinal Disord Tech. 2002;15(6):469–76.

22. Chiu CC, Chuang TY, Chang KH, Wu CH, Lin PW, Hsu WY. The probability of spontaneous regression of lumbar herniated disc: a systematic review. Clin Rehabil. 2015;29(2):184–95 PubMed PMID: 25009200.

23. Elkan P, Sten-Linder M, Hedlund R, Willers U, Ponzer S, Gerdhem P. Markers of inflammation and fibrinolysis in relation to outcome after surgery for lumbar disc herniation. A prospective study on 177 patients. Eur Spine J. 2016;25(1): 186–91. https://doi.org/10.1007/s00586-015-3998-7.

24. Onel D, Tuzlaci M, Sari H, Demir K. Computed tomographic investigation of the effect of traction on lumbar disc herniations. Spine. 1989;14(1):82–90 PubMed PMID: 2913674.

25. Hiyama A, Mochida J, Sakai D. Stem cell applications in intervertebral disc repair. Cell Mol Biol. 2008;54(1):24–32 PubMed PMID: 18954548.

26. Takada T, Nishida K, Doita M, Kurosaka M. Fas ligand exists on intervertebral disc cells: a potential molecular mechanism for immune privilege of the disc. Spine. 2002;27(14):1526–30 PubMed PMID: 12131712.

27. Green DR, Ferguson TA. The role of Fas ligand in immune privilege. Nat Rev Mol Cell Biol. 2001;2(12):917–24 PubMed PMID: 11733771.

28. Doita M, Kanatani T, Ozaki T, Matsui N, Kurosaka M, Yoshiya S. Influence of macrophage infiltration of herniated disc tissue on the production of matrix metalloproteinases leading to disc resorption. Spine. 2001;26(14):1522–7 PubMed PMID: 11462080.

29. Ikeda T, Nakamura T, Kikuchi T, Umeda S, Senda H, Takagi K. Pathomechanism of spontaneous regression of the herniated lumbar disc: histologic and immunohistochemical study. J Spinal Disord. 1996;9(2):136–40 PubMed PMID: 8793781.

30. Koike Y, Uzuki M, Kokubun S, Sawai T. Angiogenesis and inflammatory cell infiltration in lumbar disc herniation. Spine. 2003;28(17):1928–33 PubMed PMID: 12973136.

31. Rothoerl R, Woertgen C, Holzschuh M, Brehme K, Ruschoff J, Brawanski A. Macrophage tissue infiltration, clinical symptoms, and signs in patients with lumbar disc herniation. A clinicopathological study on 179 patients. Acta Neurochir. 1998;140(12):1245–8 PubMed PMID: 9932124.

32. Shamji MF, Setton LA, Jarvis W, So S, Chen J, Jing L, et al. Proinflammatory cytokine expression profile in degenerated and herniated human intervertebral disc tissues. Arthritis Rheum. 2010;62(7):1974–82 PubMed PMID: 20222111. Pubmed Central PMCID: 2917579.

33. Henson PM. Mechanisms of exocytosis in phagocytic inflammatory cells. Parke-Davis Award Lecture. Am J Pathol. 1980;101(3):494–511 PubMed PMID: 7004205. Pubmed Central PMCID: 1903647.

34. Tsuru M, Nagata K, Ueno T, Jimi A, Irie K, Yamada A, et al. Electron microscopic observation of established chondrocytes derived from human intervertebral disc hernia (KTN-1) and role of macrophages in spontaneous regression of degenerated tissues. Spine J. 2001;1(6):422–31 PubMed PMID: 14588300.

35. Haro H, Shinomiya K, Komori H, Okawa A, Saito I, Miyasaka N, et al. Upregulated expression of chemokines in herniated nucleus pulposus resorption. Spine. 1996;21(14):1647–52 PubMed PMID: 8839466.

36. Molinos M, Almeida CR, Caldeira J, Cunha C, Goncalves RM, Barbosa MA. Inflammation in intervertebral disc degeneration and regeneration. J R Soc Interface. 2015;12(108):20150429 PubMed PMID: 26040602. Pubmed Central PMCID: 4528607.

37. Burke JG, Watson RW, McCormack D, Dowling FE, Walsh MG, Fitzpatrick JM. Spontaneous production of monocyte chemoattractant protein-1 and interleukin-8 by the human lumbar intervertebral disc. Spine. 2002;27(13): 1402–7 PubMed PMID: 12131736.

38. Haro H, Komori H, Okawa A, Murakami S, Muneta T, Shinomiya K. Sequential dynamics of monocyte chemotactic protein-1 expression in herniated nucleus pulposus resorption. J Orthop Res. 1997;15(5):734–41 PubMed PMID: 9420604.

39. Kikuchi T, Nakamura T, Ikeda T, Ogata H, Takagi K. Monocyte chemoattractant protein-1 in the intervertebral disc. A histologic experimental model. Spine. 1998;23(10):1091–9 PubMed PMID: 9615359.

40. Yoshida M, Nakamura T, Kikuchi T, Takagi K, Matsukawa A. Expression of monocyte chemoattractant protein-1 in primary cultures of rabbit intervertebral disc cells. J Orthop Res. 2002;20(6):1298–304 PubMed PMID: 12472243.

41. Geiss A, Sobottke R, Delank KS, Eysel P. Plasmacytoid dendritic cells and memory T cells infiltrate true sequestrations stronger than subligamentous sequestrations: evidence from flow cytometric analysis of disc infiltrates. Eur Spine J. 2016;25(5):1417–27 PubMed PMID: 26906170.

42. Kang JD, Stefanovic-Racic M, McIntyre LA, Georgescu HI, Evans CH. Toward a biochemical understanding of human intervertebral disc degeneration and herniation. Contributions of nitric oxide, interleukins, prostaglandin E2, and matrix metalloproteinases. Spine. 1997;22(10):1065–73 PubMed PMID: 9160463.

43. Takada T, Nishida K, Doita M, Miyamoto H, Kurosaka M. Interleukin-6 production is upregulated by interaction between disc tissue and macrophages. Spine. 2004; 29(10):1089–92 discussion 93. PubMed PMID: 15131434.

44. Takada T, Nishida K, Maeno K, Kakutani K, Yurube T, Doita M, et al. Intervertebral disc and macrophage interaction induces mechanical hyperalgesia and cytokine production in a herniated disc model in rats. Arthritis Rheum. 2012;64(8):2601–10 PubMed PMID: 22392593.

45. Haro H, Crawford HC, Fingleton B, MacDougall JR, Shinomiya K, Spengler DM, et al. Matrix metalloproteinase-3-dependent generation of a macrophage chemoattractant in a model of herniated disc resorption. J Clin Invest. 2000; 105(2):133–41 PubMed PMID: 10642591. Pubmed Central PMCID: 377425.

46. Haro H, Crawford HC, Fingleton B, Shinomiya K, Spengler DM, Matrisian LM. Matrix metalloproteinase-7-dependent release of tumor necrosis factor-alpha in a model of herniated disc resorption. J Clin Invest. 2000;105(2):143–50 PubMed PMID: 10642592. Pubmed Central PMCID: 377426.

47. Kato T, Haro H, Komori H, Shinomiya K. Sequential dynamics of inflammatory cytokine, angiogenesis inducing factor and matrix degrading enzymes during spontaneous resorption of the herniated disc. J Orthop Res. 2004;22(4):895–900 PubMed PMID: 15183452.

48. Haro H, Kato T, Komori H, Osada M, Shinomiya K. Vascular endothelial growth factor (VEGF)-induced angiogenesis in herniated disc resorption. J Orthop Res. 2002;20(3):409–15 PubMed PMID: 12038611.

49. Haro H. Translational research of herniated discs: current status of diagnosis and treatment. J Orthop Sci. 2014;19(4):515–20 PubMed PMID: 24777237. Pubmed Central PMCID: 4111856.

50. Ozaki S, Muro T, Ito S, Mizushima M. Neovascularization of the outermost area of herniated lumbar intervertebral discs. J Orthop Sci. 1999;4(4):286–92 PubMed PMID: 10436276.

51. Jia CQ, Zhao JG, Zhang SF, Qi F. Stromal cell-derived factor-1 and vascular endothelial growth factor may play an important role in the process of neovascularization of herniated intervertebral discs. J Int Med Res. 2009; 37(1):136–44 PubMed PMID: 19215683.

52. Minamide A, Hashizume H, Yoshida M, Kawakami M, Hayashi N, Tamaki T. Effects of basic fibroblast growth factor on spontaneous resorption of herniated intervertebral discs. An experimental study in the rabbit. Spine. 1999;24(10):940–5 PubMed PMID: 10332782.

53. Cunha C, Lamas S, Goncalves RM, Barbosa MA. Joint analysis of IVD herniation and degeneration by rat caudal needle puncture model. J Orthop Res. 2017;35(2):258–68 PubMed PMID: 26610284.

54. Cunha C, Almeida CR, Almeida MI, Silva AM, Molinos M, Lamas S, et al. Systemic delivery of bone marrow mesenchymal stem cells for in situ intervertebral disc regeneration. Stem Cells Transl Med. 2017;6(3):1029–39 PubMed PMID: 28297581. Pubmed Central PMCID: 5442789.

55. Murai K, Sakai D, Nakamura Y, Nakai T, Igarashi T, Seo N, et al. Primary immune system responders to nucleus pulposus cells: evidence for immune response in disc herniation. Eur Cell Mater. 2010;19:13–21 PubMed PMID: 20077401.

56. Geiss A, Larsson K, Rydevik B, Takahashi I, Olmarker K. Autoimmune properties of nucleus pulposus: an experimental study in pigs. Spine. 2007; 32(2):168–73 PubMed PMID: 17224810.

57. Rand NS, Dawson JM, Juliao SF, Spengler DM, Floman Y. In vivo macrophage recruitment by murine intervertebral disc cells. J Spinal Disord. 2001;14(4):339–42 PubMed PMID: 11481557.

58. Geiss A, Larsson K, Junevik K, Rydevik B, Olmarker K. Autologous nucleus pulposus primes T cells to develop into interleukin-4-producing effector cells: an experimental study on the autoimmune properties of nucleus pulposus. J Orthop Res. 2009;27(1):97–103 PubMed PMID: 18634006.

59. Park JB, Chang H, Kim KW. Expression of Fas ligand and apoptosis of disc cells in herniated lumbar disc tissue. Spine. 2001;26(6):618–21 PubMed PMID: 11246372.

60. Virri J, Gronblad M, Seitsalo S, Habtemariam A, Kaapa E, Karaharju E. Comparison of the prevalence of inflammatory cells in subtypes of disc herniations and associations with straight leg raising. Spine. 2001;26(21):2311–5 PubMed PMID: 11679814.

61. Kawaguchi S, Yamashita T, Yokogushi K, Murakami T, Ohwada O, Sato N. Immunophenotypic analysis of the inflammatory infiltrates in herniated intervertebral discs. Spine. 2001;26(11):1209–14 PubMed PMID: 11389385.

20

The involvement of C5a in the progression of experimental arthritis with *Porphyromonas gingivalis* infection in SKG mice

Syuichi Munenaga[1], Kazuhisa Ouhara[1*] , Yuta Hamamoto[1], Mikihito Kajiya[1], Katsuhiro Takeda[1], Satoshi Yamasaki[2], Toshihisa Kawai[3], Noriyoshi Mizuno[1], Tsuyoshi Fujita[1], Eiji Sugiyama[4] and Hidemi Kurihara[1]

Abstract

Background: Epidemiological evidence to suggest that periodontal disease (PD) is involved in the progression of rheumatoid arthritis (RA) is increasing. The complement system plays a critical role in immune responses. C5a has been implicated in chronic inflammatory diseases, including PD and RA. *Porphyromonas gingivalis* is the major causative bacteria of PD and can produce C5a. Therefore, it is hypothesized that *P. gingivalis* infection is involved in the progression of RA by elevating C5a levels. In the present study, *P. gingivalis*–infected RA model mice were established to investigate the involvement of C5a.

Methods: SKG mice orally infected with *P. gingivalis* were immunized with intraperitoneal injection of laminarin (LA) to induce arthritis. Arthritis development was assessed by arthritis score (AS), bone destruction on the talus, histology, and serum markers of RA. In order to investigate the effects of serum C5a on bone destruction, osteoclast differentiation of bone marrow mononuclear cells was examined by using serum samples from each group of mice. The relationship between C5a levels and antibody titers to periodontal pathogens in patients with RA was investigated by enzyme-linked immunosorbent assay.

Results: *P. gingivalis* oral infection increased AS, infiltration of inflammatory cells, bone destruction on the talus, and serum markers of RA in mice immunized with LA. The addition of serum from LA-injected mice with the *P. gingivalis* oral infection promoted osteoclast differentiation, and the addition of a neutralization antibody against C5a suppressed osteoclast differentiation. C5a levels of serum in RA patients with positive *P. gingivalis* antibody were elevated compared with those in RA patients with negative *P. gingivalis* antibody.

Conclusions: These results suggest that *P. gingivalis* infection enhances the progression of RA via C5a.

Keywords: Arthritis, C5a, *Porphyromonas gingivalis*, SKG mice

Background

Rheumatoid arthritis (RA) is a systemic autoimmune disease that leads to synovial inflammation, cartilage damage, and bone destruction [1, 2]. In recent years, the involvement of periodontal disease (PD) in the pathogenesis of RA has attracted attention. PD is characterized by chronic inflammation due to interactions between periodonto-pathogenic bacteria and host immune responses. Periodontopathogenic bacteria are composed of a group of Gram-negative anaerobic organisms. *Porphyromonas gingivalis*, *Treponema denticola*, and *Tannerella forsythia* play a central role in the pathogenesis of PD and these bacteria are the so-called "red complex" [3]. Previous studies evaluated the systemic effects of PD [4, 5].

RA and PD have immunologically common features. Both disease conditions involve inflammatory cytokines, T helper 17 (Th17) cells, and osteoclast-mediated bone

* Correspondence: kouhara@hiroshima-u.ac.jp
[1]Department of Periodontal Medicine, Graduate School of Biomedical & Sciences, Hiroshima University, 1-2-3, Kasumi, Minami-ku, Hiroshima 734-8553, Japan
Full list of author information is available at the end of the article

destruction [6, 7]. They also show the overlap of environment and genetic factors, such as major histocompatibility complex (MHC) class II HLA-DRB1 epitopes and smoking, respectively [8]. Although epidemiological evidence to support the link between PD and RA is increasing, the underlying mechanisms remain unclear [9–11]. These two diseases are prevalent inflammatory diseases, and many patients exhibit chronic inflammation, the loss of function, and disability in daily life. Therefore, the involvement of PD in the pathogenesis of RA needs to be clarified in more detail and may lead to the development of future preventive and therapeutic strategies.

Complement plays an important role in host defenses and inflammation by affecting innate and adaptive immune cells [12]. The involvement of the complement system in the pathogenesis of both diseases seems to be important. There are three pathways of complement activation: the classic pathway, lectin pathway, and alternative pathway. All three pathways result in the generation of C3 convertase, which leads to the activation of effector molecules such as C3a and C5a. C5a mediates the recruitment and activation of myeloid cells such as neutrophils, monocytes, and macrophages via C5aR. Among complement factors, C5a is the most powerful effector molecule and has been implicated in chronic inflammatory diseases, including PD and RA [13, 14]. A large number of studies support the C5a–C5aR axis being a critical factor for both diseases.

In patients with RA, the amount of C5a and number of C5aR-positive cells were found to be increased in synovial tissues [15, 16]. C5aR-deficient mice and C5aR antagonist (C5aRA; PMX53)-treated mice in a collagen-induced arthritis (CIA) model, which is a classic model of inflammatory arthritis, were shown to be resistant to synovial inflammation and bone destruction in joints [17, 18]. In PD, when mouse models of P. gingivalis–induced periodontitis were locally treated with a C5aRA, gingival inflammation and alveolar bone destruction were significantly less severe than in the same model without C5aRA [19, 20]. P. gingivalis generates biologically active C5a by its Arg-specific gingipains that have C5 convertase-like activity [21]. Therefore, P. gingivalis can interfere with host immunity, leading to the development of PD. Furthermore, C5a is known to be involved in bone immunopathology. C5a may induce osteoclast differentiation from blood mononuclear cells, and C5aR is required for osteoclast differentiation [22, 23]. Hence, C5a may function as a key factor in the potential link between the two diseases and have important implications for therapeutic approaches against them. As such, the involvement of C5a with P. gingivalis infection in the progression of RA needs to be clarified.

SKG mice, in which a point mutation of the gene encoding ZAP-70 exists on the BALB/c background,

develop an arthritis whose features closely resemble those of human RA [24]. Our group previously reported that arthritis was exacerbated in SKG mice infected with P. gingivalis via intraperitoneal (i.p.) injection. One of the underlying mechanisms was the promotion of osteoclast differentiation [25]. Arthritis in SKG mice was induced by an injection of β-glucan, such as laminarin (LA) [26]. β-glucan activates innate immunity and the complement pathway, leading to the generation of C5a. C5a signaling induces the development of Th17 cells, which play a critical role in the development of arthritis through the induction of cytokines such as interleukin-1beta (IL-1β), IL-6, and granulocyte-macrophage colony-stimulating factor (GM-CSF) in macrophages [27]. C5aR-deficient SKG mice inhibit arthritis and Th17 cell development. Therefore, the C5a–C5aR axis plays an important role in regulating Th17-mediated autoimmune arthritis.

In the present study, we hypothesized that the C5a elevation in P. gingivalis infection is involved in the progression of RA. To test this hypothesis, SKG mice with P. gingivalis oral infection were established and investigated whether P. gingivalis oral infection affects the development of experimental arthritis via elevations in C5a levels. In addition, the association between antibody titers to P. gingivalis and C5a levels in patients with RA was examined.

Methods

Preparation of bacteria

P. gingivalis W83 was purchased from the American Type Culture Collection (Manassas, VA, USA). P. gingivalis W83 was cultured on a sheep blood agar plate at 37 °C using the Anaeropack system (Mitsubishi Gas Chemical, Tokyo, Japan). After a 2-day incubation, P. gingivalis W83 was inoculated in 40 mL of trypticase soy broth supplemented with 1% yeast extract, hemin (200 µg), and menadione (20 µg). Bacteria were harvested in the exponential growth phase and washed with phosphate-buffered saline (PBS).

Induction of arthritis and periodontitis

Female 6- to 8-week-old SKG mice (Clea Japan, Inc., Tokyo, Japan) were immunized by an i.p. injection of LA (Sigma-Aldrich, St. Louis, MO, USA, 10 mg/100 µL/mouse) to induce arthritis. Periodontitis was also induced in SKG mice by an oral inoculation of 10^8 colony-forming units P. gingivalis W83. P. gingivalis W83 was suspended in 50 µL of PBS containing 2% carboxymethylcellulose (CMC) and inoculated repeatedly every 3 days for 42 days. This term was set in accordance with a previous bone resorption mouse model infected by P. gingivalis [19]. The number of administered bacteria was determined by considering body weight and the number of bacteria in the saliva of patients with periodontitis.

Mice were divided into four groups (Ctrl group: PBS administration; Pg group: Pg inoculation; LA group: LA injection; Pg/LA group: Pg inoculation + LA injection). Animal experiments were approved by the ethics committee of Hiroshima University (approval A12–15). All experiments were performed three times ($n = 6$ per group).

Assessment of periodontitis

In order to measure alveolar bone loss (ABL), maxilla halves were assessed as described previously [28].

Measurement of antibody titers to periodontopathogenic bacteria

Antibody titers to periodontopathogenic bacteria (*P. gingivalis*, *Prevotella intermedia*, *Treponema denticola*, *Tannerella forsythia*, and *Aggregatibcter actinomycetemcomitans*) were measured by enzyme-linked immunosorbent assay (ELISA). The antigens of the fraction of outer membrane proteins from periodontopathogenic bacteria were coated onto 96-well Maxisorp Nunc Immunoplates (Nunc, Roskilde, Denmark) in sodium bicarbonate buffer, pH 9.4, overnight at room temperature (RT). After blocking each well with 1% bovine serum albumin (BSA) in PBS supplemented with 0.05% Tween 20 (PBST) at RT for 1 h, human serum (3200-fold dilution) or mouse serum (100-fold dilution) were applied to each well at RT for 2 h. Wells were washed three times by PBST and incubated with a human or mouse horseradish peroxidase (HRP)-conjugated secondary antibody (2000-fold dilution in PBST) at RT for 1 h. After the final washes, citrate-phosphate buffer, pH 5.0, containing 0.3% hydrogen peroxide and 0.25% o-phenylenediamine was added. The coloring reaction was allowed to continue for 15 min and was stopped by the addition of 25 µL of 2 N sulfuric acid. Absorbance at 405 nm was measured by using a plate reader (Bio-Rad Laboratories, Hercules, CA, USA).

Clinical assessment of experimental arthritis

Arthritis score (AS) was monitored weekly and recorded using a previously published system [24]: 0, no swelling or redness; 0.1, swelling or redness of the digits; 0.5, mild swelling or redness (or both) of the wrist or ankle joints; 1, severe swelling of the large joints. Scores of the affected joints were totaled for each mouse; the maximum total score per mouse was 6.0, and the minimum was 0.

Histological examination

Ankle joints were isolated at the end of the experiment in 4% paraformaldehyde for 24 h, decalcified in 10% ethylene diamine tetrameric acid (EDTA) for 42 days, and embedded in paraffin. Seven-micrometer-thick tissue sections were stained with hematoxylin and eosin (HE), Safranin O, and a tartrate-resistant acid phosphatase

(TRAP) staining kit (Takara Bio, Inc., Shiga, Japan). The severities of inflammation and cartilage damage were scored using published criteria [29]. The number of TRAP-positive cells in a randomly selected diseased site (three sites per picture) was counted and compared among the different groups.

Micro-computed tomography analysis

In the micro-computed tomography (micro-CT) analysis, mice were scanned by using a Skyscan 1076 (Bruker, Kontich, Belgium) to evaluate bone destruction. Joint samples were scanned and reconstructed at 18 µm³ voxels by using a micro-CT system.

Measurement of the factors in serum by ELISA

ELISAs for human C5a (#DY2037; R&D, Minneapolis, MN, USA), mouse C5a (#EK0987; Boster, Pleasanton, CA, USA), mouse IL-6 (#431304; BioLegend Inc., San Diego, CA, USA), mouse matrix metalloproteinase-3 (MMP-3, #MMP300; R&D), and mouse anti-citrullinated protein antibody (ACPA) (#ORG601 Orgentec, Chicago, IL, USA) in serum were performed in accordance with the instructions of the manufacturers. The limits of detection for each analyte were as follows: human C5a, 31.3 pg/mL; mouse C5a, 15.6 pg/mL; mouse IL-6, 7.8 pg/mL; mouse MMP-3, 0.312 ng/mL; and mouse ACPA, 0 U/mL.

Immunohistochemical analysis

Fixed tissues were embedded in paraffin wax, at a thickness of 7 µm, mounted on slides. Slides were incubated with a primary goat polyclonal antibody for C5a (#sc-21,944; Santa Cruz Biotechnology, Inc., Dallas, TX, USA) at 4 °C overnight. Slides were then washed three times in PBST and incubated with a goat HRP-conjugated secondary antibody (1:200) at RT for 1 h. After three washings, color development was achieved with 3,3′-diaminobenzidine. Photographs were taken with a Nikon Eclipse E600 (Nikon, Tokyo, Japan).

Collection of bone marrow mononuclear cells

Bone marrow mononuclear cells (BMCs) from the femurs of SKG mice were isolated by density gradient centrifugation with Histopaque-1083 (Sigma-Aldrich) in complete Dulbecco's modified Eagle's medium (DMEM) containing 10% fetal bovine serum (FBS) (Invitrogen, Carlsbad, CA, USA), antibiotics (penicillin, streptomycin, and gentamicin; Invitrogen), and L-glutamine.

Quantitative RT-PCR

Total RNA was extracted from the liver and BMCs by using RNAiso (Takara Bio, Inc.) in accordance with the protocol of the manufacturer. Briefly, one microgram of total RNA was used for reverse transcription by

ReverTra Ace˙ for reverse transcription-polymerase chain reaction (RT-PCR) (cat. no. TRT-101, Toyobo, Osaka, Japan). Real-time PCR was performed by StepOne Plus (Applied Biosystems, Carlsbad, CA, USA). Amplification conditions were described previously [30]. Template cDNA was mixed with the Core Reagent Fast SYBR˙ Master Mix system (Applied Biosystems), distilled water, and a primer (10 pmol). The following primer sets were used for real-time PCR: C5 forward, 5′-TTTC AGCACCCAAAATCCTC-3′ and C5 reverse, 5′-CGCG TTTTGGAATTTGTTTT-3′; tumor necrosis factor (TNF) receptor-associated factor 6 (TRAF6) forward, 5′-CTGCAAAGCCTGCATCAT-3′ and TRAF6 reverse, 5′-AATGTGTGTATTAACCTGGC-3′; nuclear factor of activated T cells, cytoplasmic 1 (NFATc1) forward, 5′-TCATCCTGTCCAACACCAAA-3′ and NFATc1 reverse, 5′-TTGCGGAAAGGTGGTATCTC-3′; MMP-9 forward, 5′-CTGGACAGCCAGACACTAAAG-3′ and MMP-9 reverse, 5′-CTCGCGGCAAGTCTTCAGA G-3′; 18 s rRNA forward, 5′-GTAACCCGTTGAAC CCCATT-3′ and 18 s rRNA reverse, 5′-CCATCCAAT CGGTAGTAGCG-3′. Relative expression levels were calculated by standard curve methods and ΔΔCt methods, and 18S ribosomal RNA was used as the internal control.

Osteoclast differentiation and resorption assay

BMCs were seeded on 96-well plates for osteoclast differentiation assay or osteo assay plates for resorption assay at a density of 1.0×10^5 cells per well and cultured in alpha-modified Eagle's minimum essential medium (α-MEM) with 15% FBS containing 20 ng/mL M-CSF (#315–02; Peprotech, Rocky Hill, NJ, USA) and 50 ng/ mL murine soluble recombinant receptor activation of nuclear factor kappa-B ligand (sRANKL, #315–11; Peprotech). After 2 days, BMCs were cultured in the presence of 20 ng/mL M-CSF and 50 ng/mL sRANKL with 10% FBS and 5% mouse serum for 3 days. Sera were prepared from each group of mice. In regard to the neutralization of C5a, 0.5 μg/mL anti-mouse C5a antibody (#MAB21501; R&D) or rat IgG2 isotype control (#MAB006; R&D) was added to the culture medium. After 3 days, differentiated osteoclasts were identified by TRAP staining and TRAP-positive multinucleated (more than three nuclei) cell numbers were evaluated. Resorption areas were measured by ImageJ after removal of the cells with 1 M NH₄OH.

Participants

Sera were collected from 40 patients at the Department of Clinical Immunology and Rheumatology, Hiroshima University Hospital. All of the patients with RA fulfilled the 2010 American College of Rheumatology criteria for RA.

Ethics approval

All patients provided written informed consent prior to enrollment. This study was approved by the ethics committee of Hiroshima University Hospital (#1017).

Evaluation of antibody titers of patients by ELISA units

The antibody titers to periodontal pathogens in human were expressed as ELISA units. ELISA units were measured as described previously [31]. A positive antibody response was defined as a standard deviation of more than 2 above the mean ELISA units of the age-similar healthy hospital personnel.

Statistical analysis

Data are expressed as the mean ± standard error of the mean. Statistical analyses between two groups were performed by using the Mann–Whitney U test in the case of a non-normal distribution. For multiple comparisons, the Tukey-Kramer test or Bonferroni-corrected Mann–Whitney U test was used. Pearson's or Spearman's correlation coefficient was calculated for the correlations performed. In all tests, a P value of less than 0.05 was considered significant.

Results

Periodontitis induced by *P. gingivalis* oral infection increases the severity of experimental arthritis

In order to evaluate the induction of periodontitis, ABL and antibody titers to *P. gingivalis* in SKG mice after the oral infection of *P. gingivalis* were analyzed. The severity of ABL was remarkably greater in the Pg and Pg/LA groups than in the Ctrl and LA groups (Pg group: $125 \pm 2.68\%$ increase, Pg/LA group: $130.7 \pm 7.86\%$ increase against Ctrl, respectively) (Fig. 1a, b). The inoculation of the Pg and Pg/LA groups resulted in an increase in antibody titers to *P. gingivalis* in serum (Pg group: 2.32 ± 0.34-fold increase, Pg/LA group: 2.92 ± 0.43-fold increase against the Ctrl group, respectively) (Fig. 1c). However, no significant differences were observed between the Pg and Pg/LA groups. These results indicate that *P. gingivalis* oral infection induces periodontitis in SKG mice.

In order to examine the pathophysiological role of *P. gingivalis* oral infection in experimental arthritis, arthritis development was assessed in each group. The AS and incidence of arthritis were higher in the Pg/LA group than in the other groups in a time-dependent manner (Fig. 1d–f) (Ctrl group: 0.13 ± 0.07; Pg group: 0.15 ± 0.07; LA group: 1.2 ± 0.14; Pg/LA group: 3.6 ± 0.64). In order to investigate the influence of *P. gingivalis* oral infection on bone loss in joints, the bone properties of the talus as a parameter of focal bone loss were analyzed. Bone erosion of the talus in the Pg/LA group was

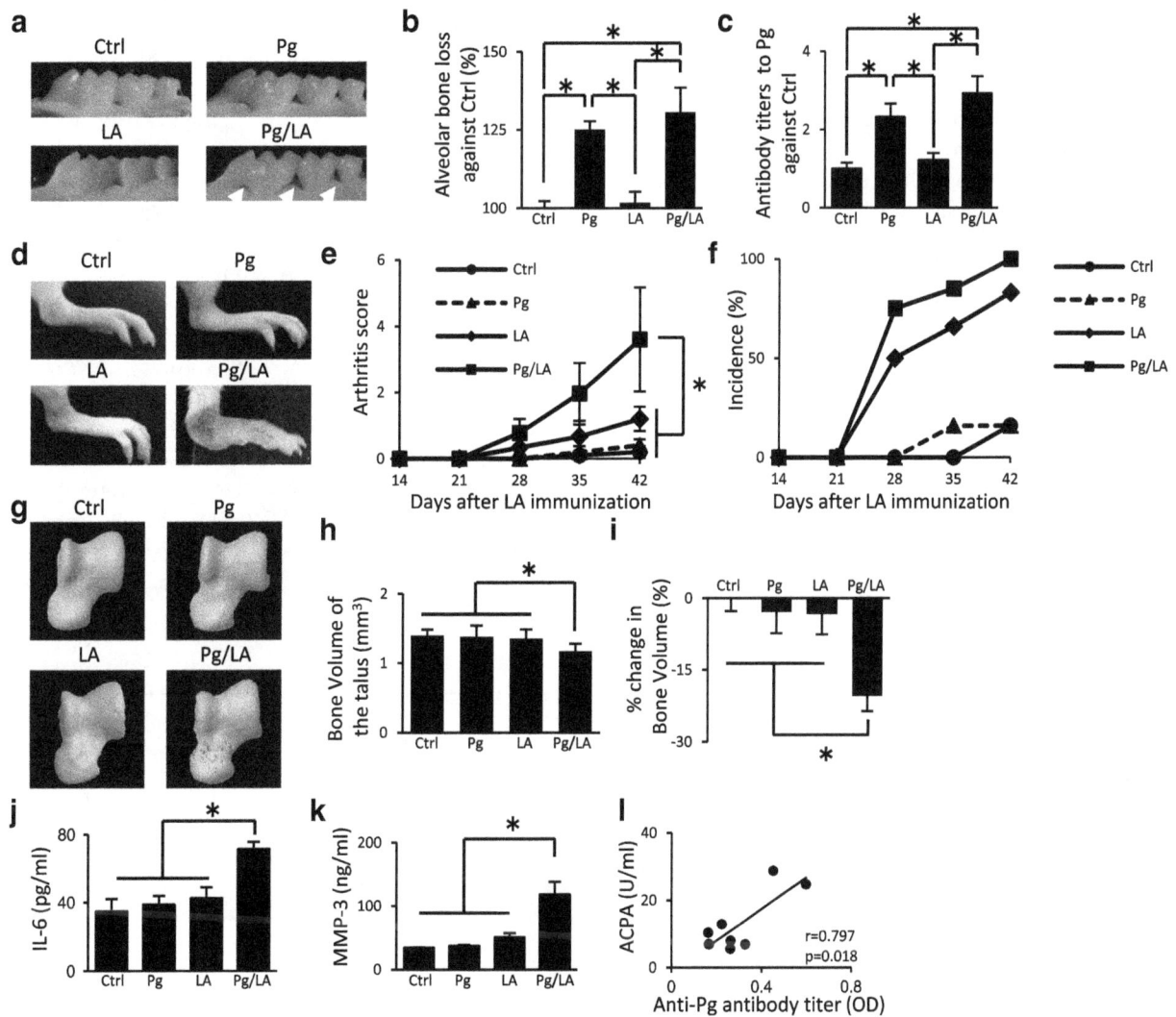

Fig. 1 SKG mice received an oral inoculation of *Porphyromonas gingivalis* (Pg) (10^8 colony-forming units per mouse) repeatedly every 3 days for 42 days after the laminarin (LA) immunization: control (Ctrl) $n = 6$, Pg $n = 6$, LA $n = 6$, Pg/LA $n = 8$. **a** Representative images of the palatal surfaces of the maxillary molars from the four groups (arrows indicate the resorption site). **b** Alveolar bone loss was analyzed by measuring the distance from the cemento-enamel junction to the alveolar bone crest on palatal surfaces. **c** Antibody titers to *P. gingivalis* in serum were measured by enzyme-linked immunosorbent assay. **d** Representative figures of hind paws for the four groups showing joint inflammation. **e, f** The severity and incidence of arthritis were scored by using Sakaguchi's arthritis score. **g** Representative micro-computed tomography images of the talus. **h, i** Bone volume of the talus and percentage changes in bone volume relative to Ctrl mice. **j, k** Serum concentrations of interleukin-6 (IL-6) and matrix metalloproteinase-3 (MMP-3) in the four groups. **l** The correlation between the serum level of anti-citrullinated protein antibody (ACPA) in the Pg/LA group and anti-Pg antibody titer. Data represent the mean ± standard deviation (**b, c**, and **d**) or mean ± standard error of the mean (**a**, and **e–k**) of 6–8 mice per group. Statistical analyses were performed by using the Tukey-Kramer test, Bonferroni-corrected Mann–Whitney U test, or Pearson's correlation coefficient (*P <0.05). Abbreviation: *OD* optical density

observed in the micro-CT analysis (Fig. 1g). Talar bone volume was lower in the Pg/LA group than in the other groups (Ctrl group: 1.4 ± 0.08 mm³; Pg group: 1.36 ± 0.13 mm³; LA group: 1.35 ± 0.13 mm³; Pg/LA group: 1.11 ± 0.09 mm³), and the percentage of reduction in bone volume relative to the Ctrl group was the highest in the Pg/LA group ($20.4 \pm 3.19\%$) (Fig. 1h, i). Although the ankle joint was inflamed in the LA group, bone erosion, which was assessed using a

micro-CT analysis, was not observed. Furthermore, increase of IL-6 and MMP-3 production in serum was greater in the Pg/LA group than in the other groups (IL-6: 54.3 ± 16.6 pg/mL; MMP-3: 118.6 ± 19.6 ng/mL) (Fig. 1j, k). The correlation between the production of ACPA in serum of Pg/LA group and anti-Pg antibody titer was analyzed. A positive correlation was observed ($r = 0.797$, $P = 0.018$) (Fig. 1l). These results suggest that *P. gingivalis* oral infection exacerbates experimental arthritis and bone destruction in SKG mice.

Impact of *P. gingivalis* oral infection on the histopathology of arthritis

Histopathological changes in the ankle joint by HE staining, Safranin O staining, and TRAP staining were not observed in the Ctrl or Pg group (Fig. 2a). Inflammation, cartilage damage, and bone destruction were more severe in the Pg/LA group than in the other groups (Fig. 2a). These evaluation points were quantified by using a histological scoring system [29]. Inflammation, cartilage damage, and bone destruction in the ankle joint were more severe in the Pg/LA group than in the other groups (inflammation score: 2.67 ± 0.45; cartilage damage score: 2.17 ± 0.28; TRAP-positive cell number: 13.8 ± 8.74) (Fig. 2b–d). These results suggest that *P. gingivalis* oral infection in SKG mice promotes arthritis and leads to the bone destruction phase.

Production of C5a in the serum and ankle joint

Previous studies indicated that C5a plays an important role in the progression of RA [17, 18]. Quantitative RT-PCR revealed that the mRNA expression levels of C5 in the liver were increased by *P. gingivalis* infection (Pg group: 2.66 ± 0.53-fold increase; Pg/LA group: 2.66 ± 0.49-fold increase against the Ctrl group, respectively) (Fig. 3a). C5a levels in serum were higher in the Pg and LA groups than in the Ctrl group. The increase of C5a levels observed in the Pg/LA group was prominent (Ctrl group: 19.4 ± 6.1 ng/mL; Pg group: 39.2 ± 3.54 ng/mL; LA group: 33.6 ± 3.57 ng/mL; Pg/LA group: 55.2 ± 1.99 ng/mL) (Fig. 3b). In the Pg/LA group, C5a levels in serum showed a positive correlation with AS and anti–*P. gingivalis* antibody titers (Fig. 3c, d).

Immunohistochemical-based quantification indicated that the positive area of C5a in the Pg/LA group was significantly increased ($4.16 \pm 0.23\%$) (Fig. 3e–m). The localization of C5a was close to the area of bone destruction in the punnus (Fig. 3h). These results support C5a

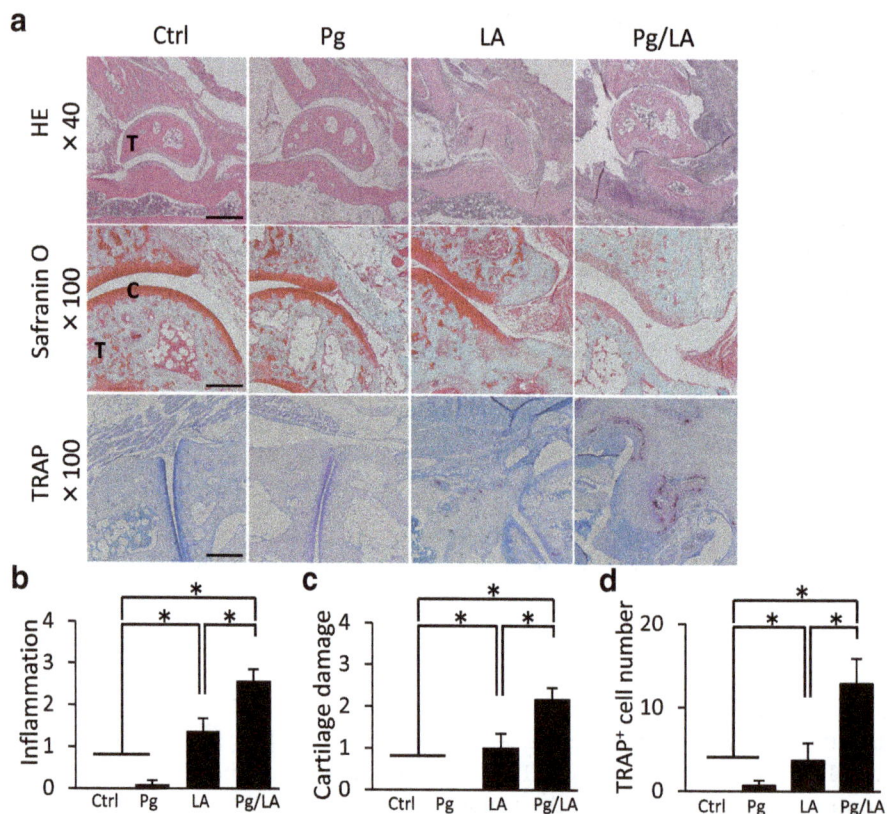

Fig. 2 Histological assessment of ankle joints on day 42 from each group of mice. **a** Representative sections of the ankle joint stained with hematoxylin and eosin (HE), Safranin O, and tartrate-resistant acid phosphatase (TRAP). **b–d** Histological scores of inflammation, cartilage damage, and TRAP-positive cell numbers from each group of mice (n = 6 per group). Data represent the mean ± standard error of the mean. Statistical analyses were performed by the Bonferroni-corrected Mann–Whitney *U* test (*P <0.05). Original magnifications: 40×; scale bar = 500 μm, 100×; scale bar = 250 μm. Abbreviations: *C* cartilage, *Ctrl* control, *LA* laminarin, *Pg* Porphyromonas gingivalis, *T* talus

The involvement of C5a in the progression of experimental arthritis with Porphyromonas gingivalis infection...

215

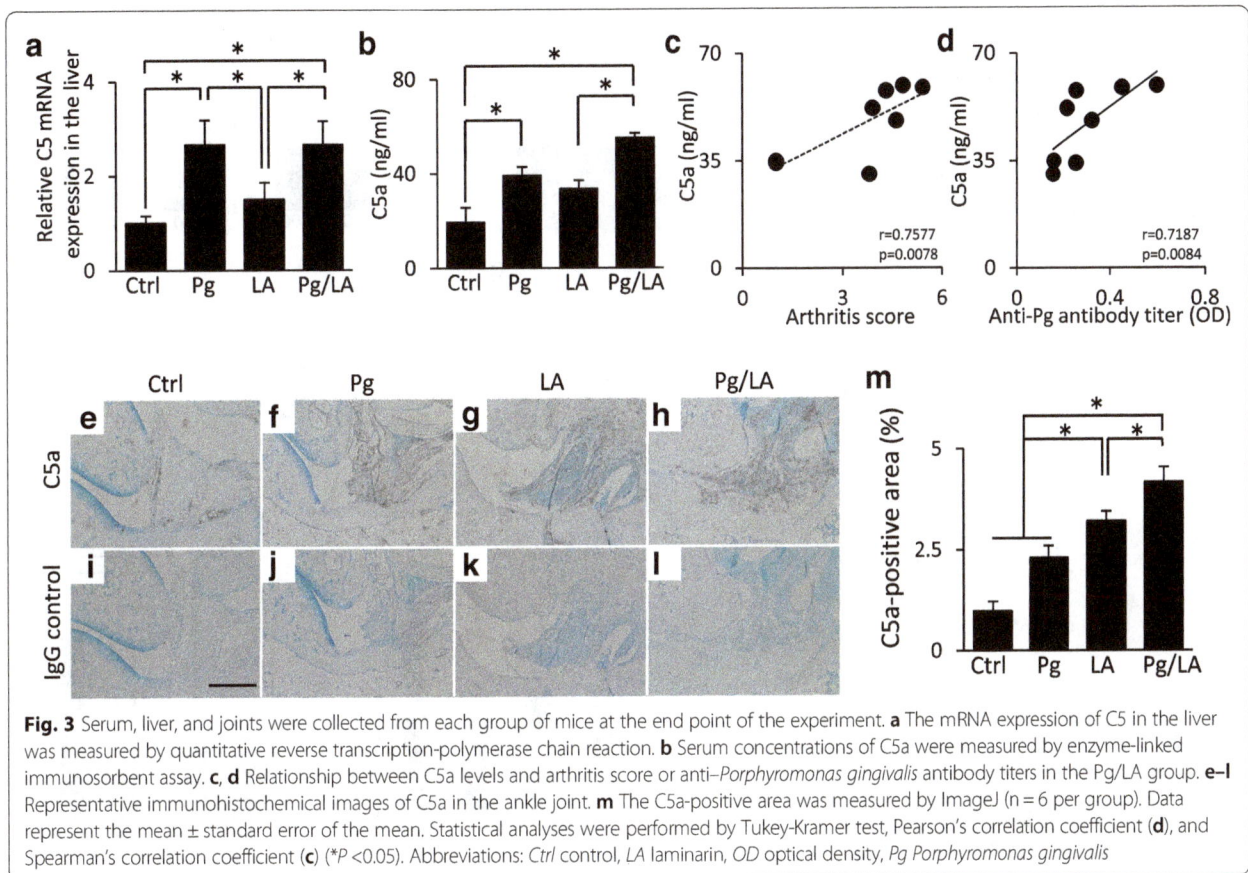

Fig. 3 Serum, liver, and joints were collected from each group of mice at the end point of the experiment. **a** The mRNA expression of C5 in the liver was measured by quantitative reverse transcription-polymerase chain reaction. **b** Serum concentrations of C5a were measured by enzyme-linked immunosorbent assay. **c, d** Relationship between C5a levels and arthritis score or anti–*Porphyromonas gingivalis* antibody titers in the Pg/LA group. **e–l** Representative immunohistochemical images of C5a in the ankle joint. **m** The C5a-positive area was measured by ImageJ (n = 6 per group). Data represent the mean ± standard error of the mean. Statistical analyses were performed by Tukey-Kramer test, Pearson's correlation coefficient (**d**), and Spearman's correlation coefficient (**c**) (*P <0.05). Abbreviations: *Ctrl* control, *LA* laminarin, *OD* optical density, *Pg Porphyromonas gingivalis*

being involved in bone destruction in inflamed joints in the Pg/LA group.

Effects of C5a derived from serum on osteoclast differentiation

In order to investigate the contribution of C5a to bone destruction, osteoclast differentiation was examined by using BMCs in the presence of C5a. C5a could induce TRAP-positive cells in a dose-dependent manner (Fig. 4a, b). It was confirmed by pit formation assay that these cells have the function of bone resorption (Fig. 4c, d). C5a induced the mRNA expression of *NFATc1*, which is a master regulator of osteoclastogenesis, in a dose-dependent manner (Fig. 4e). In addition, the mRNA expression of *TRAF6* and *MMP-9*, which are osteoclast-associated markers, were induced (Fig. 4f, g). These results suggest that C5a can induce functional osteoclasts through the elevation of osteoclast-associated transcription factors, including *NFATc1*.

Furthermore, the addition of serum collected from the Pg/LA group induced functional osteoclasts more effectively than that from the other groups. These effects were blocked by the neutralizing antibody against C5a (Fig. 4h–k), indicating that the high level of C5a in the Pg/LA group

was responsible for osteoclast differentiation. These results suggest that elevated C5a levels of serum in the Pg/LA group activate osteoclast differentiation.

Relationship between C5a levels and antibody titers to periodontal pathogens in patients with RA

The demographics of RA participants in the present study are summarized in Table 1.

Patients with RA had significantly greater mean C5a levels in serum than healthy control participants (Fig. 5a). There was no significant correlation between C5a levels and C-reactive protein (CRP) or erythrocyte sedimentation rate (ESR) in serum (Fig. 5b, c). Thus, it was suggested that C5a was not solely dependent on inflammation in patients with RA. The relationship between C5a levels and antibody titers to periodontal pathogens in patients with RA was investigated. Antibody titers to periodontal pathogens differed among patients. RA patients with positive *P. gingivalis* antibody responses had significantly elevated C5a levels in serum compared with negative *P. gingivalis* antibody (Fig. 5d). The higher tendency of the levels of C5a in serum from the group of RA patients with negative *Treponema denticola*, *Tannerella forsythia*, and *Aggregatibcter actinomycetemcomitans* antibody was observed compared with serum from the group of positive *Treponema denticola*,

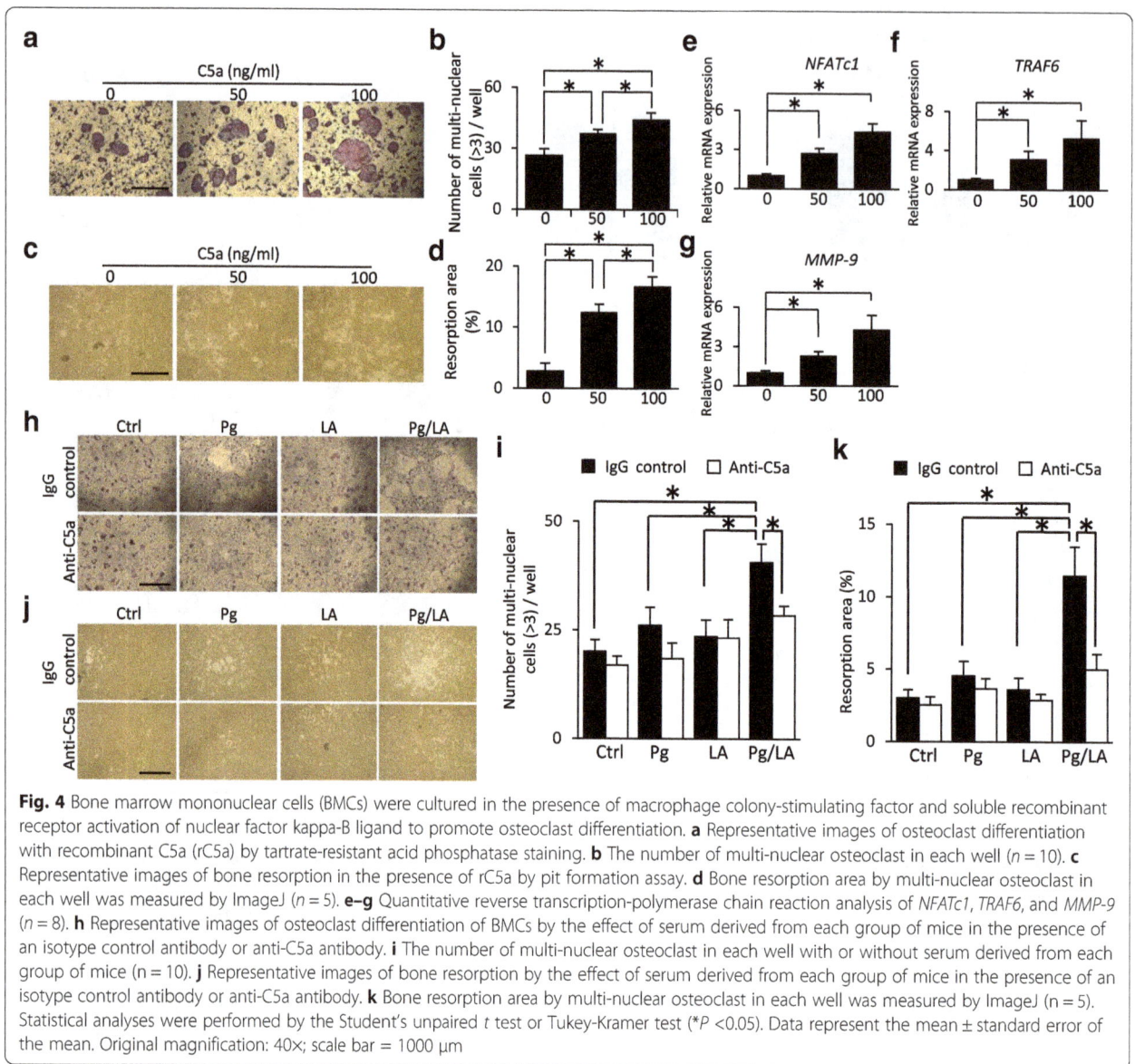

Fig. 4 Bone marrow mononuclear cells (BMCs) were cultured in the presence of macrophage colony-stimulating factor and soluble recombinant receptor activation of nuclear factor kappa-B ligand to promote osteoclast differentiation. **a** Representative images of osteoclast differentiation with recombinant C5a (rC5a) by tartrate-resistant acid phosphatase staining. **b** The number of multi-nuclear osteoclast in each well ($n = 10$). **c** Representative images of bone resorption in the presence of rC5a by pit formation assay. **d** Bone resorption area by multi-nuclear osteoclast in each well was measured by ImageJ ($n = 5$). **e–g** Quantitative reverse transcription-polymerase chain reaction analysis of *NFATc1*, *TRAF6*, and *MMP-9* ($n = 8$). **h** Representative images of osteoclast differentiation of BMCs by the effect of serum derived from each group of mice in the presence of an isotype control antibody or anti-C5a antibody. **i** The number of multi-nuclear osteoclast in each well with or without serum derived from each group of mice ($n = 10$). **j** Representative images of bone resorption by the effect of serum derived from each group of mice in the presence of an isotype control antibody or anti-C5a antibody. **k** Bone resorption area by multi-nuclear osteoclast in each well was measured by ImageJ ($n = 5$). Statistical analyses were performed by the Student's unpaired t test or Tukey-Kramer test (*$P < 0.05$). Data represent the mean ± standard error of the mean. Original magnification: 40×; scale bar = 1000 μm

Table 1 Clinical conditions of participants ($n = 40$)

Parameters	Mean ± standard error
Age, years	60.6 ± 1.8
Female, percentage	65.0
CRP, mg/dL	0.57 ± 0.14
ESR, mm/hr	27.0 ± 3.51
VAS score, mm	40.5 ± 4.9
RF levels, IU/ml	73.9 ± 13.9
ACPA, U/ml	115.0 ± 35.3

Abbreviations: *ACPA* anti-citrullinated protein antibody, *CRP* C-reactive protein, *ESR* erythrocyte sedimentation rate, *RF* rheumatoid factor, *VAS* Visual Analogue Scale

Tannerella forsythia, and *Aggregatibcter actinomycetemcomitans* antibody patients. However, there was no statistical difference between positive and negative groups (Fig. 5e–h). These results suggest that *P. gingivalis* infection increases in C5a levels in patients with RA.

Discussion

Epidemiological evidence to suggest that PD is involved in RA is increasing [32, 33]. Patients with RA show a significantly higher antibody response to *P. gingivalis* in comparison with systemically healthy individuals [34]. Serum levels of antibodies to *P. gingivalis* reflect the clinical and laboratory profiles of RA [35]. In addition, periodontal therapy was suggested to reduce the severity of RA as well as serum levels of antibodies to *P. gingivalis* [36]. Therefore, chronic *P. gingivalis* infection may

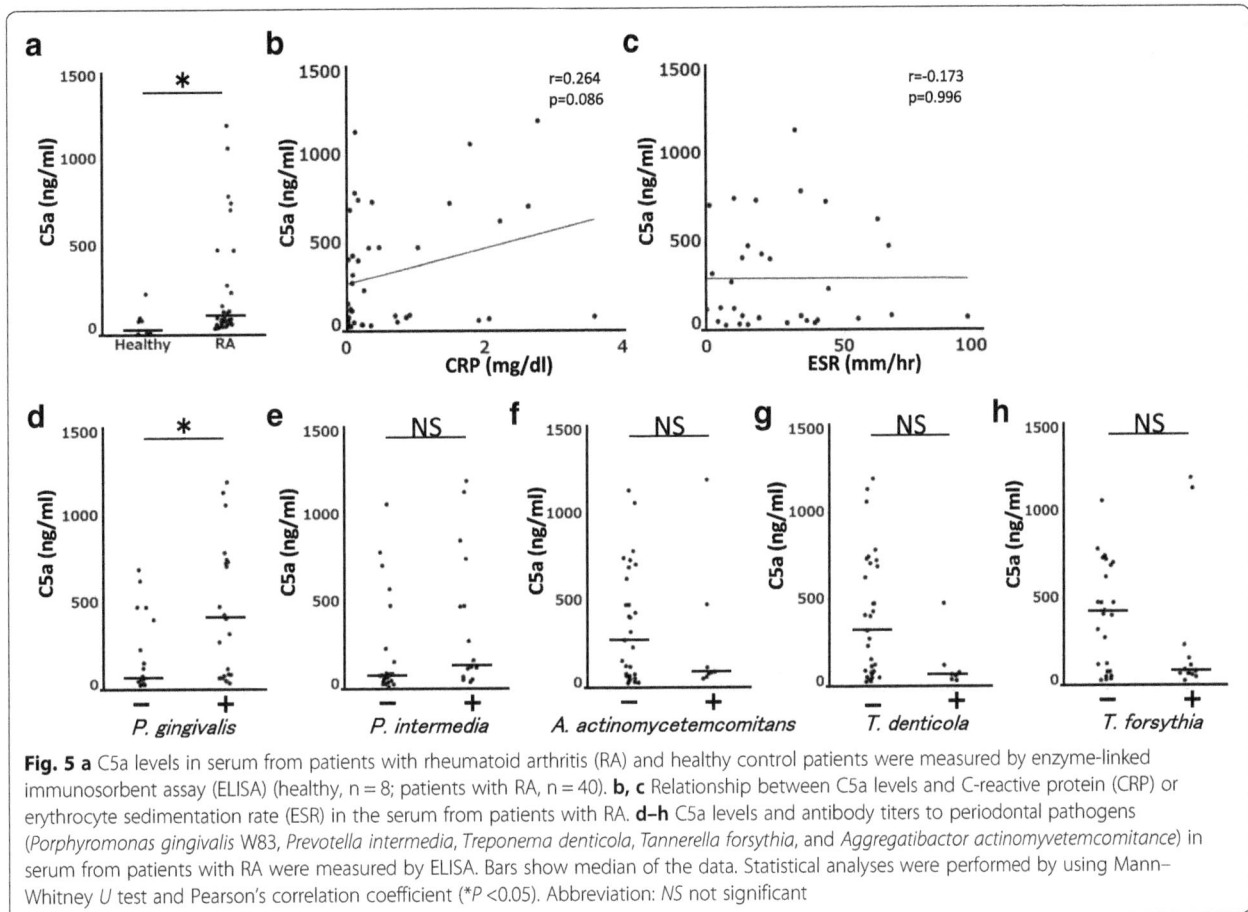

Fig. 5 a C5a levels in serum from patients with rheumatoid arthritis (RA) and healthy control patients were measured by enzyme-linked immunosorbent assay (ELISA) (healthy, n = 8; patients with RA, n = 40). **b, c** Relationship between C5a levels and C-reactive protein (CRP) or erythrocyte sedimentation rate (ESR) in the serum from patients with RA. **d–h** C5a levels and antibody titers to periodontal pathogens (*Porphyromonas gingivalis* W83, *Prevotella intermedia*, *Treponema denticola*, *Tannerella forsythia*, and *Aggregatibactor actinomyetemcomitance*) in serum from patients with RA were measured by ELISA. Bars show median of the data. Statistical analyses were performed by using Mann–Whitney *U* test and Pearson's correlation coefficient (*P <0.05). Abbreviation: *NS* not significant

influence the development of arthritis. *P. gingivalis* is the only human pathogen producing the peptidyl-arginine deiminase (PgPAD). Because of the PgPAD expression, *P. gingivalis* was considered as an important link between PD and RA [37]. However, the mechanisms responsible for this association remain unclear. *P. gingivalis* also has several virulence factors, such as fimbriae, lipopolysaccharide (LPS), and gingipain, which systemically activate immune response. *P. gingivalis* can also induce active C5a generation, which is one of the complement factors, via digestion by gingipain. Therefore, we focused on the involvement of complement in the progression of RA by *P. gingivalis* infection.

The complement system is activated by bacterial infection and inflammatory conditions, leading to the generation of anaphylatoxins such as C5a. Thus, C5a levels may be equally elevated in any of the periodontal pathogenic bacteria. However, our results showed the significantly elevated C5a levels of serum in RA patients with positive *P. gingivalis* antibody compared with that with negative *P. gingivalis* antibody. Moreover, no significant difference was observed between any of the other periodontal pathogens and C5a levels in serum (Fig. 5). Therefore, infection by *P. gingivalis* may have a greater

potential to promote the generation of C5a than other periodontal pathogens in patients with RA. In order to account for this relationship, a large-scale clinical study is needed. It currently remains unclear how *P. gingivalis* infection is involved in the activation of C5a-mediated immune responses. Complement activation occurs through three different pathways (classic, lectin, and alternative) after bacterial infection and inflammatory responses as innate immunity [38]. It is possible that a proteinase derived from *P. gingivalis* (gingipain) or the immune complex consisting of bacterial antigens activates the complement cascade [39]. There is a report about the activation of C5a by gingipain [21]. The application of gingipain knockout mutant is a good way to clarify the involvement of C5a in the progression of Pg-induced RA. However, gingipain displays a diversity of effects on host cells, including the increase of attachment to gingival epithelial cells, hemin acquisition for growth, and proteolytical inactivation of cytokine [40]. Therefore, there is a possibility that the inhibitory effect of C5a cannot be observed by knockout mutant which is weak against host immune response.

The CIA model is the most widely accepted mouse model of RA and has contributed to clarify the pathology of RA. Previous reports indicated that *P. gingivalis* affects the immune system and the gut microbiota composition, leading to the arthritis development in the CIA model [41, 42]. Our group previously reported that *P. gingivalis* infection exacerbates arthritis in SKG mice via the promotion of osteoclast differentiation [25]. The cause of RA is systemic and abnormal immune responses [43]. SKG mice develop arthritis that closely resembles human RA, and arthritis in SKG mice is induced by an injection of β-glucan through the activation of systemic immune cells. Therefore, the use of SKG mice as an RA model has the advantage of inducing systemic immune responses. An i.p. injection of *P. gingivalis* to SKG mice was previously selected in an attempt to simplify the systemic effects of *P. gingivalis* in *in vivo* experiments [25]. However, orally applied bacteria are also known to influence bacterial flora in the digestive tract such as the mouth and gut. Since *P. gingivalis* is periodontopathogenic bacteria, an oral *P. gingivalis* inoculation model needs to be analyzed in order to physiologically investigate the effects of *P. gingivalis* infection.

In the present study, we established that arthritis was augmented by *P. gingivalis* oral infection in SKG mice. Severity of swelling, inflammation, cartilage damage, and bone destruction in joints was observed in the Pg/LA group (Figs. 1 and 2), and the expression of C5a in serum and joint was increased (Fig. 3). The increased expression of C5a by *P. gingivalis* oral infection is a potential cause of the acceleration of arthritis, particularly in the involvement of osteoclast differentiation. We confirmed that C5a can induce functional osteoclasts from BMCs and the mRNA expression of *NFATc1* in a dose-dependent manner. In addition, we demonstrated that the osteoclast differentiation of BMCs was potentiated more by serum from the Pg/LA group than from the other groups (Fig. 4). These results suggest that circulating C5a promoted osteoclast genesis, leading to bone destruction in joints. However, the biological activity of C5a is potently inhibited by removal of the carboxyl-terminal Arg, which is known as C5a des Arg [44]. Although C5a des Arg has many of the same functions, higher concentrations are needed in order to induce biological effects [45]. Moreover, other cytokines in serum, such as TNF-α, may participate in osteoclast differentiation [46, 47]. In order to validate the direct effects of C5a in serum, a neutralizing antibody against C5a was used in osteoclast differentiation. The osteoclast differentiation of BMCs, which were added to serum from the Pg/LA group, was significantly inhibited by the neutralizing antibody against C5a. Therefore, C5a in serum is involved in osteoclast differentiation. In addition to these results, BMCs that were harvested from arthritic SKG mice by an i.p. injection of *P. gingivalis* differentiated into markedly larger

and multinuclear osteoclasts in our previous study [25]. There is a possibility that C5a in serum is involved in this mechanism.

In SKG mice, C5a drives Th17 cell differentiation and triggers autoimmune arthritis [27]. The number of CD4$^+$ T cells and the Th17/regulatory T (Th17/Treg) ratio in the spleen were higher in the Pg/LA group than in the other groups (data not shown). Therefore, increases in C5a levels by *P. gingivalis* infection may be involved in the exacerbation of arthritis by driving Th17 development.

Clinical findings suggest that ACPA plays an important role in the pathogenesis of RA and correlates with the severity of bone damage in patients with RA [48, 49]. ACPA activates the human complement system via classic and alternative pathways, leading to the release of C5a [50]. Previous studies indicated that elevations in antibodies to *P. gingivalis* are associated with serum levels of ACPA in patients with RA [51]. In the present study, a positive correlation was observed between antibody titers to *P. gingivalis* W83 and serum levels of ACPA, and the Pg/LA group showed an increase in ACPA levels in serum (Fig. 1l). Therefore, elevated C5a levels may have been caused by the ACPA, which was generated by PgPAD. In order to investigate this possibility, the construction of a PAD-deficient strain of *P. gingivalis* is needed. It is true that PgPAD is involved in the generation of ACPA. A previous report indicated that a PAD-deficient strain of *P. gingivalis* reduced the level of ACPA in CIA model mice [52]. However, not only the PgPAD but also other pathogenic factors produced by Pg, including gingipain, fimbriae, cupsule, and LPS, are possible ACPA-inducing factors. For these reasons, there is a limitation to clarify the involvement of PgPAD by using *P. gingivalis* knockout mutants in the progression of RA.

Previous studies indicated that, besides PD and RA, C5a is related to various diseases, including systemic lupus erythematosus, asthma and allergy, atherosclerosis, Alzheimer's disease, and glomerulonephritis [53]. PD is a highly prevalent chronic inflammatory disease, and many patients with PD are infected with *P. gingivalis* [54]. PD with *P. gingivalis* infection might affect the exacerbation of these diseases via C5a.

Conclusions

In summary, we demonstrated that oral infection with *P. gingivalis* exacerbated arthritis in the SKG model. Elevations of C5a levels in serum were confirmed in patients with RA and experimental arthritis mice. Elevated C5a levels by an infection with *P. gingivalis* may be partially involved in arthritis via bone destruction by the promotion of osteoclast differentiation. These results suggest that C5a is a target for elucidating the relationship between PD and RA. Further studies are needed in order to clarify the mechanisms by which infection with *P. gingivalis* increases C5a levels in serum as well as the effects of the control of C5a by the treatment with PD on RA.

Abbreviations

ABL: Alveolar bone loss; ACPA: Anti-citrullinated protein antibody; AS: Arthritis score; BMC: Bone marrow mononuclear cell; C5aRA: C5aR antagonist; CIA: Collagen-induced arthritis; Ctrl: Control; ELISA: Enzyme-linked immunosorbent assay; FBS: Fetal bovine serum; HE: Hematoxylin and eosin; HRP: Horseradish peroxidase; IL: Interleukin; I.p.: Intraperitoneal; LA: Laminarin; LPS: Lipopolysaccharide; M-CSF: Macrophage colony-stimulating factor; Micro-CT: Micro-computed tomography; MMP: Matrix metalloproteinase; NFATc1: Nuclear factor of activated T cells cytoplasmic 1; PAD: Peptidyl-arginine deiminase; PBS: Phosphate-buffered saline; PBST: Phosphate-buffered saline supplemented with 0.05% Tween 20; PD: Periodontal disease; Pg: *Porphyromonas gingivalis*; PgPAD: *Porphyromonas gingivalis* peptidyl-arginine deiminase; RA: Rheumatoid arthritis; RT: Room temperature; RT-PCR: Reverse transcription-polymerase chain reaction; sRANKL: Soluble recombinant receptor activation of nuclear factor kappa-B ligand; Th17: T helper 17; TNF: Tumor necrosis factor; TRAF6: Tumor necrosis factor receptor-associated factor 6; TRAP: Tartrate-resistant acid phosphatase

Acknowledgments

We would like to thank the Medical English Service (Kyoto, Japan) for the helpful support in correcting the grammar of this paper.

Funding

This research was supported by Grants-in-Aid for Scientific Research (C) (15 K11390, 18 K095990) from the Japan Society for the Promotion of Science.

Authors' contributions

KO had full access to all of the data in the study and takes responsibility for the integrity of the data and the accuracy of the data analysis. SM, KO, MK, and HK contributed to conception and design. SM and KO performed *in vivo* and *in vitro* experiments. SM, KO, MK, KT, YH, SY, TK, NM, TF, ES, and HK analyzed the results and performed interpretation of data. All authors read and approved the final manuscript.

Consent for publication

The consent of all coauthors was collected before submission.

Competing interests

The authors declare that they have no competing interests.

Author details

[1]Department of Periodontal Medicine, Graduate School of Biomedical & Sciences, Hiroshima University, 1-2-3, Kasumi, Minami-ku, Hiroshima 734-8553, Japan. [2]Division of Rheumatology, Kurume University Medical Center, 155-1 Kokubu-machi, Kurume 839-0863, Japan. [3]Department of Periodontology, Nova Southeastern University College of Dental Medicine, 3200 South University Drive, Fort Lauderdale, FL 33328, USA. [4]Department of Clinical Immunology and Rheumatology, Hiroshima University Hospital, 1-2-3 Kasumi, Minami-ku, Hiroshima 734-8553, Japan.

References

1. McInnes IB, Schett G. The pathogenesis of rheumatoid arthritis. N Engl J Med. 2011;365:2205–19.
2. Goronzy JJ, Weyand CM. Developments in the scientific understanding of rheumatoid arthritis. Arthritis Res Ther. 2009;11:249.
3. Socransky SS, Haffajee AD. Implications of periodontal microbiology for the treatment of periodontal infections. Compend Suppl. 1994:S684–5 688–693; quiz S714–687.
4. Han YW, Wang X. Mobile microbiome: oral bacteria in extra-oral infections and inflammation. J Dent Res. 2013;92:485–91.
5. Scher JU, Bretz WA, Abramson SB. Periodontal disease and subgingival microbiota as contributors for rheumatoid arthritis pathogenesis: modifiable risk factors? Curr Opin Rheumatol. 2014;26:424–9.
6. Hienz SA, Paliwal S, Ivanovski S. Mechanisms of Bone Resorption in Periodontitis. J Immunol Res. 2015;2015:615486.
7. Boissier MC. Cell and cytokine imbalances in rheumatoid synovitis. Joint Bone Spine. 2011;78:230–4.
8. de Pablo P, Chapple IL, Buckley CD, Dietrich T. Periodontitis in systemic rheumatic diseases. Nat Rev Rheumatol. 2009;5:218–24.
9. de Pablo P, Dietrich T, McAlindon TE. Association of periodontal disease and tooth loss with rheumatoid arthritis in the US population. J Rheumatol. 2008;35:70–6.
10. Chen HH, Huang N, Chen YM, Chen TJ, Chou P, Lee YL, et al. Association between a history of periodontitis and the risk of rheumatoid arthritis: a nationwide, population-based, case-control study. Ann Rheum Dis. 2013;72:1206–11.
11. Mikuls TR, Thiele GM, Deane KD, Payne JB, O'Dell JR, Yu F, et al. Porphyromonas gingivalis and disease-related autoantibodies in individuals at increased risk of rheumatoid arthritis. Arthritis Rheum. 2012;64:3522–30.
12. Ricklin D, Hajishengallis G, Yang K, Lambris JD. Complement: a key system for immune surveillance and homeostasis. Nat Immunol. 2010;11:785–97.
13. Guo RF, Ward PA. Role of C5a in inflammatory responses. Annu Rev Immunol. 2005;23:821–52.
14. Sturfelt G, Truedsson L. Complement in the immunopathogenesis of rheumatic disease. Nat Rev Rheumatol. 2012;8:458–68.
15. Jose PJ, Moss IK, Maini RN, Williams TJ. Measurement of the chemotactic complement fragment C5a in rheumatoid synovial fluids by radioimmunoassay: role of C5a in the acute inflammatory phase. Ann Rheum Dis. 1990;49:747–52.
16. Kiener HP, Baghestanian M, Dominkus M, Walchshofer S, Ghannadan M, Willheim M, et al. Expression of the C5a receptor (CD88) on synovial mast cells in patients with rheumatoid arthritis. Arthritis Rheum. 1998;41:233–45.
17. Grant EP, Picarella D, Burwell T, Delaney T, Croci A, Avitahl N, et al. Essential role for the C5a receptor in regulating the effector phase of synovial infiltration and joint destruction in experimental arthritis. J Exp Med. 2002; 196:1461–71.
18. Andersson C, Wenander CS, Usher PA, Hebsgaard JB, Sondergaard BC, Rono B, et al. Rapid-onset clinical and mechanistic effects of anti-C5aR treatment in the mouse collagen-induced arthritis model. Clin Exp Immunol. 2014;177:219–33.
19. Liang S, Krauss JL, Domon H, McIntosh ML, Hosur KB, Qu H, et al. The C5a receptor impairs IL-12-dependent clearance of Porphyromonas gingivalis and is required for induction of periodontal bone loss. J Immunol. 2011;186:869–77.
20. Abe T, Hosur KB, Hajishengallis E, Reis ES, Ricklin D, Lambris JD, et al. Local complement-targeted intervention in periodontitis: proof-of-concept using a C5a receptor (CD88) antagonist. J Immunol. 2012;189:5442–8.
21. Wingrove JA, DiScipio RG, Chen Z, Potempa J, Travis J, Hugli TE. Activation of complement components C3 and C5 by a cysteine proteinase (gingipain-1) from Porphyromonas (Bacteroides) gingivalis. J Biol Chem. 1992;267:18902–7.
22. Ignatius A, Schoengraf P, Kreja L, Liedert A, Recknagel S, Kandert S, et al. Complement C3a and C5a modulate osteoclast formation and inflammatory response of osteoblasts in synergism with IL-1beta. J Cell Biochem. 2011; 112:2594–605.
23. Tu Z, Bu H, Dennis JE, Lin F. Efficient osteoclast differentiation requires local complement activation. Blood. 2010;116:4456–63.
24. Sakaguchi N, Takahashi T, Hata H, Nomura T, Tagami T, Yamazaki S, et al. Altered thymic T-cell selection due to a mutation of the ZAP-70 gene causes autoimmune arthritis in mice. Nature. 2003;426:454–60.

25. Yamakawa M, Ouhara K, Kajiya M, Munenaga S, Kittaka M, Yamasaki S, et al. Porphyromonas gingivalis infection exacerbates the onset of rheumatoid arthritis in SKG mice. Clin Exp Immunol. 2016;186:177–89.

26. Yoshitomi H, Sakaguchi N, Kobayashi K, Brown GD, Tagami T, Sakihama T, et al. A role for fungal {beta}-glucans and their receptor Dectin-1 in the induction of autoimmune arthritis in genetically susceptible mice. J Exp Med. 2005;201:949–60.

27. Hashimoto M, Hirota K, Yoshitomi H, Maeda S, Teradaira S, Akizuki S, et al. Complement drives Th17 cell differentiation and triggers autoimmune arthritis. J Exp Med. 2010;207:1135–43.

28. Lin X, Han X, Kawai T, Taubman MA. Antibody to receptor activator of NF-kappaB ligand ameliorates T cell-mediated periodontal bone resorption. Infect Immun. 2011;79:911–7.

29. Mukai T, Gallant R, Ishida S, Kittaka M, Yoshitaka T, Fox DA, et al. Loss of SH3 domain-binding protein 2 function suppresses bone destruction in tumor necrosis factor-driven and collagen-induced arthritis in mice. Arthritis Rheumatol. 2015;67:656–67.

30. Shiba H, Tsuda H, Kajiya M, Fujita T, Takeda K, Hino T, et al. Neodymium-doped yttrium-aluminium-garnet laser irradiation abolishes the increase in interleukin-6 levels caused by peptidoglycan through the p38 mitogen-activated protein kinase pathway in human pulp cells. J Endod. 2009;35:373–6.

31. Kudo C, Naruishi K, Maeda H, Abiko Y, Hino T, Iwata M, et al. Assessment of the plasma/serum IgG test to screen for periodontitis. J Dent Res. 2012;91:1190–5.

32. Mikuls TR, Payne JB, Yu F, Thiele GM, Reynolds RJ, Cannon GW, et al. Periodontitis and Porphyromonas gingivalis in patients with rheumatoid arthritis. Arthritis Rheumatol. 2014;66:1090–100.

33. Scher JU, Ubeda C, Equinda M, Khanin R, Buischi Y, Viale A, et al. Periodontal disease and the oral microbiota in new-onset rheumatoid arthritis. Arthritis Rheum. 2012;64:3083–94.

34. Bender P, Burgin WB, Sculean A, Eick S. Serum antibody levels against Porphyromonas gingivalis in patients with and without rheumatoid arthritis - a systematic review and meta-analysis. Clin Oral Investig. 2017;21:33–42.

35. Okada M, Kobayashi T, Ito S, Yokoyama T, Komatsu Y, Abe A, et al. Antibody responses to periodontopathic bacteria in relation to rheumatoid arthritis in Japanese adults. J Periodontol. 2011;82:1433–41.

36. Al-Katma MK, Bissada NF, Bordeaux JM, Sue J, Askari AD. Control of periodontal infection reduces the severity of active rheumatoid arthritis. J Clin Rheumatol. 2007;13:134–7.

37. Maresz KJ, Hellvard A, Sroka A, Adamowicz K, Bielecka E, Koziel J, et al. Porphyromonas gingivalis facilitates the development and progression of destructive arthritis through its unique bacterial peptidylarginine deiminase (PAD). PLoS Pathog. 2013;9:e1003627.

38. Monk PN, Scola AM, Madala P, Fairlie DP. Function, structure and therapeutic potential of complement C5a receptors. Br J Pharmacol. 2007;152:429–48.

39. Hajishengallis G, Maekawa T, Abe T, Hajishengallis E, Lambris JD. Complement Involvement in Periodontitis: Molecular Mechanisms and Rational Therapeutic Approaches. Adv Exp Med Biol. 2015;865:57–74.

40. Bostanci N, Belibasakis GN. Porphyromonas gingivalis: an invasive and evasive opportunistic oral pathogen. FEMS Microbiol Lett. 2012;333:1–9.

41. Marchesan JT, Gerow EA, Schaff R, Taut AD, Shin SY, Sugai J, et al. Porphyromonas gingivalis oral infection exacerbates the development and severity of collagen-induced arthritis. Arthritis Res Ther. 2013;15:R186.

42. Sato K, Takahashi N, Kato T, Matsuda Y, Yokoji M, Yamada M, et al. Aggravation of collagen-induced arthritis by orally administered Porphyromonas gingivalis through modulation of the gut microbiota and gut immune system. Sci Rep. 2017;7:6955.

43. Hata H, Sakaguchi N, Yoshitomi H, Iwakura Y, Sekikawa K, Azuma Y, et al. Distinct contribution of IL-6, TNF-alpha, IL-1, and IL-10 to T cell-mediated spontaneous autoimmune arthritis in mice. J Clin Invest. 2004;114:582–8.

44. Campbell WD, Lazoura E, Okada N, Okada H. Inactivation of C3a and C5a octapeptides by carboxypeptidase R and carboxypeptidase N. Microbiol Immunol. 2002;46:131–4.

45. Sarma JV, Ward PA. New developments in C5a receptor signaling. Cell Health Cytoskelet. 2012;4:73–82.

46. Lam J, Takeshita S, Barker JE, Kanagawa O, Ross FP, Teitelbaum SL. TNF-alpha induces osteoclastogenesis by direct stimulation of macrophages exposed to permissive levels of RANK ligand. J Clin Invest. 2000;106:1481–8.

47. O' Gradaigh D, Ireland D, Bord S, Compston JE. Joint erosion in rheumatoid arthritis: interactions between tumour necrosis factor alpha, interleukin 1,

and receptor activator of nuclear factor kappaB ligand (RANKL) regulate osteoclasts. Ann Rheum Dis. 2004;63:354–9.

48. Kuhn KA, Kulik L, Tomooka B, Braschler KJ, Arend WP, Robinson WH, et al. Antibodies against citrullinated proteins enhance tissue injury in experimental autoimmune arthritis. J Clin Invest. 2006;116:961–73.

49. Uysal H, Bockermann R, Nandakumar KS, Sehnert B, Bajtner E, Engstrom A, et al. Structure and pathogenicity of antibodies specific for citrullinated collagen type II in experimental arthritis. J Exp Med. 2009;206:449–62.

50. Trouw LA, Haisma EM, Levarht EW, van der Woude D, Ioan-Facsinay A, Daha MR, et al. Anti-cyclic citrullinated peptide antibodies from rheumatoid arthritis patients activate complement via both the classical and alternative pathways. Arthritis Rheum. 2009;60:1923–31.

51. Lundberg K, Wegner N, Yucel-Lindberg T, Venables PJ. Periodontitis in RA-the citrullinated enolase connection. Nat Rev Rheumatol. 2010;6(12):727–30.

52. Sandal I, Karydis A, Luo J, Prislovsky A, Whittington KB, Rosloniec EF, et al. Bone loss and aggravated autoimmune arthritis in HLA-DRbeta1-bearing humanized mice following oral challenge with Porphyromonas gingivalis. Arthritis Res Ther. 2016;18:249.

53. Wagner E, Frank MM. Therapeutic potential of complement modulation. Nat Rev Drug Discov. 2010;9:43–56.

54. Puig-Silla M, Montiel-Company JM, Dasi-Fernandez F, Almerich-Silla JM. Prevalence of periodontal pathogens as predictor of the evolution of periodontal status. Odontology. 2017;105:467–76.

21

The multi-biomarker disease activity score tracks response to rituximab treatment in rheumatoid arthritis patients: a post hoc analysis of three cohort studies

Nadia M. T. Roodenrijs[1*], Maria J. H. de Hair[1], Gill Wheater[2], Mohsen Elshahaly[3], Janneke Tekstra[1], Y. K. Onno Teng[4], Floris P. J. G. Lafeber[1], Ching Chang Hwang[5], Xinyu Liu[5], Eric H. Sasso[5] and Jacob M. van Laar[1]

Abstract

Background: A multi-biomarker disease activity (MBDA) score has been validated as an objective measure of disease activity in rheumatoid arthritis (RA) and shown to track response to treatment with several disease-modifying anti-rheumatic drugs (DMARDs). The objective of this study was to evaluate the ability of the MBDA score to track response to treatment with rituximab.

Methods: Data were used from 57 RA patients from three cohorts treated with rituximab 1000 mg and methylprednisolone 100 mg at days 1 and 15. The MBDA score was assessed in serum samples obtained at baseline and 6 months. Spearman's rank correlation coefficients were calculated for baseline values, 6-month values, and change from baseline to 6 months (Δ), between MBDA score and the following measures: disease activity score assessing 28 joints (DAS28) using erythrocyte sedimentation rate (ESR) or high-sensitivity C-reactive protein (hsCRP), ESR, (hs)CRP, swollen and tender joint counts assessing 28 joints (SJC28, TJC28), patient visual analogue scale for general health (VAS-GH), health assessment questionnaire (HAQ), and radiographic progression over 12 months using Sharp/van der Heijde score (SHS), as well as six bone turnover markers. Additionally, multivariable linear regression analyses were performed using these measures as dependent variable and the MBDA score as independent variable, with adjustment for relevant confounders. The association between ΔMBDA score and European League Against Rheumatism (EULAR) response at 6 months was assessed with adjustment for relevant confounders.

Results: At baseline, the median MBDA score and DAS28-ESR were 54.0 (IQR 44.3–70.0) and 6.3 (IQR 5.4–7.1), respectively. MBDA scores correlated significantly with DAS28-ESR, DAS28-hsCRP, ESR and (hs)CRP at baseline and 6 months. ΔMBDA score correlated significantly with changes in these measures. ΔMBDA score was associated with EULAR good or moderate response (adjusted OR = 0.89, 95% CI = 0.81–0.98, $p = 0.02$). Neither baseline MBDA score nor ΔMBDA score correlated statistically significantly with ΔSHS ($n = 11$) or change in bone turnover markers ($n = 23$), although ΔSHS ≥ 5 was observed in 5 (56%) of nine patients with high MBDA scores.

Conclusions: We have shown, for the first time, that the MBDA score tracked disease activity in RA patients treated with rituximab and that change in MBDA score reflected the degree of treatment response.

Keywords: Rheumatoid arthritis, Disease activity, Treatment response, MBDA score, Biomarkers, Rituximab

* Correspondence: n.m.t.roodenrijs@umcutrecht.nl
[1]Department of Rheumatology & Clinical Immunology, University Medical Center Utrecht, Heidelberglaan 100, 3508 GA Utrecht, The Netherlands
Full list of author information is available at the end of the article

Background

Rheumatoid arthritis (RA) is the most common, chronic inflammatory joint disease, characterised by synovitis, joint damage, and systemic immune and inflammatory manifestations. Achieving remission or low disease activity is the main treatment goal in order to prevent joint damage and disability [1]. The European League Against Rheumatism (EULAR) and the American College of Rheumatology (ACR) recommend regular assessment of the level of disease activity [2, 3]. The disease activity score assessing 28 joints (DAS28) is one of the most frequently used composite scores for the assessment of disease activity in clinical studies of RA [4]. However, the DAS28 has shortcomings that hamper its use in clinical practice [5]. It does not include the ankles or feet, whereas these are common sites of inflammation in RA. Moreover, the DAS28 contains subjective components, making it highly variable between and within assessors and unreliable at the patient level. In addition, RA inflammation can be extra-articular, which is not readily detected by the DAS28. Thus, there is a need for an objective measure that reflects systemic disease activity and is sensitive to change. It would be of additional benefit if that measure could be used to predict radiographic progression.

The multi-biomarker disease activity (MBDA) score is based on biochemical markers only. It is thus more objective than the DAS28 and may potentially be a better indicator of systemic inflammation. The MBDA score is calculated with an algorithm that uses the concentrations of 12 serum protein biomarkers to produce a score, on a scale of 1 to 100, that represents the level of disease activity in patients with RA [6]. The MBDA score has been validated based on its correlation with DAS28 using C-reactive protein (CRP) and other clinical disease activity measures [7, 8]. The clinical validation of the MBDA score is supported by evidence that the MBDA score is a stronger predictor of radiographic progression than DAS28-CRP, and that it predicts radiographic progression when it is discordant with DAS28-CRP (e.g. when DAS28 is low and MBDA score is high) [9].

The MBDA score tracks response to a variety of disease-modifying anti-rheumatic drugs (DMARDs), including methotrexate [10] (with and without prednisone [11]), tumour necrosis factor (TNF) inhibitors [12–14], abatacept [13–15] and the Janus kinase (JAK) inhibitor tofacitinib [16]. The MBDA score has not yet been assessed in patients treated with rituximab.

Rituximab is an anti-CD20 monoclonal antibody. CD20 is expressed by pre-B and mature B cells, which produce a number of pro-inflammatory cytokines, such as interleukin-6 (IL-6) and TNF. By depleting CD20+ B cells, rituximab treatment leads to a decrease in these pro-inflammatory cytokines [17, 18], thereby reducing clinical disease activity. IL-6 and TNF are 2 of the 12 biomarkers of the MBDA

score. It is not known if the clinical response to rituximab is paralleled by changes in the biomarker profile of the MBDA score.

The purpose of the current study was to assess the ability of the MBDA score to measure disease activity upon and track response to treatment with rituximab and, if so, if this would be mainly explained by the objective component of the DAS28 (acute phase reactants). Furthermore, we investigated the ability of the MBDA score to predict radiographic progression and change in serum bone turnover markers upon rituximab treatment.

Methods

Study population and treatment protocol

We used data from three prospective cohort studies in which adult, refractory RA patients were treated with rituximab because of active disease despite conventional treatment (e.g. a combination of DMARDs, including maximum tolerable doses of a conventional synthetic (cs)DMARD and/or TNF inhibitor): one cohort from the Leiden University Medical Center (LUMC) [19] and one from the University Medical Center (UMC) Utrecht [20], both in the Netherlands, and the HORUS cohort in the United Kingdom [21]. All patients with available serum samples were selected from the cohorts. Patients received rituximab 1000 mg intravenously on days 1 and 15, after an infusion with intravenous methylprednisolone 100 mg. Patients were followed for at least 1 year from baseline. For the current study, we used disease activity data from the first 6 months following rituximab infusion, to avoid potentially confounding effects from repeat rituximab infusions in some patients.

Clinical assessments and serum samples

Demographics, disease duration, smoking status (no or yes) and serum status for rheumatoid factor (RF) and for autoantibodies against citrullinated peptides (ACPA) were assessed at baseline. Swollen and tender joint counts assessing 28 joints (SJC28, TJC28), patient visual analogue scale (VAS) for general health (GH), and health assessment questionnaire (HAQ) were obtained for patients at baseline and 6 months, as were erythrocyte sedimentation rate (ESR), CRP and high-sensitivity (hs)CRP (the latter only in HORUS). The DAS28 was calculated using both ESR and hsCRP. EULAR response at 6 months was determined using DAS28-ESR [22]. Radiographs of hands and feet were obtained at baseline and at 12 months (UMC Utrecht cohort) and radiographic progression was assessed using the Sharp/van der Heijde score (SHS) by one reader. Clinically important radiographic progression was defined as $\Delta SHS \geq 5$ [23]. In the HORUS cohort, serum bone formation markers (BAP (bone-specific alkaline phosphatase), P1NP (procollagen type 1 amino-terminal propeptide), DKK1 (Dickkopf-1), sclerostin) and bone resorption markers (TRAP5b (tartrate-resistant acid phosphatase isoenzyme 5b), βCTX (beta-isomerised carboxy terminal telopeptide of type I collagen)) were determined at baseline and at 6 months (Additional file 1).

Determination of the MBDA score

Serum samples were collected at baseline in all three cohorts, and at 6 months in the UMC Utrecht and HORUS cohorts. Samples were shipped frozen to Crescendo Bioscience, Inc. (South San Francisco, CA, USA) for measurement of the 12 MBDA biomarkers. The biomarkers represent inflammatory and destructive processes: vascular cell adhesion molecule-1 (VCAM-1), epidermal growth factor (EGF), vascular endothelial growth factor A (VEGF-A), IL-6, TNF receptor type 1 (TNF-R1), matrix metalloproteinase 1 (MMP-1), MMP-3, human cartilage glycoprotein-39 (YKL-40), leptin, resistin, serum amyloid A (SAA) and CRP. The MBDA biomarkers were measured by

electrochemiluminescence-based multiplexed sandwich immunoassays (Meso Scale Discovery, Rockville, MD, USA) using the same types of reagents and instrument and the same algorithm as described previously [6, 7].

Statistical analyses

Baseline characteristics were assessed using descriptive statistics. Differences between the three cohorts were analysed using one-way analysis of variance, Kruskal-Wallis test or chi-square test, as appropriate.

Spearman's rank correlations (r) were analysed for values at baseline, at 6 months and for change from baseline to 6 months (Δ) between MBDA score and the following measures: DAS28-ESR, DAS28-hsCRP, ESR, CRP, hsCRP, SJC28, TJC28, VAS-GH, HAQ, SHS (UMC Utrecht cohort), bone turnover markers (HORUS cohort). Multivariable linear regression analyses were performed using these measures as dependent variable and the MBDA score as independent variable, with adjustment by age, gender,

Table 1 Patient characteristics at baseline

	All, n = 57	HORUS, n = 26	UMC Utrecht, n = 20	LUMC, n = 11	p value
Female, n (%)	41 (72)	22 (85)	12 (60)	7 (64)	0.15[1]
Age in years, mean (SD)	56.6 (11.2)	59.3 (10.8)	56.7 (11.6)	50.1 (9.5)	0.07[2]
Disease duration in years, median (IQR)	11.5 (6.3–16.4)	9.9 (4.1–14.4)	13.4 (8.4–17.6)	13.0 (5.2–15.5)	0.46[3]
Smoking status, number (%)					
No	37 (65)	16 (62)	12 (60)	9 (82)	0.42[1]
Yes	20 (35)	10 (38)	8 (40)	2 (18)	
RF positive, number (%)	51 (90)	23 (89)	19 (95)	9 (82)	0.51[1]
ACPA positive, number (%)	44 (80)	19 (79), n = 24	17 (85)	8 (73)	0.71[1]
Menopausal status, females (%)					
Pre-menopausal	14 (25)	6 (23)	5 (25)	3 (27)	0.30[1]
Post-menopausal	27 (47)	16 (62)	7 (35)	4 (36)	
SJC28, median (IQR)	9 (4–16)	9 (4–15)	12 (8–19), n = 19	4 (1–10), n = 8	0.02[3]
TJC28, median (IQR)	15 (10–23)	16 (11–25)	14 (8–17), n = 19	13 (5–24), n = 8	0.35[3]
VAS-GH, 0–100 mm (worst), median (IQR)	64 (45–73)	69 (40–78)	57 (46–69), n = 19	65 (53–84), n = 8	0.36[3]
ESR, mm/h, median (IQR)	37 (21–51)	32 (12–41), n = 24	52 (21–91), n = 18	32 (29–44), n = 7	0.02[3]
CRP, mg/L, median (IQR)	15 (6–34)	11 (5–25), n = 25	29 (11–50), n = 18	13 (5–56), n = 5	0.02[3]
hsCRP, mg/L, median (IQR)	NA	10 (3–26)	NA	NA	NA
DAS28-ESR, median (IQR)	6.3 (5.4–7.1)	6.2 (5.0–7.2), n = 25	6.6 (5.8–7.1), n = 18	6.1 (3.8–7.3), n = 8	0.64[3]
DAS28-hsCRP, median (IQR)	NA	5.8 (4.6–6.8)	NA	NA	NA
MBDA score, median (IQR)	54 (44–70)	51 (44–67), n = 25	64 (49–74)	55 (34–71), n = 7	0.15[3]
HAQ, median (IQR)	1.8 (1.4–2.1)	1.9 (1.7–2.1)	1.5 (1.1–1.9), n = 11	1.3 (1.3–1.9), n = 7	0.02[3]
SHS, median (IQR)	44 (24–128)	NA	61 (29–142), n = 19	25 (21–94), n = 8	0.34[3]

SD standard deviation, IQR interquartile range, RF rheumatoid factor, ACPA anti-citrullinated protein antibodies, SJC28 swollen joint count assessing 28 joints, TJC28 tender joint count assessing 28 joints, VAS-GH patient visual analogue scale for general health, ESR erythrocyte sedimentation rate, mm/h millimetre/hour, CRP C-reactive protein, mg/L milligram/litre, hsCRP high-sensitivity CRP, DAS28 disease activity score assessing 28 joints, MBDA multi-biomarker disease activity, HAQ health assessment questionnaire, SHS Sharp/van der Heijde score, NA not applicable
[1]Differences between cohorts were analysed using chi-square test
[2]Differences between cohorts were analysed using one-way analysis of variance
[3]Differences between cohorts were analysed using Kruskal-Wallis test

smoking status (no or yes), RF status, ACPA status, and cohort. Bone turnover markers were additionally adjusted for menopausal status (pre-menopausal or post-menopausal) [24]. Logistic regression analysis was performed to assess the association between baseline MBDA score or ΔMBDA score and EULAR response (good or moderate) at 6 months, with adjustment by the same covariates.

Two-sided p values < 0.05 were considered statistically significant. All statistical analyses were performed using IBM SPSS Statistics 21 software (IBM Corp, Armonk, NY, USA).

Results

Patient characteristics at baseline

Baseline characteristics were generally typical of those for patients with established RA starting rituximab treatment and were mostly similar between the three cohorts. SJC28, ESR, CRP and HAQ were statistically significantly different between the three cohorts (Table 1). Overall, 90% and 80% of patients were seropositive for RF or ACPA, respectively.

MBDA score and DAS28 at baseline and 6 months

At baseline the median MBDA score was 54 (interquartile range (IQR) 44–70, $n = 52$), with high (> 44), moderate (30–44) or low (< 30; [7]) scores observed in 40 (77%), 7 (13%) and 5 (10%) patients, respectively. At 6 months the

median MBDA score was 51 (IQR 39–58, $n = 42$), with high, moderate or low scores observed in 26 (62%), 11 (26%) and 5 patients (12%), respectively. The median ΔMBDA score was –7 (IQR –19–3, $n = 42$).

At baseline and at 6 months, the median values for DAS28-ESR were 6.3 (IQR 5.4–7.1, $n = 51$) and 5.0 (IQR 4.2–6.2, $n = 45$), respectively, and the median ΔDAS28-ESR was –1.0 (IQR –2.0 to –0.1, $n = 42$). At baseline and at 6 months, the median values for DAS28-hsCRP were 5.8 (IQR 4.6–6.8, $n = 26$) and 4.7 (IQR 3.8–6.2, $n = 26$), respectively, and the median ΔDAS28-hsCRP was – 0.9 (IQR –1.6–0.1, $n = 26$).

Correlation between MBDA score and disease activity measures

Correlations between MBDA score and DAS28 and their changes over time are shown in Fig. 1. A significant Spearman's correlation was found between MBDA score and DAS28-ESR at baseline ($r = 0.52$, $p < 0.01$) and at 6 months ($r = 0.49$, $p < 0.01$). ΔMBDA score from baseline to 6 months was significantly correlated with ΔDAS28-ESR ($r = 0.60$, $p < 0.01$).

Similarly, the MBDA score was significantly correlated with DAS28-hsCRP at baseline ($r = 0.51$, $p < 0.01$) and at 6 months ($r = 0.45$, $p = 0.03$). ΔMBDA score from baseline to 6 months was significantly correlated with ΔDAS28-hsCRP ($r = 0.48$, $p = 0.02$).

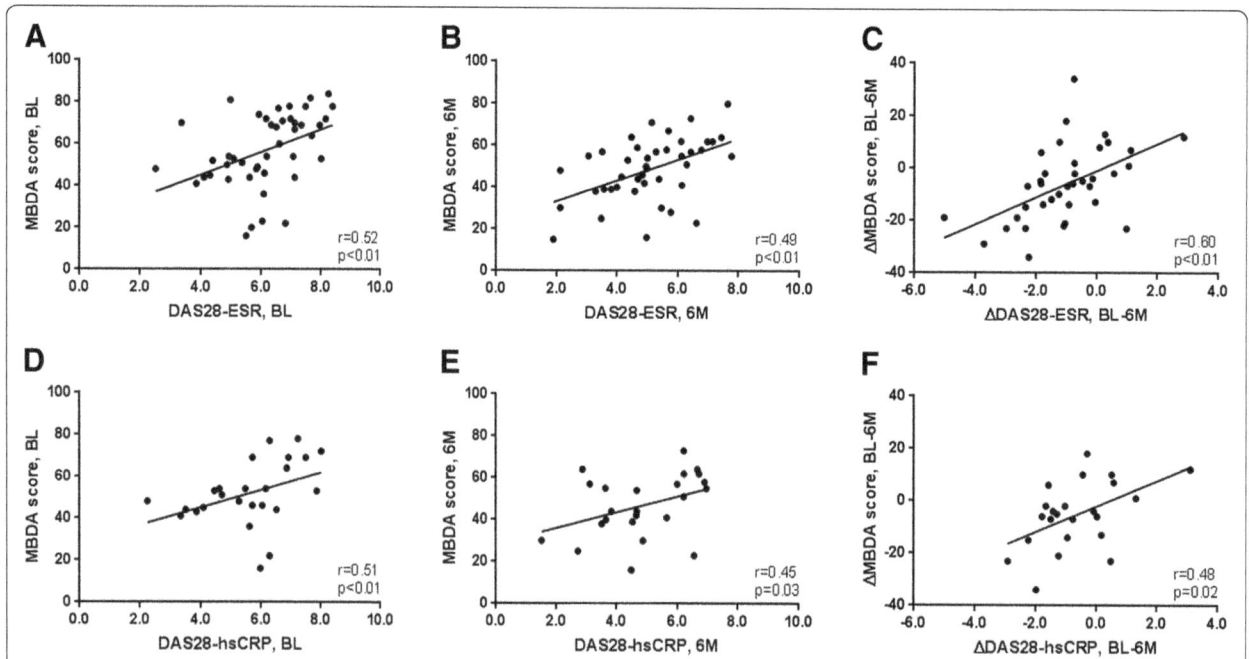

Fig. 1 Correlation between MBDA score and DAS28. **a** MBDA score versus DAS28-ESR at baseline ($n = 46$). **b** MBDA score versus DAS28-ESR at 6 months ($n = 42$). **c** ΔMBDA score versus ΔDAS28-ESR, from baseline to 6 months ($n = 38$). **d** MBDA score versus DAS28-hsCRP at baseline ($n = 25$). **e** MBDA score versus DAS28-hsCRP at 6 months ($n = 24$). **f** ΔMBDA score versus ΔDAS28-hsCRP, from baseline to 6 months ($n = 23$). Negative change values represent improvement over 6 months

MBDA score was significantly correlated with ESR, hsCRP and CRP, as was also true for their changes from baseline to 6 months (Table 2).

Correlations were not significant between the MBDA score and SJC28, TJC28, VAS-GH or HAQ, except for ΔSJC28 and ΔVAS-GH from baseline to 6 months (Table 2).

The results of the multivariable regression analysis resembled those of the correlation analyses, except that the associations between ΔMBDA score versus ΔESR and ΔSJC28 were not statistically significant and the association between MBDA score versus TJC28 at baseline was statistically significant (Table 2).

Association between MBDA score and EULAR response

At 6 months, 21 patients (48%) were classified as non-, 19 patients (43%) as moderate and 4 patients (9%) as good EULAR responders. The distribution of values for ΔMBDA score within each EULAR response category is shown in Fig. 2. ΔMBDA score from baseline to 6 months was significantly associated with EULAR response (good or moderate) versus non-response at 6 months (odds ratio (OR): 0.93 (95% CI = 0.88–0.98, $p = 0.01$) per unit change in MBDA score, Fig. 2). Adjusted by age, gender, smoking status, RF status, ACPA status, and cohort, this association remained statistically significant (OR: 0.89 (95% CI = 0.81–0.98, $p = 0.02$) per unit change in MBDA score).

Table 2 Correlations and associations between the MBDA score and disease activity measures

Measure	Time point or period for comparison with MBDA score	Number of available samples	r	p value	β (95% CI)[1]	p value
DAS28-ESR	BL	46	0.52	< 0.01	0.05 (0.02–0.07)	< 0.01
	6 M	42	0.49	< 0.01	0.06 (0.02–0.09)	0.01
	Δ	38	0.60	< 0.01	0.05 (0.01–0.08)	0.02
ESR	BL	44	0.75	< 0.01	1.20 (0.71–1.70)	< 0.01
	6 M	42	0.66	< 0.01	0.81 (0.36–1.26)	< 0.01
	Δ	37	0.48	< 0.01	0.57 (−0.03–1.17)	0.06
DAS28-hsCRP[2]	BL	25	0.51	< 0.01	0.06 (0.02–0.10)	0.01
	6 M	24	0.45	0.03	0.06 (0.02–0.10)	< 0.01
	Δ	23	0.48	0.02	0.05 (0.00–0.09)	< 0.05
hsCRP[2]	BL	25	0.80	< 0.01	1.24 (0.72–1.76)	< 0.01
	6 M	24	0.80	< 0.01	0.75 (0.41–1.10)	< 0.01
	Δ	23	0.71	< 0.01	0.90 (0.60–1.21)	< 0.01
CRP	BL	46	0.75	< 0.01	1.07 (0.62–1.52)	< 0.01
	6 M	40	0.76	< 0.01	0.82 (0.58–1.06)	< 0.01
	Δ	37	0.59	< 0.01	0.68 (0.18–1.19)	< 0.01
SJC28	BL	48	0.15	0.32	0.10 (−0.06–0.26)	0.22
	6 M	42	0.26	0.10	0.14 (−0.01–0.28)	0.06
	Δ	40	0.42	< 0.01	0.12 (−0.04–0.29)	0.14
TJC28	BL	48	0.23	0.12	0.17 (0.02–0.32)	0.03
	6 M	42	0.25	0.11	0.17 (−0.01–0.34)	0.06
	Δ	40	0.28	0.08	0.04 (−0.15–0.23)	0.67
VAS-GH	BL	48	0.20	0.18	0.34 (−0.12–0.79)	0.14
	6 M	42	0.27	0.09	0.46 (−0.08–0.99)	0.09
	Δ	40	0.36	0.02	0.74 (0.08–1.40)	0.03
HAQ	BL	39	0.02	0.91	0.06 (−0.06–0.02)	0.30
	6 M	41	−0.03	0.85	−0.01 (− 0.01–0.01)	0.84
	Δ	34	0.19	0.28	0.00 (−0.01–0.01)	0.77

DAS28 disease activity score using 28 joints, *ESR* erythrocyte sedimentation rate, *hsCRP* high-sensitivity C-reactive protein, *SJC28* swollen joint count assessing 28 joints, *TJC28* tender joint count assessing 28 joints, *VAS-GH* patient visual analogue scale for general health, *HAQ* health assessment questionnaire, *MBDA* multi-biomarker disease activity, *BL* MBDA score and measure both at baseline, *6 M* MBDA score and measure both at month 6, Δ change in MBDA score and measure, both from baseline to month 6, *r* Spearman's rank correlation, *CI* confidence interval
[1]β: regression coefficient from multivariable linear regression analysis, after adjustment by age, gender, smoking status, RF status, ACPA status, and cohort
[2]HORUS cohort only

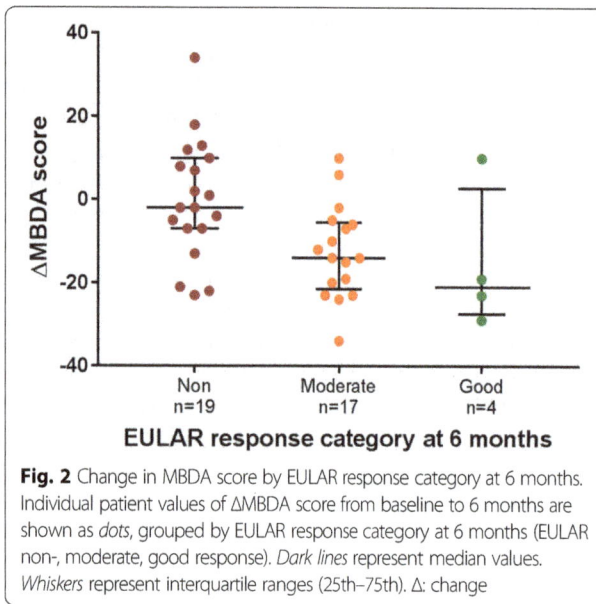

Fig. 2 Change in MBDA score by EULAR response category at 6 months. Individual patient values of ΔMBDA score from baseline to 6 months are shown as *dots*, grouped by EULAR response category at 6 months (EULAR non-, moderate, good response). *Dark lines* represent median values. *Whiskers* represent interquartile ranges (25th–75th). Δ: change

The MBDA score at baseline was not associated with EULAR response (good or moderate) versus non-response at 6 months, with OR of 1.01 (95% CI = 0.98–1.05, $p = 0.35$) per unit MBDA score, even after adjustment by age, gender, smoking status, RF status, ACPA status, and cohort (OR: 1.03 (95% CI = 0.98–1.08, $p = 0.27$) per unit MBDA score).

Correlation between MBDA score and radiographic progression or bone turnover markers

For the 11 patients with radiographs available at baseline and 12 months, all from the UMC Utrecht cohort, the median ΔSHS was 3 (IQR –1–12). At baseline, low, moderate and high MBDA scores were observed in 1, 1 and 9 patients, respectively. Radiographic progression (ΔSHS ≥ 5) in patients with low, moderate and high MBDA scores was observed in 0 (0%), 0 (0%) and 5 (56%) patients, respectively.

No significant Spearman's correlation was found between MBDA score or ΔMBDA score and ΔSHS over 12 months, nor bone turnover markers (Table 3). Similar findings were obtained with multivariable regression analysis adjusted by age, gender (menopausal status for bone turnover markers), smoking status, RF status and ACPA status (Table 3).

Discussion

The MBDA score has been shown to track response to a variety of DMARDs. We found significant correlations between the MBDA score and DAS28-ESR as well as DAS28-hsCRP at baseline and at 6 months, and between ΔMBDA score and ΔDAS28-ESR and ΔDAS28-hsCRP from baseline to 6 months in patients treated with rituximab. Moreover, ΔMBDA score was significantly associated with EULAR response to rituximab treatment. This is the first time it has been shown that the MBDA score

can be used to track disease activity in RA patients upon treatment with rituximab and that change in the MBDA score reflects response to rituximab treatment.

Our findings on the MBDA score are consistent with several previous studies in RA patients upon treatment with other cs-, biological, or targeted synthetic DMARDs [6–8, 10–16].

In our study, we additionally investigated if the MBDA score correlated with the individual components of the DAS28. We found correlations between the MBDA score or ΔMBDA score and ESR, hsCRP or their changes, but found limited correlations between the MBDA score and the other DAS28 components. The correlation between the MBDA score and the DAS28 thus seems predominantly dependent on the biochemical components of the DAS28, the ESR or (hs)CRP. It would be of interest to assess the additional value of the MBDA score above ESR or CRP alone, but the present study was not powered to analyse this. A larger study has reported that an increase in TJC, SJC and patient global assessment was paralleled by an increase in MBDA score; and that, in patients positive for either RF and/or ACPA, an MBDA score excluding CRP was a significant predictor of both DAS28-CRP, and of DAS28 without any CRP or ESR component [7].

In addition, MBDA score appeared to be more sensitive for detecting inflammation than ESR or CRP. A study of 9135 RA patients with active disease found that ESR and CRP were normal in the majority [25]. In other studies, MBDA score was often elevated in such patients [26] and, when it was, risk of radiographic progression was increased [9, 27]. In patients with disproportionally high subjective disease activity components (e.g. high tender joint counts with low ESR or CRP) the MBDA score might be an important alternative disease activity measure. We could not address this hypothesis, as no patients with normal ESR or normal CRP (defined as ≤ 1 mm/h or mg/L) were included in this study.

Previous studies have shown that the MBDA score was a significant predictor of radiographic progression, both in early and established RA [9, 27–30]. In the present study, all patients with clinically important radiographic progression (ΔSHS ≥ 5) had a high MBDA score at baseline. This result resembles the findings in previous studies [9, 27–30]. We did not find a significant Spearman's correlation between baseline MBDA score and ΔSHS in patients treated with rituximab, possibly due to the small number of patients ($n = 11$) and the limited observation period.

B-cell depletion upon rituximab treatment has been shown to be most effective in RF-positive patients [31], and has been suggested to be associated with ACPA positivity [32]. In future studies, it would be of interest to stratify the performance of the MBDA score in rituximab-treated RA patients according to RF and ACPA status.

Table 3 Correlations and associations between the MBDA score and radiographic progression or bone turnover markers

Measure	Time point or period for comparison with MBDA score	Number of available samples	r	p value	β (95% CI)[1]	p value
ΔSHS (baseline-12 months)[2]	BL	11	0.19	0.57	0.34 (−0.33–1.01)	0.23
	6 M	11	0.18	0.60	0.18 (−0.72–1.08)	0.62
	Δ	11	0.19	0.57	−0.38 (−1.35–0.60)	0.34
Bone turnover markers[3]						
βCTX	Δ	23	0.22	0.31	1.10 (−6.79–8.99)	0.77
P1NP	Δ	23	−0.14	0.54	−0.31 (−2.05–1.42)	0.70
BAP	Δ	23	−0.01	0.98	−0.01 (−0.17–0.15)	0.88
TRAP5b	Δ	23	−0.20	0.37	0.00 (−0.03–0.03)	0.99
DKK1	Δ	23	0.27	0.22	0.15 (−0.40–0.69)	0.57
Sclerostin	Δ	23	0.11	0.63	0.10 (−0.37–0.56)	0.66

SHS Sharp/van der Heijde score, βCTX beta-isomerised carboxy terminal telopeptide of type I collagen, P1NP procollagen type 1 amino-terminal propeptide, TRAP5b tartrate-resistant acid phosphatase isoenzyme 5b, DKK1 Dickkopf-1, BAP bone-specific alkaline phosphatase, MBDA multi-biomarker disease activity, BL MBDA score at baseline, 6 M MBDA score at month 6, Δ change (for SHS: ΔMBDA score from baseline to month 6 and ΔSHS from baseline to month 12; for bone turnover markers: both Δ from baseline to month 6), r Spearman's rank correlation, CI confidence interval
[1]β: regression coefficient from multivariable linear regression analysis, after adjustment by age, gender and/or menopausal status, smoking status, RF status, and ACPA status
[2]UMC Utrecht cohort only
[3]HORUS cohort only

Other studies have shown that rituximab treatment increases bone formation and decreases bone resorption in RA patients [33, 34]. For example, a significant correlation was found between the changes of DAS28 and βCTX [34], showing that the anti-inflammatory therapeutic response with rituximab and the anti-resorptive effect on bone might be related. In future, in larger studies with longer follow-up, it may be of interest to investigate the relationship between the MBDA score and bone turnover.

Conclusions

In conclusion, we have shown, for the first time, that the MBDA score correlated with DAS28 following treatment with the B-cell depleting agent rituximab and that ΔMBDA score reflected the treatment response. Our findings are consistent with previous research in RA patients treated with other DMARDs.

Abbreviations
ACPA: Autoantibodies against citrullinated peptides; ACR: American College of Rheumatology; BAP: Bone-specific alkaline phosphatase; CI: Confidence interval; CRP: C-reactive protein; DAS28: Disease activity score assessing 28 joints; DKK1: Dickkopf-1; DMARDs: Disease modifying anti-rheumatic drugs; EGF: Epidermal growth factor; ESR: Erythrocyte sedimentation rate; EULAR: European League Against Rheumatism; HAQ: Health assessment questionnaire; hsCRP: High-sensitivity C-reactive protein; IL-6: Interleukin 6; JAK: Janus kinase; MBDA: Multi-biomarker disease activity; MMP-1: Matrix metalloproteinase 1; MMP-3: Matrix metalloproteinase 3; OR: Odds ratio;

P1NP: Procollagen type 1 amino-terminal propeptide; RA: Rheumatoid arthritis; RF: Rheumatoid factor; SAA: Serum amyloid A; SD: Standard deviation; SHS: Sharp/van der Heijde score; SJC28: Swollen joint count assessing 28 joints; TJC28: Tender joint count assessing 28 joints; TNF: Tumour necrosis factor; TNF-R1: TNF receptor type 1; TRAP5b: Tartrate-resistant acid phosphatase isoenzyme 5b; VAS-GH: Visual analogue scale measuring general health; VCAM-1: Vascular cell adhesion molecule-1; VEGF-A: Vascular endothelial growth factor A; YKL-40: Human cartilage glycoprotein-39; βCTX: Beta-isomerised carboxy terminal telopeptide of type I collagen

Acknowledgements
Not applicable.

Funding
Not applicable.

Authors' contributions
NMTR contributed to the data analysis, interpretation of data and manuscript preparation. MJHdH contributed to the design of the study, data analysis, interpretation of data and manuscript preparation. GW, ME, JT and YKOT contributed to the acquisition of data, interpretation of data and manuscript preparation. FPJGL contributed to interpretation of data and manuscript preparation. CCH, XL and EHS contributed to the design of the study, data analysis, interpretation of data and manuscript preparation. JMvL contributed to the design of the study, interpretation of data and manuscript preparation. All authors read and approved the final manuscript.

Consent for publication
Not applicable.

Competing interests
YKOT is supported by the Dutch Kidney Foundation (KJPB12.028 and 17OKG04), Clinical Fellowship from the Netherlands Organization for Scientific Research (90713460). CCH and XL are employees of Crescendo Bioscience. EHS is an employee of Crescendo Bioscience and holds stock shares in Myriad Genetics. JMvL received fees from Arthrogene, MSD, Pfizer, Eli Lilly, and BMS and research grants from Astra Zeneca, Roche-Genentech. The other authors declare that they have no competing interests.

Author details

[1]Department of Rheumatology & Clinical Immunology, University Medical Center Utrecht, Heidelberglaan 100, 3508 GA Utrecht, The Netherlands. [2]Department of Biochemistry, The James Cook University Hospital, Marton Road, Middlesborough TS4 3BW, UK. [3]Department of Rheumatology and Rehabilitation, Suez Canal University, Suez Canal University Circular Road, Ismailia 411522, Egypt. [4]Department of Nephrology, Leiden University Medical Center, Albinusdreef 2, 2333 ZA Leiden, The Netherlands. [5]Crescendo Bioscience, 341 Oyster Point Blvd, South San Franscisco, CA 94080, USA.

References

1. Smolen JS, Aletaha D, McInnes IB. Rheumatoid arthritis. Lancet. 2016;388: 2023–38.
2. Smolen JS, Landewé R, Bijlsma J, Burmester G, Chatzidionysiou K, Dougados M, et al. EULAR recommendations for the management of rheumatoid arthritis with synthetic and biological disease-modifying antirheumatic drugs: 2016 update. Ann Rheum Dis. 2017;76:960–77.
3. Singh JA, Saag KG, Bridges SL, Akl EA, Bannuru RR, Sullivan MC, et al. American College of Rheumatology guideline for the treatment of rheumatoid arthritis. Arthritis Rheumatol. 2016. 2015;68:1–26.
4. Gaujoux-Viala C, Mouterde G, Baillet A, Claudepierre P, Fautrel B, Le Loët X, et al. Evaluating disease activity in rheumatoid arthritis: Which composite index is best? A systematic literature analysis of studies comparing the psychometric properties of the DAS, DAS28, SDAI and CDAI. Joint Bone Spine. 2012;79:149–55.
5. Jacobs JWG, Ten Cate DF, van Laar JM. Monitoring of rheumatoid arthritis disease activity in individual patients: still a hurdle when implementing the treat-to-target principle in daily clinical practice. Rheumatology. 2015;54: 959–61.
6. Centola M, Cavet G, Shen Y, Ramanujan S, Knowlton N, Swan KA, et al. Development of a Multi-Biomarker Disease Activity Test for Rheumatoid Arthritis. PLoS One. 2013;8:e60635.
7. Curtis JR, Van Der Helm-Van Mil AH, Knevel R, Huizinga TW, Haney DJ, Shen Y, et al. Validation of a novel multibiomarker test to assess rheumatoid arthritis disease activity. Arthritis Care Res. 2012;64:1794–803.
8. Hirata S, Dirven L, Shen Y, Centola M, Cavet G, Lems WF, et al. A multi-biomarker score measures rheumatoid arthritis disease activity in the best study. Rheumatology. 2013;52:1202–7.
9. Li W, Sasso EH, van der Helm-van Mil AHM, Huizinga TWJ. Relationship of multi-biomarker disease activity score and other risk factors with radiographic progression in an observational study of patients with rheumatoid arthritis. Rheumatology. 2016;55:357–66.
10. Bakker MF, Cavet G, Jacobs JW, Bijlsma JWJ, Haney DJ, Shen Y, et al. Performance of a multi-biomarker score measuring rheumatoid arthritis disease activity in the CAMERA tight control study. Ann Rheum Dis. 2012;71:1692–7.
11. Jurgens MS, Jacobs JW, Bijlsma JW, Bakker MF, Welsing PMJ, Tekstra J. The multi-biomarker disease activity test for assessing response to treatment strategies using methotrexate with or without prednisone in the CAMERA trial-II; 2014. p. 81–98.
12. Hirata S, Li W, Defranoux N, Cavet G, Bolce R, Yamaoka K, et al. A multi-biomarker disease activity score tracks clinical response consistently in patients with rheumatoid arthritis treated with different anti-tumor necrosis factor therapies: A retrospective observational study. Mod Rheumatol. 2015;25:344–9.
13. Fleischmann R, Connolly SE, Maldonado MA, Schiff M. Brief report: estimating disease activity using multi-biomarker disease activity scores in rheumatoid arthritis patients treated with abatacept or adalimumab. Arthritis Rheumatol. 2016;68:2083–9.
14. Curtis JR, Wright GC, Strand V, Davis CS, Hitraya E, Sasso EH. Reanalysis of the multi-biomarker disease activity score for assessing disease activity in the abatacept versus adalimumab comparison in biologic-naive rheumatoid arthritis subjects with background methotrexate study: Comment on the article by Fleischmann. Arthritis Rheumatol. 2017;69:863–5.
15. Haney D, Cavet G, Durez P, Alten R, Burmester G, Tak PP, et al. Correlation of a multi-biomarker disease activity response assessment to disease activity

16. Yamaoka K, Kubo S, Li W, Sonomoto K, Hirata S, Sasso EH, et al. FRI0333 effects of tofacitinib treatment on leptin and other components of the multi-biomarker disease activity score in patients with rheumatoid arthritis. Ann Rheum Dis. 2014;73:507–8.
17. Shaw T, Quan J, Totoritis MC. B cell therapy for rheumatoid arthritis: the rituximab (anti-CD20) experience. Ann Rheum Dis. 2003;62(Suppl 2):ii55–9.
18. Mok CC. Rituximab for the treatment of rheumatoid arthritis: an update. Drug Des Devel Ther. 2013;8:87.
19. Teng YO, Wheater G, Hogan VE, Stocks P, Levarht EN, Huizinga TWJ, et al. Induction of long-term B-cell depletion in refractory rheumatoid arthritis patients preferentially affects autoreactive more than protective humoral immunity. Arthritis Res Ther. 2012;14:57.
20. Teng YKO, Tekstra J, Breedveld FC, Lafeber F, Bijlsma JWJ, Van Laar JM. Rituximab fixed retreatment versus on-demand retreatment in refractory rheumatoid arthritis: comparison of two B cell depleting treatment strategies. Ann Rheum Dis. 2009;68:1075–7.
21. Elshahaly M, Wheater G, Naraghi K, Tuck SP, Datta HK, Ng W-F, et al. Changes in bone density and bone turnover in patients with rheumatoid arthritis treated with rituximab, a B cell depleting monoclonal antibody (HORUS TRIAL). BMC Musculoskelet Disord. 2013;14:A10.
22. van Riel PL, van Gestel AM, van de Putte LB. Development and validation of response criteria in rheumatoid arthritis: steps towards an international consensus on prognostic markers. Br J Rheumatol. 1996;35(Suppl 2):4–7.
23. Bruynesteyn K, Der HV, Boers M, Saudan A, Peloso P, Paulus H, et al. Determination of the minimal clinically important difference in rheumatoid arthritis joint damage of the Sharp/van der Heijde and Larsen/ Scott scoring methods by clinical experts and comparison with the smallest detectable difference. Arthritis Rheum. 2002;46:913–20.
24. Curtis JR, Greenberg JD, Harrold LR, Kremer JM, Palmer JL. Influence of obesity, age, and comorbidities on the multi-biomarker disease activity test in rheumatoid arthritis. Semin Arthritis Rheum. 2018;47:472–7.
25. Kay J, Morgacheva O, Messing SP, Kremer JM, Greenberg JD, Reed GW, et al. Clinical disease activity and acute phase reactant levels are discordant among patients with active rheumatoid arthritis: acute phase reactant levels contribute separately to predicting outcome at one year. Arthritis Res Ther. 2014;16:R40.
26. Lee YC, Hackett J, Frits M, Iannaccone CK, Shadick NA, Weinblatt ME, et al. Multibiomarker disease activity score and C-reactive protein in a cross-sectional observational study of patients with rheumatoid arthritis with and without concomitant fibromyalgia. Rheumatology. 2016;55:640–8.
27. van der Helm-van Mil AHM, Knevel R, Cavet G, Huizinga TWJ, Haney DJ. An evaluation of molecular and clinical remission in rheumatoid arthritis by assessing radiographic progression. Rheumatology. 2013;52:839–46.
28. Markusse IM, Dirven L, Van Den Broek M, Bijkerk C, Han KH, Ronday HK, et al. A multibiomarker disease activity score for rheumatoid arthritis predicts radiographic joint damage in the best study. J Rheumatol. 2014;41:2114–9.
29. Hirata S, Li W, Kubo S, Fukuyo S, Mizuno Y, Hanami K, et al. Association of the multi-biomarker disease activity score with joint destruction in patients with rheumatoid arthritis receiving tumor necrosis factor-alpha inhibitor treatment in clinical practice. Mod Rheumatol. 2016;26:850–6.
30. Hambardzumyan K, Bolce R, Saevarsdottir S, Cruickshank SE, Sasso EH, Chernoff D, et al. Pretreatment multi-biomarker disease activity score and radiographic progression in early RA: Results from the SWEFOT trial. Ann Rheum Dis. 2015;74:1102–9.
31. Benucci M, Manfredi M, Sarzi-Puttini P, Atzeni F. Predictive factors of response to rituximab therapy in rheumatoid arthritis: What do we know today? Autoimmun Rev. 2010;9:801–3.
32. Cuppen BVJ, Welsing PMJ, Sprengers JJ, Bijlsma JWJ, Marijnissen ACA, van Laar JM, et al. Personalized biological treatment for rheumatoid arthritis: a systematic review with a focus on clinical applicability. Rheumatology. 2016;55:826–39.
33. Zerbini CAF, Clark P, Mendez-Sanchez L, Pereira RMR, Messina OD, Uña CR, et al. Biologic therapies and bone loss in rheumatoid arthritis. Osteoporos Int. 2017;28:429–46.
34. Wheater G, Hogan VE, Teng YKO, Tekstra J, Lafeber FP, Huizinga TWJ, et al. Suppression of bone turnover by B-cell depletion in patients with rheumatoid arthritis. Osteoporos Int. 2011;22:3067–72.

22

Psychometric validation of an empowerment scale for Spanish-speaking patients with rheumatoid arthritis

Irazú Contreras-Yáñez[1], Emmanuel Ruiz-Medrano[1], Luz del Carmen R. Hernández[2] and Virginia Pascual-Ramos[1]* ⓘ

Abstract

Background: Rheumatoid arthritis (RA) knowledge has been constructed with studies performed in Caucasians patients; Latin American patients present unique characteristics. Empowerment is a social multidimensional construct that has been associated to better health-related quality of life in RA. There is no validated instrument for use with Spanish-speaking patients. The objective of the study was to adapt the Spanish version of the Health Empowerment Scale (S-HES), which was selected for its psychometric properties and suitability for low-literacy populations, for RA Hispanic patients (RAEH), and to perform its psychometric validation.

Methods: RAEH adaptation, pilot testing, and psychometric validation were performed. Three convenience samples of RA outpatients from a national tertiary care level center were used. For RAEH adaptation, the word "health" was substituted with "RA" in the original S-HES, integrated by 8 items. Pilot testing (in 50 patients) assessed feasibility. Psychometric validation included content validity (nine experts rated item convenience, clarity, and cultural semantic accuracy), internal consistency (in 200 patients, Cronbach's alpha) and test–retest (in a subsample of 50 patients, ICC and 95% CI), construct validity (factor analysis), and face validity (in 20 patients, % of agreement). Patients gave written informed consent.

Results: Patients were primarily middle-aged females and had typical long-standing disease, although early disease was represented. In the psychometric validation sample, the majority of the outpatients had autoantibodies; meanwhile, half of them had no evidence of disease activity, with acute reactants phase determinations within normal range. Patients with comorbidities and joint replacement were also included.

Experts agreed upon the attributes of content validity: 83–100% considered the item was essential, 100% agreed on the item's clarity and 80–100% on the cultural semantic accuracy. In the pilot sample, ≥ 80% of the patients agreed with the item's clarity and format.

In the psychometric validation sample, mean RAEH was 34 (maximum possible score: 40 = highest score). RAEH had a good internal consistency, Cronbach's α = 0.86, and moderately good reliability (ICC [95% CI] test–retest: 0.79 [0.62–0.88]). Factor analysis for construct validity showed a single factor explaining 52% of the variance.

Patients agreed with each item content validity (85–100%) and clarity (75–100%).

Conclusions: RAEH was valid and reliable to evaluate empowerment in Spanish-speaking RA patients.

Keywords: Rheumatoid arthritis, Empowerment scale, Psychometric validation

---

* Correspondence: virtichu@gmail.com
[1]Department of Immunology and Rheumatology, Instituto Nacional de Ciencias Médicas y Nutrición Salvador Zubirán, Vasco de Quiroga 15, Colonia Belisario Domínguez Sección XVI, México City, Mexico
Full list of author information is available at the end of the article

Background

Patient empowerment is a social multidimensional construct [1], largely accomplished by individuals themselves. Most empowerment definitions focus on the individual's capacity to make decisions about their health-related behavior and to have or take control over aspects of their lives that relate to health [2, 3]. Empowerment has been conceived as a health-enhancing process [3, 4], as a measurable health-related psychosocial outcome [2, 5] and even as an aspect of health-related quality of life (HRQoL) [6]. Currently, there is not a universal definition of empowerment and it has been argued that the construct may be context- and population-specific [7]; culture, age and socioeconomic resources influence empowerment level and the degree to which the different social groups can be and wish to be empowered differ [2]. A study performed in 33 developing countries, 21 of them African, demonstrated considerable variation between countries with regard to the relationship between women's empowerment and their use of maternal health services; the authors highlighted the need to develop locally sensitive and meaningful measures of (women's) empowerment [8]. In the field of chronic (non-rheumatic) diseases, empowerment facilitates patients' involvement in their care and has been related to treatment safety and effectiveness [9, 10], to lower dependence on health services [9, 11], to better treatment adherence, and to improvement in specific health outcomes [9, 10].

Rheumatoid arthritis (RA) is a worldwide chronic inflammatory disease that impacts patients' HRQoL and may result in increased mortality. Early and aggressive treatment with disease modifying anti-rheumatic drugs (DMARDs) improves outcomes [12]. The 2013 European League against Rheumatism (EULAR) treatment-recommendations for RA emphasizes that treatment must be based on a shared decision between the patient and the rheumatologist [12]. In order to have patients form a partnership with their primary physician in optimizing their health-related disease, patients require knowledge about their disease, skills to self-manage their disease and participate in medical decision making, and power [13]; all of them reflect empowerment attributes.

RA patients from Latin American countries present distinctive characteristics; the literature highlights a lower prevalence [14], a younger age at presentation [14, 15], and a higher female:male ratio [14, 15] in this population, compared with Caucasians. In addition, patients from Latin America present individual and situational sources of vulnerability [14–16] that affect compliance with medications and negatively impact outcomes [15, 17]. Two studies assessed empowerment in RA patients and its association with patient-related outcomes. In the first one, performed in the USA, RA patients found an association between enhancing patients' empowerment (no validated scale was used) and improvement in some 36-item Short Form (SF-36) categories [18]. The second one was performed in Swedish patients with rheumatic diseases (including RA) and showed an association between patients' empowerment, as assessed according to a scale that was validated in the same study, and better self-reported health [19]. Few additional studies described empowerment-enhancing approaches in RA patients, although no validated scales were used [20–23]. None of these studies had been performed in Latin American populations, which limits the comprehensiveness of the topic.

Assessment of empowerment requires the use of validated tools with appropriate psychometric properties. A recent systematic review detailed 19 measures with varying quality, 6 of them generic and 13 developed for a specific condition [24]. In addition, a Spanish questionnaire to assess empowerment for self-care has been described, although limited to climacteric women [25]. The Swedish Rheumatic Disease Empowerment Scale (SWE-RES-23) is the only questionnaire adapted for rheumatic diseases and was developed in Swedish [19]. The scale, adapted from the Swedish version of a Diabetes Empowerment Scale, showed adequate psychometric properties in Swedish patients with rheumatic diseases; there is no Spanish version. The Spanish version of the Elders Health Empowerment Scale (S-HES) is a generic scale that reflects the attributes of empowerment construct; its psychometric properties were tested in urban senior citizens (men and women) from Rosario, Argentina [26]. The literature highlights important differences between Hispanic and non-Hispanic Whites, particularly in regard to health-related decision making [27], which is conceptually close to empowerment construct. In addition, the S-HES has shown good validity and reliability (in Spanish-speaking people), is easy to apply as the instrument includes 8 items, and is considered simple to understand according to an elementary literacy level [26, 28], which is relevant for Latin American countries. Based on those considerations, we selected the S-HES, adapted the scale as an RA Empowerment Scale for Hispanic patients (RAEH), and perform its psychometric validation. We present herein the results.

Methods

The study was conducted in three steps: (1) RAEH adaptation, (2) pilot testing, and (3) psychometric validation.

Description of samples

Three different convenience samples of consecutive RA patients were considered; patients included in each sample belonged to the outpatient clinic of the Instituto Nacional de Ciencias Médicas y Nutrición Salvador-Zubirán (INCMyN-SZ), a tertiary care level and national referral center for rheumatic diseases. All the patients had RA diagnosis, which was established according to their primary physician criteria (rheumatologist or trainee in rheumatology, no validated classification criteria were used), who additionally classified each patient as in remission or with active disease (no standard definition was used). In addition, all the patients had major comorbidity assessed according to the Charlson score [29]. In the three samples, the patients' selection was directed to have age, gender (female preponderance), disease duration, and disease activity quotes represented.

The first sample included 50 patients and was used to evaluate feasibility; the second one included 200 patients and was used for the psychometric validation; the last sample included 20 patients and was used for face validity.

Sample size calculation for psychometric validation

Considering the number of RAEH items (8 items), a sample size of at least 80 RA outpatients was required as the exploratory factor analysis recommends 5 to 10 respondents per item [30]. However, taking into account additional published recommendations (at least 150 to 200 patients), we decided to include 200 RA patients (fair sample size) in the final sample [31].

Step (1) RAEH adaptation (see Additional file 1)

The S-HES author was contacted in order to have him involved in the process. The RAEH was adapted from the S-HES, that retained 8 items (one per subscale), with 8 subscales: satisfaction and dissatisfaction related to health, identification and achievement of personally meaningful goals, application of a systematic problem-solving process, coping with the emotional aspects of living with health, stress management, appropriate social support, self-motivation and making cost/benefit decisions about making behavior changes. Each item is scored on a 5-point Likert scale, ranging from 5 (strongly agree) to 1 (strongly disagree). In the scale, higher scores indicate stronger level of health-related empowerment, with scale scores ranging from 1 to 5.

First, in each item of the S-HES, the word "health" was substituted by "rheumatoid arthritis". Then, each of three researchers (one rheumatologist, one trainee in rheumatology and one social worker, a PhD candidate in Health Sciences) suggested one sentence per item, in order to have different perspectives represented; researchers were blinded to each other proposals. After a consensus was obtained, the three researchers selected one sentence per item and integrated a preliminary version of the RAEH. RAEH was scored as in the original scale, but the sum of individual item-scores was provided; accordingly, RAEH score ranged from 8 to 40.

Step (2) Pilot testing

Feasibility was tested (in 50 patients) according to the following criteria: time required to fill the scale, patients' perceived item's clarity, and patients' format acceptance.

Step (3) Psychometric validation
Content validity

Content validity was tested by a Validation Expert Committee (VEC) that was integrated by six rheumatologists and two psychiatrists who received relevant literature related to empowerment construct, and the author of the original S-HES (a geriatrist and psychiatrist). Content validity was examined by asking members of the VEC to rate each of the eight sentences (one per item) according to three categories: unnecessary, important but not necessary or essential. In addition, the VEC rated the item's clarity and cultural semantic accuracy.

Reliability

Internal consistency (assessed in 200 patients) and test–retest (assessed in a subsample of 50 patients, by the same researcher, with an interval of 3 ± 1 weeks) were evaluated to determine the reliability of the scale.

Construct validity

Construct validity was determined with factor analysis.

Face validity

Previously, a brief explanation of the empowerment concept was offered to 20 patients, who were, in a second step, directed to rate each item as a valid measure of the respective empowerment dimension (Yes/No) along with each sentence's clarity (Yes/No).

Statistical analysis

Descriptive statistics was performed to estimate the frequencies and percentages (for categorical variables), means and standard deviation (SD) or medians and 25th–75th interquartile (IQ) ranges (for continuous variables) of sociodemographic- and disease characteristics-related variables.

RAEH construct validity was evaluated by confirmatory factor analysis (maximum likelihood) with Varimax rotation. Sampling adequacy was confirmed by the Kaiser-Mayer-Olkin (KMO) measure (appropriate value ≥ 0.5); use of factor analysis was supported by the Bartlett's test of sphericity (significant value $p < 0.05$), eigenvalue > 1 and correlations coefficients > 0.30 [32]. Floor and ceiling effects were determined as the percentage of patients who achieved the lowest and highest score of the scale, respectively.

Cronbach's α and inter-item correlation for the complete scale and for each dimension was used to assess RAEH internal consistency of the questionnaire. Cronbach's alpha interpretation was as follows: < 0.70

indicates that individual items provide an inadequate contribution to the overall scale and values of > 0.90 suggest redundancy, [33].

RAEH test–retest reliability was evaluated by the t test comparison between total test scores and by between partial test dimension score. In addition, intra-class correlation coefficients (ICC) and their 95% confident intervals (CI) were calculated based on a single measurement, absolute-agreement, two-way mixed-effects model. According to the ICC, values < 0.5 indicate poor reliability, between 0.5–0.75 moderate reliability, between 0.75 and 0.9 good reliability and values > 0.9 indicate excellent reliability. Finally, 95% CI estimates between 0.83 and 0.94 were considered as good reliability level and those between 0.95 and 0.99 estimates, as excellent reliability level [34].

All statistical analyses were performed with Statistical Package for the Social Sciences version 21.0 (IBM Corp., Armonk, NY, USA). A value of $p \leq 0.05$ (two tails) was considered to be statistically significant.

Ethical considerations

The study received ethical approval from the Comité de Ética en Investigación of the INCMyN-SZ (reference number: 2226-17/ 18-1. Written informed consent was obtained from all the patients who agreed to participate.

Results

Description of the population characteristics of the three samples

During the study, there were 270 RA outpatients recruited; they were divided in three samples. Table 1 summarizes their characteristics. Patients were primarily middle-aged females, married, had basic education and medium-low socioeconomic status. The population had long-standing disease although patients with ≤ 5 years of disease duration were also represented.

In the sample for the psychometric validation, more than half of the patients were in remission and had acute reactants phase determinations (erythrocyte sedimentation rate [ESR] and C-reactive protein [CRP]) within normal range; also, the majority of the patients had disease-specific autoantibodies, particularly rheumatoid factor (RF) and antibodies to cyclic citrullinated peptides (ACCP).

Finally, in the three samples, patients with a major comorbid condition and patients with a surgical joint replacement were also represented.

Patients and disease characteristics were similar in the three samples, but patients from the face validation sample were more frequently married and had more disease duration ≤ 5 years ($p = 0.02$ and $p = 0.03$, respectively).

Table 1 Description of the population characteristics of the three samples

Population characteristics	N = 50 (Feasibility)	N = 200 (Psychometric validation)	N = 20 (Face validity)
Females, N (%)	46 (92)	184 (92)	19 (95)
Age, years	55 (47–63)	52 (41–61)	52 (32–61)
Marital status, patients married, N (%)	27 (54)	113 (56.5)	19 (95)
Formal education, years	9 (9–11)	9 (9–12)	12 (9–17)
Patients with medium-low SE level, N (%)	47 (94)	186 (98)	16 (80)
Disease duration, years	12 (6.8–19)	12 (6–18)	11 (3–5)
Patients with disease duration ≤5 years, N (%)	10 (5)	44 (22)	7 (35)
Patients with remission, N (%)	NA	107 (53.5)	NA
CRP, mg/dL	NA	0.57 (0. 18–1.5)	NA
ESR, mm/H	NA	12 (5–24)	NA
Patients with RF, N (%)	NA	179 (89.5)	NA
Patients with ACCP, N (%)	NA	134 (72.4)*	NA
Patients with major comorbidities, N (%)	11 (22)	38 (19)	4 (10)
Patients with joint replacement, N (%)	5 (10)	30 (15)	2 (10)

Data as presented as median (25th–75th interquartile range) unless otherwise indicated *ACCP* antibodies to cyclic citrullinated peptides, *CRP* C-reactive protein, *ESR* erythrocyte sedimentation rate, *N* number, *NA* not available, *SE* socioeconomic, *RF* rheumatoid factor. *Data limited to 185 patients with sample available

Feasibility

Early during pilot testing (five patients enrolled), patients manifested a preference for a different order in the item's disposition; the suggestion was adopted and maintained in the final version of the RAEH used during the validation process (see Additional file 2).

(Mean) time required to fill the scale was 7 min and all the patients agreed the time was convenient. Eighty-five percent of the patients agreed on the item's clarity and 95% of them agreed on the scale format.

Content validity

The preliminary version of the RAEH was integrated by 8 items, one per subscale. This version was submitted the VEC who agreed that each sentence/item was essential (83–100%), and about each item clarity (100%) and cultural semantic accuracy (100%), as summarized in Table 2.

Reliability

The median RAEH score for the sample was 34 (31–37), with a minimum possible score of 8 and a maximum possible score of 40. Coefficient of Kurtosis (4.5) and skewness (1.29) showed non-normal data distribution. RAEH exhibited good internal consistency, with Cronbach's α = 0.86 for the full scale. Floor and ceiling effects were of 0.5% and 7.5%, respectively; for individual items, the percentage of patients scoring at the floor was 0.5–2% and the percentage of patients scoring at the ceiling was 26. 5–52.5%. Details of statistics, Cronbach's α,

inter-item correlation and floor and ceiling effects for each particular item are summarized in Table 3.

Mean (±SD) time between the two measurements in the test–retest analysis was of 19.3 (±6.9) days; ICC was of 0.79 (95% CI: 0.62–0.88, $p \leq 0.001$). Finally, comparison of means of the total score and each dimension-score between the two measurements did not significantly differed (data not shown).

Construct validity

Construct validity was demonstrated by KMO = 0.884 and Barlett's test of sphericity ($X^2 = 610.93$, $p \leq 0.001$) which confirmed the adequacy of the sample size for conducting factor analysis. A single factor structure was extracted, accounting for 52% of the variance. Table 3 summarizes results for items construct validity.

Patients' RAEH face validity

Table 4 summarizes results from this process; the majority of the patients agreed that the items were a valid measure of the corresponding dimension (85–100%) and that items were clear (75–100%).

Handling of incomplete questionnaires

Only 10 scales (5% of the psychometric validation sample) had ≤ 1 missing response/item. There was no consistency

Table 2 RAEH content validity according to the Validation Expert Committee (VEC)

Empowerment subscales	Items	VEC*		
		Essential	Clarity	CS accuracy
Self-control	I know what parts of taking care of my rheumatoid arthritis that I am dissatisfied with.	83	100	100
Self-efficacy	I am able to achieve my rheumatoid arthritis goals through concrete actions.	100	100	100
Problem solving	I can try out different ways of overcoming barriers to achieve my rheumatoid arthritis goals.	83	100	100
Psychosocial coping/Coping with emotional aspects	I can find ways to feel good having rheumatoid arthritis.	100	100	100
Psychosocial coping/Stress management	I can use positive ways to cope with rheumatoid arthritis-related stress.	100	100	80
Support	I can find support to care for my rheumatoid arthritis.	83	100	100
Motivation	I recognize what helps me stay motivated to care for my rheumatoid arthritis.	83	100	100
Decision making	I know enough about myself to make rheumatoid arthritis care choices that are the most convenient to me.	83	100	100

CS cultural semantic (accuracy), *RAEH* Rheumatoid Arthritis Empowerment Scale for Hispanic patients
*% of agreement among members of the VEC

Table 3 Statistics, corrected item-total correlation, floor and ceiling effects, and factorial loading for RAEH items (N = 200)

Item	Median (25th–75th IQ) score	Corrected item-total correlation	Floor effect (% scoring 1)	Ceiling effect (% scoring 5)	α if item delete	Factorial loading
1	4 (4–5)	0.544	0.5	26.5	0.854	0.594
2	4 (4–5)	0.566	1	41.5	0.851	0.612
3	4 (4–5)	0.636	0.5	40	0.844	0.674
4	5 (4–5)	0.671	0.5	52.5	0.840	0.719
5	4 (3–5)	0.508	1.5	27	0.860	0.566
6	4 (4–5)	0.670	0.5	38.5	0.839	0.729
7	4 (4–5)	0.666	2	40	0.839	0.735
8	4 (4–5)	0.673	0.5	42.5	0.839	0.735

Item 1 = I can use positive ways to cope with rheumatoid arthritis-related stress
Item 2 = I can find support to care for my rheumatoid arthritis
Item 3 = I recognize what helps me stay motivated to care for my rheumatoid arthritis
Item 4 = I know enough about myself to make rheumatoid arthritis care choices that are the most convenient to me
Item 5 = I know what parts of taking care of my rheumatoid arthritis that I am dissatisfied with
Item 6 = I am able to achieve my rheumatoid arthritis goals through concrete actions
Item 7 = I can try out different ways of overcoming barriers to achieve my rheumatoid arthritis goals
Item 8 = I can find ways to feel good having rheumatoid arthritis
IQ interquartile, *RAEH* Rheumatoid Arthritis Empowerment Scale for Hispanic patients

Table 4 Patients' RAEH face validity (*N* = 20)

Items	Valid measure*	Clarity/readability*
I can use positive ways to cope with rheumatoid arthritis-related stress.	19 (95)	19 (95)
I can find support to care for my rheumatoid arthritis.	20 (100)	20 (100)
I recognize what helps me stay motivated to care for my rheumatoid arthritis.	20 (100)	19 (95)
I know enough about myself to make rheumatoid arthritis care choices that are the most convenient to me.	19 (95)	20 (100)
I know what parts of taking care of my rheumatoid arthritis that I am dissatisfied with.	17 (85)	15 (75)
I am able to achieve my rheumatoid arthritis goals through concrete actions.	18 (90)	19 (95)
I can try out different ways of overcoming barriers to achieve my rheumatoid arthritis goals.	20 (100)	20 (100)
I can find ways to feel good having rheumatoid arthritis.	20 (100)	20 (100)

RAEH Rheumatoid Arthritis Empowerment Scale for Hispanic patients
*N (%) of patients with agreement

in the items with omitted response. In all cases, patients stated that they skipped it by mistake. No item was considered objectionable or did not apply to the patient. Incomplete scales were returned back to the patients, who filled them in.

Discussion

In the present study, we performed a psychometric validation of the RAEH, which was adapted from a generic scale that assessed health-related empowerment. RAEH psychometric properties were adequate in terms of construct, content and face validity, and reliability, which were evaluated with internal consistency and test–retest, as recommended [30]. In addition, RAEH was also feasible based on users' evaluation. Importantly, different samples of consecutive RA outpatients were used to perform analysis. We suggest that RAEH can be used to evaluate empowerment in Hispanic RA patients; the scale is simple and suitable for low-literacy patients and its use could be generalized to Spanish-speaking RA patients from other countries. Although ethnic heterogeneity is characteristic of the Latin American population, RA patients from this geographic area present distinctive characteristics when compared to white populations from the United States and Europe [35].

The RAEH showed adequate internal consistency reliability; Cronbach's α coefficient for the total scale and the eight empowerment dimensions were good, with α value of 0.86 [33]. The test–retest reliability assessed in 50 patients by the same researcher showed an ICC of 0.79, indicating good reliability [34], with 95% CI of 0.62–0.88. The construct validity was demonstrated by KMO sampling and Barlett's test of sphericity, both confirming the adequacy of the sample size for conducting factor analysis [33], and a single factor structure was extracted, accounting for 52% of the variance. Face and content validity were examined by patients, and a multidisciplinary committee of health care providers involved in RA management. Patients (RAEH face validity) agreed that items were a valid measure of the corresponding dimension and that items were clear; additional patients confirmed RAEH feasibility. Patients involvement may be particularly relevant as one would expect the indicators of empowerment to be defined by the patients themselves, rather than (or in addition to) by health care professionals. Finally, the RAEH (total score) did not show neither floor nor ceiling effect, which had been defined when more than 15% of the patients achieved the lowest or highest score, respectively [30]. Both, floor and ceiling effects can reduce the possibility of detecting change over time.

This is the first scale validated in the Hispanic population that measures empowerment in patients with RA. There is only one additional scale, the SWE-RES-23, which assessed empowerment in patients with rheumatic diseases [19]. The scale was developed in Swedish and psychometric properties were evaluated in a population primarily represented by middle-aged females; in addition, although patients with different rheumatic diagnosis were included, 74% of them were classified with inflammatory joint diseases, which include RA diagnosis. The RAEH and the SWE-RES-23 showed similar psychometric properties in terms of construct validity, internal consistency and reliability although stability reliability was not tested in the SWE-RES-23, meanwhile the RAEH showed good ICC. Regarding RAEH ceiling effects, it should be mentioned there were ceiling effects in all the individual's dimensions, which indicates that patients start with higher empowerment skills than the average and may lack room for improvement [30]. Arvidsson et al. also found ceiling effects in two subscales of the SWE-RES-23 and the total score [19], as did Serrani in six out of eight subscales of the S-HES [25] (see Additional file 3).

The median RAEH score for our target population was 34, which confirms that our patients showed an empowerment level above medium values, as has been found in other studies [19, 25]. The average of the empowerment measurement cannot be compared between the RAEH and the SEW-RES-23, because they had different number of reagents and dimensions. Nonetheless, total RAEH mean value (4.2 ± 0.57) was superior to that from either the SWE-RES-23 (vs. 3.53 ± 0.57, $p = 0.001$) or the S-HES (vs. 3.51 ± 0.73, $p = 0.001$). Our higher scale mean value may be considered unexpectedly high for a population with limited literacy, but could be explained by the long-term RA duration present in our patients (12 years of disease duration).

Additional studies have tried to measure the level of empowerment in patients with RA; however, empowerment has been measured in a subjective manner. Geller et al. [18] used an empowerment program for 6 months in patients with chronic pain (six of them had RA) and assessed the quality of life, but did not quantitatively measure the level of empowerment. Allam et al. [36] tested the effects of online social support and gamification on health outcomes in 157 RA patients; empowerment levels changed over time, more so in the groups having access to online support or a gamified experience of the website. van der Vaart et al. [37] applied questionnaires and measured use, satisfaction and impact of a web portal, which provided patients with home access to their electronic medical records, in 360 RA patients; only 54% of the respondents (to the questionnaires) had viewed their electronic medical records; among those who had logged in, 44% reported feeling more involved in their treatment, 37% felt they had more knowledge about their treatment, but differences over time were not found on the empowerment-related instruments. Different empowerment-enhancing approaches had been described in RA patients in order to support the patients [20] and promote patient independence [21]. Clinical trials may be considered complex systems, and patients enrolled explained their participation as an experience that substantially improved their control and adaptation by a better understanding of their disease, which may ultimately enhance empowerment [22]. Similarly, alternative models of RA patients' follow-up, whereby patients initiate appointments themselves, may offer greater self-management of the underlying rheumatic disease [23].

The study has some limitations. First, we did not assess RAEH response to change, neither had indication of minimal important change nor minimal important difference, and without such information, it is impossible to understand if changes in levels of empowerment matters to patients [24]. Second, the RAEH was adapted and validated in a particular population of Hispanic RA outpatients from México and, given cultural differences in Latin America, results present here need to be reproduced in other Spanish-speaking countries. Nonetheless, the RAEH is simple and easy to apply particularly in populations with poor levels of literacy. Third, the RAEH questionnaire assessed empowerment skills at the individual level, but did not account for organizational and community levels that may additionally impact empowerment, particularly in patients with chronic conditions [7]. Finally, the RAEH evaluates empowerment limited to RA; nonetheless, empowerment is a complex construct and it may be necessary to set up a disease-specific context to understand empowerment implications, in terms of outcomes relevant to patients.

Conclusions

In conclusion, RAEH is valid, reliable, and feasible to evaluate empowerment in Spanish-speaking RA patients. Patients from Latin America present unique characteristics and research needs to focus on such populations in order to complete the picture of RA, knowledge of which has been constructed based on studies performed primarily in Caucasians patients. There is (qualitative) evidence in non-rheumatic diseases suggesting that enhancing patient empowerment over their health is highly valued and enables patients to better manage their lives. These, if reproduced in patients with rheumatic diseases, in particular RA, should be conceived as a valuable outcome. The RAEH could be applied in a practical way in studies that use empowerment-enhancing programs in Spanish-speaking RA patients.

Abbreviations
ACCP: Antibodies to cyclic citrullinated peptide; C-RP: C-reactive protein; ESR: Erythrocyte sedimentation rate; HRQoL: Health-related quality of life; ICC: Intra-class correlation coefficient; INCMyN-SZ: Instituto Nacional de Ciencias Médicas y Nutrición Salvador Zubirán; KMO: Kaiser-Meyer-Olkin sampling; RA: Rheumatoid arthritis; RAEH: Rheumatoid Arthritis Empowerment Scale for Hispanic patients; RF: Rheumatoid factor; SD: Standard deviation; S-HES: Spanish-Health Empowerment Scale; SWE-RES-23: Swedish Rheumatic Disease Empowerment Scale; VEC: Validation Expert Committee

Acknowledgements
None.

Funding
This work was carried out with a grant from UCB Mexico Biopharmaceutical Company.

Availability of data and materials
The data that support the findings of this study are available on request from the corresponding author (VPR). The data are not publicly available due to them containing information that could compromise research participant consent.

Authors' contributions
ICY participated in the conception and design of the study and performed the statistical analysis. ERM participated in the conception of the study and reviewed the manuscript. LCHR participated in the conception of the study and reviewed the manuscript. VPR participated in the conception and design of the study; performed the statistical analysis, and drafted the manuscript. All authors read and approved the final manuscript.

Authors' information
All authors read and approved this manuscript.

Consent for publication
Not applicable.

Competing interests
The authors declare that they have no financial interests that could create a potential conflict of interest with regard to the work.

Author details
[1]Department of Immunology and Rheumatology, Instituto Nacional de Ciencias Médicas y Nutrición Salvador Zubirán, Vasco de Quiroga 15, Colonia Belisario Domínguez Sección XVI, México City, Mexico. [2]External collaborator, Mexico City, Mexico.

References
1. Tengland P-A. Empowerment: A conceptual discussion. Health Care Anal. 2008;16:77–96.
2. McAllister M, Dunn G, Payne K, Davies L, Todd C. Patient empowerment: The need to consider it as a measurable patient-reported outcome for chronic conditions. BMC Health Serv Res. 2012;12:157.
3. Aujoulat I, d'Hoore W, Deccache A. Patient empowerment in theory and practice: Polysemy or cacophony? Patient Educ Counseling. 2007;66:13–20.
4. Bergsma LJ. Empowerment education: the link between media literacy and health promotion. Am Behav Sci. 2004;48:152–64.
5. Anderson RM, Funnell MM. Patient empowerment: Myths and misconceptions. Patient Educ Couns. 2010;79:277–82.
6. Tengland P-A. Empowerment: A goal or a means of health promotion? Med Health Care and Philosophy. 2007;10:197–207.
7. Zimmerman MA. Empowerment theory: psychological, organizational and community levels of analysis. In: Rappaport J, Seldman E, editors. Handbook of Community Psychology. New York: Plenum; 2000.
8. Ashmed S, Creanga AA, Gillespie DG, Tsui AO. Economic status, education and empowerment: implications for maternal health service utilization in developing countries. PLoS One. 2010;6:e11190.
9. Voshaar MJH, Nota I, van der Laar MAFJ, van der Bemt BJF. Patient-centred care in established rheumatoid arthritis. Best Pract and Res Clin Rheumatol. 2015;29:643–63.
10. Elwyn G, Laitner S, Coulter A, Walker E, Watson P, Thomson R. Implementing share decision-making in the NHS. British Med J. 2010;341:c5146.
11. Counter A, Ellins J. Effectiveness of strategies for informing, educating, and involving patients. Br Med J. 2007;335:24–7.
12. Smolen JS, Landerwe R, Breedveld FC, Buch M, Burmester G, Dougados M, et al. EULAR recommendations for the management of rheumatoid arthritis with synthetic and biologic disease modifying anti-rheumatic drugs: 2013 update. Ann Rheum Dis. 2014;73(3):492–509.
13. Hibbard JH. Moving toward a more patient-centred health care delivery system. Health Aff (Millwood) 2004 Suppl Variation: var 133–5.
14. Mody GM, Cardiel MH. Challenges in the management of rheumatoid arthritis in developing countries. Best Pract Clin Rheumatol. 2008;22:621–41.
15. Contreras-Yáñez I, Pascual-Ramos V. Window of opportunity to achieve major outcomes in early rheumatoid arthritis patients: How persistence with therapy matters. Arthritis Res Ther. 2015;17:177. https://doi.org/10.1186/s13075-015-0697-z.
16. Pérez-Román DI, Ortiz-Haro AB, Ruiz-Medrano E, Contreras-Yáñez I, Pascual-Ramos V. Outcomes after rheumatoid arthritis patients complete their participation in a long-term observational study with tofacitinib combined with methotrexate: Practical and ethical implications in vulnerable populations after tofacitinib discontinuation. Rheumatol Int. 2018;38(4):599–606.
17. Van Den Bemt BJF, Zwikker HE, Van Den Ende CH. Medication adherence in patients with rheumatoid arthritis: a critical appraisal of the existing literature. Expert Rev Clin Immunol. 2012;8:337–51.
18. Geller JS, Kulla J, Shoemaker A. Group medical visits using empowerment based model as treatment for women with chronic pain in an underserved community. Global Adv Health Med. 2015;4:27–31.
19. Arvidsson S, Bergman S, Arvidsson B, Fridlund B, Tingström P. Psychometric properties of the Swedish rheumatic disease empowerment scale, SWE-RES-23. Musculoskeletal Care. 2012;10:101–9.
20. Arvidsson SB, Petersson A, Nilsson I, Andersson B, Arvidsson B, Petersson IF, et al. A nurse led rheumatology clinic's impact on empowering patients with rheumatoid arthritis: A qualitative study. Nurs Health Sci. 2006;8:133–9.
21. De la Torre-Aboki J. Aportación de la consulta de enfermería en el manejo del paciente con artritis reumatoide. Reumatol Clin. 2011;6(S3):S16–9.
22. De Jorge M, Parra S, De la Torre-Aboki J, Herrero-Beaumont G. Randomized clinical trials as reflexive-interpretative process in patients with rheumatoid arthritis: a qualitative study. Rheumatol Int. 2015;35(8):1423–30. https://doi.org/10.1007//S00296-015-3218-0.
23. Child S, Goodwin VA, Perry MG, Gericke C, Byng R. Implementing a patient-initiative review system in rheumatoid arthritis: a qualitative evaluation. BMC Health Serv Res. 2015;15:157.
24. Barr PJ, Scholl I, Bravo P, Faber MJ, Elwyn G, McAllister M. Assessment of patient empowerment: A systematic review of measures. PLoS One. 2015;10(5):e0126553. https://doi.org/10.1371/journal.pone.0126553.
25. Doubova SV, Espinosa-Alarcón P, Infante C, Aguirre-Hernández R, Rodríguez-Aguilar R, Olivares-Santos R, et al. Adaptation and validation of scales to measure self-efficacy and empowerment for self-care in Mexican climateric stage women. Salud Pública Mex. 2013;55(3):257–66.
26. Serrani Azcurra DJL. Elders health empowerment scale. Spanish adaptation and psychometric analysis. Columbia Médica. 2014;45:179–85.
27. Katz JN, Lyons N, Wolff LS, Silverman J, Emrani P, Holt HL, et al. Medical-decision making among Hispanics and non-Hispanics with chronic back and knee pain: A qualitative study. BMC Musculoskelet Disord. 2011;12:78.
28. Barrio-Cantalejo IM, Simón-Lorda P, Melguizo M, Escalona I, Marijuán MI, Hernando P. Validación de la escala INFLESZ para evaluar la legibilidad de los textos dirigidos a pacientes. Anales Sis San Navarra. 2008;31(2):135–52.
29. Charlson ME, Pompei P, Ales KL, Mackenzie CR. A new method of classifying prognostic comorbidity in longitudinal studies: Development and validation. J Chronic Dis. 1987;40:373–83.
30. Terwee CB, Bot SD, de Boer MR, van der Windt DA, Knol DL, Dekker J, et al. Quality criteria were proposed for measurement properties of health status questionnaires. J Clin Epidemiol. 2007;60:34–42.
31. Fleiss J. The design and analysis of clinical experiments. New York: Wiley; 1986.
32. Pett MA, Lackey NR, Sullivan JJ. Making sense of factor analysis: The use of factor analysis for instrument development in health care research. Thousand Oaks: Sage Publications Inc; 2003.
33. Bland J, Altman D. Statistics notes: Cronbach's alpha. BMJ. 1997;314:275.
34. Koo TK, Li MY. A guideline of selecting and reporting intraclass correlation coefficients for reliability research. J Chiropr Med. 2016;15:155–63.
35. Cardiel MH, Latin American Rheumatology Associations of the Pan American League of Associations for Rheumatology (PANLAR); Grupo Latino Americano de Estudio de Artritis Reumatoide GLADAR. First Latin-American position paper on the pharmacological treatment of rheumatoid arthritis. Rheumatology (Oxford). 2006;45(Suppl 2):ii7–ii22.
36. Allam A, Kostova z NK, Schulz PJ. The effect of social support features and gamification on a web-based intervention for rheumatoid arthritis patients: Randomized controlled trial. J Med Intern Res. 2015;17(1):e14.
37. van der Vaart R, Drossaert CHC, Taal E, Drossaers-Bakker KW, Vonkeman HE, van der Laar MAFJ. Impact on patient-accessible electronic medical records in rheumatology: use, satisfaction and effects on empowerment among patients. BMC Musculoskeletal Dis. 2014;15:102.

23

Comorbidities in polymyalgia rheumatica: a systematic review

Richard Partington *[ID], Toby Helliwell, Sara Muller, Alyshah Abdul Sultan and Christian Mallen

Abstract

Background and aim: Comorbidities are known to exist in many rheumatological conditions. Polymyalgia rheumatica (PMR) is a common inflammatory rheumatological condition affecting older people which, prior to effective treatment, causes severe disability. Our understanding of associated comorbidities in PMR is based only on case reports or series and small cohort studies. The objective of this study is to review systematically the existing literature on the comorbidities associated with PMR.

Methods: MEDLINE, EMBASE, PsycINFO and CINAHL databases were searched for original observational research from inception to November 2016. Papers containing the words 'Polymyalgia Rheumatica' OR 'Giant Cell Arteritis' OR the terms 'PMR' OR 'GCA' were included. Article titles were reviewed based on pre-defined criteria by two reviewers. Following selection for inclusion, studies were quality assessed using the Newcastle–Ottawa tool and data were extracted.

Results: A total of 17,329 papers were reviewed and 41 were incorporated in this review, including three published after the search took place. Wide variations were found in study design, comorbidities reported and populations studied. Positive associations were found between PMR diagnosis and stroke, cardiovascular disease, peripheral arterial disease, diverticular disease and hypothyroidism. Two studies reported a positive association between PMR and overall malignancy rate. Seven studies reported an association between PMR and specific types of cancer, such as leukaemia, lymphoma, myeloproliferative disease and specified solid tumours, although nine studies found either no or negative association between cancer and PMR.

Conclusion: Quantification of the prevalence of comorbidities in PMR is important to accurately plan service provision and enable identification of cases of PMR which may be more difficult to treat. This review highlights that research into comorbidities in PMR is, overall, methodologically inadequate and does not comprehensively cover all comorbidities. Future studies should consider a range of comorbidities in patients with a validated diagnosis of PMR in representative populations.

Keywords: Polymyalgia rheumatica, Giant cell arteritis, Systematic review, Comorbidities, Multimorbidity, Epidemiology

Introduction

Polymyalgia rheumatica (PMR) is the most common inflammatory rheumatological condition affecting people over the age of 50 years [1]. Symptoms include muscle stiffness and pain, predominantly around the neck or shoulder and pelvic girdles [2], as well as a low-grade fever, depression, fatigue, anorexia and weight loss [3, 4]. Raised inflammatory markers (erythrocyte sedimentation rate (ESR) or C-reactive protein (CRP)) are a hallmark of this condition. PMR is usually treated with medium/low dose oral glucocorticoids (GCs) which are gradually reduced and stopped over several years [5].

Patients with common inflammatory rheumatological conditions, for example gout [6] and rheumatoid arthritis (RA) [7], are predisposed to developing cardiovascular disease (CVD). In patients with RA, this risk has been attributed to an increased prevalence of arterial atherosclerotic plaques [8, 9], the quantity of which are correlated with levels of systemic inflammation [10] and duration of

* Correspondence: r.partington@keele.ac.uk
Arthritis Research UK Primary Care Centre, Primary Care Sciences, Keele University, Keele ST5 5BG, UK

rheumatological disease [11]. Patients with RA are also known to have a higher risk of lung diseases [12] and certain types of cancers, particularly haematological cancers [13]. PMR, like RA, is a rheumatological condition characterised by increased levels of inflammation, and therefore patients with PMR may have a similar predisposition to increased risks of certain conditions.

In order to diagnose PMR, guidelines endorsed by the American College of Rheumatology and the European League Against Rheumatism advise the exclusion of conditions which may cause similar symptoms [14]. These include core exclusion conditions (GCA, cancer and infections) as well as RA, fibromyalgia, hypothyroidism and drug-induced myalgia. The guidelines also suggest an evaluation of whether patients have comorbidities that put them at greater risk of side effects from GC treatment [14]. Quantifying the burden of comorbidities in this group of patients is therefore important.

The age group (typically over 50 years) most commonly affected by PMR frequently has more than one comorbidity. Aging is an important predictor of multimorbidity; a recent Scottish study found the number of adults with two or more chronic conditions increased from 30.4% between age 45 and 64 years, to 64.9% in those aged 65–84 years, to greater than 80% in those aged over 85 years [15]. This systematic review aims to summarise the available evidence of the comorbidity profile of people with PMR, and will be the first review to assess comprehensively the evidence for all comorbidities and whether there is evidence for multiple comorbidities existing together. If the evidence shows that patients with PMR commonly have multiple comorbidities then these may no longer be viewed as exclusion criteria precluding a diagnosis of PMR, potentially revealing the true burden of PMR to be higher than currently recognised.

Methods

We conducted a systematic review and narrative synthesis of research literature. We searched medical bibliographic databases to identify articles containing data on any comorbidity either preceding or following a diagnosis of PMR.

Data sources, searches and study selection

The search was conducted in MEDLINE, EMBASE, PsyciINFO and CINAHL from their inception until the date of search in November 2016. Additional articles were found by examining reference lists of included studies and an updated search was run in June 2018 which led to the inclusion of a further study. The exploded MeSH terms 'polymyalgia rheumatica' and 'giant cell arteritis' were used in combination with text word searches for the same as well as for 'PMR' and 'Giant Cell Arteritis' (GCA). GCA is a vasculitis which very commonly co-occurs with PMR; around 10–30% of patients with PMR develop GCA during the course of their illness [16, 17]. Given this overlap in conditions, GCA was included

to increase the likelihood of ensuring that all studies in which PMR comorbidities were considered were included in the review. PRISMA guidelines were followed throughout the review process [18].

All article titles identified were screened by a single reviewer (RP) against the inclusion and exclusion criteria. A random sample of 100 of these titles was reviewed by a second reviewer (TH) and agreement between decisions was assessed using adjusted κ calculation [19]. All selected abstracts were then assessed by two reviewers (RP and TH). Any citation thought to be eligible by either reviewer was carried forward to full text review. Reasons for exclusion were recorded. Finally, the remaining full texts were reviewed by the same two authors and a list of papers to be included in the narrative synthesis was created.

Inclusion and exclusion criteria

The inclusion criteria for this review included: a sample of patients with PMR and at least one comorbidity; and the study design must be either cross-sectional, case–control or a prospective or retrospective cohort study. Exclusion criteria were: patients under the age of 40 years; randomised control trials (RCTs); and review articles or conference abstracts. PMR is a disease of older adults. In order to make a diagnosis of PMR, clinical guidelines suggest patients must be aged over 50 years [20], therefore patients under 40 years old are likely to represent misdiagnosis. RCTs were excluded as we wished to look at representative samples of patients with PMR drawn from real-world, observational data. Review articles and conference abstracts were not included to ensure all articles were peer reviewed and fully referenced. In order to ensure that all conditions represented true comorbidities, rather than secondary complications of GC treatment in PMR, we excluded trials which reported only complications of GC therapy [3, 21–27].

There were no date or language restrictions although all included studies were in English. Potentially relevant studies that contained data on GCA were included until full text review due to the overlap between PMR and GCA. If, at that point, the paper only contained data about GCA, it was excluded. The reference lists of other systematic reviews that had assessed individual comorbidities related to PMR were also reviewed to reduce the chance of missing relevant studies.

Quality assessment

Both reviewers, using the Newcastle–Ottawa Scale for case–control and/or cohort studies [28], evaluated the quality of studies. This scale was chosen as it is endorsed for use in systematic reviews of non-randomised trials by the Cochrane Collaboration [29].

Data extraction

A standardised form was developed and used by both reviewers independently to ensure the accuracy of data extraction (Additional file 1). The primary outcome of interest was the total number of patients with PMR who developed a comorbidity of interest compared to controls (without PMR). Other data extracted included clinical criteria used to diagnose PMR, study design, comorbidity under investigation and its temporal relationship to PMR. Meta-data from each study, such as lead author name, publication year, sex, age, country and healthcare setting, were also extracted. Comorbidities were categorised into four groups: malignant disease, particularly haematological malignancies; vascular disease, including coronary, cerebroarterial and peripheral arterial disease; mortality; and other comorbidities (e.g. endocrine, psychiatric and neurological diseases).

Data analysis

Using the total number of patients with PMR and, if present, their controls we attempted to aggregate data to obtain pooled estimates of prevalence of comorbidities and odds ratios to quantify the strength of any apparent association.

Results

Search results

A total of 27,698 articles were identified in this search with a further seven identified following review of references of other articles. Of this total, 10,376 were removed due to duplications, leaving 17,329 unique articles. Following application of inclusion and exclusion criteria during screening of titles, 17,042 further citations were excluded. Of the random selection of 100 of these articles which were reviewed by a second author, agreement between authors was excellent ($\kappa = 0.86$).

The abstracts of 287 studies were assessed for eligibility, and 131 were excluded at this stage. The full texts of articles were reviewed and 41 were retained for data extraction [30–70]. This process, which followed PRISMA guidelines, including reasons for exclusion of studies [18], is illustrated in Fig. 1.

Articles included in the review

Of the 41 included studies, 32 were cohort studies [30–61] and nine were case–control studies [62–70]. Eighteen of the cohort studies did not use a formal comparator group. Of the 14 cohort studies with controls, six were based on national datasets, whereas eight were based either on local datasets or on patients presenting to clinics at the same hospital. PMR cases were defined from medical records in 16 studies, national registries in 19 studies and national databases in the remaining six studies. Co-existent GCA cases were formally excluded in six studies and included, or not explicitly excluded, in 35 studies. All but one study was

from Europe (predominantly Scandinavia) or the United States. Included studies are tabulated in Additional file 2.

PMR and cancer

Seven studies, reporting 12 outcome measures, have assessed the risk of cancer diagnosis prior to PMR onset (Table 1). All of these studies excluded PMR diagnoses made in the year prior to diagnosis of cancer, to reduce the risk of reverse causality (i.e. cancer causing PMR or PMR symptoms). Of these, the rate of haematogenous cancers was significantly higher among patients with PMR in five cases, while the other seven were non-significantly different.

Six studies reported prospective rates of any cancer diagnosis after diagnosis with PMR (Table 2); two showed an increase in the proportion of people with PMR who developed cancer compared to controls, two were equivocal and the remaining two found the opposite.

In six prospective cohort studies the risk of 17 types of cancer following diagnosis with PMR was considered. Two studies showed an increase in the risk of Hodgkin's lymphoma [55] and non-Hodgkin's lymphoma [56]. Of the remaining four studies, three reported no difference in the rates of female cancers [51], upper gastrointestinal cancers [47] or myeloma [54]. The final study reported no difference in mortality following diagnosis with gastrointestinal cancers [50] among people with or without PMR.

PMR and vascular disease

A number of studies ($n = 8$) have assessed a variety of different vascular diseases in patients with PMR (Table 3). Fifteen outcome measures were reported, although only seven gave comparable figures for patients without PMR. In each study with a comparator group the proportion of people with PMR who developed vascular disease was higher compared to controls.

PMR and mortality

Few studies have assessed the association between PMR and mortality ($n = 4$). Three studies reported reduced mortality among patients diagnosed with PMR [35, 38, 39] while one study found an increase, but this study did not differentiate between patients with PMR and GCA [36].

PMR and other comorbidities

An association between thyroid disease and PMR is unproven. Bowness et al. [31] found an increase in the risk of hypothyroid disease (RR 3.2 (95% confidence interval 1.71, 5.91)), but Juchet et al. [33] did not. One recent case–control study found a significantly increased rate of diverticular disease prior to a diagnosis with PMR (OR 4.06 (95% CI 1.76–9.35)) [70].

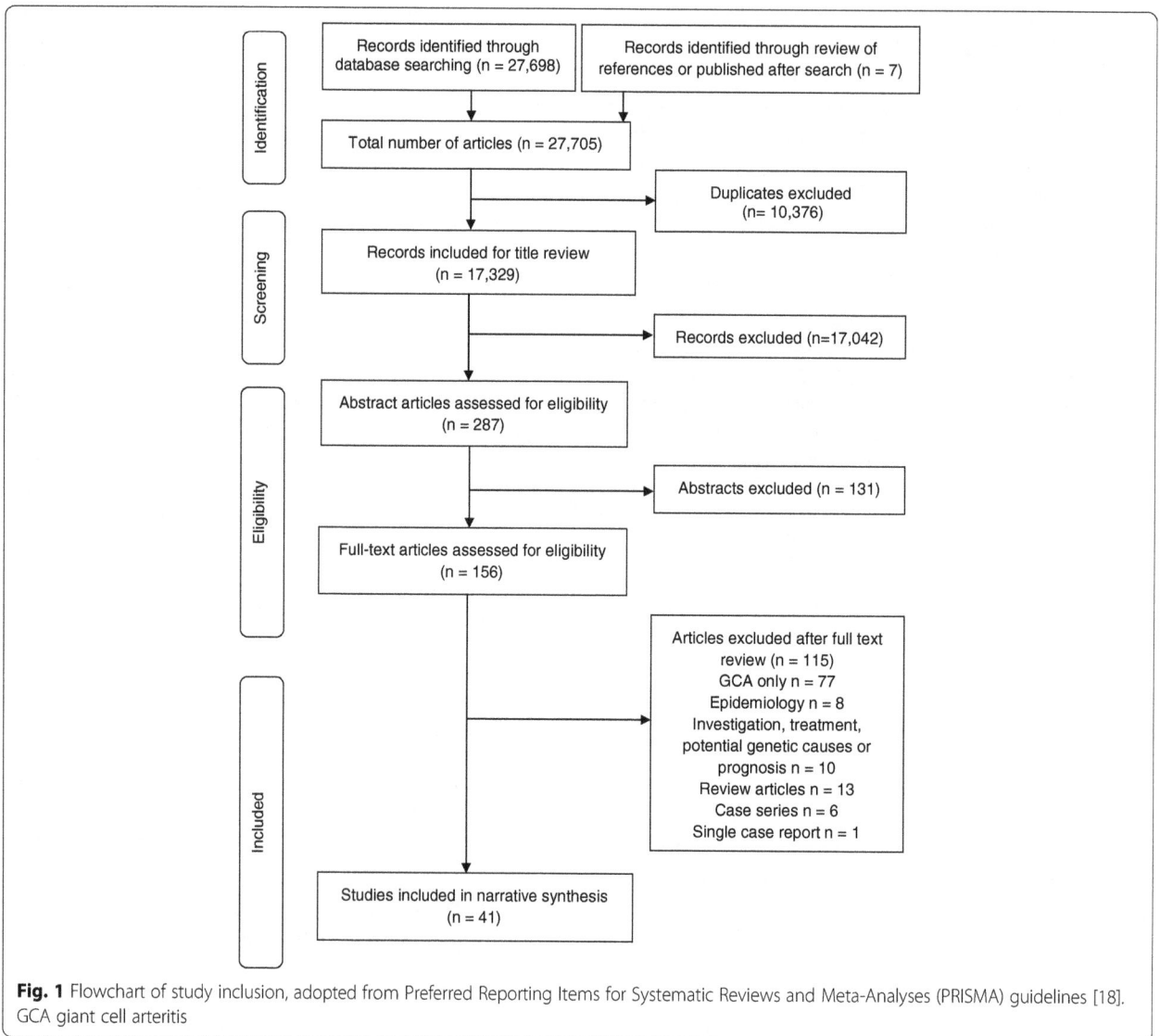

Fig. 1 Flowchart of study inclusion, adopted from Preferred Reporting Items for Systematic Reviews and Meta-Analyses (PRISMA) guidelines [18]. GCA giant cell arteritis

No evidence has been found to associate PMR with psychiatric comorbidities, including schizophrenia [44, 69] and bipolar disease [44]. Li et al. [49] found a potential association between PMR and Parkinson's disease (SIR 1.25 (95% CI 1.01, 1.53)). Hemminki et al. [53] also reported an association between PMR and hospitalisation due to obesity (SIR 1.65 (95% CI 1.22, 2.19)).

A small number of studies from the United States (n = 2) [40, 59] looked at wide ranges of different comorbidities but their sample size was insufficient to find significant associations for the majority of the comorbidities.

Quality assessment

All of the articles in this study used medical records or nationwide registries (based on medical records) to corroborate diagnosis of PMR and the comorbidity; therefore, they were awarded three or four stars for cohort or case selection using the Newcastle–Ottawa criteria. All

studies also achieved at least two stars for outcome measurement. However, many of the studies failed to recruit a comparator group, instead using the population as a reference, and therefore comparability scores were low (Additional file 2).

Many of the cohort studies identified failed to include comparison groups (n = 18), instead using indirect standardisation to calculate incidence or mortality ratios. The lack of comparison groups limits the generalisability of many of the studies. Further to this, almost half of the studies (n = 19) sourced their sample of patients with PMR based on hospital discharge data. This may be an appropriate approach for some autoimmune conditions, but the majority of patients with PMR are managed in primary care settings [71, 72].

Aggregation of data to calculate pooled odds and hazard ratios was attempted for vascular disease and cancer diagnoses; however, high levels of heterogeneity were

Table 1 Cancer prior to diagnosis with PMR

Retrospective case–control study

Study	Diagnosis	Cases (n)	PMR cases (n)	Controls (n)	PMR controls (n)	Odds ratio (95% CI)	Case rate (%)	Control rate (%)
Anderson et al. [64]	Lymphoid malignancies	33,721	344	122,531	1244	0.9 (0.8–1.0)	1.02	1.02
Anderson et al. [63]	Myeloid malignancy	9998	125	160,086	1288	1.7 (1.4–2.1)	1.25	0.80
	Myelodysplastic malignancy	3758	55	42,886	518	1.5 (1.1–2)	1.46	1.21
Anderson et al. [67]	HCL	418	9	160,086	2721	1.5 (0.5–3.9)	2.15	1.70
Askling et al. [62]	All lymphoma	42,676	114	78,487	250	0.8 (0.7–1.0)	0.27	0.32
	NHL	28,355	88	52,164	187	0.9 (0.7–1.1)	0.31	0.36
	HL	4037	3	7394	15	0.4 (0.1–1.3)	0.07	0.2
	CLL	10,555	24	19,391	52	0.8 (0.5–1.4)	0.23	0.27
Kristinsson et al. [66]	Any MPN	11,039	46	43,550	104	1.7 (1.2–2.5)	0.42	0.24
Lanoy and Engels [65]	Cutaneous NHL	2652	19	178,452	1731	0.7 (0.5–1.1)	0.72	0.97
Lindqvist et al. [68]	MM	19,112	56	75,408	116	1.9 (1.4–2.6)	0.29	0.15
	MGUS	5403	58	21,209	79	2.9 (2.1–4.1)	1.07	0.37

PMR polymyalgia rheumatica, *HCL* hairy cell leukaemia, *NHL* non-Hodgkin's lymphoma, *HL* Hodgkin's lymphoma, *CLL* chronic lymphocytic leukaemia, *MM* multiple myeloma, *MPN* myeloproliferative neoplasm, *MGUS* monoclonal gammopathy of undetermined significance

found between the studies (88–100%) and therefore this was not reported.

Many of the studies limited themselves to a small number of comorbid conditions, thus not allowing a picture of the overall health of patients with PMR to develop. Two studies [34, 40] did attempt to look at a range of comorbidities but they were underpowered.

Discussion

Statement of principle findings

This review found some evidence of an association between PMR and vascular disease, and possibly cancer,

Table 2 Cancer following diagnosis with PMR

Prospective cohort with combined cancer cases

Study	PMR patients			Control patients		
	PMR cases (n)	Cancer cases (n)	Proportion (%)	Controls (n)	Cancer cases (n)	Proportion (%)
Muller et al. [57]	2877	667	23.18	9942	1938	19.49
Bellan et al. [61]	100	24	24.00	702	41	5.84
Ji et al. [45]	35,918	3941	10.97	–	–	–
Myklebust et al. [37]	366	34	9.29	1324	143	10.80
Haga et al. [32]	91	10	10.99	794	131	16.50
Pfeifer et al. [59]	359	66	18.38	357	62	17.37
Total[a]	39,711	4742	21.12	13,119	2315	17.65

PMR polymyalgia rheumatica

[a]Ji et al. [45] not included in calculation as no control group

particularly in the first 6 months following diagnosis. However, the evidence for this is not robust.

The concentration of the apparent association between PMR and cancer in the first 6 months following diagnosis suggests the possibility of an element of misdiagnosis. This could occur as some of the features of PMR (myalgia, fatigue, weight loss, raised inflammatory markers) are also non-specific early features of some cancers. Furthermore, as time passed, the rate of diagnosis of cancer was found to drop down to the background population rate.

Regarding specific types of cancer, some studies have proposed there could be associations between PMR and haematological cancers. This includes Hodgkin's and non-Hodgkin's lymphoma [56], myeloma [68] and other myeloid malignancies [63, 66]. An increase in the risk of lymphoma has been observed with RA, which has been postulated to be due to higher accumulated inflammatory activity in RA [73]; a similar mechanism may lie behind the apparent increase in patients with PMR.

The overall trend of results suggests that PMR may be associated with an increased risk of the development of vascular disease. Knowing that both PMR and RA are inflammatory conditions, there is biological plausibility that PMR and vascular disease could be associated. However, the two largest studies, both based on population data from the UK, reported conflicting results: Hancock et al. [58] stated that PMR was significantly associated with vascular disease, while Pujades-Rodriguez et al. [60] reported a reduction in the risk (incidence rate ratio 0.88 (95% CI 0.83–, 0.94)). However, in the latter study when only patients with PMR were included, there was a slight increase in the proportion of patients with the condition who went on to have a vascular event compared to controls (23.24% compared to 20.43%).

These two studies employed similar approaches selecting with PMR from linked UK databases. However, a number of differences existed between the studies, including the age of participants (> 50 years only for Hancock et al. [58] and > 18 years for Pujades-Rodriguez et al. [60]), average years of follow up (7.8 and 3.13 years respectively) as well as the total number of patients found with PMR (3249 compared to 11,320 patients). Potentially, the variation in risk of vascular events between these studies could be explained by the differences in follow up or the age distribution of the study population.

Another reason for inconsistent evidence of an increase in vascular risk for patients with PMR may be the modulating effect that GCs have upon levels on inflammation. If the risk of vascular disease correlates with the presence of inflammation in the body, GC therapy would reduce this, which may then also reduce vascular risk. The study by Kremers et al. [42] appears to bear this out. In this study, the risk of vascular events was lower in patients with PMR who were treated with GCs compared to those who were not. Further to this, Hancock et al. [58] reported that the excess vascular risk in PMR

reduced over time; this could reflect declining levels of inflammation.

Overall, although some studies dissent from this view, it appears that a diagnosis of PMR increases an individual's risk of vascular disease. However, further research in this area is needed to add clarity.

Conversely, it appears that a diagnosis with PMR is associated with a reduction in mortality. This was demonstrated in three out of the four studies that reported it as an independent outcome. A possible explanation for this could again be surveillance bias. Patients with chronic illness (and especially PMR where regular assessment, follow up and monitoring are advised) are more likely to be under active follow up for their condition and any developing morbidity, particularly if related to well-recognised adverse effects of treatment, is likely to be identified and managed earlier.

There is a small amount of evidence that patients with PMR may be more likely to develop hypothyroidism [31] and Parkinson's disease [49]. PMR and hypothyroidism both preferentially affect females, and therefore a similar autoimmune pathway may be present in both conditions. However, as has been pointed out, PMR does not share all of the characteristics of traditional autoimmune conditions, for example it lacks specific autoantibodies [74].

Table 3 Vascular disease and PMR

Study	PMR patients			Control patients		
	PMR cases (n)	Comorbid condition (n)	Proportion (%)	Controls (n)	Comorbid condition (n)	Proportion (%)
Stroke						
Kang et al. [46]	781	113	14.47	3905	273	6.99
Zoller et al. [48]	16,496	1981	12.01			
Kremers et al. [42]	276	58	21.01			
Hancock et al. [58]	3249	397	12.22	12,735	556	4.37
Myocardial infarction						
Kremers et al. [42]	276	47	17.03			
Hancock et al. [58]	3249	460	14.16	12,735	575	4.52
Zoller et al. [48]	21,351	5669	26.55			
Heart failure						
Kremers et al. [42]	276	68	24.64			
Peripheral vascular disease						
Kremers et al. [42]	276	35	12.68			
Hancock et al. [58]	3249	140	4.31	12,735	151	1.19
Warrington et al. [43]	353	38	10.76	705	28	3.97
Combined						
Kremers et al. [42]	276	208	75.36			
Hancock et al. [58]	3249	918	28.25	12,735	1150	9.03
Pujades-Rodriguez et al. [60]	9776	2272	23.24	105,504	21,559	20.43
Bengtsson and Malmvall [30]	73	16	21.92			

PMR polymyalgia rheumatica

Furthermore, it seems that PMR is not associated as strongly with other autoimmune conditions as would be expected if it was a pure autoimmune disease. Parkinson's disease is a condition which predominantly affects older people, as does PMR, and therefore this association may just be a result of clustering of diagnoses in an older population.

Strengths and weaknesses

The main strength of the study was its deliberately broad scope and aim to include any study in which the risk of any comorbidity either before or after diagnosis with PMR was to be reviewed. Following the initial broad search, articles from the 'grey literature' were excluded and only articles fully published in peer-reviewed journals were included.

The potential limitations in this study arose not due to the protocol but rather because the majority of studies were of relatively poor quality. These risks included selection bias, surveillance bias and a lack of adequate control groups.

Selection bias within the included studies is a possibility in this review, as the majority of studies drew PMR cases from secondary care, either from hospital discharge data or from rheumatology outpatient clinics. Current UK guidelines suggest only referring atypical cases, cases of diagnostic uncertainty or treatment predicaments [5, 14], meaning that in the UK 71–84% of patients with PMR are treated in the community by primary care physicians [71, 72]. Therefore, the patient population in these studies may not accurately reflect the majority of those who are diagnosed with PMR. This may have artificially inflated the apparent differences in development of comorbidities between patients with and without PMR.

Another limitation is the risk of surveillance bias as discussed earlier around the apparent reduction in mortality [75]. Some case–control studies attempted to deal with this by excluding comorbid disease found in the year prior to diagnosis [63, 64, 67, 68], while in two observational cohort studies [58, 60], controls were selected that had contacted a primary care service in the year the index cases were diagnosed. Finally, many of these studies assessed multiple variables, often > 30 different autoimmune conditions, increasing the likelihood of a chance finding (type II error).

Furthermore, we also noted that the range of comorbidities reported in the literature was more limited than we expected; for example, there were no studies which explicitly examined the risks of important and common conditions such as diabetes mellitus and asthma or other chronic respiratory conditions.

A further potential bias is the effect of GC therapy and the impact of this on the risks of comorbidities. As GC is the only widely accepted treatment for PMR, we could not exclude studies where patients were treated with GC. To reduce the impact of potential bias from GC treatment, we excluded studies in which direct complications of GC therapy were assessed. However, as discussed previously in relation to vascular risk, GC therapy is inevitable in PMR and therefore we could not completely mitigate this effect.

Conclusion

This review has found the overall standard of evidence regarding the association of comorbidities with PMR to be weak. There may be an increased risk of vascular disease and possibly cancer in patients with PMR. Weaker quality evidence also suggests that patients with PMR have a reduced mortality rate. Currently, there is little evidence around the wider health of patients with PMR either at the time of diagnosis or in the period following.

This lack of firm evidence around which comorbidities exist alongside or are potentially associated with PMR presents a problem for the pragmatic clinician. Current clinical guidelines suggest that in order to diagnose PMR, a large number of other conditions which may mimic the symptoms of PMR should be excluded. This list includes, but is not limited to, rheumatoid arthritis and endocrine, infective and neoplastic conditions [14]. However, comorbidities are very common in the age group affected by PMR [76], and therefore the coexistence of one of these comorbidities with PMR should not necessarily prevent or invalidate the diagnosis of PMR.

The uncertainty around the general health of patients with PMR and comorbidities that may coexist with it presents a challenge for healthcare practitioners who deal most with this condition, be they from primary or secondary care. A rigorous diagnostic and follow-up process is crucial to ensure this uncertainty does not translate into misdiagnosis. In the future, it is important to confirm whether, and if so to what extent, a diagnosis of PMR imparts an excess risk of vascular disease or cancer.

Further research in the form of large observational studies, based in primary care, of the health of patients with PMR, including the prevalence of comorbidities before and after diagnosis, would allow clinicians to better monitor for these outcomes.

Abbreviations

CRP: C-reactive protein; CVD: Cardiovascular disease; ESR: Erythrocyte sedimentation rate; GC: Glucocorticoid; GCA: Giant cell arteritis;

PMR: Polymyalgia rheumatica; RA: Rheumatoid arthritis; RCT: Randomised control trial

Acknowledgements
Thanks to Opeyemi Babatunde (Research Associate: Systematic Reviews, Keele University) and Jo Jordan (Research Information Manager, Keele University) for assistance with the protocol and search strategy.

Funding
RP is funded by NHS Research and Infrastructure funds. CM is funded by the NIHR Collaborations for Leadership in Applied Health Research and Care West Midlands, the NIHR School for Primary Care Research and an NIHR Research Professorship in General Practice, which also supports AAS (NIHR-RP-2014-04-026). TH is funded by an NIHR Clinical Lectureship in General Practice. The views expressed are those of the authors and not necessarily those of the NHS, the NIHR or the Department of Health and Social Care. The funder was not involved in the study design; in the collection, analysis and interpretation of data; in the writing of the report; or in the decision to submit the article for publication.

Authors' contributions
RP, TH, SM, CM and AAS contributed to study design. RP performed the literature search, RP and TH the title, abstract and full text review. RP produced the first draft of the manuscript and the tables. SM, TH, CM and AS performed critical revision of the manuscript drafts. All authors read and approved the final manuscript.

Competing interests
The authors declare that they have no competing interests.

References

1. Michet CJ, Matteson EL. Polymyalgia rheumatica. Br Med J. 2008;336:765–9. https://doi.org/10.1016/S0140-6736(97)05001-0.
2. Salvarani C, Cantini F, Hunder GG. Polymyalgia rheumatica and giant-cell arteritis. Lancet. 2008;372(9634):234–45. https://doi.org/10.1016/S0140-6736(08)61077-6.
3. Chuang TY, Hunder GG, Ilstrup DM, Kurland LT. Polymyalgia rheumatica: a 10-year epidemiologic and clinical study. Ann Intern Med. 1982;97(5):672–80.
4. Salvarani C, Macchioni PL, Tartoni PL, et al. Polymyalgia rheumatica and giant cell arteritis: a 5-year epidemiologic and clinical study in Reggio Emilia, Italy. Clin Exp Rheumatol. 1987;5(3):205–15.
5. Dasgupta B, Borg FA, Hassan N, et al. BSR and BHPR guidelines for the management of polymyalgia rheumatica. Rheumatology. 2010;49(1):186–90. https://doi.org/10.1093/rheumatology/kep303a.
6. Clarson L, Chandratre P, Hider S, et al. Increased cardiovascular mortality associated with gout: a systematic review and meta-analysis. Eur J Prev Cardiol. 2013;22(3):335–43. https://doi.org/10.1177/2047487313514895.
7. Avina-Zubieta JA, Thomas J, Sadatsafavi M, Lehman AJ, Lacaille D. Risk of incident cardiovascular events in patients with rheumatoid arthritis: a meta-analysis of observational studies. Ann Rheum Dis. 2012;71(9):1524–9. https://doi.org/10.1136/annrheumdis-2011-200726.
8. Pamuk ÖN, Ünlü E, Çakir N. Role of insulin resistance in increased frequency of atherosclerosis detected by carotid ultrasonography in rheumatoid arthritis. J Rheumatol. 2006;33(12):2447–52.
9. Jonsson SW, Backman C, Johnson O, et al. Increased prevalence of atherosclerosis in patients with medium term rheumatoid arthritis. J Rheumatol. 2001;28(12):2597 602 pmid: 11764203.
10. Kumeda Y, Inaba M, Goto H, et al. Increased thickness of the arterial intima-media detected by ultrasonography in patients with rheumatoid arthritis. Arthritis Rheum. 2002;46(6):1489–97. https://doi.org/10.1002/art.10269.
11. Dessein PH, Norton GR, Woodiwiss AJ, Joffe BI, Wolfe F. Influence of nonclassical cardiovascular-risk factors on the accuracy of predicting subclinical atherosclerosis in rheumatoid arthritis. J Rheumatol. 2007;34(5):943–51.
12. Brown K. Rheumatoid lung disease. Proc Am Thorac Soc. 2007;4:443–8. https://doi.org/10.1513/pats.200703-045MS.
13. Chen Y-J, Chang Y-T, Wang C-B, Wu C-Y. The risk of cancer in patients with rheumatoid arthritis: A nationwide cohort study in Taiwan. Arthritis Rheum. 2011;63(2):352–8. https://doi.org/10.1002/art.30134.
14. Dejaco C, Singh YP, Perel P, et al. 2015 Recommendations for the management of polymyalgia rheumatica: a European League Against Rheumatism/American College of Rheumatology collaborative initiative. Ann Rheum Dis. 2015;74:1799–807. https://doi.org/10.1136/annrheumdis-2015-207492.
15. Barnett K, Mercer SW, Norbury M, Watt G, Wyke S, Guthrie B. Epidemiology of multimorbidity and implications for health care, research, and medical education: a cross-sectional study. Lancet. 2012;380(9836):37–43. https://doi.org/10.1016/S0140-6736(12)60240-2.
16. Salvarani C, Cantini F, Boiardi L, Hunder GG. Polymyalgia rheumatica and giant-cell arteritis. N Engl J Med. 2002;347(4):261–71.
17. Weyand CM, Goronzy J. Giant-cell arteritis and polymyalgia rheumatica. Ann Intern Med. 2003;139:505–16.
18. Moher D, Liberati A, Tetzlaff J, Altman DG, Grp P. Preferred Reporting Items for Systematic Reviews and Meta-Analyses: the PRISMA statement (reprinted from Annals of Internal Medicine). PLoS ONE. 2009;6(7):1-6. https://doi.org/10.1371/journal.pmed.1000097.
19. Byrt T, Bishop J, Carlin JB. Bias, prevalence and kappa. J Clin Epidemiol. 1993;46(5):423–9. https://doi.org/10.1016/0895-4356(93)90018-V.
20. Dasgupta B, Cimmino MA, Kremers HM, et al. 2012 Provisional classification criteria for polymyalgia rheumatica: a European League Against Rheumatism/American College of Rheumatology collaborative initiative. Arthritis Rheum. 2012;64(4):943–54. https://doi.org/10.1002/art.34356.
21. Behn AR, Perera T, Myles AB. Polymyalgia rheumatica and corticosteroids: how much for how long? Ann Rheum Dis. 1983;42(4):374–8. https://doi.org/10.1136/ard.42.4.374.
22. Gabriel SE, Sunku J, Salvarani C, O'Fallon WM, Hunder GG. Adverse outcomes of antiinflammatory therapy among patients with polymyalgia rheumatica. Arthritis Rheum. 1997;40(10):1873–8. https://doi.org/10.1002/art.1780401022.
23. Mazzantini M, Torre C, Miccoli M, et al. Adverse events during longterm low-dose glucocorticoid treatment of polymyalgia rheumatica: a retrospective study. J Rheumatol. 2012;39(3):552–7. https://doi.org/10.3899/jrheum.110851.
24. Proven A, Gabriel SE, Orces C, O'Fallon WM, Hunder GG. Glucocorticoid therapy in giant cell arteritis: duration and adverse outcomes. Arthritis Rheum. 2003;49(5):703–8. https://doi.org/10.1002/art.11388.
25. Paskins Z, Whittle R, Sultan AA, et al. Risk of fracture among patients with polymyalgia rheumatica and giant cell arteritis: a population-based study. BMC Med. 2018;16(4):1–9. https://doi.org/10.1186/s12916-017-0987-1.
26. Shbeeb I, Challah D, Raheel S, Crowson CS, Matteson EL. Comparable rates of glucocorticoid associated adverse events in patients with polymyalgia rheumatica and comorbidities in the general population. Arthritis Care Res. 2018;70(4):643–7. https://doi.org/10.1002/acr.23320.
27. Albrecht K, Huscher D, Buttgereit F, et al. Long-term glucocorticoid treatment in patients with polymyalgia rheumatica, giant cell arteritis, or both diseases: results from a national rheumatology database. Rheumatol Int. 2018;38(4):569–77. https://doi.org/10.1007/s00296-017-3874-3.
28. Wells G, Shea B, O'Connell D, Peterson J, Welch V, Losos M. The Newcastle-Ottawa Scale (NOS) for assessing the quality if nonrandomized studies in meta-analyses. Available from: http://www.ohri.ca/programs/clinical_epidemiology/oxford.htm. Accessed 1 Nov 2016.
29. Higgins JPT, Green S. Cochrane Handbook for Systematic Reviews of Interventions. Version 5.1.0 [updated March 2011]. The Cochrane Collaboration; 2011. Available from http://handbook.cochrane.org.

30. Bengtsson BA, Malmvall BE. The epidemiology of giant cell arteritis including temporal arteritis and polymyalgia rheumatica. Incidences of different clinical presentations and eye complications. Arthritis Rheum. 1981; 24(7):899–904.

31. Bowness P, Shotliff K, Middlemiss A, Myles AB. Prevalence of hypothyroidism in patients with polymyalgia rheumatica and giant cell arteritis. Br J Rheumatol. 1991;30(5):349–51.

32. Haga H, Eide G, Brun J, Johansen A, Langmark F. Cancer in association with polymyalgia rheumatica and temporal arteritis. J Rheumatol. 1993;20(8): 1335–9.

33. Juchet H, Labarthe M, Ollier S, Vilain C, Arlet P. Prevalence of hypothyroidism and hyperthyroidism in patients with giant cell arteritis or polymyalgia rheumatica: a controlled study in one hundred and four cases. Rev du Rhum English Ed. 1993;60(7–8):406–11.

34. Schaufelberger C, Bengtsson BA, Andersson R. Epidemiology and mortality in 220 patients with polymyalgia rheumatica. Br J Rheumatol. 1995;34(3): 261–4. https://doi.org/10.1093/rheumatology/34.3.261.

35. Gran JT, Myklebust G, Wilsgaard T, Jacobsen BK. Survival in polymyalgia rheumatica and temporal arteritis: a study of 398 cases and matched population controls. Rheumatology. 2001;40(11):1238–42 http://www.ncbi. nlm.nih.gov/pubmed/11709607.

36. Uddhammar A, Eriksson A-L, Nyström L, et al. Increased mortality due to cardiovascular disease in patients with giant cell arteritis in northern Sweden. J Rheumatol. 2002;29(4):737–42.

37. Myklebust G, Wilsgaard T, Jacobsen BK, Gran TJ. No increased frequency of malignant neoplasms in polymyalgia rheumatica and temporal arteritis. A prospective longitudinal study of 398 cases and matched population controls. J Rheumatol. 2002;29(10):2143–7.

38. Doran MF, Crowson CS, O'Fallon WM, Hunder GG, Gabriel SE. Trends in the incidence of polymyalgia rheumatica over a 30 year period in Olmsted County, Minnesota, USA. J Rheumatol. 2002;29(8):1694–7.

39. Myklebust G, Wilsgaard T, Jacobsen BK, Gran JT. Causes of death in polymyalgia rheumatica. A prospective longitudinal study of 315 cases and matched population controls. Scand J Rheumatol. 2003;32(1):38–41. https:// doi.org/10.1080/03009740310000382.

40. Kremers HM, Reinalda MS, Crowson CS, Zinsmeister AR, Hunder GG, Gabriel SE. Direct medical costs of polymyalgia rheumatica. Arthritis Rheum. 2005; 53(4):578–84. https://doi.org/10.1002/art.21311.

41. Eaton WW, Rose NR, Kalaydjian A, Pedersen MG, Mortensen PB. Epidemiology of autoimmune diseases in Denmark. J Autoimmun. 2007; 29(1):1–9.

42. Kremers HMH, Reinalda MMS, Crowson CCS, Davis JMJ, Hunder GGG, Gabriel SES. Glucocorticoids and cardiovascular and cerebrovascular events in polymyalgia rheumatica. Arthritis Care Res. 2007;57(2):279–86. https://doi. org/10.1002/art.22548.

43. Warrington KJ, Jarpa EP, Crowson CS, et al. Increased risk of peripheral arterial disease in polymyalgia rheumatica: a population-based cohort study. Arthritis Res Ther. 2009;11(2):R50. https://doi.org/10.1186/ar2664.

44. Eaton WW, Byrne M, Ewald H, et al. Association of schizophrenia and autoimmune diseases: linkage of Danish national registers. Am J Psychiatry. 2006;163(3):521–8. https://doi.org/10.1176/appi.ajp.163.3.521.

45. Ji J, Liu X, Sundquist K, Sundquist J, Hemminki K. Cancer risk in patients hospitalized with polymyalgia rheumatica and giant cell arteritis: a follow-up study in Sweden. Rheumatology. 2010;49(6):1158–63.

46. Kang J-H, Sheu J-J, Lin H-C. Polymyalgia rheumatica and the risk of stroke: a three-year follow-up study. Cerebrovasc Dis. 2011;32(5):497–503. https://doi. org/10.1159/000332031.

47. Hemminki K, Liu X, Ji J, Sundquist J, Sundquist K. Autoimmune disease and subsequent digestive tract cancer by histology. Ann Oncol. 2012;23(4):927–33. https://doi.org/10.1093/annonc/mdr333.

48. Zoller B, Li X, Sundquist J, Sundquist K. Risk of subsequent ischemic and hemorrhagic stroke in patients hospitalized for immune-mediated diseases: a nationwide follow-up study from Sweden. BMC Neurol. 2012;12:41. https://doi.org/10.1186/1471-2377-12-41.

49. Li X, Sundquist J, Sundquist K. Subsequent risks of Parkinson disease in patients with autoimmune and related disorders: a nationwide epidemiological study from Sweden. Neurodegener Dis. 2012;10(1–4):277–84. https://doi.org/10.1159/000333222.

50. Hemminki K, Liu X, Ji J, Sundquist J, Sundquist K. Effect of autoimmune diseases on mortality and survival in subsequent digestive tract cancers. Ann Oncol. 2012;23(8):2179–84. https://doi.org/10.1093/annonc/mdr590.

51. Hemminki K, Liu X, Ji J, Forsti A, Sundquist J, Sundquist K. Effect of autoimmune diseases on risk and survival in female cancers. Gynecol Oncol. 2012;127(1):180–5. https://doi.org/10.1016/j.ygyno.2012.07.100.

52. Zöller B, Li X, Sundquist J, Sundquist K. Risk of subsequent coronary heart disease in patients hospitalized for immune-mediated diseases: a nationwide follow-up study from Sweden. PLoS One. 2012;7(3):1–8. https:// doi.org/10.1371/journal.pone.0033442.

53. Hemminki K, Li X, Sundquist J, Sundquist K. Risk of asthma and autoimmune diseases and related conditions in patients hospitalized for obesity. Ann Med. 2012;44(3):289–95.

54. Hemminki K, Liu X, Forsti A, Ji J, Sundquist J, Sundquist K. Effect of autoimmune diseases on incidence and survival in subsequent multiple myeloma. J Hematol Oncol. 2012;5:59.

55. Fallah M, Liu X, Ji J, Forsti A, Sundquist K, Hemminki K. Hodgkin lymphoma after autoimmune diseases by age at diagnosis and histological subtype. Ann Oncol. 2014;25(7):1397–404. https://doi.org/10.1093/annonc/mdu144.

56. Fallah M, Liu X, Ji J, Forsti A, Sundquist K, Hemminki K. Autoimmune diseases associated with non-Hodgkin lymphoma: a nationwide cohort study. Ann Oncol. 2014;25:2025–30. https://doi.org/10.1093/annonc/mdu365.

57. Muller S, Hider SLS, Belcher J, Helliwell T, Mallen CD. Is cancer associated with polymyalgia rheumatica? A cohort study in the General Practice Research Database. Ann Rheum Dis. 2014;73:1769–73. https://doi.org/10. 1136/annrheumdis-2013-203465.

58. Hancock AT, Mallen CD, Muller S, et al. Risk of vascular events in patients with polymyalgia rheumatica. Can Med Assoc J. 2014;186(13):495–501.

59. Pfeifer EC, Crowson CS, Major BT, Matteson EL. Polymyalgia Rheumatica and its Association with Cancer. Rheumatology (Sunnyvale). 2015;(Suppl 6):003. https://doi.org/10.4172/2161-1149.S6-003.Polymyalgia.

60. Pujades-Rodriguez M, Duyx B, Thomas SL, Stogiannis D, Smeeth L, Hemingway H. Associations between polymyalgia rheumatica and giant cell arteritis and 12 cardiovascular diseases. Heart. 2016;102(5):383–9.

61. Bellan M, Boggio E, Sola D, et al. Association between rheumatic diseases and cancer: results from a clinical practice cohort study. Intern Emerg Med. 2017;12(5):621-7. https://doi.org/10.1007/s11739-017-1626-8.

62. Askling J, Klareskog L, Hjalgrim H, Baecklund E, Bjorkholm M, Ekbom A. Do steroids increase lymphoma risk? A case-control study of lymphoma risk in polymyalgia rheumatica/giant cell arteritis. Ann Rheum Dis. 2005;64(12): 1765–8.

63. Anderson LA, Pfeiffer RM, Landgren O, Gadalla S, Berndt SI, Engels EA. Risks of myeloid malignancies in patients with autoimmune conditions. Br J Cancer. 2009;100(5):822–8.

64. Anderson LA, Gadalla S, Morton LM, et al. Population-based study of autoimmune conditions and the risk of specific lymphoid malignancies. Int J Cancer. 2009;125(2):398–405.

65. Lanoy E, Engels EA. Skin cancers associated with autoimmune conditions among elderly adults. Br J Cancer. 2010;103(1):112–4.

66. Kristinsson SY, Landgren O, Samuelsson J, Bjorkholm M, Goldin LR. Autoimmunity and the risk of myeloproliferative neoplasms. Haematologica. 2010;95(7):1216–20. https://doi.org/10.3324/haematol.2009.020412.

67. Anderson LA, Engels EA. Autoimmune conditions and hairy cell leukemia: an exploratory case-control study. J Hematol Oncol. 2010;3:35.

68. Lindqvist EK, Goldin LR, Landgren O, et al. Personal and family history of immune-related conditions increase the risk of plasma cell disorders: a population-based study. Blood. 2011;118(24):6284–91.

69. Chen SJ, Chao YL, Chen CY, et al. Prevalence of autoimmune diseases in in-patients with schizophrenia: nationwide population-based study. Br J Psychiatry. 2012;200:374–80. https://doi.org/10.1192/bjp.bp.111.092098.

70. Scrivo R, Gerardi MC, Rutigliano I, et al. Polymyalgia rheumatica and diverticular disease: just two distinct age-related disorders or more? Results from a case-control study. Clin Rheumatol. 2018;37(9):2573-7. https://doi. org/10.1007/s10067-018-4137-8.

71. Yates M, Graham K, Watts R, MacGregor A. The prevalence of giant cell arteritis and polymyalgia rheumatica in a UK primary care population. BMC Musculoskelet Disord. 2016;17:285.

72. Barraclough K, Liddell WG, du Toit J, et al. Polymyalgia rheumatica in primary care: a cohort study of the diagnostic criteria and outcome. Fam Pract. 2008;25(5):328–33.

73. Hellgren K, Baecklund E, Backlin C, Sundstrom C, Smedby KE, Askling J. Rheumatoid Arthritis and risk of malignant lymphoma: is the risk still increased? Arthritis Rheumatol. 2017;69(4):700–8. https://doi.org/10.1002/art. 40017.

74. Floris A, Piga M, Cauli A, Salvarani C, Mathieu A. Polymyalgia rheumatica: zn autoinflammatory disorder? RMD Open. 2018;4(1):2–6. https://doi.org/10.1136/rmdopen-2018-000694.

75. Haut ER, Pronovost PJ. Surveillance bias in outcomes reporting. JAMA. 2011;305(23):2462–3. https://doi.org/10.1001/jama.2011.822.

76. Piccirillo JF, Vlahiotis A, Barrett LB, Flood KL, Spitznagel EL, Steyerberg EW. The changing prevalence of comorbidity across the age spectrum. Crit Rev Oncol Hematol. 2008;67(2):124–32. https://doi.org/10.1016/j.critrevonc.2008.01.013.

24

Risk of chronic kidney disease in patients with gout and the impact of urate lowering therapy: a population-based cohort study

Matthew Roughley[1]* ⓘ, Alyshah Abdul Sultan[2], Lorna Clarson[2], Sara Muller[2], Rebecca Whittle[2], John Belcher[3], Christian D. Mallen[2] and Edward Roddy[2,4]

Abstract

Background: An association between gout and renal disease is well-recognised but few studies have examined whether gout is a risk factor for subsequent chronic kidney disease (CKD). Additionally, the impact of urate-lowering therapy (ULT) on development of CKD in gout is unclear. The objective of this study was to quantify the risk of CKD stage ≥ 3 in people with gout and the impact of ULT.

Methods: This was a retrospective cohort study using data from the Clinical Practice Research Datalink (CPRD). Patients with incident gout were identified from general practice medical records between 1998 and 2016 and randomly matched 1:1 to patients without a diagnosis of gout based on age, gender, available follow-up time and practice. Primary outcome was development of CKD stage ≥ 3 based on estimated glomerular filtration rate (eGFR) or recorded diagnosis. Absolute rates (ARs) and adjusted hazard ratios (HRs) were calculated using Cox regression models. Risk of developing CKD was assessed among those prescribed ULT within 1 and 3 years of gout diagnosis.

Results: Patients with incident gout (n = 41,446) were matched to patients without gout. Development of CKD stage ≥ 3 was greater in the exposed group than in the unexposed group (AR 28.6 versus 15.8 per 10,000 person-years). Gout was associated with an increased risk of incident CKD (adjusted HR 1.78 95% CI 1.70 to 1.85). Those exposed to ULT had a greater risk of incident CKD, but following adjustment this was attenuated to non-significance in all analyses (except on 3-year analysis of women (adjusted HR 1.31 95% CI 1.09 to 1.59)).

Conclusions: This study has demonstrated gout to be a risk factor for incident CKD stage ≥ 3. Further research examining the mechanisms by which gout may increase risk of CKD and whether optimal use of ULT can reduce the risk or progression of CKD in gout is suggested.

Keywords: Gout, Chronic kidney disease, Urate-lowering therapy, Cohort

Background

Gout is the most prevalent inflammatory arthritis, affecting 2.5% of adults in the UK and 3.9% in the USA [1, 2]. Chronic kidney disease (CKD) is also a common problem, with the global prevalence of CKD stages 3–5 (estimated glomerular filtration rate (eGFR) < 60 mL/min/1.73m^2) estimated to be 10.6% [3]. An association between gout and CKD has been recognised for many years [4–6].

CKD can progress to end-stage renal disease (ESRD) and can lead to premature mortality [7]. The rate of progression to renal replacement therapy (RRT) or death over 5 years in patients with CKD stage 3 is 1.3% and 24.3%, respectively, and with stage 4 it is 19.9% and 45.7%, respectively [8]. In our recent systematic review and meta-analysis, 24% of people with gout had CKD stage ≥ 3 [9]. The association between hyperuricaemia, gout and CKD is thought to be bidirectional, with CKD known to be an independent risk factor for gout [10–13] and gout potentially predisposing to CKD by a number of mechanisms including hyperuricaemia, chronic inflammation and drug therapy with non-steroidal anti-inflammatory

* Correspondence: mattjroughley@gmail.com
[1]East London NHS Foundation Trust, Trust Headquarters, 9 Alie Street, London E1 8DE, UK
Full list of author information is available at the end of the article

drugs (NSAIDs). In addition, hypertension, diabetes mellitus and obesity are highly prevalent in gout [14] and CKD, and are risk factors for CKD [15]. Our systematic review identified only two cohort studies investigating the risk of CKD in people with gout. Although large, both examined risk of ESRD rather than the earlier stages of CKD and neither used data from Europe [16, 17]. Better understanding of the risk of earlier stages of CKD in people with gout would help guide screening and the management of associated comorbidities and could aid the early identification or possible prevention of CKD in gout.

Urate-lowering therapy (ULT) should be considered for all patents with gout, in particular those with recurrent flares or tophi [18–20]. Data from randomised trials suggests that ULT in patients with CKD can slow the rate of decline of eGFR and reduce risk of progression to ESRD [21]. However, these trials were largely conducted in individuals without gout and the impact of ULT on development of CKD in people with gout remains unclear. The aim of this study was to quantify the risk of developing CKD stage ≥ 3 among patients with incident gout and assess the impact of ULT on this risk.

Methods

Data source and study population

This retrospective cohort study utilised data from the Clinical Practice Research Datalink (CPRD). The CPRD is a large database containing anonymised UK primary care medical records [22]. Approximately 98% of the population of England and Wales is registered with a general practitioner (GP), who is responsible for the majority of a patient's medical care [23]. The CPRD covers more than 7% of the UK population and is representative of the general UK population in terms of age and gender distribution [23]. More than 58% of CPRD practices are linked to hospital episode statistics (HES). HES holds data items including admissions, diagnoses and operative procedures for all patients treated in hospitals in England [24]. The linkage is performed by a trusted third party based on National Health Service number, date of birth and gender. As HES only covers England; practices from Scotland, Wales and Northern Ireland were excluded from this analysis.

In this cohort study the exposed group consisted of individuals with a first-ever recorded diagnosis of gout and these were identified from general practice between 1998 and 2016 using previously published methods [25]. Ascertainment of gout was based on a medical (Read) code assigned by the GP. Gout diagnoses have been validated in the CPRD and have a positive predictive value of 90% [26]. Each patient with gout was assigned an index date corresponding to the date of gout diagnosis and randomly matched to one patient without a gout diagnosis or evidence of ULT, on age (± 5 years), gender, available follow-up time (± 3 years)

and practice. Matching on follow up is a common approach when using the CPRD as patients with chronic illness typically have longer follow up compared to those without, and gout is associated with several comorbidities [25], it is a proxy method of minimising the potential bias this may induce. For both exposed and unexposed patients, follow up commenced from the index date. Those with evidence of CKD stage ≥ 3 or RRT before the index date or < 1 year after the index date were excluded from the study.

The primary outcome was developing CKD stage ≥ 3 and was based on two consecutive measurements of eGFR< 60 mL/min/1.73m^2 at least 3 months apart. eGFR was calculated using serum creatinine values recorded in patients' medical records using the Chronic Kidney Disease Epidemiology Collaboration equation [27]. For those considered to have CKD stage ≥ 3, the date of the first eGFR measurement was taken as the first occurrence of CKD. We also identified patients with CKD stage ≥ 3 or more based on a recorded diagnosis of CKD stages 3–5, ESRD or having evidence of renal replacement therapy (RRT (kidney transplant or dialysis)) in their primary or secondary care medical record.

Covariates

To assess the independent association between gout and CKD stage ≥ 3, information on various baseline characteristics was extracted. These included body mass index (BMI), smoking status, index of multiple deprivation (IMD), and specific comorbidities. The comorbidities included were; myocardial infarction, systemic lupus erythematosus (SLE), rheumatoid arthritis, congestive heart failure, cerebrovascular disease, peripheral vascular disease, hospitalisations and treated hypertension or diabetes mellitus before the index date. Information was extracted on NSAID use (two or more prescriptions) in the 6 months before gout diagnosis. In addition, baseline serum uric acid (SUA) level was adjusted for in the analyses examining risk of CKD associated with ULT prescription. Finally, for each subject we calculated the visit rate on unique calendar dates with a medical diagnosis code over the observation time to estimate how often they visited their general practitioner. The visit rate was then categorised into tertiles.

Landmark analysis is routinely used to assess the impact of treatment where there is a potential lag between disease occurrence and initiation of therapy [28]. As the timing of initiation of ULT varies after gout diagnosis, we utilised landmark analysis to examine the effect of ULT on the risk of CKD. Landmark analysis deals with the issue of immortal time bias, which biases the results in favour of the treatment under study by granting a spurious survival advantage to the treated group [28]. In the case of gout, patients receiving ULT must have at least survived from time of diagnosis to time of treatment whereas no such requirement is necessary for the unexposed group (individuals with gout not receiving ULT). Bias would be introduced by ignoring this, as ULT exposure status may be dependent on the length of follow up. In landmark analysis, a fixed time after the initiation of therapy is selected a priori for conducting survival analysis [29]. Only those alive, event-free and contributing data at the landmark time were included in the analysis. Exposure to ULT was evaluated between the index date (diagnosis of gout) and the landmark time, whereas development of CKD stage ≥ 3 was only considered after the landmark time point. Two landmark points were considered in the analysis (1 and 3 years after diagnosis) based on a previously published study [30]. Only patients initiated on and prescribed more than 6 months of ULT were considered to be exposed (Fig. 1). This was based on previous literature [30] and expert consensus, as allopurinol is started at a low dose and increased gradually and it can take several months to escalate the dose sufficiently to lower serum urate to below the biochemical target level. The duration of ULT was calculated based on quantity prescribed and numeric daily dose.

Statistical analysis

Absolute rates (ARs) of CKD stage ≥ 3 per 10,000 person-years and 95% confidence intervals (CI) were calculated for the exposed and unexposed groups. These were stratified by age, gender, IMD and time after diagnosis. Hazard ratios (HRs) were modelled using Cox proportional hazards regression adjusting for the stated confounding factors. Those with missing body mass index (BMI) status were categorised separately and included in the analysis, as BMI was assumed not to be missing at random. Similarly, we compared the risk of CKD stage ≥ 3 among those prescribed ULT within 1 and 3 years after diagnosis to patients with gout who were not prescribed ULT. The HRs were additionally adjusted for baseline serum creatinine and uric acid levels. Baseline serum creatinine and uric acid level was considered before the ULT exposure or landmark date for those not prescribed ULT. For those with missing laboratory values, an indicator

variable was included in the regression analysis. All missing values were imputed using a constant to ensure that all data were included in the analysis. This study was approved by the CPRD in-house Independent Scientific Advisory Committee (ISAC) reference number 15_214RA.

Sample size calculations: based on previous literature, we anticipated at least 30,000 cases of incident gout in HES-linked CPRD matched to a similar number of unexposed individuals [31]. Given the annual incidence of stage 3 CKD is 15% (aged 65–74 years) in the UK, our sample size provided more than 99% power to detect a HR of 1.5 using Cox proportional hazards model at 5% level of significance. For the landmark analysis, assuming that 10% of patients with gout are treated with ULT within the first year, we had approximately 82% power to detect a HR of 1.35 between ULT users and non-users, using a Cox proportional hazards model at 5% level of significance.

Results

Patients with incident gout (n = 41,446) were identified and matched to 41,446 patients without gout. At baseline, mean participant age was 57 years and 81% were male. The median duration of follow up was 6 years with a total of 484,455 person-years of follow up. At baseline, patients with gout had a higher prevalence of diabetes mellitus, hypertension, vascular disease and obesity. In addition, patients with gout attended their GP more frequently and received more NSAID prescriptions than patients without gout (Table 1).

During follow up, 6694 patients (16.2%) with gout developed CKD stage ≥ 3 compared to 3953 (9.5%) patients without gout (absolute rate 28.6 versus 15.8 per 10,000 person-years respectively). A diagnosis of gout was associated with increased risk of development of CKD stage ≥3 compared to patients without gout (unadjusted HR 1.79 95% CI 1.72 to 1.86). Adjustment for age, gender, comorbidities, deprivation, NSAID use, frequency of hospital admission and GP attendance, had a minimal effect and the association remained statistically significant (adjusted HR 1.78 95% CI 1.70 to 1.85) (Table 2).

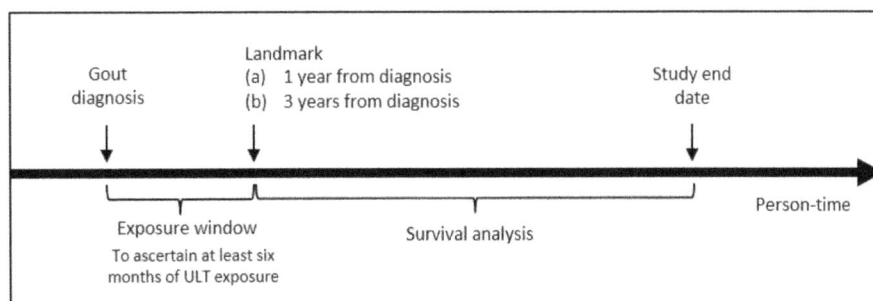

Fig. 1 Graphical illustration of landmark analysis. ULT, urate-lowering therapy

Table 1 Basic characteristics of the study population

Variable	Gout		Non-gout	
	Number	Percentage	Number	Percentage
Total number	41,446		41,446	
Mean age (SD)	57.2	(13.6)	57.1	(13.7)
Median follow up (IQR)	6.0	(3.3, 9.5)	5.9	(3.2, 9.4)
Male	33,574	81.0	33,574	81.0
Body mass index				
Normal	7394	17.8	12,341	29.8
Underweight	349	0.8	681	1.6
Overweight	15,537	37.5	14,760	35.6
Obese	15,311	36.9	8417	20.3
Missing	2855	6.9	5247	12.7
Smoking status				
Never/ex-smoker	36,153	87.2	34,406	83.0
Current smoker	5293	12.8	7040	17.0
Comorbidities				
Diabetes mellitus	2686	6.5	2417	5.8
Treated hypertension	11,982	28.9	6648	16.0
Rheumatoid arthritis	276	0.7	302	0.7
SLE	25	0.1	24	0.1
Heart failure	1342	3.2	482	1.2
Myocardial infarction	1660	4.0	1166	2.8
Cerebrovascular disease	1537	3.7	1241	3.0
Peripheral vascular disease	901	2.2	670	1.6
Anti-diabetic drugs	1847	4.5	1881	4.5
NSAIDs	5852	14.1	1619	3.9
Previous hospitalisations	11,016	26.6	9129	22.0
GP consultation rates (tertiles)				
1	10,375	25.0	17,256	41.6
2	14,609	35.2	13,022	31.4
3	16,462	39.7	11,168	26.9
IMD quintiles				
1 (least deprived)	10,526	25.4	10,485	25.3
2	10,220	24.7	10,232	24.7
3	8411	20.3	8330	20.1
4	7034	17.0	7164	17.3
5 (most deprived)	5216	12.6	5206	12.6

SLE systemic lupus erythematosus, *NSAID* non-steroidal anti-inflammatory drug, *GP* general practitioner, *IMD* Index of multiple deprivation

In the stratified analyses, for both exposed and unexposed patients, the absolute rate of development of CKD stage ≥ 3 was greater in women and increased with age. The adjusted HRs remained largely consistent between genders and across all age groups and IMD quintiles (Table 2). Risk of development of CKD stage ≥ 3 was found to be higher within the first 2 years of gout diagnosis (adjusted HR 2.20 95% CI 2.07 to 2.36) compared to 6–10 years following diagnosis (adjusted HR 1.45 95% CI 1.29 to 1.63). Figure 2 describes the development of CKD stage ≥ 3 in patients with gout and patients without gout during follow up.

In the landmark analysis, patients with gout were excluded due to either death, developing CKD or transfer from general practice within 1 year (n = 1962) or 3 years (n = 12,947) of gout diagnosis. Of the remaining

Table 2 Absolute rate of CKD per 10,000 person-years and hazard ratios

Variable	Gout			Non-gout			Unadjusted		Adjusted*	
	n	Rate[‡]	95% CI	n	Rate[‡]	95% CI	Hazard ratio	95% CI	Hazard ratio	95% CI
Overall	6694	28.6	27.9, 29.3	3953	15.8	15.3, 16.3	1.79	1.72, 1.86	1.78	1.70, 1.85
Male	4608	23.6	22.9, 24.3	2681	13.0	12.5, 13.5	1.80	1.71, 1.89	1.78	1.69, 1.87
Female	2086	53.8	51.5, 56.1	1272	28.7	27.1, 30.3	1.82	1.70, 1.95	1.79	1.66, 1.93
Age at index in years										
< 55 years	690	5.8	5.4, 6.30	279	2.3	2.1, 2.6	2.52	2.19, 2.89	1.78	1.54, 2.07
55–65	1581	24.6	23.4, 25.8	844	12.3	11.5, 13.2	1.99	1.83, 2.16	1.76	1.61, 1.92
65–75	2506	66.2	63.6, 68.8	1498	33.8	32.1, 35.5	1.91	1.79, 2.04	1.87	1.75, 2.00
> 75	1917	141.0	134.8, 147.5	1332	78.1	74.0, 82.4	1.75	1.63, 1.88	1.71	1.59, 1.84
IMD (quintiles)										
1 (least deprived)	1579	25.6	24.3, 26.9	914	13.9	13.0, 14.8	1.81	1.67, 1.97	1.84	1.69, 2.01
2	1689	29.2	27.9, 30.7	1008	16.2	15.2, 17.2	1.78	1.65, 1.92	1.79	1.65, 1.94
3	1439	30.9	29.3, 32.5	831	16.7	15.6, 17.9	1.83	1.68, 1.99	1.77	1.62, 1.94
4	1143	29.4	27.8, 31.2	698	16.6	15.4, 17.8	1.76	1.60, 1.93	1.78	1.61, 1.97
5 (most deprived)	841	29.1	27.2, 31.2	501	16.5	15.1, 18.0	1.76	1.57, 1.96	1.67	1.49, 1.88

CKD chronic kidney disease, *IMD* index of multiple deprivation
*Adjusted for age, gender, body mass index, smoking status, diabetes mellitus, treated hypertension, rheumatoid arthritis, systemic lupus erythematosus, heart failure, IMD, myocardial infraction, cerebrovascular disease, peripheral vascular disease, history of hospitalisation, consultation rates, and non-steroidal anti-inflammatory drug exposure, when not stratified by them, [‡] per 10,000 person-years

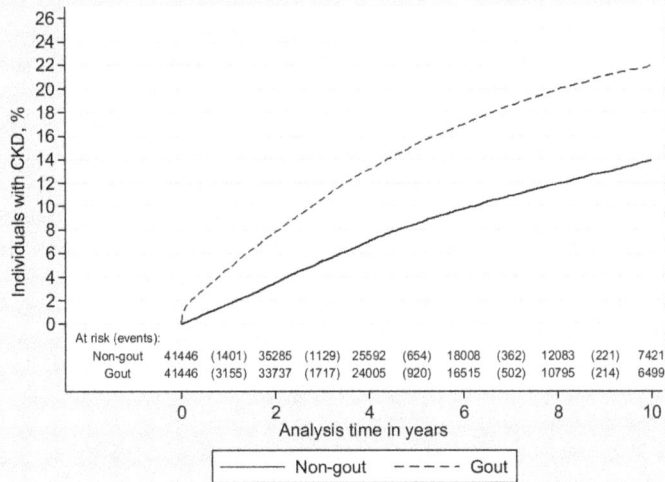

	<2years	3-5 years	6-10 years
Non-gout rate (95%CI)	17.7 (16.8-18.7)	17.2 (16.4-18.0)	11.9 (10.9-12.9)
Gout rate (95%CI)	41.1 (39.7-42.6)	27.0 (26.0-28.1)	16.2 (15.1-17.5)
Adjusted HR* (95%CI)	2.20 (2.07-2.36)	1.58 (1.49-1.69)	1.45 (1.29-1.63)

*Adjusted for age, gender, BMI, smoking status, diabetes mellitus, treated hypertension, rheumatoid arthritis, SLE, heart failure, index of multiple deprivation, myocardial infraction, cerebrovascular disease, peripheral vascular disease, history of hospitalisation, no. of consultations and NSAIDs exposure.
‡per 10,000 person-years

Fig. 2 Development of chronic kidney disease (CKD) stage ≥ 3 in patients with gout and patients without gout (non-gout) during follow up

patients with gout, 4198 (10.6%) in the 1-year landmark analysis and 4793 (16.8%) in the 3-year landmark analysis were receiving ULT (Additional file 1: Figure S1).

Those receiving ULT were older, more frequently hypertensive and diabetic and had higher baseline serum urate levels compared to those unexposed to ULT (Table 3). Those exposed to at least 6 months of ULT within 1 and 3 years of gout diagnosis had a greater risk of development of CKD stage ≥ 3, compared to those not exposed (1-year unadjusted HR 1.47 95% CI 1.35 to 1.59, 3-year unadjusted HR 1.35 95% CI 1.23 to 1.49). This risk however, following

adjustment, was attenuated to non-significance in all analyses apart from the 3-year landmark analysis in women only (adjusted HR 1.31 95% CI 1.09 to 1.59) (Table 4).

Discussion

This retrospective cohort study, set in a large UK primary care population, compared the risk of developing CKD stage ≥ 3 in those with gout versus those without gout. Following adjustment for age, gender, comorbidities, deprivation, NSAID use, frequency of hospital admission and GP attendance, patients with gout had 78% increased

Table 3 Basic characteristics of gout cases by ULT exposure with 1 and 3 years after gout diagnosis

Variable	1-Year landmark				3-Year landmark			
	Exposed n = 4198		Unexposed n = 35,286		Exposed n = 4793		Unexposed n = 23,706	
	N	%	N	%	N	%	N	%
Mean age (SD)	58.2	(12.8)	56.3	(13.5)	56.1	(12.1)	55.1	(12.9)
Male	3485	83.0	28,809	81.6	4151	86.6	19,526	82.4
Body mass index								
Normal	530	12.6	6385	18.1	575	12.0	4335	18.3
Underweight	22	0.5	292	0.8	15	0.3	196	0.8
Overweight	1504	35.8	13,294	37.7	1781	37.2	9036	38.1
Obese	1893	45.1	12,801	36.3	2177	45.4	8581	36.2
Missing	249	5.9	2514	7.1	245	5.1	1558	6.6
Smoking status								
Never/ex-smoker	3808	90.7	30,501	86.4	4355	90.9	20,459	86.3
Current smoker	390	9.3	4785	13.6	438	9.1	3247	13.7
Comorbidities								
Diabetes mellitus	357	8.5	2114	6.0	338	7.1	1259	5.3
Treated hypertension	1539	36.7	9509	26.9	1625	33.9	5856	24.7
Rheumatoid arthritis	40	1.0	213	0.6	39	0.8	122	0.5
Heart failure	200	4.8	900	2.6	166	3.5	372	1.6
Myocardial infraction	219	5.2	1247	3.5	216	4.5	685	2.9
Cerebrovascular disease	176	4.2	1172	3.3	143	3.0	627	2.6
Peripheral vascular disease	118	2.8	663	1.9	85	1.8	351	1.5
Anti-diabetic drugs	233	5.6	1462	4.1	208	4.3	860	3.6
NSAIDs	1082	25.8	4455	12.6	1143	23.8	2887	12.2
Previous hospitalisations	1256	29.9	8964	25.4	1200	25.0	5392	22.7
IMD quintiles								
1	871	20.7	9211	26.1	1089	22.7	6338	26.7
2	1021	24.3	8700	24.7	1178	24.6	5894	24.9
3	889	21.2	7076	20.1	977	20.4	4733	20.0
4	764	18.2	5935	16.8	827	17.3	3915	16.5
5	647	15.4	4332	12.3	717	15.0	2810	11.9
Mean serum urate (SD) µmol/L	478.4	(90.8)	432.2	(98.1)	476.5	(95.7)	427.3	(99.1)
Mean serum creatinine (SD)* µmol/L	89.5	(16.7)	87.2	(16.1)	90.3	(15.2)	86.4	(15.4)

NSAID non-steroidal anti-inflammatory drug, IMD Index of multiple deprivation
*Missing serum creatinine value = 10,335 (1-year landmark), 5872 (3-year landmark), missing serum urate: 15,638 (1-year landmark), 10,176 (3-year landmark)

Table 4 Absolute rate of CKD by ULT exposure

Variable	Exposed			Unexposed			Unadjusted		Adjusted*	
	n	Rate‡	95% CI	n	Rate‡	95% CI	Hazard ratio	95% CI	Hazard ratio	95% CI
1-Year landmark										
Overall	674	34.3	31.8, 37.0	4058	23.3	22.6, 24.0	1.47	1.35, 1.59	1.09	0.99, 1.18
Male	450	26.4	24.1, 28.9	2878	19.8	19.1, 20.5	1.33	1.21, 1.47	1.08	0.98, 1.20
Female	224	86.7	76.1, 98.9	1180	41.0	38.7, 43.4	2.01	1.74, 2.32	1.11	0.96, 1.29
3-Year landmark										
Overall	549	26.1	24.0, 28.4	2027	19.3	18.4, 20.1	1.35	1.23, 1.49	1.03	0.94, 1.14
Male	390	20.7	18.8, 22.9	1538	17.5	16.6, 18.4	1.19	1.06, 1.33	0.96	0.85, 1.07
Female	159	71.1	60.9, 83.1	489	28.3	25.9, 31.0	2.43	2.03, 2.90	1.31	1.09, 1.59

CKD chronic kidney disease, *ULT* urate-lowering therapy
*Adjusted for age, gender, body mass index, smoking status, diabetes mellitus, treated hypertension, rheumatoid arthritis, heart failure, index of multiple deprivation, myocardial infarction, cerebrovascular disease, peripheral vascular disease, history of hospitalisation, non-steroidal anti-inflammatory drug exposure and baseline serum creatine and uric acid, when not stratified by them. ‡ per 10,000 person-years

risk of development of CKD stage ≥ 3 compared to patients without gout. Risk of CKD development was highest in the first 2 years following gout diagnosis. Following adjustment patients with gout exposed to at least 6 months ULT had no increased risk of developing CKD compared to those not exposed, in all analyses apart from analysis in women receiving ULT within 3 years of diagnosis.

This study has a number of strengths. Participants were from primary care where the majority of patients with gout are managed, thus aiding generalisability. The sample size was large and the median follow up was 6 years, which should be sufficient for development and ascertainment of CKD stage ≥ 3. Ascertainment of the primary outcome required either a clinical diagnostic code or two consecutive eGFR measurements < 60 mL/min/1.73m². Utilising biochemical data and Read codes should aid completeness compared to using codes alone, as GP coding of CKD has been shown to capture only 72% of those with biochemically evident disease [32]. Previous cohort studies examining gout and renal disease used either record linkage or diagnostic codes alone and examined either the severest form of CKD (ESRD) [16, 17] or "renal diseases" [25], which would include a large number of heterogenous conditions. This is the first study to the best of our knowledge to examine risk of earlier stages of CKD and to use biochemical data, which is an additional strength. Immortal time bias, which could have resulted in lower observed risk of CKD associated with ULT exposure, was addressed with the use of landmark analysis, which is also a strength of this study.

An important caveat is gout ascertainment based on GP-coded diagnoses alone, risking misclassification bias, although gout diagnoses have been validated in CPRD and have a positive predictive value of 90% [26]. Ascertainment bias is a possible limitation of this study as patients with gout presented more frequently to their GP and hospital and had higher prevalence of hypertension and

diabetes mellitus, which could have prompted more frequent renal function testing. GP consultation rates during follow up were adjusted for in the statistical analysis but may not completely address this issue. Furthermore, it was not possible to account for patient ethnicity or the severity of comorbidities. Regarding ULT prescription data, prescriptions do not necessarily equate to dispensing of ULT and it was not possible assess adherence.

In this study, those with CKD stage ≥ 3 or RRT occurring pre-index or within 1 year of gout diagnosis were excluded. Despite this, the possibility of reverse causation could still potentially underlie an association between gout and CKD e.g. undiagnosed or mild renal dysfunction leading to hyperuricaemia, thus conferring risk of gout development, with later progression to CKD [33]. It is possible that our finding of the risk of CKD development being highest within 2 years of gout diagnosis reflects this. It is also of note that nine genetic loci associated with both CKD and serum urate concentration, with varying direction of effect, have been identified by genome-wide association studies, which could further complicate the relationship between gout and CKD [34].

The prevalence of CKD stage ≥ 3 in gout was found to be 24% in our recent systematic review and meta-analysis [9]. We identified only two other prospective studies examining the risk of CKD associated with gout. These studies reported an increased risk of ESRD of 57% [17] and 80% [16], in keeping with our risk estimate for CKD stage ≥ 3. One study published subsequent to our systematic review found three times increased risk of "renal diseases" (defined using Read codes rather than eGFR) following gout diagnosis but did not differentiate between acute or chronic forms [25]. In our study allopurinol accounted for 99% of all ULT prescriptions. We did not find clear evidence that ULT exposure influenced the risk of developing CKD. Risk was greater in those exposed to ULT, but those exposed were older and more frequently had diabetes mellitus and hypertension and these factors appeared to explain the ULT-CKD association in our data. In previous studies examining the association between ULT and renal disease, benefits were noted to be greatest in those taking higher doses of ULT [35] or reaching target SUA levels [36]. It is of note, however, that patients with gout often remain on lower doses of allopurinol and the majority do not reach target SUA levels [37, 38]. This study has not explored whether target SUA levels were reached and our finding of no association may reflect suboptimal urate-lowering rather than the true effect of ULT.

Women who develop gout are typically older, have more comorbidities such as hypertension, diabetes mellitus and obesity and receive ULT less frequently than men [39]. Possible explanations for our finding of increased risk of CKD associated with ULT in women in the 3-year analysis include women prescribed ULT potentially having more severe gout and therefore possibly conferring greater risk of CKD, incomplete adjustment for comorbidities or medications or ascertainment bias, as comorbid women taking allopurinol may have more frequent renal function testing. It is possible that allopurinol has deleterious effects on renal function in women with gout but to the best of our knowledge this has not been found in previous studies. The finding of increased risk was not replicated in the 1-year analysis, however, suggesting the finding in the 3-year analysis could be related to chance.

Whilst it is not possible to make causal inferences from this observational study, it is worth considering the potentially plausible mechanisms for the association between gout and CKD. Renal damage could result from comorbid hypertension, diabetes mellitus, obesity or use of nonsteroidal anti-inflammatory drugs. Hyperuricaemia-mediated endothelial dysfunction has been suggested to lead to renovascular disease [40], although Mendelian randomisation studies have not found an association between urate and CKD [34]. Inflammation in gout is increasingly recognised to persist in the intercritical period between acute attacks [41, 42], raising the possibility that inflammatory mechanisms contribute to increased risk. Activation of the NLRP3 inflammasome and subsequent production of interleukin-1β is a key inflammatory process in gout [43]. This is of note as renal NLRP3 expression is significantly increased in CKD and it has been suggested that this and interleukin-1β contribute to progression of CKD [44, 45]. We are unable to make comparisons to previous cohort studies, as they have used different outcome measures and, as discussed above, the possibility of reverse causation complicates temporal inferences from this study. As also noted previously, a number of conditions associated with gout are also risk factors for CKD and incomplete adjustment for these could result in residual confounding.

Conclusion

This study has demonstrated gout to be a risk factor for incident CKD stage ≥ 3, after adjustment for age, gender, comorbidities, deprivation, NSAID use, frequency of hospital admission and GP attendance. In clinical practice, renal function monitoring is often suboptimal in gout [36] suggesting an area for improvement. Further research examining the mechanisms by which gout may increase risk of CKD is suggested, including the role of hyperuricaemia and possible linked inflammatory processes. Due to high prevalence of CKD in gout, further research into whether optimal use of ULT can reduce the risk or progression of CKD in patients with gout would also be of value.

Abbreviations

AR: Absolute rate; BMI: Body mass index; CKD: Chronic kidney disease; CPRD: Clinical practice research datalink; eGFR: Estimated glomerular filtration rate; ESRD: End-stage renal disease; GP: General practitioner; HES: Hospital episode statistics; HR: Hazard ratio; IMD: Index of multiple deprivation; ISAC: Independent scientific advisory committee; NSAIDs: Non-steroidal anti-inflammatory drugs; RRT: Renal replacement therapy; SLE: Systemic lupus erythematosus; SUA: Serum uric acid; ULT: Urate-lowering therapy

Acknowledgements

Not applicable.

Funding

MJR received a bursary from the Jean Shanks Foundation to fund his intercalated MPhil. CDM is funded by the National Institute for Health Research (NIHR) Collaborations for Leadership in Applied Health Research and Care West Midlands, the NIHR School for Primary Care Research and a NIHR Research Professorship in General Practice, which also supports AAS and RW (NIHR-RP-2014-04-026). LC is funded by an NIHR Clinical Lectureship in General Practice. The views expressed are those of the author(s) and not necessarily those of the National Health Service (NHS), the NIHR or the Department of Health or Social Care. The funder was not involved in the study design; in the collection, analysis, and interpretation of data; in the writing of the report; and in the decision to submit the article for publication.

Authors' contributions

ER, LC and CDM conceived the study. Analysis was undertaken by AAS, SM and RW. All authors were involved in the design, interpretation of data, and drafting, revising and final approval of the manuscript. ER is guarantor and affirms that the manuscript is an honest, accurate and transparent account of the study being reported, and that no important aspects of the study have been omitted. There are no discrepancies from the study as planned. All authors had full access to all of the data (including statistical reports and tables) in the study and can take responsibility for the integrity of the data and the accuracy of the data analysis.

Competing interests

All authors have completed the Unified Competing Interest form at www.icmje.org/coi_disclosure.pdf (available on request from the corresponding author) and declare that: the authors do not have any support from any company for the submitted work; the authors do not have any relationships with any companies that might have an interest in the submitted work in the previous 3 years; their spouses, partners, or children do not have any financial relationships that may be relevant to the submitted work; and the authors do not have any non-financial interests that may be relevant to the submitted work.

Author details

[1]East London NHS Foundation Trust, Trust Headquarters, 9 Alie Street, London E1 8DE, UK. [2]Research Institute for Primary Care and Health Sciences, Keele University, Keele, Staffordshire ST5 5BG, UK. [3]School of Computing and Mathematics, Keele University, Keele, Staffordshire ST5 5BG, UK. [4]Haywood Academic Rheumatology Centre, Midland Partnership NHS Foundation Trust, Haywood Hospital, Burslem, Staffordshire ST6 7AG, UK.

References

1. Kuo CF, Grainge MJ, Mallen C, Zhang W, Doherty M. Rising burden of gout in the UK but continuing suboptimal management: a nationwide population study. Ann Rheum Dis. 2015;74:661–7.

2. Zhu Y, Pandya BJ, Choi HK. Prevalence of gout and hyperuricemia in the US general population: The National Health and Nutrition Examination Survey 2007-2008. Arthritis Rheum. 2011;63:3136–41.

3. Hill NR, Fatoba ST, Oke JL, Hirst JA, O'Callaghan CA, Lasserson D, et al. Global prevalence of chronic kidney disease - a systematic review and meta-analysis. PLoS One. 2016;11:e0158765.

4. Yu TF, Berger L. Impaired renal function gout: its association with hypertensive vascular disease and intrinsic renal disease. Am J Med. 1982;72:95–100.

5. Berger L, Yu TF. Renal function in gout. IV. An analysis of 524 gouty subjects including long-term follow-up studies. Am J Med. 1975;59:605–13.

6. Fessel WJ. Renal outcomes of gout and hyperuricemia. Am J Med. 1979;67:74–82.

7. Chronic Kidney Disease Prognosis Consortium. Association of estimated glomerular filtration rate and albuminuria with all-cause and cardiovascular mortality in general population cohorts: a collaborative meta-analysis. Lancet. 2010;12:2073–81.

8. Keith DS, Nichols GA, Gullion CM, Brown JB, Smith DH. Longitudinal follow-up and outcomes among a population with chronic kidney disease in a large managed care organization. Arch Intern Med. 2004;164:659–63.

9. Roughley MJ, Belcher J, Mallen CD, Roddy E. Gout and risk of chronic kidney disease and nephrolithiasis: meta-analysis of observational studies. Arthritis Res Ther. 2015;17:1–12.

10. Cea Soriano L, Rothenbacher D, Choi HK, Garcia Rodriguez LA. Contemporary epidemiology of gout in the UK general population. Arthritis Res Ther. 2010;13:R39.

11. Wang W, Bhole VM, Krishnan E. Chronic kidney disease as a risk factor for incident gout among men and women: retrospective cohort study using data from the Framingham Heart Study. BMJ Open. 2015;5:e006843.

12. Krishnan E. Chronic kidney disease and the risk of incident gout among middle-aged men: a seven-year prospective observational study. Arthritis Rheum. 2013;65:3271–8.

13. Choi HK, Atkinson K, Karlson EW, Curhan G. Obesity, weight change, hypertension, diuretic use, and risk of gout in men: The Health Professionals Follow-up Study. Arch Intern Med. 2005;165:742–8.

14. Roddy E, Choi HK. Epidemiology of gout. Rheum Dis Clin N Am. 2014;40:155–75.

15. Kazancioglu R. Risk factors for chronic kidney disease: an update. Kidney Int Suppl. 2013;3:368–71.

16. Hsu C, Iribarren C, McCulloch CE, Darbinian J, Go AS. Risk factors for end-stage renal disease - 25-year follow-up. Arch Intern Med. 2009;169:342–50.

17. Yu KH, Kuo CF, Luo SF, See LC, Chou IJ, Chang HC, et al. Risk of end-stage renal disease associated with gout: a nationwide population study. Arthritis Res Ther. 2012;14:R83.

18. Richette P, Doherty M, Pascual E, Barskova V, Becce F, Castaneda-Sanabria J, et al. 2016 Updated EULAR evidence-based recommendations for the management of gout. Ann Rheum Dis. 2017;76:29–42.

19. Hui M, Carr A, Cameron S, Davenport G, Doherty M, Forrester H, et al. The British Society For Rheumatology guideline for the management of gout. Rheumatology. 2017;56:e1–e20.

20. Khanna D, Fitzgerald JD, Khanna PP, Bae S, Singh MK, Neogi T, et al. 2012 American College of Rheumatology guidelines for management of gout. Part 1: Systematic nonpharmacologic and pharmacologic therapeutic approaches to hyperuricemia. Arthritis Care Res. 2012;64:1431–46.

21. Su X, Xu B, Yan B, Qiao X, Wang L. Effects of uric acid-lowering therapy in patients with chronic kidney disease: a meta-analysis. PLoS One. 2017;12:e0187550.

22. Clinical Practice Research Database. Available at: https://www.cprd.com/. Accessed 25 Oct 2018.

23. Herrett E, Gallagher AM, Bhaskaran K, Forbes H, Mathur R, Staa T, et al. Data resource profile: Clinical Practice Research Datalink (CPRD). Int J Epidemiol. 2015;44:827–36.

24. Royal College of Physicians & UHCE. HES for physicians: a guide to the use of information derived from Hospital Episode Statistics. London: Royal College of Physicians & UHCE; 2007.

25. Kuo CF, Grainge MJ, Mallen C, Zhang W, Doherty M. Comorbidities in patients with gout prior to and following diagnosis: case-control study. Ann Rheum Dis. 2016;75:210–7.

26. Meier CR, Jick H. Omeprazole, other antiulcer drugs and newly diagnosed gout. Br J Clin Pharmacol. 1997;44:175–8.

27. Levey AS, Stevens LA, Schmid CH, Zhang Y, Castro AF III, Feldman HI, et al. A new equation to estimate glomerular filtration rate. Ann Intern Med. 2009;150:604–12.

28. Dafni U. Landmark analysis at the 25-year landmark point. Circ Cardiovasc Qual Outcomes. 2011;4:363–71.

29. Giobbie-Hurder A, Gelber RD, Regan MM. Challenges of guarantee-time bias. J Clin Oncol. 2013;31:2963–9.

30. Kuo CF, Grainge MJ, Mallen C, Zhang W, Doherty M. Effect of allopurinol on all-cause mortality in adults with incident gout: propensity score-matched landmark analysis. Rheumatology. 2015;54:2145–50.

31. Abdul Sultan A, Mallen C, Hayward R, Muller S, Whittle R, Hotston M, et al. Gout and subsequent erectile dysfunction: a population-based cohort study from England. Arthritis Res Ther. 2017;19:123.

32. Jain P, Calvert M, Cockwell P, McManus RJ. The need for improved identification and accurate classification of stages 3-5 chronic kidney disease in primary care: retrospective cohort study. PLoS One. 2014;9:e100831.

33. Bardin T, Richette P. Impact of comorbidities on gout and hyperuricaemia: an update on prevalence and treatment options. BMC Med. 2017;15:123.

34. Johnson RJ, Bakris GL, Borghi C, Chonchol MB, Feldman D, Lanaspa MA, et al. Hyperuricemia, acute and chronic kidney disease, hypertension, and cardiovascular disease: report of a scientific workshop organized by the National Kidney Foundation. Am J Kidney Dis. 2018;71:851–65.

35. Singh JA, Yu S. Are allopurinol dose and duration of use nephroprotective in the elderly? A Medicare claims study of allopurinol use and incident renal failure. Ann Rheum Dis. 2017;76:133–9.

36. Levy GD, Rashid N, Niu F, Cheetham TC. Effect of urate-lowering therapies on renal disease progression in patients with hyperuricemia. J Rheumatol. 2014;41:955–62.

37. Cottrell E, Crabtree V, Edwards JJ, Roddy E. Improvement in the management of gout is vital and overdue: an audit from a UK primary care medical practice. BMC Fam Pract. 2013;14:170.

38. Roddy E, Zhang W, Doherty M. Concordance of the management of chronic gout in a UK primary-care population with the EULAR gout recommendations. Ann Rheum Dis. 2007;66:1311–5.

39. Harrold LR, Etzel CJ, Gibofsky A, Kremer JM, Pillinger MH, Saag KG, et al. Sex differences in gout characteristics: tailoring care for women and men. BMC Musculoskelet Disord. 2017;18:108.

40. Jin M, Yang F, Yang I, Yin Y, Luo JJ, Wang H, et al. Uric acid, hyperuricemia and vascular diseases. Front Biosci. 2012;17:656–69.

41. Pascual E. Persistence of monosodium urate crystals and low-grade inflammation in the synovial fluid of patients with untreated gout. Arthritis Rheum. 1991;34:141–5.

42. Roddy E, Menon A, Hall A, Datta P, Packham J. Polyarticular sonographic assessment of gout: a hospital-based cross-sectional study. Joint Bone Spine. 2013;80:295–300.

43. Kingsbury SR, Conaghan PG, McDermott MF. The role of the NLRP3 inflammasome in gout. J Inflamm Res. 2011;4:39–49.

44. Vianna HR, Soares CM, Tavares MS, Teixeira MM, Silva AC. Inflammation in chronic kidney disease: the role of cytokines. J Bras Nefrol. 2011;33:351–64.

45. Vilaysane A, Chun J, Seamone ME, Wang W, Chin R, Hirota S, et al. The NLRP3 inflammasome promotes renal inflammation and contributes to CKD. J Am Soc Nephrol. 2010;21:1732–44.

Permissions

Contributors

João J. Oliveira and Pamela Clarke
Department of Medical Genetics, JDRF/Wellcome Diabetes and Inflammation Laboratory, NIHR Cambridge Biomedical Research Centre, Cambridge Institute for Medical Research, University of Cambridge, Cambridge, UK

Daniel B. Rainbow, Arcadio Rubio García, Linda S. Wicker, Ricardo C. Ferreira and John A. Todd
Department of Medical Genetics, JDRF/Wellcome Diabetes and Inflammation Laboratory, NIHR Cambridge Biomedical Research Centre, Cambridge Institute for Medical Research, University of Cambridge, Cambridge, UK
JDRF/Wellcome Diabetes and Inflammation Laboratory, Wellcome Centre for Human Genetics, Nuffield Department of Medicine, NIHR Oxford Biomedical Research Centre, University of Oxford, Roosevelt Drive, Oxford, UK

Sarah Karrar, Christopher L. Pinder and Tim J. Vyse
Division of Genetics and Molecular Medicine and Division of Immunology, Infection and Inflammatory Disease, King's College London, Great Maze Pond, London, UK

Osama Al-Assar
3JDRF/Wellcome Diabetes and Inflammation Laboratory, Wellcome Centre for Human Genetics, Nuffield Department of Medicine, NIHR Oxford Biomedical Research Centre, University of Oxford, Roosevelt Drive, Oxford, UK.

Keith Burling
NIHR Cambridge Biomedical Research Centre, Core Biochemical Assay Laboratory, Cambridge, UK

Sian Morris and Richard Stratton
UCL Centre for Rheumatology and Connective Tissue Diseases, UCL Medical School, Royal Free Hospital Campus, Rowland Hill Street, London, UK

Weiyu Han
Clinical Research Centre, Zhujiang Hospital, Southern Medical University, Guangzhou, Guangdong, China

Zhaohua Zhu
Clinical Research Centre, Zhujiang Hospital, Southern Medical University, Guangzhou, Guangdong, China
Menzies Institute for Medical Research, University of Tasmania, Hobart, TAS, Australia

Changhai Ding
Clinical Research Centre, Zhujiang Hospital, Southern Medical University, Guangzhou, Guangdong, China
Menzies Institute for Medical Research, University of Tasmania, Hobart, TAS, Australia
Department of Epidemiology and Preventive Medicine, Monash University, Melbourne, VIC, Australia

Shuang Zheng and Graeme Jones
Menzies Institute for Medical Research, University of Tasmania, Hobart, TAS, Australia

Tania Winzenberg
Menzies Institute for Medical Research, University of Tasmania, Hobart, TAS, Australia
Faculty of Health, University of Tasmania, Hobart, TAS, Australia

Flavia Cicuttini
Department of Epidemiology and Preventive Medicine, Monash University, Melbourne, VIC, Australia

Guo-yi Su, Yu Hou and Shu-dong Chen
The Department of Spinal Surgery, The Second Affiliated Hospital of Guangzhou University of Chinese Medicine, No. 111, Dade Road, Yuexiu District, Guangzhou 510120, China
The Laboratory Affiliated to Orthopaedics and Traumatology of Chinese Medicine of Linnan Medical Research Center of Guangzhou University of Chinese Medicine, No. 12, Jichang Road, Baiyun District, Guangzhou 510405, China
Guangzhou University of Chinese Medicine, No. 12, Jichang Road, Baiyun District, Guangzhou 510405, China

Zhi-feng Xiao, Jian-bo He, Mei-hui Chen and Ding-kun Lin
The Department of Spinal Surgery, The Second Affiliated Hospital of Guangzhou University of Chinese Medicine, No. 111, Dade Road, Yuexiu District, Guangzhou 510120, China

The Laboratory Affiliated to Orthopaedics and Traumatology of Chinese Medicine of Linnan Medical Research Center of Guangzhou University of Chinese Medicine, No. 12, Jichang Road, Baiyun District, Guangzhou 510405, China
Guangzhou University of Chinese Medicine, No. 12, Jichang Road, Baiyun District, Guangzhou 510405, China

Dong-Jin Park and Shin-Seok Lee
Division of Rheumatology, Department of Internal Medicine, Chonnam National University Medical School and Hospital, 42 Jebong-ro, Dong-gu, Gwangju 61469, Republic of Korea

Seong-Ho Kim
Department of Internal Medicine, Inje University Haeundae Paik Hospital, Busan, Korea

Seong-Su Nah
Department of Internal Medicine, Soonchunhyang University, College of Medicine, Cheonan, Korea

Ji Hyun Lee
Department of Internal Medicine, Maryknoll Medical Center, Busan, Korea

Seong-Kyu Kim
Department of Internal Medicine, Catholic University of Daegu, School of Medicine, Daegu, Korea

Yeon-Ah Lee, Seung-Jae Hong
Department of Internal Medicine, School of Medicine, Kyung Hee University, Seoul, Korea

Hyun-Sook Kim
Department of Internal Medicine, Soonchunhyang University Seoul Hospital, Seoul, Korea

Hye-Soon Lee
Hanyang University College of Medicine and the Hospital for Rheumatic Diseases, Seoul, Korea

Hyoun Ah Kim
Department of Allergy and Rheumatology, Ajou University Hospital, Ajou University School of Medicine, Suwon, Korea

Chung-Il Joung
Department of Internal Medicine, Konyang University Medical School, Daejeon, Korea

Sang-Hyon Kim
Departments of Internal Medicine, School of Medicine, Keimyung University, Daegu, Korea

Hyoung Rae Kim, Sung-Hwan Park and Ji Hyeon Ju
Division of Rheumatology, Department of Internal Medicine, College of Medicine, The Catholic University of Korea, Seoul, South Korea

Yeon Sik Hong and Kwi Young Kang
Division of Rheumatology, Department of Internal Medicine, Incheon St. Mary's Hospital, College of Medicine, The Catholic University of Korea, #56,Dongsu-Ro, Bupyung-Gu, Incheon, South Korea

Zeki Soypaçacı
Department of Internal Medicine, Division of Nephrology, Izmir Katip Celebi University School of Medicine, Karabağlar, 35360 İzmir, Turkey

Zeynep Zehra Gümüş
Dogubeyazit Public Hospital, Internal Medicine, Agri, Turkey

Fulya Çakaloğlu
Department of Pathology, Izmir Katip Celebi University, Izmir, Turkey

Mustafa Özmen, Dilek Solmaz, Sercan Gücenmez, Önay Gercik and Servet Akar
Department of Internal Medicine, Division of Rheumatology, Izmir Katip Celebi University, Izmir, Turkey

Yuichi Ishikawa, Shigeru Iwata, Kentaro Hanami, Mingzeng Zhang, Kaoru Yamagata, Yasuyuki Todoroki, Kazuhisa Nakano, Shingo Nakayamada and Yoshiya Tanaka
The First Department of Internal Medicine, School of Medicine, University of Occupational and Environmental Health, Japan, 1-1 Iseigaoka, Yahatanishi-ku, Kitakyushu City 807-8555, Japan

Aya Nawata
The First Department of Internal Medicine, School of Medicine, University of Occupational and Environmental Health, Japan, 1-1 Iseigaoka, Yahatanishi-ku, Kitakyushu City 807-8555, Japan
Department of Pathology and Cell Biology, School of Medicine, University of Occupational and Environmental Health, Japan, Kitakyushu City, Japan

Shintaro Hirata
The First Department of Internal Medicine, School of Medicine, University of Occupational and Environmental Health, Japan, 1-1 Iseigaoka, Yahatanishi-ku, Kitakyushu City 807-8555, Japan
Department of Clinical Immunology and Rheumatology, Hiroshima University Hospital, Hiroshima, Japan

Kei Sakata
The First Department of Internal Medicine, School of Medicine, University of Occupational and Environmental Health, Japan, 1-1 Iseigaoka, Yahatanishi-ku, Kitakyushu City 807-8555, Japan Mitsubishi Tanabe Pharma Corporation, Yokohama, Japan

Minoru Satoh
Department of Clinical Nursing, School of Health Sciences, University of Occupational and Environmental Health, Japan, Kitakyushu City, Japan

Xavier M Teitsma, Johannes W G Jacobs, Jacob M van Laar, Johannes W J Bijlsma and Floris P J G Lafeber
Department of Rheumatology and Clinical Immunology, University Medical Center Utrecht, Heidelberglaan 100, 3584 CX Utrecht, Netherlands

Wei Yang
Leiden Academic Center for Drug Research, Leiden University, 2300 RA Leiden, Netherlands

Amy C Harms and Thomas Hankemeier
Leiden Academic Center for Drug Research, Leiden University, 2300 RA Leiden, Netherlands Netherlands Metabolomic Centre, Einsteinweg 55, 2333 CC Leiden, Netherlands

Attila Pethö-Schramm
F. Hoffmann-La Roche, Grenzacherstrasse 124, 4070 CH Basel, Switzerland

Michelle E A Borm
Roche Nederland BV, Beneluxlaan 2a, 3446 GR Woerden, Netherlands

Yushiro Endo, Tomohiro Koga, Midori Ishida, Yuya Fujita, Sosuke Tsuji, Ayuko Takatani, Toshimasa Shimizu, Remi Sumiyoshi, Takashi Igawa, Masataka Umeda, Shoichi Fukui, Ayako Nishino, Shinya Kawashiri, Naoki Iwamoto, Kunihiro Ichinose, Mami Tamai, Hideki Nakamura, Tomoki Origuchi and Atsushi Kawakami
Department of Immunology and Rheumatology, Unit of Advanced Preventive Medical Sciences, Nagasaki University Graduate School of Biomedical Sciences, 1-7-1 Sakamoto, Nagasaki 852-8501, Japan

Kazunaga Agematsu
Department of Infection and Host Defense, Graduate School of Medicine, Shinshu University, 3-1-1 Asahi, Matsumoto 390-8621, Japan

Akihiro Yachie
Department of Pediatrics, School of Medicine, Kanazawa University, 13-1 Takaramachi, Kanazawa 920-8641, Japan

Junya Masumoto
Proteo-Science Center, Ehime University, 3 Bunkyo-cho, Matsuyama 790-8577, Japan

Kiyoshi Migita
Department of Rheumatology, Fukushima Medical University School of Medicine, 1 Hikarigaoka, Fukushima 960-1295, Japan

Karin Hjorton, Niklas Hagberg, Olof Berggren, Johanna K. Sandling, Maija-Leena Eloranta and Lars Rönnblom
Department of Medical Sciences, Rheumatology, Science for Life Laboratory, Uppsala University, Rudbecklaboratoriet, Dag Hammarskjölds v 20, C11, 751 85 Uppsala, Sweden

Elisabeth Israelsson, Lisa Jinton, Kristofer Thörn and John Mo
Respiratory, Inflammation and Autoimmunity, IMED Biotech Unit, AstraZeneca, Gothenburg, Sweden

Maurizio Cutolo, Stefano Soldano, Paola Montagna, Amelia Chiara Trombetta, Barbara Ruaro, Alberto Sulli, Sabrina Paolino, Carmen Pizzorni and Renata Brizzolara
Research Laboratory and Academic Division of Clinical Rheumatology, Department of Internal Medicine, University of Genoa, IRCCS San Martino Polyclinic Hospital, Viale Benedetto XV, 616132 Genoa, Italy

Paola Contini
Division of Clinical Immunology, Department of Internal Medicine, University of Genoa, Genoa, Italy

Stefano Scabini and Emanuela Stratta
Oncologic Surgery, Department of Surgery, IRCCS San Martino Polyclinic, Genoa, Italy

Vanessa Smith
Department of Rheumatology, Ghent University Hospital, Ghent University, Ghent, Belgium

Philip Helliwell
Leeds Institute of Rheumatic and Musculoskeletal Medicine, University of Leeds, 2nd Floor Chapel Allerton Hospital, Chapeltown Road, Leeds LS7 4SA, UK

Laura C. Coates
Nuffield Department of Orthopaedics Rheumatology and Musculoskeletal Sciences, University of Oxford, Windmill Road, Oxford OX3 7LD, UK

Oliver FitzGerald
Department of Rheumatology, St Vincent's University Hospital, 196 Merrion Road, Elm Park, Dublin D04 T6F4, Ireland

Peter Nash
Department of Medicine, University of Queensland, St Lucia, Brisbane QLD 4072, Australia

Enrique R. Soriano
El Hospital Italiano se encuentra ubicado en Tte. Gral. Juan Domingo Perón 4190, C.A.B.A, Buenos Aires, Argentina

M. Elaine Husni
Cleveland Clinic Lerner Research Institute, N building, 9620 Carnegie Avenue, Cleveland, OH 44106, USA

Ming-Ann Hsu, Keith S. Kanik, Joseph Wu and Elizabeth Kudlacz
Pfizer Inc, 280 Shennecossett Rd, Groton, CT 06340, USA

Thijs Hendrikx
Pfizer Inc, 500 Arcola Rd, Collegeville, PA 19426, USA

Marion Hückel, Mieczyslaw Gajda, Peter K. Petrow and Rolf Bräuer
Institute of Pathology, University Hospital, Jena, Germany

Oliver Frey
Institute of Pathology, University Hospital, Jena, Germany
Institute of Clinical Chemistry and Laboratory Medicine, University Hospital, Am Klinikum 1, D-07743 Jena, Germany
Present address: Institute of Medical Diagnostics, Berlin, Germany

Elena Raschi and Laura Cesana
Experimental Laboratory of Immunological and Rheumatologic Researches, IRCCS Istituto Auxologico Italiano, Via Zucchi 18, 20095 Cusano Milanino, Milan, Italy

Daniela Privitera and Maria Orietta Borghi
Experimental Laboratory of Immunological and Rheumatologic Researches, IRCCS Istituto Auxologico Italiano, Via Zucchi 18, 20095 Cusano Milanino, Milan, Italy
Department of Clinical Sciences and Community Health, University of Milan, Via Festa del Perdono 7, 20122 Milan, Italy

Cecilia Beatrice Chighizola
Experimental Laboratory of Immunological and Rheumatologic Researches, IRCCS Istituto Auxologico Italiano, Via Zucchi 18, 20095 Cusano Milanino, Milan, Italy
Department of Clinical Sciences and Community Health, University of Milan, Via Festa del Perdono 7, 20122 Milan, Italy
Allergology, Clinical Immunology and Rheumatology Unit, IRCCS Istituto Auxologico Italiano, Piazzale Brescia 20, 20149 Milan, Italy

Pier Luigi Meroni
Experimental Laboratory of Immunological and Rheumatologic Researches, IRCCS Istituto Auxologico Italiano, Via Zucchi 18, 20095 Cusano Milanino, Milan, Italy
Department of Clinical Sciences and Community Health, University of Milan, Via Festa del Perdono 7, 20122 Milan, Italy
Division of Rheumatology, ASST G. Pini, Piazza C Ferrari 1, 20122 Milan, Italy

Francesca Ingegnoli
Department of Clinical Sciences and Community Health, University of Milan, Via Festa del Perdono 7, 20122 Milan, Italy
Division of Rheumatology, ASST G. Pini, Piazza C Ferrari 1, 20122 Milan, Italy

Claudio Mastaglio
Rheumatology Unit, Ospedale Moriggia-Pelascini, Via Pelascini 3, 22015 Gravedona, Como, Italy

Erika Mosor, Maisa Omara, Romualdo Ramos and Tanja Alexandra Stamm
Section for Outcomes Research, Centre for Medical Statistics, Informatics, and Intelligent Systems, Medical University of Vienna, Spitalgasse 23, 1090 Vienna, Austria

Valentin Ritschl
Section for Outcomes Research, Centre for Medical Statistics, Informatics, and Intelligent Systems, Medical University of Vienna, Spitalgasse 23, 1090 Vienna, Austria
Division of Rheumatology, Department of Medicine 3, Medical University of Vienna, Vienna, Austria
Division of Occupational Therapy, University of Applied Sciences FH Campus Wien, Vienna, Austria

Michaela Lehner and Paul Studenic
Division of Rheumatology, Department of Medicine 3, Medical University of Vienna, Vienna, Austria

Josef Sebastian Smolen
Division of Rheumatology, Department of Medicine 3, Medical University of Vienna, Vienna, Austria

Department of Internal Medicine, Centre for Rheumatic Diseases, Hietzing Hospital, Vienna, Austria

Angelika Lackner
Department of Rheumatology, Medical University of Graz, Styria, Austria

Carina Boström
Division of Physiotherapy, Department of Neurobiology, Karolinska Institute, Care Sciences and Society (NVS), Huddinge, Sweden
Karolinska University Hospital, Stockholm, Sweden

Sonia Pezet, Anne Cauvet, Carole Nicco and Frédéric Batteux
Université Paris Descartes, Sorbonne Paris Cité, INSERM U1016, Institut Cochin, CNRS UMR8104, Paris, France

Gonçalo Boleto, Yannick Allanore and Jérôme Avouac
Université Paris Descartes, Sorbonne Paris Cité, INSERM U1016, Institut Cochin, CNRS UMR8104, Paris, France
Université Paris Descartes, Sorbonne Paris Cité, Service de Rhumatologie A, Hôpital Cochin, 27 rue du Faubourg Saint Jacques, 75014 Paris, France

Christophe Guignabert and Ly Tu
INSERM UMR_S 999, Le Plessis-Robinson, France
Université Paris-Sud, Université Paris-Saclay, Le Kremlin-Bicêtre, France

Jérémy Sadoine
EA 2496 Pathologie, Imagerie et Biothérapies Orofaciales, UFR Odontologie, Université Paris Descartes and PIDV, PRES Sorbonne Paris Cité, Montrouge, France

Camille Gobeaux
Clinical Chemistry Laboratory, Cochin and Hôtel-Dieu Hospitals, Paris, France

Giuliana Guggino, Giovanni Triolo and Francesco Ciccia
Dipartimento Biomedico di Medicina Interna e Specialistica, Sezione di Reumatologia, Università di Palermo, Palermo, Italy

Valentina Orlando and Marco Pio La Manna
Central Laboratory of Advanced Diagnosis and Biomedical Research (CLADIBIOR), Azienda Ospedaliera Universitaria Policlinico P. Giaccone, Palermo, Italy

Francesco Dieli and Nadia Caccamo
Central Laboratory of Advanced Diagnosis and Biomedical Research (CLADIBIOR), Azienda Ospedaliera Universitaria Policlinico P. Giaccone, Palermo, Italy

Laura Saieva and Riccardo Alessandro
Dipartimento di Biopatologia e Biotecnologie Mediche, Università di Palermo, Palermo, Italy

Piero Ruscitti, Paola Cipriani and Roberto Giacomelli
Division of Rheumatology, Department of Biotechnological and Applied Clinical Science, School of Medicine, University of L'Aquila, L'Aquila, Italy

Hui-Chun Yu
Division of Allergy, Immunology and Rheumatology, Dalin Tzu Chi Hospital, Buddhist Tzu Chi Medical Foundation, No. 2, Minsheng RoadDalin, Chiayi 62247, Taiwan

Ning-Sheng Lai, Chien-Hsueh Tung, Kuang-Yung Huang and Ming-Chi Lu
Division of Allergy, Immunology and Rheumatology, Dalin Tzu Chi Hospital, Buddhist Tzu Chi Medical Foundation, No. 2, Minsheng RoadDalin, Chiayi 62247, Taiwan
School of Medicine, Tzu Chi University, Hualien City, Taiwan

Hsien-Bin Huang
Department of Life Science and Institute of Molecular Biology, National Chung Cheng University, Minxiong, Chiayi, Taiwan

Carla Cunha and Ana J. Silva
i3S—Instituto de Investigação e Inovação em Saúde, Universidade do Porto, Rua Alfredo Allen 208, 4200-135 Porto, Portugal
INEB—Instituto de Engenharia Biomédica, Universidade do Porto, Rua do Campo Alegre 823, 4150-180 Porto, Portugal

Raquel M. Gonçalves and Mário A. Barbosa
i3S—Instituto de Investigação e Inovação em Saúde, Universidade do Porto, Rua Alfredo Allen 208, 4200-135 Porto, Portugal
INEB—Instituto de Engenharia Biomédica, Universidade do Porto, Rua do Campo Alegre 823, 4150-180 Porto, Portugal
ICBAS—Instituto de Ciências Biomédicas Abel Salazar, Universidade do Porto, Rua Jorge Viterbo Ferreira 228, 4050-313 Porto, Portugal

Rui Vaz
i3S—Instituto de Investigação e Inovação em Saúde, Universidade do Porto, Rua Alfredo Allen 208, 4200-135 Porto, Portugal
Department of Neurosurgery, Centro Hospitalar São João, Porto, Portugal

Department of Clinical Neurosciences and Mental Health, Faculty of Medicine, University of Porto, Porto, Portugal
Neurosciences Center, CUF Porto Hospital, Porto, Portugal

Paulo Pereira
Department of Neurosurgery, Centro Hospitalar São João, Porto, Portugal
Department of Clinical Neurosciences and Mental Health, Faculty of Medicine, University of Porto, Porto, Portugal
Neurosciences Center, CUF Porto Hospital, Porto, Portugal

Syuichi Munenaga, Kazuhisa Ouhara, Yuta Hamamoto, Mikihito Kajiya, Katsuhiro Takeda, Noriyoshi Mizuno, Tsuyoshi Fujita and Hidemi Kurihara
Department of Periodontal Medicine, Graduate School of Biomedical and Sciences, Hiroshima University, 1-2-3, Kasumi, Minami-ku, Hiroshima 734-8553, Japan

Satoshi Yamasaki
Division of Rheumatology, Kurume University Medical Center, 155-1 Kokubu-machi, Kurume 839-0863, Japan

Toshihisa Kawai
Department of Periodontology, Nova Southeastern University College of Dental Medicine, 3200 South University Drive, Fort Lauderdale, FL 33328, USA

Eiji Sugiyama
Department of Clinical Immunology and Rheumatology, Hiroshima University Hospital, 1-2-3 Kasumi, Minami-ku, Hiroshima 734-8553, Japan

Nadia M. T. Roodenrijs, Maria J. H. de Hair, Janneke Tekstra, Floris P. J. G. Lafeber and Jacob M. van Laar
Department of Rheumatology and Clinical Immunology, University Medical Center Utrecht, Heidelberglaan 100, 3508 GA Utrecht, The Netherlands

Gill Wheater
Department of Biochemistry, The James Cook University Hospital, Marton Road, Middlesborough TS4 3BW, UK

Mohsen Elshahaly
Department of Rheumatology and Rehabilitation, Suez Canal University, Suez Canal University Circular Road, Ismailia 411522, Egypt

Y. K. Onno Teng
Department of Nephrology, Leiden University Medical Center, Albinusdreef 2, 2333 ZA Leiden, The Netherlands

Ching Chang Hwang, Xinyu Liu and Eric H. Sasso
Crescendo Bioscience, 341 Oyster Point Blvd, South San Franscisco, CA 94080, USA

Irazú Contreras-Yáñez, Emmanuel Ruiz-Medrano and Virginia Pascual-Ramos
Department of Immunology and Rheumatology, Instituto Nacional de Ciencias Médicas y Nutrición Salvador Zubirán, Vasco de Quiroga 15, Colonia Belisario Domínguez Sección XVI, México City, Mexico

Luz del Carmen R. Hernández
External collaborator, Mexico City, Mexico

Richard Partington, Toby Helliwell, Sara Muller, Alyshah Abdul Sultan and Christian Mallen
Arthritis Research UK Primary Care Centre, Primary Care Sciences, Keele University, Keele ST5 5BG, UK

Matthew Roughley
East London NHS Foundation Trust, Trust Headquarters, 9 Alie Street, London E1 8DE, UK

Alyshah Abdul Sultan, Lorna Clarson, Sara Muller, Rebecca Whittle and Christian D. Mallen
Research Institute for Primary Care and Health Sciences, Keele University, Keele, Staffordshire ST5 5BG, UK

Edward Roddy
Research Institute for Primary Care and Health Sciences, Keele University, Keele, Staffordshire ST5 5BG, UK
Haywood Academic Rheumatology Centre, Midland Partnership NHS Foundation Trust, Haywood Hospital, Burslem, Staffordshire ST6 7AG, UK

John Belcher
School of Computing and Mathematics, Keele University, Keele, Staffordshire ST5 5BG, UK

Index